Tumors
of the
Lower Respiratory Tract

Atlas
of
Tumor Pathology

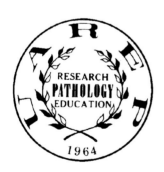

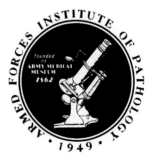

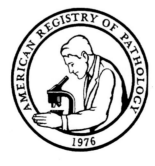

ATLAS OF TUMOR PATHOLOGY

Third Series
Fascicle 13

TUMORS OF THE LOWER RESPIRATORY TRACT

by

THOMAS V. COLBY, M.D.
Laboratory of Medicine and Pathology
Mayo Clinic Scottsdale
Scottsdale, Arizona 85259

MICHAEL N. KOSS, M.D.
Co-Chairman
Department of Pulmonary and Mediastinal Pathology
Armed Forces Institute of Pathology
Washington, D.C. 20306-6000
and
Department of Pathology
University of Southern California
Los Angeles, California 90033

WILLIAM D. TRAVIS, M.D.
Co-Chairman
Department of Pulmonary and Mediastinal Pathology
Armed Forces Institute of Pathology
Washington, D.C. 20306-6000

Published by the
ARMED FORCES INSTITUTE OF PATHOLOGY
Washington, D.C.

Under the Auspices of
UNIVERSITIES ASSOCIATED FOR RESEARCH AND EDUCATION IN PATHOLOGY, INC.
Bethesda, Maryland
1995

Accepted for Publication
1994

Available from the American Registry of Pathology
Armed Forces Institute of Pathology
Washington, D.C. 20306-6000
ISSN 0160-6344
ISBN 1-881041-17-4

ATLAS OF TUMOR PATHOLOGY

EDITOR
JUAN ROSAI, M.D.
Department of Pathology
Memorial Sloan-Kettering Cancer Center
New York, New York 10021-6007

ASSOCIATE EDITOR
LESLIE H. SOBIN, M.D.
Armed Forces Institute of Pathology
Washington, D.C. 20306-6000

EDITORS' NOTE

The Atlas of Tumor Pathology has a long and distinguished history. It was first conceived at a Cancer Research Meeting held in St. Louis in September 1947 as an attempt to standardize the nomenclature of neoplastic diseases. The first series was sponsored by the National Academy of Sciences-National Research Council. The organization of this Sisyphean effort was entrusted to the Subcommittee on Oncology of the Committee on Pathology, and Dr. Arthur Purdy Stout was the first editor-in-chief. Many of the illustrations were provided by the Medical Illustration Service of the Armed Forces Institute of Pathology, the type was set by the Government Printing Office, and the final printing was done at the Armed Forces Institute of Pathology (hence the colloquial appellation "AFIP Fascicles"). The American Registry of Pathology purchased the Fascicles from the Government Printing Office and sold them virtually at cost. Over a period of 20 years, approximately 15,000 copies each of nearly 40 Fascicles were produced. The worldwide impact that these publications have had over the years has largely surpassed the original goal. They quickly became among the most influential publications on tumor pathology ever written, primarily because of their overall high quality but also because their low cost made them easily accessible to pathologists and other students of oncology the world over.

Upon completion of the first series, the National Academy of Sciences-National Research Council handed further pursuit of the project over to the newly created Universities Associated for Research and Education in Pathology (UAREP). A second series was started, generously supported by grants from the AFIP, the National Cancer Institute, and the American Cancer Society. Dr. Harlan I. Firminger became the editor-in-chief and was succeeded by Dr. William H. Hartmann. The second series Fascicles were produced as bound volumes instead of loose leaflets. They featured a more comprehensive coverage of the subjects, to the extent that the Fascicles could no longer be regarded as "atlases" but rather as monographs describing and illustrating in detail the tumors and tumor-like conditions of the various organs and systems.

Once the second series was completed, with a success that matched that of the first, UAREP and AFIP decided to embark on a third series. A new editor-in-chief and an associate editor were selected, and a distinguished editorial board was appointed. The mandate for the third series remains the same as for the previous ones, i.e., to oversee the production of an eminently practical publication with surgical pathologists as its primary audience, but also aimed at other workers in oncology. The main purposes of this series are to promote a consistent, unified, and biologically sound nomenclature; to guide the surgical pathologist in the diagnosis of the various tumors and tumor-like lesions; and to provide relevant histogenetic, pathogenetic, and clinicopathologic information on these entities. Just as the second series included data obtained from ultrastructural (and, in the more recent Fascicles, immunohistochemical) examination, the third series will, in addition, incorporate pertinent information obtained with the newer molecular biology techniques. As in the past, a continuous attempt will be made to correlate, whenever possible, the nomenclature used in the Fascicles with that proposed by the World Health Organization's International Histological Classification of Tumors. The format of the third series has been changed in order to incorporate additional items and to ensure a consistency of style throughout. This includes the dropping of the 's possessive in eponymic terms, in accordance with the WHO and the International Nomenclature of Diseases. Close cooperation between the various authors and their respective liaisons from the editorial board will be emphasized to minimize unnecessary repetition and discrepancies in the text and illustrations.

To its everlasting credit, the participation and commitment of the AFIP to this venture is even more substantial and encompassing than in previous series. It now extends to virtually all scientific, technical, and financial aspects of the production.

The task confronting the organizations and individuals involved in the third series is even more daunting than in the preceding efforts because of the ever-increasing complexity of the matter at hand. It is hoped that this combined effort—of which, needless to say, that represented by the authors is first and foremost—will result in a series worthy of its two illustrious predecessors and will be a suitable introduction to the tumor pathology of the twenty-first century.

Juan Rosai, M.D.
Leslie H. Sobin, M.D.

PREFACE AND ACKNOWLEDGEMENTS

Any work of this type requires many more individuals than the authors alone, and there are many whom we would like to thank and acknowledge. First and foremost, we would all like to dedicate this work to our wives (Pamela Colby, Linda Koss, Ph.D, and Lois Travis, M.D., Sc.D.), and thank them for their support during its writing.

A number of our figures have been previously published, and the publishers have been acknowledged. We would also like to thank the following individuals who provided advice, gross photographs, or glass slides to photograph. Particular thanks is given to Dr. Constantine Axiotis, Albany, New York; Dr. William Bennett, Bethesda, Maryland; Dr. Klaus Bensch, Stanford, California; Dr. Jerome Burke, Berkeley, California; Dr. J.A. Carney, Rochester, Minnesota; Dr. Andrew Churg, Vancouver, British Columbia; Dr. R. Curran, Birmingham, England; Dr. E. Drilcek, Vienna, Austria, and colleagues; Dr. William Edwards, Rochester, Minnesota; Dr. Richard Fraser, Montreal, Canada; Dr. Michael Gaffey, Charlottesville, Virginia; Dr. Anthony Gal, Atlanta, Georgia; Dr. Kaoru Hamada, Nara, Japan; Dr. Samuel Hammar, Bremerton, Washington; Dr. Curtis Harris, Bethesda, Maryland; Dr. M. Higashiyama, Osaka, Japan; Dr. Liselotte Hochholzer, Washington, D.C.; Dr. Hiroshi Ishikura, Sapporo, Japan; Dr. E. Jones, Birmingham, England; Dr. Spencer Kerley, Kansas City, Missouri; Dr. Ilona Linnoila, Bethesda, Maryland; Dr. Lance Liotta, Bethesda, Maryland; Dr. Bruce Mackay, Houston, Texas; Dr. Carlos Manivel, Minneapolis, Minnesota; Mr. H. Miller, Birmingham, England; Dr. Cesar Moran, Washington, D.C.; Dr. Jeffrey Myers, Rochester, Minnesota; Dr. June Olson, Portland, Oregon; Dr. Geno Sacccammanno, Grand Junction, Colorado; Dr. G. Sterrett, Nedlands, Western Australia; Dr. Thomas Stocker, Washington, D.C.; Dr. Maria Tsokos, Bethesda, Maryland; Dr. Samuel Yousem, Pittsburgh, Pennsylvania.

For excellent photographic assistance the authors thank: Richard Dreyfus, Bethesda, Maryland; Robin-Anne V. Ferris, MFS; and Luther Ducket, Washington, D.C.

Special acknowledgement is given to Charles B. Carrington, M.D., whose untimely death in 1985 foreshortened his career in pulmonary pathology. Many of the illustrations in this Fascicle come from some of the 13,000 cases in the Charles B. Carrington Memorial Pulmonary Pathology teaching collection which is housed in Scottsdale, Arizona, and available for interested individuals to study.

Thomas V. Colby, M.D.
Michael N. Koss, M.D.
William D. Travis, M.D.

Permission to use copyrighted illustrations has been granted by:

American College of Chest Physicians:
    Chest 1991;100:826–37. For figure 8-8.

American Medical Association:
    Arch Path Lab Med 1989;113:1166–9. For figure 4-9.
    Arch Path Lab Med 1970;90:577–82. For figure 24-1.

American Society of Roentgenology:
    AJR Am J Roentgenol 1985;144:687–94. For figure 4-6.

Kinpodo Publishing Company:
    Lymphatic System of the Human Lung, 1989. For figures 2-4, 2-5, and 8-9.

JB Lippincott Company:
    Am J Clin Path 1987;87:1–6. For figure 24-11.
    Cancer 1972;30:836–47. For figure 19-21.
    Cancer 1987;60:1346–52. For figures 6-3, 6-8, 6-9, and 6-13.
    Cancer 1987;60:2532–41. For figures 19-21 and 19-24.
    Cancer 1993;71:1368–83. For figure 3-4.
    Pediatric Pathology 1992. For figures 21-15, 21-16, and 21-17.

McGraw-Hill, Inc.:
    Pulmonary Diseases and Disorders, 2nd ed. 1988. For figures 2-2 and 2-6.

Mosby-Year Book, Inc.:
    Curr Probl Surg 1986;23:251–314. For figures 2-8, 2-9, and 2-14.
    Essentials of Human Embryology, 1988. For figure 2-1.

New England Journal of Medicine:
    N Engl J Med 1983;308:1466–72. For figure 24-26.

Oxford University Press:
    Tumours: Structure and Diagnosis, 1991. For figure 23-34.

Raven Press:
    Am J Surg Pathol 1977;1:5–16. For figure 10-3.
    Am J Surg Pathol 1991;15:529–53. For figure 14-18.
    Am J Surg Pathol 1992;16:1039–50. For figures 16-35 and 16-36.

Springer-Verlag:
    International Union Against Cancer: TNM Atlas. 3rd ed. 1989. For figure 8-10.

WB Saunders:
    Human Pathol 1977;8:155–72. For figure 2-17.
    Human Pathol 1986;17:1066–71. For figure 5-4.
    Human Pathol 1990;21:1097–107. For figures 21-9 and 21-10.
    Semin Oncol 1988;15:215–25. For figure 7-1.
    Semin Oncol 1988;15:236–45. For figures 8-12, 8-13, 8-14, 8-15.

Williams & Wilkins:
    Molecular Foundations of Oncology. 1st ed. 1991. For table 3-5.

Urban & Schwarzenberg:
    Cell and Tissue Biology: A Textbook of Histology, 1988. For figure 2-7.

TUMORS OF THE LOWER RESPIRATORY TRACT

Jose Costa

Contents

TUMORS OF THE LOWER RESPIRATORY TRACT

1

INTRODUCTION AND CLASSIFICATION

Since tumors of the lung are common, most practicing pathologists are experienced with routine primary lung carcinomas and have no problems recognizing them. However, there are many histologic variations of the common tumors as well as unusual tumors that occur in the lung. While many of these less common tumors are recognized and classified on routine histologic sections, in others the diagnosis, classification, and prognosis are aided by recently developed immunohistochemical and molecular techniques. Therefore, the purpose of this atlas is to: 1) describe and illustrate common tumors of the lung with emphasis on less common histologic variations; 2) describe and illustrate the many uncommon tumors; 3) describe and illustrate lesions that are part of the differential diagnosis of both common and uncommon tumors of the lung and describe the features distinguishing one lung tumor from another; 4) present an approach to the classification of lung tumors based on histologic and ancillary studies within the context of the World Health Organization (WHO) classification; and 5) outline and describe recent studies, such as molecular genetics, which may be of prognostic and diagnostic significance in the study of tumors of the lung.

WHO HISTOLOGIC TYPING OF LUNG TUMORS

In 1956 the WHO Director General was asked to help in the organization, development, and standardization of histologic definitions and terminology for tumors from various sites. This effort was descriptive rather than histogenetic and was meant to facilitate comparison of scientific studies of tumors from various parts of the world by use of standardized nomenclature.

The first edition of the *WHO Histological Typing of Lung Tumours* appeared in 1967 (1). This monograph was reviewed and revised in 1977, and the second, and current, edition was published in 1981 (2). This classification system for lung tumors is shown in Table 1-1.

We generally adhere to the WHO outline, although we vary the order of presentation and make some modifications (see the Table of Contents) to allow inclusion of recently described tumors, and newer techniques and histogenetic considerations. We include a number of newly described or unusual variants of recognized tumors not described in the WHO classification (for example, mucinous tumors, signet ring carcinomas, and pleomorphic carcinomas). A separate category is added for salivary type tumors of the lung and major airways as distinct from other benign and low-grade malignant lung tumors. We include a separate discussion of neuroendocrine carcinomas of the lung. Pleural and mesothelial tumors are excluded. These do not generally present as pulmonary parenchymal tumors. The second series Fascicle, *Tumors of the Serous Membranes*, by McCaughey, Kannerstein, and Churg is devoted to them, and the third series of this fascicle will be available shortly.

REFERENCES

1. Histological typing of lung tumours. International Histological Classification of Tumours No. 1. Geneva: World Health Organization, 1967.

2. Histological typing of lung tumours, Vol 1. 2nd ed. International Histological Classification of Tumours No. 1. Geneva: World Health Organization, 1981.

Table 1-1

HISTOLOGIC CLASSIFICATION OF LUNG TUMORS*

I. Epithelial Tumors
   A. Benign
      1. Papillomas
         a. Squamous cell papilloma
         b. "Transitional" papilloma
      2. Adenomas
         a. Pleomorphic adenoma ("mixed" tumor)
         b. Monomorphic adenoma
         c. Others
   B. Dysplasia/carcinoma in situ
   C. Malignant
      1. Squamous cell carcinoma (epidermoid carcinoma)
         Variant:
         a. Spindle cell (squamous carcinoma)
      2. Small cell carcinomas
         a. Oat cell carcinoma
         b. Intermediate cell type
         c. Combined oat cell carcinoma
      3. Adenocarcinomas
         a. Acinar adenocarcinoma
         b. Papillary adenocarcinoma
         c. Bronchioloalveolar carcinoma
         d. Solid carcinoma with mucus formation
      4. Large cell carcinoma
         Variants:
         a. Giant cell carcinoma
         b. Clear cell carcinoma
      5. Adenosquamous carcinoma
      6. Carcinoid tumor
      7. Bronchial gland carcinomas
         a. Adenoid cystic carcinoma
         b. Mucoepidermoid carcinoma
         c. Others
      8. Others
II. Soft Tissue Tumors Primary in the Lung
III. Mesothelial Tumors (Pleural Tumors)
   A. Benign mesothelioma (solitary fibrous tumor, localized fibrous mesothelioma)
   B. Malignant mesothelioma
      1. Epithelial
      2. Fibrous (spindle cell, sarcomatous including desmoplastic)
      3. Biphasic
IV. Miscellaneous Tumors
   A. Benign
   B. Malignant
      1. Carcinosarcoma
      2. Pulmonary blastoma
      3. Malignant melanoma
      4. Malignant lymphoma
      5. Others
V. Secondary Metastatic Tumors
VI. Unclassified Tumors
VII. Tumor-like Lesions
   A. Hamartoma
   B. Lymphoproliferative lesions
   C. Tumorlet
   D. Eosinophilic granuloma
   E. "Sclerosing hemangioma"
   F. Inflammatory pseudotumor
   G. Others

---

*From reference 2.

2

EMBRYOLOGY, ANATOMY, AND CONGENITAL, DEVELOPMENTAL, AND RELATED LESIONS

EMBRYOLOGY

The phases of lung development are summarized in Table 2-1 and figure 2-1 (1–5). In the embryo, the developing lower respiratory tract is first seen as a groove in the floor of the primitive pharynx, caudal to the pharyngeal pouches. The groove evaginates into a distinct laryngotracheal diverticulum, which elongates caudally into the primitive mesenchyme as the primitive lung bud. Bronchial buds arise by progressive dichotomous division and the segmental, subsegmental, and more distal airways are formed. Bronchial cartilage, musculature, and connective tissues are derived from the mesenchyme surrounding the bronchial buds. The development of the major airways, termed the embryonic phase, occurs between 3 and 6 weeks of gestation.

From approximately the 6th to 16th week of gestation, the small airways, including the terminal bronchioles, are formed; 16 weeks after conception, the formation of the conducting airways is complete. This is the pseudoglandular phase (fig. 2-2).

The next stage of development, the canalicular phase, occurs between 16 and 28 weeks; the acinus and its accompanying vascular supply develop. Terminal bronchioles give rise to respiratory bronchioles with terminal sacs representing primitive alveoli. Some respiratory function may be possible toward the end of this phase because of the presence of these vascularized terminal sacs.

The saccular phase is identifiable by the 28th week and extends to the 36th week of gestation. Saccules form and become lined by flattened type 1 alveolar epithelial cells. The associated capillary network develops in the surrounding mesenchyme, and lymphatics are formed.

The alveolar phase begins at approximately 36 weeks' gestation and extends to as late as 8 years of age. Vascularized alveoli are formed and are lined by type 1 alveolar lining cells.

The visceral and parietal pleura arise within the primordial mesenchyme surrounding the developing lung.

ANATOMY AND HISTOLOGY

The anatomy and histology of the lung are well described (6–12). Segmental lung anatomy is important for both bronchoscopists and pathologists in designating tumor location. Bronchial segmental anatomy and supplied pulmonary segments are shown in figure 2-3.

The lung has a dual vascular supply. Pulmonary arteries accompany airways into the lung periphery where they progressively divide into a ramifying capillary network in the alveolar

Table 2-1

PHASES OF LUNG DEVELOPMENT*

Phase	Gestation	Major Events
Embryonic	26 days to 6 weeks	Development of major airways
Pseudoglandular	6 to 16 weeks	Development of airways to terminal bronchioles
Canalicular	16 to 28 weeks	Development of the acinus and its vascularization
Saccular	28 to 36 weeks	Subdivision of saccules by secondary crests
Alveolar	36 weeks to term (and up to 4 years of age)	Acquisition of alveoli

*Modified from reference 2.

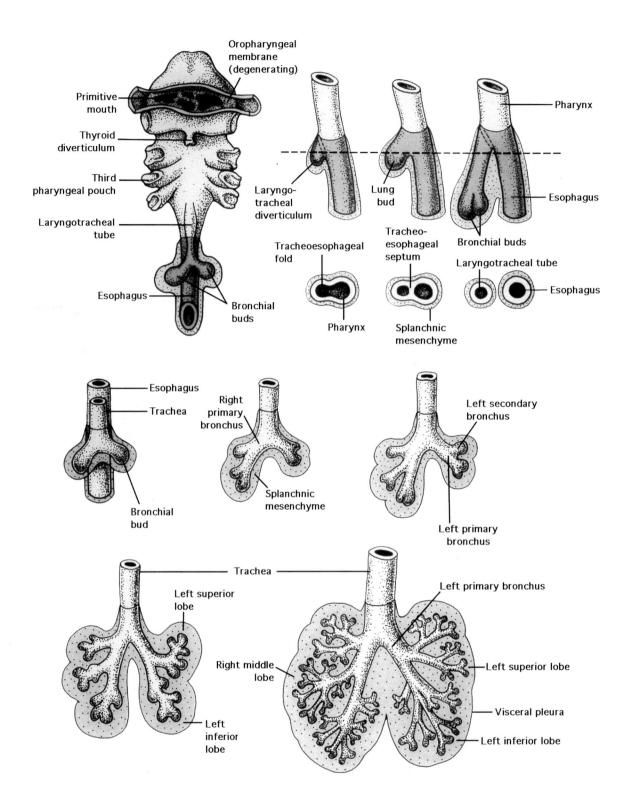

Figure 2-1
EARLY EMBRYOLOGIC DEVELOPMENT OF THE LUNG
The embryonic lungs first arise as the laryngotracheal diverticulum in the primitive gut. This elongates and forms bronchial buds which progressively divide dichotomously within the splanchnic mesenchyme. (Figs. 10-1 and 10-4 from Moore KL, Herbst M, Thompson M. Essentials of human embryology. St. Louis: Mosby-Year Book, 1988.)

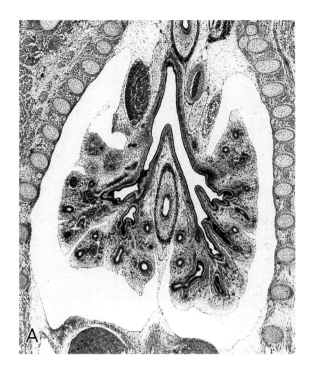

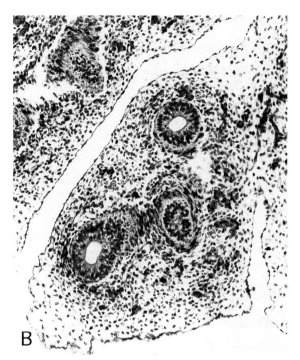

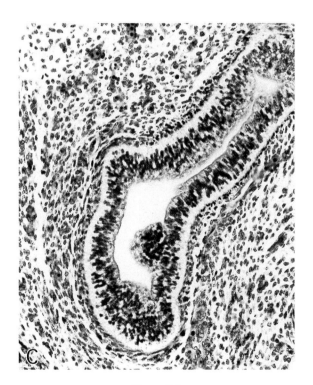

Figure 2-2
EARLY PSEUDOGLANDULAR PHASE OF LUNG DEVELOPMENT

In these histologic sections from a 7-week-old human fetus, the tracheal bifurcation into right and left main stem bronchi can be seen within the embryonic lung in the chest cavity (A). The right middle lobe is identifiable at this stage, with primitive bronchial buds, surrounded by splanchnic mesenchyme, and visceral pleural investment (B). Lung tissue in the pseudoglandular phase of development is surprisingly reminiscent of early secretory endometrium (C).

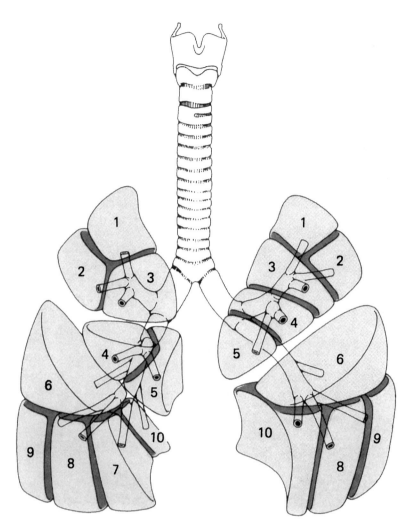

Figure 2-3
BRONCHOPULMONARY SEGMENTS OF THE HUMAN LUNG
Left and right upper lobes: 1, apical; 2, posterior; 3, anterior; 4, superior lingular; and 5, inferior lingular segments. Right middle lobe: 4, lateral and 5, medial segments. Lower lobes: 6, superior apical; 7, medial basal; 8, anterior basal; 9, lateral basal; and 10, posterior basal segments. The medial basal segment (7) is absent in the left lung. (Fig. 2-2 from Weibel ER, Taylor CR. Design and structure of the human lung. In: Fishman AP, ed. Pulmonary diseases and disorders, Vol. 1, 2nd ed. New York: McGraw-Hill, 1988.)

walls. Bronchial arteries are systemic, arising from the aorta or intercostal arteries; they form a plexus in the bronchial wall which extends peripherally as far as the respiratory bronchioles. Proximally, bronchial arteries anastomose with those supplying the trachea which derive from branches of the inferior thyroid artery. Branches of the bronchial arteries also supply the visceral pleura and some of the interstitial connective tissue. The pulmonary venous system arises from the efferent blood flow through the alveolar capillary network

in the periphery of the lobules where small veins can be seen entering pulmonary septa. Bronchopulmonary segments are often drained by more than one pulmonary vein.

The lymphatic drainage of the lung is quite complex (figs. 2-4, 2-5). In general, the lymphatics follow the bronchovascular structures and are found in the pleura and septa. They can be identified along pulmonary arteries and airways to the level of respiratory bronchioles, and along venules in the periphery of lobules and veins in

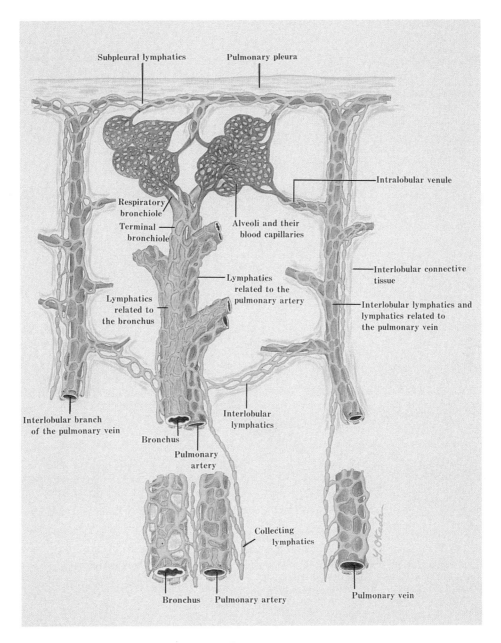

Figure 2-4
HISTOLOGIC DIAGRAM OF THE PULMONARY LYMPHATICS
The pulmonary lymphatics are located along bronchovascular structures, pulmonary veins, and within the septa and pleura. (Fig. 1 from Okada Y. Lymphatic system of the human lung. Kyoto, Japan: Kinpodo Publishing, 1989.)

the septa. A rich lymphatic network is also seen in the visceral pleura. Lymphoid tissue can be found along lymphatics, particularly at sites of branching of larger airways where inhaled particulate antigens are likely to settle and where there is respiratory epithelium specialized for absorption. This lymphoid tissue is termed bronchus-associated lymphoid tissue. It is organized into discrete lymph nodes around the larger bronchi (intrapulmonary peribronchial lymph nodes) and in the hilum. Lymphatic drainage from the pulmonary lymphatics is cephalad, primarily through lymph node groups in the chest, but is also to lymph nodes in the abdomen (fig. 2-5).

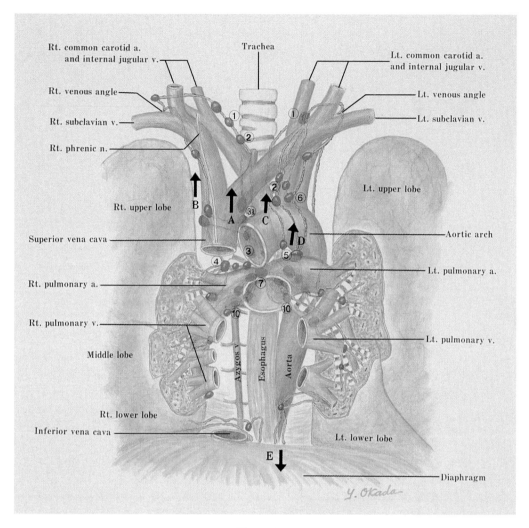

Figure 2-5
LYMPHATIC DRAINAGE OF THE LUNG
The drainage is primarily cephalad along the right paratracheal route (A), right brachial cephalic route (B), left paratracheal route (C), and para-aortic route (D). Some deep drainage into the abdomen (E) takes place from the inferior thoracic cavity. (Fig. 4 from Okada Y. Lymphatic system of the human lung. Kyoto, Japan: Kinpodo Publishing, 1989.)

The cells lining the airways and alveoli are endodermally derived and have a number of specialized modifications. The respiratory tract is organized to facilitate gas transfer distally (hence large numbers of attenuated type 1 alveolar lining cells) and for airflow and clearance along the mucociliary escalator proximally (hence larger numbers of ciliated and mucus cells) (fig. 2-6). Figure 2-7 is a schematic representation of bronchial lining epithelium; the major cell types found in the lower respiratory tract are summarized in Table 2-2.

Submucosal glands of minor salivary type are found in the submucosa of the trachea and bronchi (but not the bronchioles). Anatomically, three regions are recognized in these glands: the ciliated duct, the connecting duct, and the secretory tubules lined by serous and mucous cells. These seromucous glands are invested by a myoepithelial cell layer which probably functions in secretion. Particularly in older individuals, oncocytes (oncocytic metaplasia) may be found in the connecting duct, or replacing serous or mucous cells in the secretory tubules.

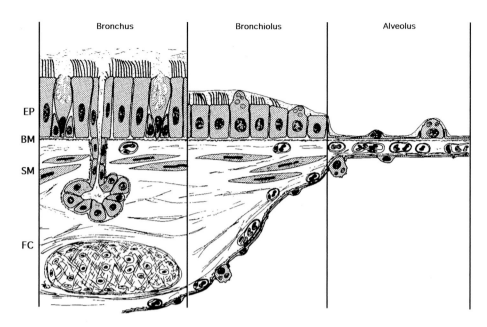

Figure 2-6
SCHEMATIC REPRESENTATION OF THE SURFACE EPITHELIUM OF THE RESPIRATORY TRACT

Columnar ciliated cells are most prominent in the bronchus whereas cuboidal-shaped cells and Clara cells with apical protrusions containing granules are more prominent in the bronchiole. The alveolus contains primarily membranous pneumocytes to facilitate gas transfer, interspersed with type 2 cells that protrude into the alveolar lumen. (Fig. 2-6 from Weibel ER, Taylor CR. Design and structure of the human lung. In: Fishman AP, ed. Pulmonary diseases and disorders, Vol. 1. 2nd ed. New York: McGraw-Hill, 1988.)

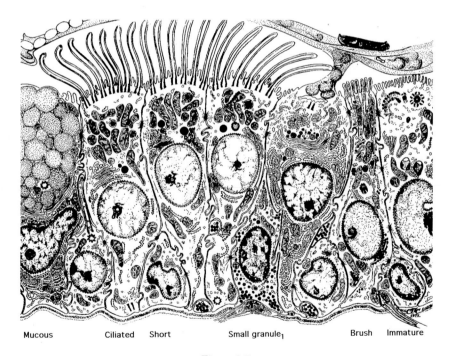

Figure 2-7
ULTRASTRUCTURAL SCHEMATIC REPRESENTATION OF RESPIRATORY
TRACT EPITHELIUM IN A LARGE AIRWAY

The various cell types comprising this epithelium are illustrated along with their ultrastructural features. Brush cells have been primarily recognized in animals. (Fig. 25-11 from Sorokin SP. The respiratory system. In: Weiss L, ed. Cell and tissue biology: a textbook of histology. Baltimore: Urban & Schwarzenberg, 1988.)

Table 2-2

MAJOR CELLS OF THE LOWER RESPIRATORY TRACT

Cell Type	Main Features	Functions	Location	Comments
Ciliated	Columnar, cuboidal, ciliated bronchial lining cells; each cell has approximately 250 cilia at the apical surface and each cilium is approximately 6 μm long	Proximal transport of mucus stream (mucociliary escalator)	Bronchi and bronchioles	Decreased number and morphologic abnormalities seen with chronic irritation
Goblet	Columnar mucus-secreting cells; contain mucus glycoprotein which discharges apically	Contribute to airway mucus	Bronchi, more numerous proximally; small numbers in bronchioles	Increased number in chronic airway irritation
Basal	Short cells with relatively little cytoplasm oriented along the basement membrane; do not reach the luminal surface of the epithelium	Precursor cell of ciliated and goblet cells	Bronchi; rare in bronchioles	——————-
Neuroendocrine (Kulchitsky or K cells)	Basal-oriented cells with numerous dense core (neurosecretory) granules; single or in groups (neuroepithelial bodies), the latter near sites of airway bifurcation	Specific functions not known in detail; considered part of the diffuse neuroendocrine system	Bronchi; rare in bronchioles	——————-
Oncocytic	Eosinophilic mitochondrial-rich cells in submucosal gland ducts	Ion secretory functions	Submucosal glands	Increasing number with aging
Squamous	Stratified squamous epithelium as an abnormal reaction replacing normal pseudostratified respiratory epithelium	Protective, reparative	Bronchi and bronchioles	Metaplastic response to irritation or repair
Clara	Columnar nonciliated bronchiolar cells; protuberant apical cytoplasm with large ovoid electron dense granules; comprise the majority of nonciliated bronchiolar cells	Secretory functions contributing to the mucus pool and maintaining extracellular lining fluid; progenitor for other bronchiolar cells; role in surfactant production	Predominantly in bronchioles	———-
Type 1 alveolar pneumocyte	Large, flat, squamous alveolar lining cells; cover some 93 percent of alveolar surface area; incapable of division	Provide a thin air/blood interface for gas transfer	Alveoli	———-
Type 2 alveolar pneumocyte	Columnar alveolar lining cells comprising 16 percent of the lung parenchyma; microvillous surface; synthesize and secrete surfactant (lamellar ultrastructural inclusions); capable of division	Maintain alveolar stability; stem cell alveoli acting as progenitor for type 1 pneumocytes	Alveoli	Increased in reparative states and as a response to chronic injury

Other cells found in the lung:
Endothelial cells and pericytes
Interstitial fibrocytes, fibroblasts, and myofibroblasts
Macrophages
Lymphoid cells
Mast cells
Mesothelial pleural lining
Cartilage and bone
Smooth muscle
Peripheral nerve
Myoepithelial cells

Table 2-3

PULMONARY DEVELOPMENTAL CYSTS, CONGENITAL ANOMALIES, AND RELATED LESIONS*

Tracheobronchial
    Tracheal atresia and agenesis
    Tracheal bronchi and diverticula
    Bronchial atresia
    Congenital bronchiectasis
    Tracheobronchial communication with other foregut derivatives (tracheoesophageal fistulae, bronchobiliary fistulae, etc.)

Sequestrations (lung tissue without tracheobronchial connection)
    Extralobar sequestration
    Intralobar sequestration

Bronchopulmonary foregut malformations (tracheobronchial or pulmonary parenchymal, including sequestered tissue with communication with the alimentary tract)

Pulmonary agenesis, aplasia, hypoplasia

Bronchogenic cysts

Congenital cystic adenomatoid malformation/congenital lung cysts

Infantile lobar emphysema (overinflation)

Interstitial pulmonary emphysema

Vascular anomalies
    Scimitar syndrome (venous drainage from right lung into inferior vena cava)
    Arteriovenous fistula(e)
    Congenital pulmonary lymphangiectasia
    Pulmonary artery agenesis

Tissue ectopias
    Intratracheal thyroid tissue
    Adrenal, pancreatic, glial, endometriosis, cardiac muscle, skeletal muscle

*Modified from references 13–18.

CONGENITAL ANOMALIES AND RELATED LESIONS

Most congenital anomalies and related lesions present within the first year of life. Notable exceptions include bronchogenic cysts and intralobar sequestrations; the latter are acquired lesions and usually present in young adults (13–18). Some anomalies are incompatible with life and are identified in stillborn infants. Many of these lesions simulate neoplasms and cannot be distinguished from them without tissue evaluation.

Table 2-3 lists major developmental cysts, congenital anomalies, and related lesions. A number of these present in neonates and young children as cystic lung lesions (Table 2-4).

Table 2-4

CYSTIC LESIONS IN NEONATES AND CHILDREN*

Sequestration/bronchopulmonary foregut malformations

Bronchogenic cyst

Congenital cystic adenomatoid malformation

Infantile lobar emphysema

Interstitial emphysema

Lymphangiectasia (lymphangiomas, lymphangiomatosis; see chapter 20)

Cystic mesenchymal neoplasms (some pleuropulmonary blastomas; see chapter 21)

Other cystic lesions
    Cystic bronchiectasis
    Post-traumatic or postinfarction cysts
    Pneumatoceles
    Late stages of bronchopulmonary dysplasia

*Modified from reference 14.

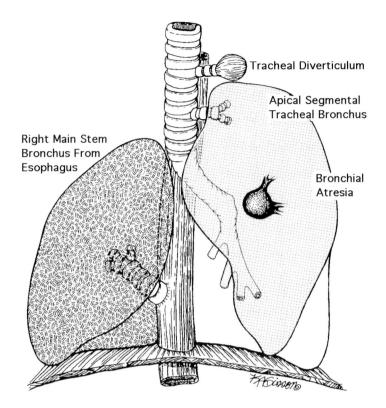

Figure 2-8
VARIOUS ANOMALIES OF THE
TRACHEA AND LARGE AIRWAYS
In bronchial atresia there is a mucus-filled bronchus with distal hyperinflation of alveoli. (Fig. 5 from Luck SR, Reynolds M, Raffensperger JG. Congenital broncho-pulmonary malformations. Curr Probl Surg 1986;23:251–314.)

Bronchial Atresia (Regional or Segmental Pulmonary Overinflation)

Bronchial atresia refers to loss of normal bronchial communication due to atresia of the segmental bronchus (19,20). The bronchus distal to the obstruction becomes filled with mucus, and the surrounding lung tissue overinflates, resulting in a radiodense mass surrounded by hyperlucency on the chest radiograph. Bronchial atresia and other tracheobronchial anomalies are illustrated in figure 2-8.

There is a slight male predominance, with an average age at presentation of 17 years (range, birth to 44 years). Sixty percent of patients are asymptomatic; those with symptoms most commonly present with recurrent pneumonia. The left upper lobe is affected in two thirds of the cases. A vascular accident early in embryologic development has been postulated as the pathogenetic cause of bronchial atresia.

In the classic case, a radiographic diagnosis is possible: there is a hilar mass with surrounding hyperaerated lung tissue which may compress adjacent lung tissue. Computerized tomography (CT) can be used to distinguish bronchial atresia from bronchogenic cysts and lobar emphysema, which are the main lesions in the differential diagnosis.

The pathologic findings depend on whether there was infection in the tissue distal to the atresia. In the absence of infection, there is a mucus-filled bronchus with surrounding lung tissue that appears grossly normal or over-inflated. If the lesion is infected, acute and chronic inflammation and fibrosis are apparent.

Pulmonary Sequestration (Intralobar Sequestration, Extralobar Sequestration)

Pulmonary sequestrations are characterized by a lack of communication with the normal tracheobronchial tree, often associated with an anomalous blood supply, particularly from the systemic circulation (fig. 2-9) (21). The various permutations in individual cases, including a variable arterial supply, variable venous drainage, or both, and the possible communication with the alimentary tract (bronchopulmonary foregut malformation) can result in a confusing picture. Nevertheless, the key feature remains a lack of communication with the normal tracheobronchial tree. Stocker (21) proposed pulmonary

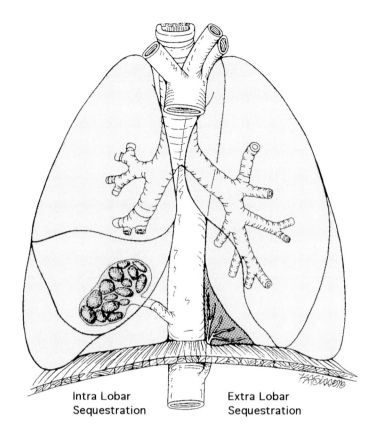

Intra Lobar
Sequestration

Extra Lobar
Sequestration

Figure 2-9
SCHEMATIC DIAGRAM
OF INTRALOBAR VERSUS
EXTRALOBAR SEQUESTRATION
Secondary changes including inflammation, fibrosis, and dilated mucus-filled spaces are typical of intralobar sequestrations. In this schematic both derive their blood supply from the descending aorta. (Fig. 14 from Luck SR, Reynolds M, Raffensperger JG. Congenital bronchopulmonary malformations. Curr Probl Surg 1986;23:251–314.)

sequestrations be defined simply as pulmonary parenchyma not in continuity with the upper respiratory tract (via the normal tracheobronchial tree). This allows classification by etiology (congenital, inflammatory, traumatic), site (abdominal, mediastinal, thoracic, intralobar), and vascular connections (pulmonary or systemic arterial, pulmonary or systemic venous) (21).

This broad definition may lead to confusion with other recognized entities (such as bronchial atresia), but it is simple and easy to apply. One must confirm the lack of a tracheobronchial communication and define the arterial supply and venous drainage in each individual case.

Sequestrations are separated into two groups: intralobar and extralobar. The major differences between these two are summarized in Table 2-5.

Extralobar sequestrations (accessory lung, Rokitanzky lobe) are true congenital anomalies in which accessory (extrapulmonary) lung tissue with its own pleural investment occurs within the thorax, diaphragm, or abdomen. Most cases are identified in male infants under 6 months of age, but some have been seen in adults as old as

81 years. Most infants present with dyspnea, cyanosis, and problems feeding. Older individuals may have a history of recurrent pneumonia, especially if there is a communication with the alimentary tract. About 10 percent of patients are asymptomatic.

The left lung is more commonly affected (65 percent). Two thirds of lesions are found between the lower lobe and the diaphragm; less than 15 percent are within or below the diaphragm.

Radiographically, extralobar sequestrations present as radiodense masses, and angiographic studies often identify anomalous vascular communications. If there is a communication with the foregut, air-fluid levels may be seen.

Extralobar sequestrations are generally single, between 0.5 and 15 cm in diameter (usually 3 to 6 cm), and pyramidal or oval. Although they lack a connection with the bronchial tree, remnants of cartilaginous bronchi may be identified in approximately half the cases, and the arterial supply should be sought and identified. Those that have been secondarily infected are grossly fibrotic and the pleural covering may be thickened

Table 2-5

INTRALOBAR SEQUESTRATION VERSUS EXTRALOBAR SEQUESTRATION*

Feature	Intralobar Sequestration	Extralobar Sequestration
Age at diagnosis	50 percent over age 20 years (15 percent asymptomatic)	60 percent less than 6 months (10 percent asymptomatic)
Sex (M:F)	1:1	4:1
Side affected	Left, 55 percent	Left, 65 percent
Arterial supply	Systemic	Systemic (rarely pulmonary)
Venous drainage	Pulmonary (rarely systemic)	Systemic or portal (25 percent wholly or in part via pulmonary veins)
Associated anomalies	Uncommon (6 to 12 percent)	Over 60 percent (e.g., pectus excavatum, diaphragmatic defects)
Pathogenesis	Majority acquired	Congenital anomaly

*Modified from references 14,17,18,21.

and covered by exudate. Cut sections show normal lung tissue or, when infected, cystic change, fibrosis, and purulent material.

The microscopic findings depend on whether or not secondary infection is present (figs. 2-10, 2-11). In uninfected cases, dilated airways are lined by bronchiolar type epithelium and dilated airspaces are lined by type 1 and type 2 pneumocytes with intra-alveolar macrophages. Well-formed bronchi may be seen. In premature infants, the tissue is immature appearing, with interstitial thickening. Extramedullary hematopoiesis may be identified, especially in premature infants. The subpleural lymphatics are typically dilated. Thick-walled vessels reflecting systemic vascular supply should be sought grossly as well as microscopically. In infected cases, there is nonspecific acute and chronic inflammation, fibrosis, and purulent exudate. Some extralobar sequestrations contain foci that are histologically indistinguishable from congenital cystic adenomatoid malformation.

Intralobar sequestrations are found within the normal pleural investment of the lung, lack a tracheobronchial communication, and have a systemic arterial supply. Stocker (21) has postulated that intralobar sequestrations are acquired lesions with inflammatory obstruction of the bronchial tree and secondary systemic arterial supply from hypertrophied pulmonary ligament arteries. This explains the propensity for intralobar sequestrations to occur in the medial lower lobes.

There is an equal sex incidence; most patients present over the age of 20 years. Symptoms typically include cough, sputum production, and a history of recurrent pneumonia. Fifteen percent of patients are asymptomatic.

In most cases, radiographs show a mass or infiltrate, usually in the medial aspect of the lower lobes, more commonly on the left. The lower lobes are affected in 95 to 98 percent of cases. Bilateral involvement may occur. An accurate clinical diagnosis can often be made based on the history and chest radiographic and angiographic findings.

Grossly, intralobar sequestrations usually show the effects of chronic inflammation: pleural thickening, adhesions, and fibrotic parenchyma with cysts up to 5 cm in diameter (fig. 2-12). The cysts often contain mucinous or frankly purulent material. Large feeder arteries may be found.

Histologically, the pulmonary parenchyma shows the effects of chronic inflammation and fibrosis (fig. 2-13). Bronchial remnants may be dilated and contain mucus or purulent material, and the alveoli are characteristically filled with alveolar macrophages, many of which are foamy. Epithelial metaplasia is common. Thick-walled vessels reflecting systemic vascular supply can be highlighted with elastic tissue stains (fig. 2-13). The border between sequestered tissue and normal lung parenchyma may be abrupt or indistinct. The development of squamous carcinoma in an intralobar sequestration has been described (21).

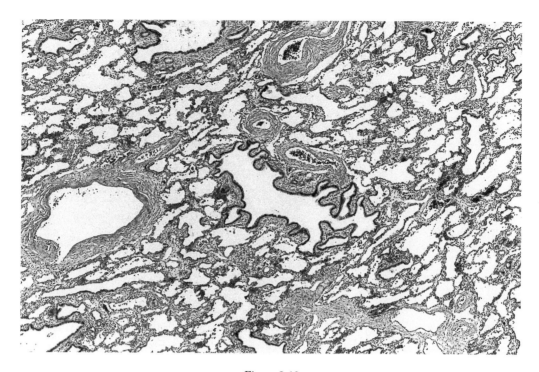

Figure 2-10
EXTRALOBAR SEQUESTRATION
This case shows immature lung tissue without inflammatory changes. Some of the irregularity in the bronchiolar structures is reminiscent of that seen in congenital cystic adenomatoid malformation.

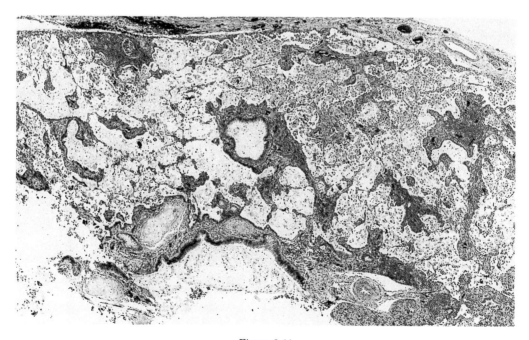

Figure 2-11
EXTRALOBAR SEQUESTRATION
This figure shows extralobar sequestration with secondary inflammatory changes including alveolar septal thickening and inflammation, and mucus stasis.

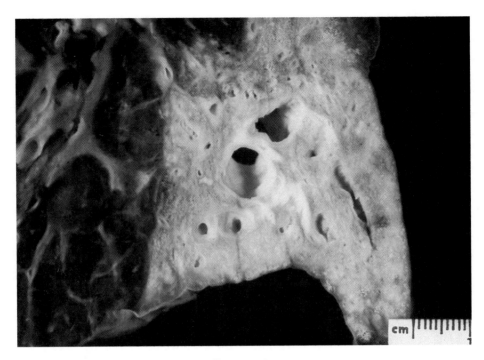

Figure 2-12
INTRALOBAR SEQUESTRATION
The lesions tend to be well demarcated from the adjacent lung parenchyma and may show secondary inflammatory changes and dilated airspaces containing mucus.

Congenital Bronchopulmonary Foregut Malformations

This is an all-encompassing term for sequestrations and bronchopulmonary foregut communications (22,23). According to this concept, all pulmonary sequestrations have a common embryologic origin and can be categorized together as bronchopulmonary foregut malformations. This conclusion is based on the observation of hybrid or mixed intralobar and extralobar sequestrations that communicate with the foregut (24). It is a useful concept for a variety of anomalies of the respiratory and alimentary tracts with associated communications between them and several clinicopathologically recognized lesions are included.

Bronchogenic Cysts (Bronchial Cysts)

Bronchogenic cysts are generally extrapulmonary and probably the residue of supernumerary foregut buds that separated from the tracheobronchial tree (fig. 2-14) (25–28). They rarely contain distal lung parenchyma or communicate with the tracheobronchial tree.

Bronchogenic cysts usually present in children or young adults, although infants and older adults may be affected. There is no sex predilection. Affected infants present with respiratory distress whereas older patients may develop symptoms secondary to infection of the cyst. Fifteen percent of patients are asymptomatic.

Radiographically, there is a mass that is sharply defined and smoothly contoured, with a water-dense center. Most bronchogenic cysts are subcarinal or midmediastinal; however, supraclavicular and infradiaphragmatic bronchogenic cysts are known to occur.

Bronchogenic cysts are usually unilocular and filled with mucus. If infected, they contain grossly purulent material (fig. 2-15).

In noninfected cysts there is a columnar to cuboidal respiratory (ciliated) epithelial lining surrounded by a fibromuscular wall which contains islands of cartilage and nests of bronchial glands (fig. 2-16). Glands and cartilage may require multiple sections for identification. If the lesion has been infected, squamous metaplasia, purulent exudate, and inflammatory changes are common.

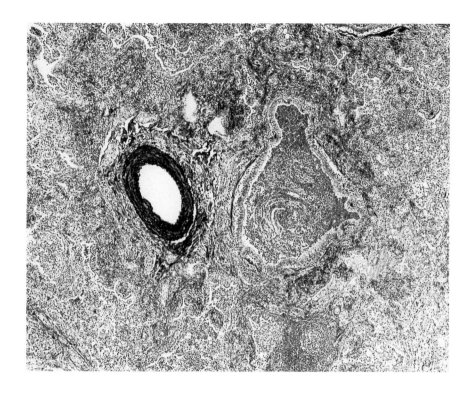

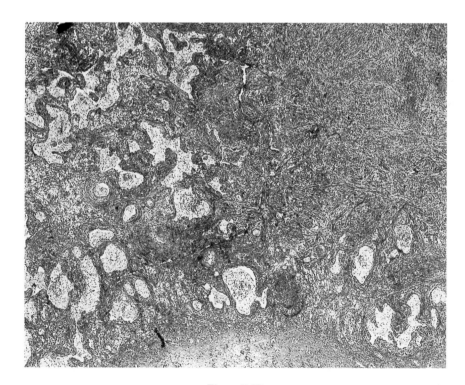

Figure 2-13
INTRALOBAR SEQUESTRATION
Arteriolar thickening is common as are inflammatory changes including purulent exudate within bronchioles (top) and parenchymal fibrosis with distortion of airspaces (bottom). (Top: Elastic tissue stain)

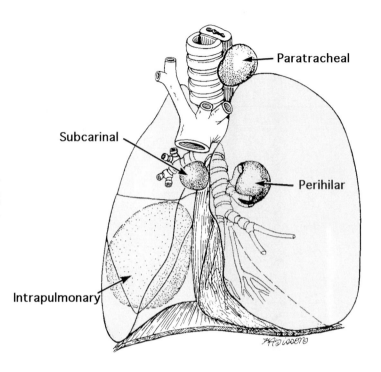

Figure 2-14
SCHEMATIC ILLUSTRATION
OF VARIOUS FORMS
OF BRONCHOGENIC CYSTS

These are located generally toward the midline and usually within the thoracic cavity. (Fig. 27 from Luck SR, Reynolds M, Raffensperger JG. Congenital bronchopulmonary malformations. Curr Probl Surg 1986;23:251–314.)

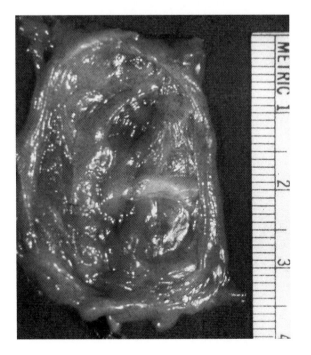

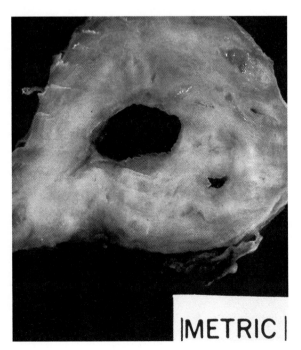

Figure 2-15
BRONCHOGENIC CYSTS

Bronchogenic cysts are grossly nondescript, usually unilocular cavities containing mucus or mucopurulent material with a wall that varies in thickness and may contain cartilage.

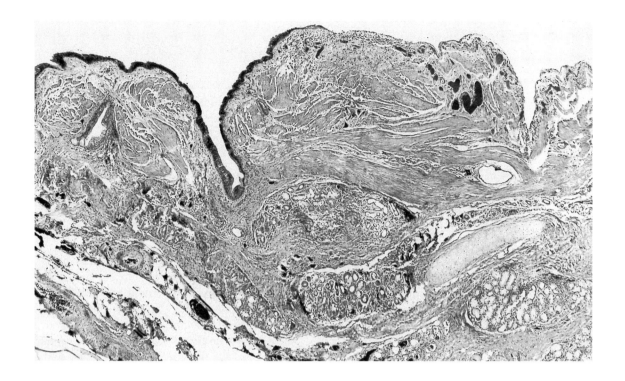

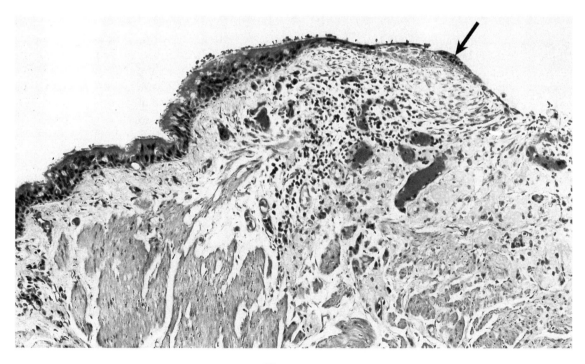

Figure 2-16
INTRATHORACIC BRONCHOGENIC CYST

Top: Histologically, smooth muscle bundles, minor salivary gland type tissue, and cartilage can be seen in the wall of the cyst.
Bottom: The lining is typically pseudostratified ciliated columnar epithelium which may show foci of squamous metaplasia at sites of inflammation (arrow).

Table 2-6

DIFFERENTIAL DIAGNOSIS OF BRONCHOGENIC CYST

Lesion	Features
Abscess	Intrapulmonary; bronchial communication (often multiple); purulent inflammation
Enteric cyst	Posterior mediastinal location; lined by gastric epithelium; may be associated with vertebral malformations
Esophageal cyst	Squamous lining; double muscle layer characteristic of esophageal wall
Pericardial cyst	Location in right or left cardiophrenic angle; unilocular (resembling a hernia sac) with a mesothelial lining
Cystic teratoma	Anterior mediastinal location; multiloculated; endodermal and ectodermal derivatives in addition to bronchial type epithelium; cartilage and bronchial type glands

The differential diagnosis includes abscesses, enteric cysts, esophageal cysts, pericardial cysts, and cystic teratomas. An abscess or other chronic cavity (for example, an infected sequestration) may be impossible to distinguish from a bronchogenic cyst on morphologic grounds alone. Location and type of bronchial and vascular communications may be extremely helpful. The presence of cartilage is necessary for a diagnosis of bronchogenic cyst; when cartilage is lacking, the designation of undifferentiated foregut cyst is appropriate. Key features of the lesions in the differential diagnosis are shown in Table 2-6 (14).

The treatment of bronchogenic cyst is surgical resection. Some cases have been treated by transtracheal needle aspiration, but it is not clear whether this is an effective long-term therapy.

Congenital Cystic Adenomatoid Malformation

Congenital cystic adenomatoid malformation (CCAM) refers to an abnormal mass of lung tissue that appears immature and malformed and may have varying degrees of cystic change (29–31). It is also known as *congenital cystic disease of the lungs and infantile hamartoma*. Compared to normal lung, there is an increase in the number of structures resembling terminal bronchioles, often with polypoid growths of cuboidal epithelium and an increase in underlying stromal elastica and smooth muscle. Cystic change varies with the subtype, and there is generally an absence of inflammation. Cartilage is only rarely present.

CCAMs usually occur in stillborn infants or newborn infants with respiratory distress. Rarely, older children and adults present with an expansile cystic mass. There is a slight male predominance with equal occurrence in the right and left lung. The lesions are usually unilateral and affect only one lobe. Recently, Moerman et al. (30) suggested that segmental bronchial atresia or absence is the primary pathogenetic defect that results in the development of a CCAM distal to the defect. Chest radiographs show a mass, often cystic, which may contain fluid levels or radiolucent foci.

The treatment is resection if other congenital anomalies do not preclude it; CCAMs are thought to predispose to recurring infections if not resected. The prognosis is favorable with resection. CCAM may be complicated by the development of carcinoma (see chapter 16).

Three types of CCAM (types I, II, and III) have been described, based on a combination of gross and microscopic features and the presence or absence of associated anomalies (figs. 2-17–2-20) (31). The three types are outlined in Table 2-7, although there is some overlap among them.

CCAMs may blend imperceptibly with normal-appearing alveolar parenchyma, and communicate with the bronchial tree and be aerated (fig. 2-20). The large spaces are lined by cuboidal or columnar respiratory epithelium, and the smaller alveolus-like spaces are lined by type 1 or type 2 cells; the latter are common in younger patients with more immature lung tissue. Mucinous cells are seen in approximately one third of patients with type I CCAM as scattered clusters and tufts of well-differentiated goblet cells. The smaller cysts in type I lesions and the cysts in type II lesions resemble markedly dilated terminal bronchioles. Type III lesions are bulky masses which histologically resemble the early canalicular stage of lung development.

TYPE I   TYPE II   TYPE III

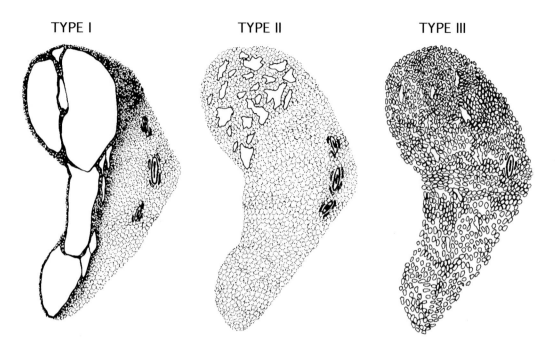

Figure 2-17
CONGENITAL CYSTIC ADENOMATOID MALFORMATION
Diagramatic representation of the three types of congenital cystic adenomatoid malformation. (Fig. 1 from Stocker JT, Madewell JE, Drake RM. Congenital cystic adenomatoid malformation of the lung: classification and morphologic spectrum. Hum Pathol 1977;8:155–72.)

Table 2-7
TYPES OF CONGENITAL CYSTIC ADENOMATOID MALFORMATIONS*

Type (% of cases)	Gross Features	Microscopic Features	Comments
I (65)	Large cysts (up to 10 cm); multilocular with broad septa	Mucinous cells identifiable in one third of cases; marked increase in elastic tissue and smooth muscle in cyst walls; broad fibrous septa; cartilage in 5 to 10 percent	Approximately 15 percent in stillborns; other anomalies rare; this type seen in older children and adults; curable with resection
II (25)	Small cysts (up to 2.5 cm)	Moderate increase in elastic tissue and smooth muscle in cyst walls; skeletal muscle tissue identifiable in 5 percent; mucinous cells rarely seen	One third in stillborns; other anomalies in over 50 percent; poor prognosis
III (10)	Essentially solid with cysts less than 0.5 cm	Mild increase in elastica and smooth muscle in septa; resembles the early canalicular state of lung development (16 to 28 weeks)	One third in stillborns; associated anomalies rare; bulky mass with mediastinal shift; poor prognosis

*Modified from references 14,16,18,31.

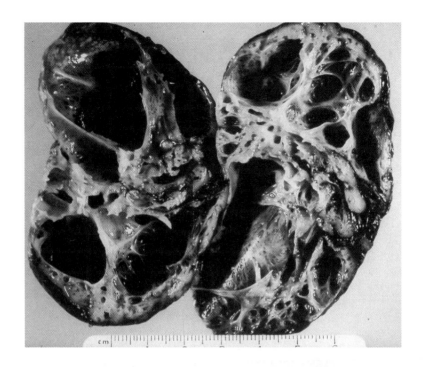

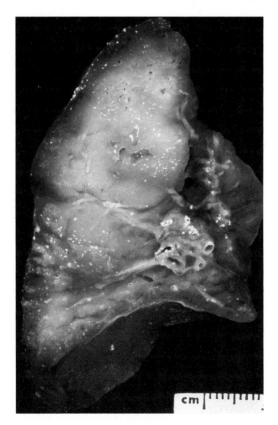

Figure 2-18

GROSS FEATURES FROM TWO CASES OF CONGENITAL CYSTIC ADENOMATOID MALFORMATION

Histologically and clinically both were considered type I although the amount of cystic change is quite variable. Both are surgical resection specimens.

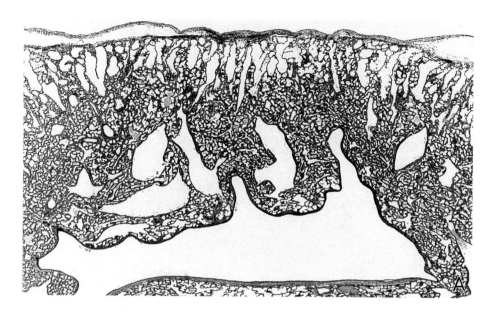

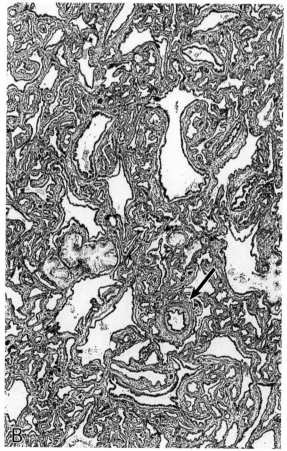

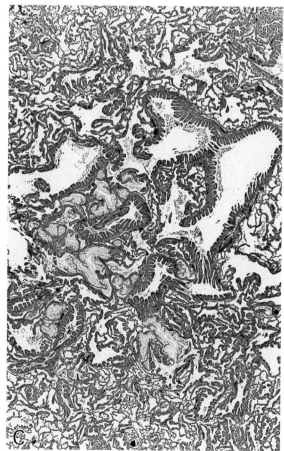

Figure 2-19
CONGENITAL CYSTIC ADENOMATOID MALFORMATION
Scanning power microscopy of three lesions show cystic spaces and peculiar dilated bronchial-like structures, often with papillary epithelial proliferation. In two cases, mucinous epithelium is identifiable. In one (arrow) there is a surprisingly normal-appearing bronchiole among the surrounding abnormally formed lung tissue.

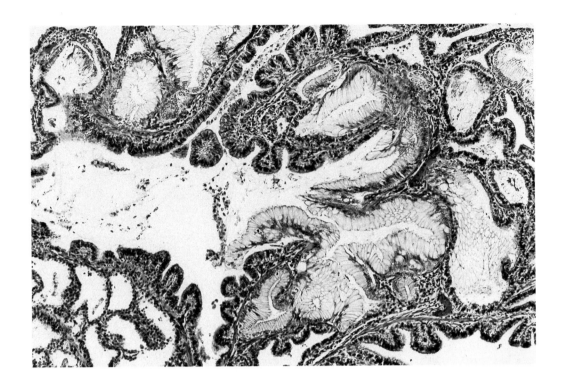

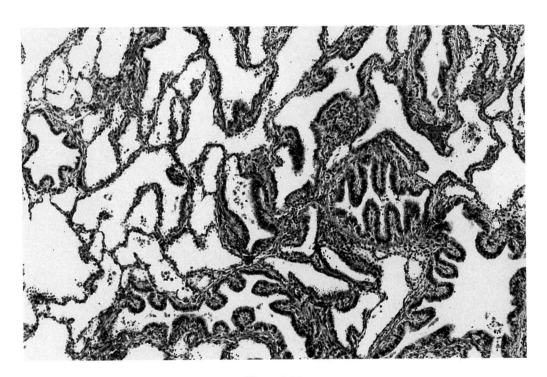

Figure 2-20
CONGENITAL CYSTIC ADENOMATOID MALFORMATION

Top: Higher power microscopy reveals remarkably abnormal-appearing lung tissue, with bronchiolar-like structures containing papillary epithelial proliferations and foci of mucinous metaplasia.

Bottom: Other foci in the same case show more normal-appearing lung parenchyma, although subtle abnormalities in the bronchioles and alveolar-like spaces can be appreciated.

Infantile Lobar Emphysema/Polyalveolar Lobe

Infantile lobar emphysema (congenital lobar overinflation) and polyalveolar lobe are not generally part of the differential diagnosis of childhood neoplasia (14,16–18). They are seen as lobar overinflation within the first 6 months of life in infants with respiratory distress. Chest radiographs show an expansile hyperlucency, usually involving an upper lobe.

Infantile lobar emphysema may be caused by extrinsic or intrinsic obstruction of a bronchus; in some cases no obstruction can be identified. Grossly and microscopically, the tissue appears normal for an adult lung, however, for an infant lung it is in fact overinflated (figs. 2-21, 2-22). In polyalveolar lobe, there is an absolute increase in the number of alveoli (14).

The treatment is surgical resection to avoid further respiratory compromise. Some mild cases have been managed conservatively, with apparent good results (14).

Pulmonary Interstitial Emphysema

Pulmonary interstitial emphysema (14–18) is usually not confused with a lung tumor. It is an acquired condition caused by a rent in the airway wall with dissection of air into the interstitium along bronchovascular structures, septa, and pleura. The interstitial air expands and compresses the normal lung parenchyma, compromising pulmonary function (figs. 2-23–2-25).

Pulmonary interstitial emphysema may be localized or diffuse and is usually associated with a history of mechanical ventilation, often in premature infants. Affected patients often have concomitant pneumothoraces.

Localized forms may be resected because of a presumptive diagnosis of infantile lobar emphysema or congenital cystic adenomatoid malformation. Unless attention is given to the abnormal spaces in the interstitium, which may appear as torn tissue in a poorly prepared slide, the lesions can easily be overlooked or confused with lymphangiectasis or congenital cystic adenomatoid malformation. With chronicity, pulmonary interstitial emphysema is associated with fibrosis and giant cell reaction in the walls (fig. 2-25).

Diffuse Pulmonary Lymphangiectasia

Diffuse pulmonary lymphangiectasia is a rare condition that is usually fatal (13–18,32,33). Occasional patients survive past infancy (32,33). There is diffuse dilatation of the pulmonary lymphatics. Diffuse pulmonary lymphangiectasia may be primary, secondary to associated cardiovascular anomalies, or associated with generalized lymphangiectasis.

Diffuse pulmonary lymphangiectasia is generally not in the differential diagnosis of lung tumors; however, cases diagnosed as lymphangiectasia may actually be localized or diffuse lymphangiomas (lymphangiomatosis) affecting the lung (see chapter 20). Diffuse pulmonary lymphangiectasis is often confused with interstitial emphysema since the interstitial air-filled spaces in the latter condition may be misinterpreted as dilated lymphatics.

Ectopic Tissues in the Lung

Tissue ectopias in the lung are rare. Thyroid tissue has been reported in the trachea (15) and lungs (35), and pancreatic tissue (40,42), neuroglial tissue (fig. 2-26) (37,39,43), and adrenocortical tissue (34,36) have been described in the lung, usually in infants. We have seen cardiac muscle in the walls of the pulmonary artery in the hilus of the lung. Skeletal muscle is also seen in the lung, sometimes associated with other anomalies (38,44).

Endometriosis occurs in the lung and pleura (41), but whether that should be considered a congenital or acquired tissue ectopia is a matter of controversy.

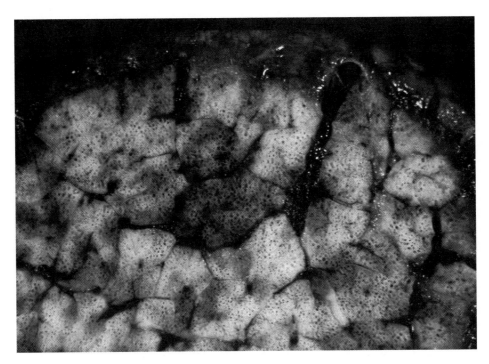

Figure 2-21
INFANTILE LOBAR EMPHYSEMA
Grossly, the lung tissue is remarkably normal appearing although some accentuation of septa can be seen.

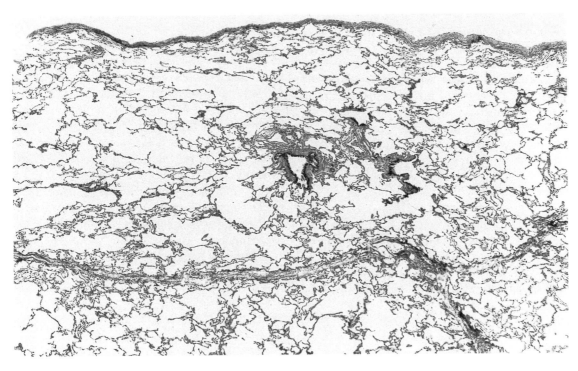

Figure 2-22
INFANTILE LOBAR EMPHYSEMA
Histologically, the lung tissue resembles normal adult lung. Compared to normal lung tissue from an individual of similar age, the alveolar septa are thinner and the alveolar space is more dilated.

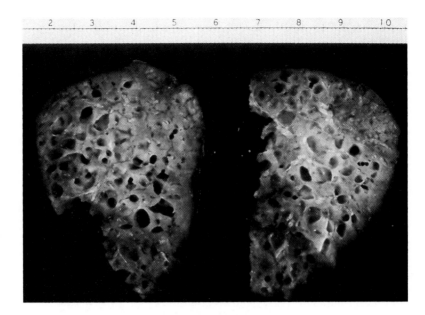

Figure 2-23
PERSISTENT INTERSTITIAL PULMONARY EMPHYSEMA

This lobe was resected for suspected infantile lobar emphysema. The lung tissue is markedly distorted by the massive expansion of interstitial air-containing spaces with associated compression of the lung tissue, which is actually anatomically normal although severely atelectatic. (Courtesy of Dr. Andrew Churg, Vancouver, Canada.)

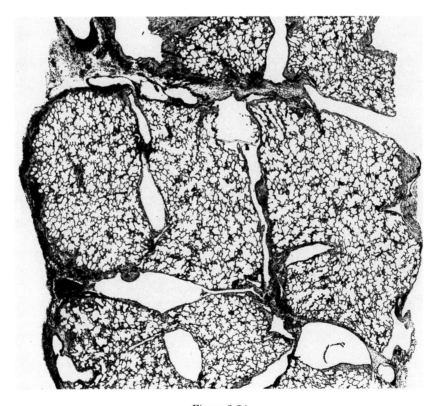

Figure 2-24
EARLY INTERSTITIAL EMPHYSEMA

Early interstitial emphysema results in dilated air-filled spaces within septa and extending into the pleura.

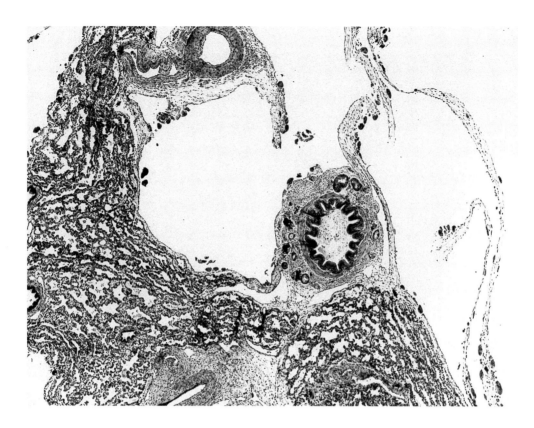

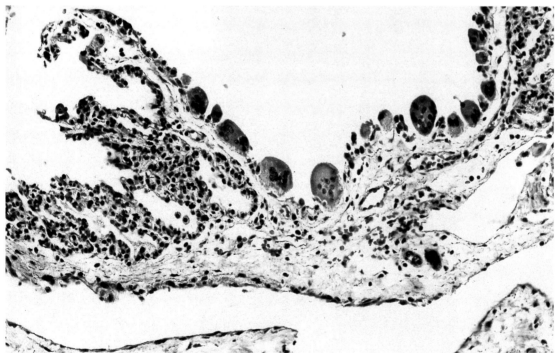

Figure 2-25
PERSISTENT INTERSTITIAL PULMONARY EMPHYSEMA
Top: Persistent interstitial pulmonary emphysema with dissecting air-containing interstitial spaces around a small bronchiole.
Bottom: The reaction has histologic evidence of chronicity in the form of giant cells.

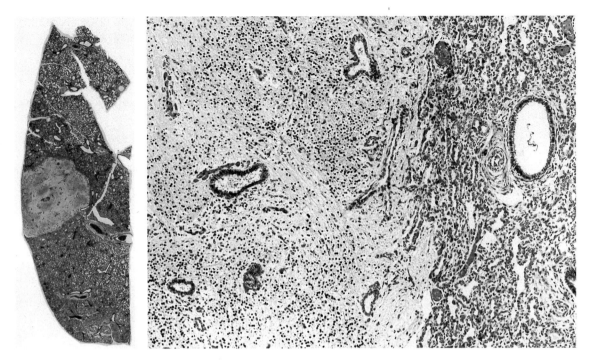

Figure 2-26
NEUROGLIAL HETEROTOPIA
A neuroglial heterotopia found in the lung of a stillborn infant with multiple central nervous system anomalies. The circumscribed subpleural nodule (left) is composed of fibrillar glial tissue surrounding airspaces lined by metaplastic cells (right).

REFERENCES

Embryology

1. Inselman LS, Mellins RB. Growth and development of the lung. J Pediatr 1981;98:1–15.
2. Langston C, Kida K, Reed M, Thurlbeck WM. Human lung growth in late gestation and in the neonate. Am Rev Respir Dis 1984;129:607–13.
3. Moore KL. The developing human. 3rd ed. Philadelphia: WB Saunders, 1982.
4. _____. Essentials of human embryology. Philadelphia: BC Decker, 1988.
5. Thurlbeck WM. Growth, aging, and adaptation. In: Murray JF, Nadel, eds. Textbook of respiratory disease. Philadelphia: WB Saunders, 1988:37–46.

Anatomy and Histology

6. Breeze RG, Wheeldon EB. The cells of the pulmonary airways. Am Rev Respir Dis 1977;116:705–77.
7. Gail DB, Lenfant CJM. Cells of the lung: biology and clinical implications. Am Rev Respir Dis 1983;127:366–87.
8. Kuhn C. Normal anatomy and histology. In: Thurlbeck WM, ed. Pathology of the lung. New York: Thieme, 1988:11–51.
9. Okada Y. Lymphatic system of the human lung. Kyoto-shi, Japan: Kinpodo, 1989.
10. Sorokin SP. The respiratory system. In: Weiss L, ed. Cell and tissue biology. 6th ed. Baltimore: Urban and Schwarzenberg, 1988:753–814.
11. Weibel ER. Design and structure of the human lung. In: Fishman AP, ed. Pulmonary diseases and disorders. 2nd ed. New York: McGraw Hill, 1988:11–60.
12. _____. Lung cell biology. In: Fishman AP, Fisher AB, eds. Handbook of physiology. Bethesda, Md: American Physiological Society, 1985:47–91.

Congenital Anomalies and Related Lesions

13. Gerle RD, Jaretzki A III, Ashley CA, Berne AS. Congenital bronchopulmonary foregut malformation: pulmonary sequestration communicating with the gastrointestinal tract. N Engl J Med 1968;278:1413–9.
14. Katzenstein AA, Askin FB. Surgical pathology of nonneoplastic lung disease. 2nd ed. Philadelphia: WB Saunders, 1990:468–506.
15. Landing BH, Dixon LG. Congenital malformations and genetic disorders of the respiratory tract (larynx, trachea, bronchi, and lungs). Am Rev Respir Dis 1979;120:151–85.
16. Luck SR, Reynolds M, Raffensberger JG. Congenital bronchopulmonary malformations. Curr Probl Surg 1986;23:245–314.

17. Stocker JT. Congenital and developmental diseases. In: Dail DH, Hammer SP, eds. Pulmonary pathology. 2nd ed. New York: Springer-Verlag, 1994:155–90.

18. _____, Drake RM, Madewell JE. Cystic and congenital lung disease in the newborn. Perspect Pediatr Pathol 1978;4:93–154.

Bronchial Atresia

19. Jederlinic PJ, Sicilian LS, Baigelman W, Gaensler EA. Congenital bronchial atresia. A report of four cases and a review of the literature. Medicine (Baltimore) 1987;66:73–83.

20. Meng RL, Jensik RJ, Faber P, Matthew GR, Kittle CF. Bronchial atresia. Ann Thor Surg 1978;25:184–92.

Sequestrations

21. Stocker JT. Sequestrations of the lung. Semin Diagn Pathol 1986;3:106–21.

Bronchopulmonary Foregut Malformations

22. Gerle RD, Jaretzki A III, Ashley CA, Berne AS. Congenital bronchopulmonary foregut malformation. Pulmonary sequestration communicating with the gastrointestinal tract. N Engl J Med 1968;278:1413–9.

23. Heithoff KB, Sane SM, Williams HJ, Jarvis CJ, Carter J, Brennon W. Bronchopulmonary foregut malformations. A unifying etiological concept. Am J Roentgenol 1976;126:46–55.

24. Hruban RH, Shumway SJ, Orel SB, Dumler JS, Baker RR, Hutchins GM. Congenital bronchopulmonary foregut malformations. Intralobar and extralobar pulmonary sequestrations communicating with the foregut. Am J Clin Pathol 1989;91:403–9.

Bronchogenic Cysts

25. Coselli MP, de Ipolyi P, Bloss RS, Diaz RF, Fitzgerald JB. Bronchogenic cysts above and below the diaphragm. Report of eight cases. Ann Thorac Surg 1987;44:491–4.

26. Reed JC, Sobonya RE. Morphologic analysis of foregut cysts in the thorax. Am J Roentgen Rad Ther Nucl Med 1976;120:851–60.

27. Rogers LF, Osmer JC. Bronchogenic cyst. A review of 46 cases. Am Roentgen Rad Ther Nucl Med 1964;91:273–83.

28. Salyer DC, Salyer WR, Eggleston JC. Benign developmental cysts of the mediastinum. Arch Pathol Lab Med 1977;101:136–9.

Congenital Cystic Adenomatoid Malformation

29. Miller RK, Sieber WK, Yunis EJ. Congenital adenomatoid malformation of the lung. A report of 17 cases and review of the literature. Pathol Annu 1980;15(Pt 1):387–402.

30. Moerman P, Fryns JP, Vandenberghe K, Devlieger H, Lauweryns JM. Pathogenesis of congenital cystic adenomatoid malformation of the lung. Histopathology 1992;21:315–21.

31. Stocker JT, Madewell JE, Drake RM. Congenital cystic adenomatoid malformation of the lung. Classification and morphologic spectrum. Hum Pathol 1977;8:155–71.

Diffuse Pulmonary Lymphangiectasia

32. Case records of the Massachusetts General Hospital (Case 13-1992). New Engl J Med 1992;326:875–84.

33. Hernandez RJ, Stern AM, Rosenthal A. Pulmonary lymphangiectasis in Noonan syndrome. AJR Am J Roentgenol 1980;134:75–80.

Ectopic Tissues in the Lung

34. Armin A, Castelli M. Congenital adrenal tissue in the lung with adrenal cytomegaly. Case report and review of the literature. Am J Clin Pathol 1984;82:225–8.

35. Bando T, Genka K, Ishikawa K, Kuniyoshi M, Kuda T. Ectopic intrapulmonary thyroid. Chest 1993;103:1278–9.

36. Bozic C. Ectopic fetal adrenal cortex in the lung of a newborn. Virchows Arch [A] 1974;363:371–4.

37. Campo E, Bombi JA. Central nervous system heterotopia in the lung of a fetus with cranial malformation. Virchows Arch [A] 1981;391:117–22.

38. Chen MF, Onerheim R, Wang NS, Huttner I. Rhabdomyomatosis of newborn lung: a case report with immunohistochemical and electronmicroscopic characterization of striated muscle cells in the lung. Pediatr Pathol 1991;11:123–9.

39. Chen WJ, Kelly MM, Shaw CM, Mottet NK. Pathogenic mechanisms of heterotopic neural tissue associated with anencephaly. Hum Pathol 1982;13:179–82.

40. Corrin B, Danel C, Allaway A, Warner J, Lenney W. Intralobar pulmonary sequestration of ectopic pancreatic tissue with gastropancreatic duplication. Thorax 1985;40:637–8.

41. Hibbard LT, Schumann WR, Goldstein GE. Thoracic endometriosis: a review and report of two cases. Am J Obstet Gynecol 1981;140:227–32.

42. Kellett HS, Lipphard D, Willis RA. Two unusual examples of heteroplasia in the lung. J Pathol Bacteriol 1962;84:421–5.

43. Kershisnik MM, Kaplan C, Craven CM, Carey JC, Townsend JJ, Knisely AS. Intrapulmonary neuroglial heterotopia. Arch Pathol Lab Med 1992;116:1043–6.

44. Vilanova JR, Burgos-Bretones J, Aguirre JM, Rivera-Pomar JM. Rhabdomyomatous dysplasia of lung and congenital diaphragmatic hernia. J Pediatr Surg 1983;18:201–3.

3
SPECIMEN HANDLING AND SPECIAL TECHNIQUES

ROUTINE HANDLING OF LUNG SPECIMENS

The lung is the source of a large number of cytologic and histologic specimens (Table 3-1). From these specimens, the pathologist must make a diagnosis, and participate in the clinical and pathologic staging of the tumor (2,27,30,45,53, 58,75,81).

The pathologist's first priority in the evaluation of a lung tumor, making a specific histologic diagnosis, can usually be accomplished with routine cytologic or histologic preparations. These may be supplemented as necessary with ancillary histochemical or immunohistochemical studies. If adequate diagnostic tissue is available, special studies such as electron microscopy, frozen section immunostaining, cytogenetics, and molecular studies can be done. In the case of small specimens, all the tissue should be routinely processed; if a diagnosis cannot be made, then subsequent biopsies can be prospectively triaged for the necessary and appropriate special studies. This is commonly the case with malignant lymphoma, in which biopsy specimens may be too small for definitive diagnosis without the aid of immunophenotypic studies.

The pathologic staging of a primary lung tumor is contingent on appropriate gross and microscopic examination of resection specimens. Standardized and unified staging schemes are necessary for comparative and collaborative studies of lung tumors (2,45,53). The staging criteria for bronchogenic carcinomas are outlined in chapter 8.

The following approach can be applied to segmentectomy, lobectomy, pneumonectomy, en bloc resections, and tracheal or bronchial sleeve resections. Lung tumor specimens are examined either fresh or after formalin fixation; each method of examination has advantages and disadvantages. Formalin inflation and fixation is achieved by cannulation of the bronchus (or a pulmonary artery) and inflation with 10 percent buffered formalin at a pressure close to 20 cm of water, or from a formalin reservoir 1 to 2 feet above the specimen. Normal lung parenchyma is

Table 3-1

SPECIMENS FROM LUNG TUMORS

Cytologic specimens
    Sputum (+/- aerosol induction)
    Transtracheal aspirate
    Bronchial brushing
    Bronchial washing/secretion
    Bronchoalveolar lavage (BAL)
    Pulmonary arterial blood cytologies
    Transbronchial and transtracheal needle aspirates
    Fine needle aspirations, smears, and touch preparations made from histologic specimens
    Effusion (especially pleural)

Histologic specimens
    Biopsies
        Tracheal/bronchial biopsy
        Transbronchial biopsy
        Thoracoscopic biopsy
        Transthoracic drill or cutting needle biopsy
        Mediastinoscopic biopsies (lymph node metastases)
        Thoracotomy with biopsy
    Resection specimens*
        Open lung biopsy
        Wedge resection
        Segmentectomy
        Lobectomy
        Bilobectomy
        Pneumonectomy
        Radical and en bloc resections including adjacent structures
        Sleeve resections of large airways
    Autopsy tissue

*Any of these specimens may include portions of adjacent structures such as the parietal pleura, chest wall, mediastinal structures, etc.

usually adequately fixed for gross sectioning in a few hours, but overnight fixation is necessary for fixation of tumor masses and extensively consolidated lung tissue. Inflated specimens are sliced at regular intervals at any selected plane; traditionally, sagittal sectioning has been used, although the use of computerized tomography (CT) has made sectioning in the transverse or horizontal plane (cross sections) preferable for correlation with CT images.

The sectioned lung tissue slices are kept in order, to reconstruct the anatomy and not lose specific relationships and landmarks needed to provide necessary information. Fresh uninflated specimens are obtained by carefully cutting out along the major airways, with particular attention to tumor location and relationship to airways and vessels. Before this is done, the bronchial margin is sectioned and often examined at frozen section. The use of probes may be helpful in selecting which of the intermediate-sized and smaller airways should be sectioned, depending on their proximity to the tumor.

The Surgical Pathology Report

Regardless of the gross evaluation method, the following information should be recorded in the pathology report for both diagnostic and staging purposes.

1. General external appearance of the resection specimen including dimensions, weight, color, appearance of pleura, and other structures included (pericardium, chest wall, etc.).

2. Tumor histologic subtype and grade; location (by segment if possible, see figure 2-5); color; consistency; secondary changes (such as cavitation); size in three dimensions; endobronchial or intravascular growth; relationship to bronchial mucosa, bronchial wall, pleura, fissures, and dissected surgical margins (inking the specimen and elastic tissue stains are helpful in determining these relationships); distance from bronchial margin and pleura; secondary changes (especially obstructive pneumonia); vascular invasion; invasion of adjacent structures (pleura, chest wall) and margins thereof; and associated dysplasia/carcinoma in situ in the proximal bronchial mucosa. The pleura includes both an internal and a common elastic lamina and invasion of either (best assessed by elastic tissue stain) is significant (27).

3. Assessment of nontumorous lung tissue for associated conditions such as chronic bronchitis, emphysema, asbestosis, and respiratory (smoker's) bronchiolitis. Tissue showing secondary effects of the tumor, as with obstructive pneumonia, should be avoided in these evaluations.

4. Examination of all lymph nodes, including those dissected off the main specimen, as well as all other intrathoracic nodes submitted separately by the surgeon. The nodes

Table 3-2

APPORTIONING LUNG TISSUE FOR SPECIAL STUDIES

Fresh tissue
    Flow cytometry
    Cytogenetics
    Cell culture

Snap frozen tumor and nontumor lung tissue saved
    at -80° C
    Frozen section immunostains including lymphoid
      marker studies
    Molecular genetics/gene rearrangements
    Quantitative biochemistry (e.g., peptide hormones)

Glutaraldehyde-fixed tumor tissue for electron
    microscopy
    1 mm cubes or
    tissue flakes 1 mm or less in thickness

Nontumorous lung tissue for microprobe or quantitative analysis
    (e.g., for asbestos)

should be kept separate according to their location for staging purposes (see chapter 8). For those on the main specimen, their relationship to the tumor should be noted.

5. Examination and description of separately submitted tissue (such as pericardium).

6. Selection of tumor and nontumorous lung tissue for special studies (see next section) in certain cases (Table 3-2).

7. Photographic documentation of above features and pictorial location of tissue blocks taken for microscopy in complicated cases. Drawings and xerographs of actual specimens are useful in illustrating the site of tissue blocks taken for microscopy.

A minimum of three sections of tumor and one section of nontumorous lung tissue should be examined in routine cases. These blocks should allow assessment of the relationship of the tumor to bronchial mucosa, bronchial wall, and pleura. A histologic section of the bronchial margin should be taken. All lymph nodes, separately submitted tissues, and margins of attached tissues should be histologically examined. For clinically occult lesions, especially squamous carcinoma in situ, microinvasive squamous carcinoma, and cases with extensive dysplasia, serial blocking and sectioning of the airways are often necessary.

Examination and description of lung tumor specimens should provide information for TNM staging

Table 3-3

PATHOLOGIC INFORMATION FROM RESECTION SPECIMENS NECESSARY FOR TNM STAGING

Features of the tumor (T):
    Histologic type (WHO) and grade*
    Size (greatest dimension)
    Distance from and status of bronchial margin
    Invasion of pleura (visceral or parietal; fissures) and adjacent structures (and margins thereof)
    Associated obstructive pneumonia

Lymph nodes (N):
    Total number of involved nodes for each separately submitted lymph node station including lymph nodes
        dissected from the specimen

*Histologic grading:
    (1) Well differentiated
    (2) Moderately differentiated
    (3) Poorly differentiated
    (4) Undifferentiated

*From reference 2.

(see chapter 8). The minimum information needed in the pathology report is shown in Table 3-3.

Protocols for the evaluation of lung carcinomas are currently being assembled by a number of groups. An example of the synoptic report used at Memorial Sloan Kettering Cancer Center was recently published by Rosai et al. (76).

SPECIAL TECHNIQUES

Remarkable advances have taken place in the diagnosis and study of lung tumors due to an explosion in the development of special techniques in the fields of immunohistochemistry, flow cytometry, in situ hybridization, and molecular biology. These developments have revolutionized the approach to the diagnosis of certain lung tumors and our thinking with regard to histogenesis and pathogenesis. This Fascicle would not be complete without highlighting some of these new developments as they apply to lung tumors. Some of the important diagnostic or prognostic information provided by these techniques is also mentioned in the discussion of specific tumors throughout the text.

Immunohistochemistry

Remarkable developments in immunohistochemical methods have revolutionized the pathologic research and diagnosis of lung tumors. The technical aspects of this subject have been reviewed in detail (18). In lung tumors, immunohistochemistry is a powerful diagnostic tool used for detecting a wide range of epithelial, mesenchymal, lymphoid, melanocytic, hormonal, neuroendocrine, and molecular markers. Since specific applications of immunohistochemistry for particular tumors are included in other chapters, this section is restricted to a brief discussion of the few markers for lung carcinoma not addressed elsewhere: immunohistochemical demonstration of cell proliferation markers, carbohydrate antigens, and histocompatibility locus antigens (HLA).

Cell Proliferation Markers. There are several methods for staining nuclei to determine cell proliferative activity including immunohistochemical staining for proliferating cell nuclear antigen (PCNA) and Ki-67, and silver staining for nucleolar organizing regions (AgNORs). PCNA is a 36kD acid nuclear protein involved in DNA synthesis. In formalin-fixed, paraffin-embedded tissues the monoclonal antibody PC10 against PCNA stains the nuclei of cells in S phase, late G1 phase, and early G2 phase. Higher PCNA immunoreactivity scores correlate with aneuploidy, Ki-67 labeling, S-phase fraction of aneuploid tumors, and mitotic counts in peripheral lymph node–negative nonsmall cell lung carcinoma (25). PCNA is also a significant predictor of survival by both univariate and multivariate analysis (24,25).

One study shows that Ki-67 labeling holds promise as a possible indicator of short-term survival in operable nonsmall cell lung carcinoma (90). However, multiparameter flow cytometry in 15 nonsmall cell lung carcinomas showed no correlation between Ki-67 staining and DNA ploidy, S-phase fraction, or histologic type (64).

Although not an immunohistochemical technique, AgNORs are used as a measure of cell proliferative activity. In lung cancer, AgNORs correlate with survival in patients with stage I nonsmall cell lung carcinoma (41). A high inverse correlation was found with the doubling time as measured by growth rates in chest radiographs in patients with lung adenocarcinomas (67) and squamous cell carcinomas (1), suggesting a correlation with the rate of tumor growth. One study of 138 cases of squamous cell carcinoma found that AgNORs are not of prognostic value (8). Another study of 58 lung adenocarcinomas found AgNOR counts not related to either the degree of histologic differentiation or the pathologic staging (67).

A study correlating Ki-67 indices and AgNOR scores showed that the kinetic data obtained by the AgNOR technique was less discriminating than with Ki-67 (85). Therefore, use of the monoclonal antibody Ki-67 may be a more reliable method of assessing proliferative activity in lung tumors (85).

Carbohydrate Antigens. The major types of carbohydrate antigens evaluated in lung carcinomas include blood group antigens (particularly Le^x) (56,61), the neural cell adhesion molecule (NCAM) (66), neoglycoproteins (44), and fucosyl-G_{m1} ganglioside (Fuc-GM1) (66). Different carbohydrate profiles correspond to different histologic subtypes. NCAM and Fuc-GM1 are frequently expressed in small cell lung carcinoma (66), while α-fucosyl-, α-mannosyl-, and α-glucosyl-specific receptors are frequently found in adenocarcinomas and squamous cell carcinomas but not in small cell lung carcinoma (44). Several studies have shown that carbohydrate expression predicts survival (56,61). Metastatic potential and survival were found to correlate with expression of 4C9 antigen (an Le^x antigen) and the *Dolichos biflorus* agglutinin (DBA) binding site (an N-acetylgalactosamine marker) (56). Loss of expression of blood group A

and H/Le^y/Le^b expression detected by the monoclonal antibody MIA-15-5 have been shown to correlate with poor survival (61).

Histocompatibility Antigens. Histocompatibility antigen expression (human leukocyte antigen, HLA) in lung carcinoma specimens has been examined by immunohistochemistry (16) and other techniques (55,73). Studies have shown variation in HLA-A,B,C expression according to histologic type and degree of differentiation (16). These differences may correlate with the variation in stromal infiltrates, which may reflect host immunologic defense mechanisms against the tumors. In small cell lung carcinoma, marked decreases of HLA-A,B,C and β-2-microglobulin have been demonstrated (55). This may allow small cell lung carcinoma to evade host immune responses, providing one potential explanation for its very malignant behavior.

Flow Cytometry

Flow cytometry is a useful tool for measuring ploidy (DNA content) and proliferative capacity in lung tumors. Other biological parameters analyzed by flow cytometry include cell size, cell viability, cytoplasmic granularity, and surface and intracellular antigens (95). Multiparameter flow cytometry allows correlation of multiple biological measurements on normal and neoplastic cells. The technical aspects of flow cytometry and other methods of analyzing DNA content are beyond the scope of this discussion and are reviewed elsewhere.

The frequency of aneuploidy in nonsmall cell lung carcinoma has been reported as low as 21 percent (22), but in most studies it is about 70 to 80 percent (17,33,62,80). Aneuploidy has been reported in 49 to 85 percent of cases of small cell lung carcinoma (11).

Many studies have shown aneuploidy to correspond to an unfavorable prognosis in patients with nonsmall cell lung carcinoma (22,62). A high proliferation index has also been found to be a negative prognostic factor (17). In several studies, multivariate analysis showed aneuploidy to be an independent predictor of survival (97); in other studies, however, aneuploidy had no prognostic value (12,15). For small cell lung carcinoma, some studies found a correlation between aneuploidy and survival (11) while others did not (69). These differences in the significance of aneuploidy may reflect variation in technique, types of specimen (paraffin-embedded, fresh, or cytologic; surgical resection or bronchoscopic biopsy), the patient population studied (distribution of stage or histologic subtype of carcinoma), study design, and data analysis. Further data are needed in this area.

The importance of tumor heterogeneity and multiple site sampling of lung cancer specimens for flow cytometry has been emphasized (10,87). In one study of 20 lung tumors, 19 (95 percent) were shown to have aneuploidy by systematic sampling of multiple tissue blocks; when only one block was studied, the percent of cases with aneuploidy was 45 (10). In addition, if the tumor tissue was specifically selected, aneuploidy could be found in 90 percent of the cases, while it was present in only 75 percent of the cases in which the entire tissue block was analyzed. Another study analyzing samples from the tumor center and edge in 59 nonsmall cell lung cancers found DNA heterogeneity (in terms of different number of DNA stem lines or different DNA indices) in 50 percent of cases (87). A third study indicated identical DNA content in 3 samples from 28 nonsmall cell lung carcinomas for all 5 diploid tumors and 82 percent of aneuploid tumors; only 17 percent of aneuploid tumors showed regional DNA heterogeneity, expressed as additional stem lines in at least one sample (78).

Flow cytometry was also used to assess the DNA ploidy pattern in each carcinomatous component of 12 adenosquamous carcinomas (38). In 8 of the 12 (67 percent) tumors, both the adenocarcinoma and squamous cell carcinoma components either showed diploid or aneuploid populations, with at least one identical abnormal clone based upon DNA index in both components. These results indicated that the DNA content was related in the two histologic tumor components.

In addition, flow cytometry has been used to determine whether two synchronous lung tumors are separate primaries or intrapulmonary metastases (37). Tumors with different patterns of DNA ploidy were regarded as synchronous primaries if both tumors showed diploidy; if at least one DNA index of abnormal clones from two aneuploid tumors was the same or similar, the cases were regarded as intrapulmonary metastases.

Flow cytometry can be used to analyze lung carcinomas with antibodies to oncoproteins such as P53, c-*myc*, and epidermal growth factor receptor (EGFR) (17,65,88) as well as the cell proliferation markers Ki-67 and PCNA (62,64,88). Multiparameter flow cytometry analyzing tumors for more than one of these markers can provide insights into the relationship between different markers in a given tumor cell population. One study simultaneously measured p53 and DNA content. The S-phase fraction was significantly greater in p53-positive cases, indicating a correlation of p53 with proliferative activity (65). One study of 15 nonsmall cell lung carcinomas showed that DNA ploidy did not correlate with accumulation of p53 protein, c-*myc* overexpression, or Ki-67 staining (64). Dazzi et al. (17) found that a high proliferation index in nonsmall cell carcinoma was a poor prognostic factor and was found more often in tumors where the majority of cells expressed EGFR.

Miyamoto et al. (62) immunohistochemically analyzed *ras* oncogene expression in 91 nonsmall cell lung carcinomas using anti-*ras* M_r 21,000 protein (p21) monoclonal antibody rp-35. Univariate analysis showed that p21 expression was a significant poor prognostic factor. By multivariate analysis, DNA ploidy, *ras* p21 expression, and the stage of the disease were significant independent prognostic factors.

Molecular Biology

Application of techniques in molecular biology has resulted in a better understanding of the genetic events that contribute to carcinogenesis, tumor growth, invasion, and metastasis of lung cancer (6,39). Normal cell proliferation is controlled by a group of coordinated cellular events regulated by a balanced expression of multiple genes and gene products. Carcinogenesis is a multistep process by which a series of genetic events results in an imbalance of activated proto-oncogenes and suppressor genes, leading to cellular transformation and autonomous, uncontrolled cellular growth (fig 3-1). These carcinogenic events may occur under the influence of carcinogen exposure, host genetic factors, or both over a period of many years in successive steps involving multiple genes.

Molecular markers are potentially useful for early detection, monitoring response to therapy,

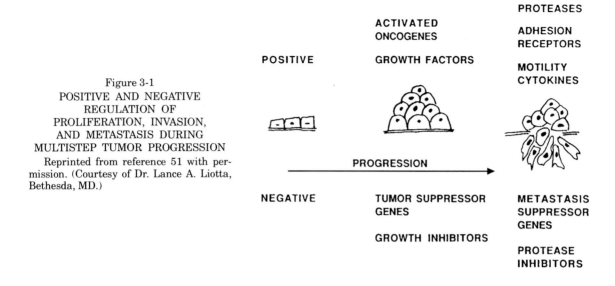

Figure 3-1
POSITIVE AND NEGATIVE
REGULATION OF
PROLIFERATION, INVASION,
AND METASTASIS DURING
MULTISTEP TUMOR PROGRESSION
Reprinted from reference 51 with permission. (Courtesy of Dr. Lance A. Liotta, Bethesda, MD.)

predicting metastatic potential and prognosis, and furthering the understanding of the etiology and carcinogenesis of lung cancer. As the molecular events of lung carcinogenesis, and invasion and metastasis are understood, innovative therapeutic approaches are being developed (59).

The molecular biology of lung cancer is divided into 1) carcinogenesis and 2) invasion and metastasis.

Carcinogenesis. Two major categories of genes are recognized in lung carcinogenesis: oncogenes (dominant) and suppressor genes (recessive oncogenes). Only a single mutation is necessary for a dominant oncogene to cause cancer while suppressor genes are considered recessive since mutations have to affect both copies of the gene for carcinogenesis to occur (59). Molecular mechanisms of oncogene activation include amplification, point mutation, translocation, and overexpression of a transcript or protein. With suppressor genes, the initial mutation is often a point mutation or another small alteration, resulting in inactivation or alteration of one copy of the gene. The second genetic change is a larger alteration, such as a deletion or translocation in the DNA of the complimentary chromosome, resulting in loss of heterozygosity (LOH) for the suppressor gene. As a result, the product of the suppressor gene is either rendered nonfunctional or is completely lost. The ultimate effect is loss of tumor suppression which enhances carcinogenesis (59).

Oncogenes. An oncogene is a gene that is normally involved with control of cellular proliferation and differentiation in which an alteration can trigger carcinogenesis. These genes are present in normal cells (proto-oncogenes) and code for cellular proteins such as growth factors, protein kinases, proteins involved in membrane signaling, and nuclear proteins which regulate gene expression. Many oncogenes, such as K-*ras* (Kirsten murine sarcoma virus), were first identified as the normal cellular homologues of the acute transforming genes of RNA tumor viruses. Other oncogenes, such as L-*myc* in small cell carcinoma, are not related to viruses but are identified because they are consistently amplified in naturally occurring tumors (59). The dominant oncogenes identified in lung cancer are listed in Table 3-4. For the purposes of this discussion, only *ras* and *myc* oncogenes will be addressed.

The *ras* family of oncogenes includes three genes: K-*ras*, H-*ras*, and N-*ras*. These code for 21-kilodalton proteins localized to the inner side of the cell membrane, which bind to guanosine triphosphate (GTP) and are implicated in signal transduction (59). Mutations in K-*ras* predominate in lung cancer, particularly in codons 12 and 13 (59). Most mutations are guanine (G) to thymidine (T) transversions and lead to changes in the amino acid sequence. K-*ras* mutations are found in 20 to 30 percent of adenocarcinomas, 21 percent of large cell carcinomas, and 5 percent of

Table 3-4

MOLECULAR MARKERS ASSOCIATED WITH LUNG CANCER

Activated proto-oncogenes (59,93)
  c-*myc*, L-*myc*, N-*myc* (deregulated expression)
  Ki-*ras*, Ha-*ras*, N-*ras* (activating mutation)
  c-*erb*-B2 (Her-2/*neu*) (EGF receptor gene;
      deregulated expression)
  c-*raf*-1
  c-*jun*
  c-*myb*
  c-*fms*
  fur
  bcl-1, *bcl*-2 (71)

Tumor suppressor genes (50,93)
  17 (*nm*23) (36)
  3p14
  3p21
  3p24-25 (von Hippel-Lindau gene)
  5q (FAP, MCC gene cluster)
  9p (interferon gene cluster)
  11;15, ~11p13
  13q14 (retinoblastoma gene [*Rb*])
  17p13 (p53)

Autocrine growth factors (70)
  Transforming growth factor-α (77) and β
  Epidermal growth factor/receptor, *erb*B-2
      (HER-2/*neu*) (77)
  Insulin-like growth factor/receptor (3)
  Gastrin-releasing peptide/receptor (small cell
      carcinoma) (59)
  μ, σ, κ opioids/receptors (59)
  Transferrin/receptor (14,29)
  Nicotine/receptor (59)
  Stem cell factor/c-kit (small cell carcinoma)
  Platelet-derived growth factor (4)

squamous cell carcinomas; they are rare in small cell lung carcinoma (59). K-*ras* mutations are correlated with cigarette smoking and a poor prognosis in patients with lung adenocarcinoma (74). Mutations in all three *ras* oncogenes are significant indicators of poor prognosis in non-small cell lung carcinoma (60), as is the immunohistochemical detection of enhanced *ras* p21 expression (62).

The *myc* oncogenes (c-*myc*, N-*myc*, and L-*myc*), which code for nuclear phosphoproteins that regulate transcription and control cell growth by binding to specific DNA sequences, are also important in lung cancer (59). In contrast to *ras*, the best known *myc* alterations include gene amplification and protein over-expression. Overexpression of one of the *myc* oncogenes occurs in 10 to 40 percent of small cell lung carcinomas; amplification of *myc* oncogenes is rare in untreated nonsmall cell lung carcinoma but can be found in up to 28 percent of nonsmall cell lung carcinomas in combination chemotherapy–treated patients.

Tumor Suppressor Genes. Tumor suppressor genes (recessive oncogenes) are genes whose normal function is to restrain cellular proliferation and tumorigenesis. The tumor suppressor genes recognized in lung cancer are listed in Table 3-4. These are often detected by restriction fragment length polymorphism (RFLP) analysis which shows allelic loss in tumor tissues: the retinoblastoma gene and p53 are tumor suppressor genes important in lung cancer. Multiple loci in the short arm of chromosome 3 also appear to contain tumor suppressor genes that are important in the pathogenesis of both small cell and non-small cell carcinoma, but the specific genes remain to be identified (49,59).

Located in the short arm of chromosome 17, p53 is a tumor suppressor gene that encodes a nuclear phosphoprotein with known functions as a transcription factor and cell cycle checkpoint (59). Loss of the p53 gene is the most frequently occurring gene mutation in human cancer. The p53 protein is thought to act in complex with other proteins as a transcription factor which may activate an entire panel of growth regulatory or tumor suppressor genes (59). Mutations in the p53 gene are common in both small cell carcinomas (more than 80 percent) and non-small cell carcinomas (60 percent) (59). Similar to *ras*, the most common mutation consists of guanine:cytosine (G:C) to thymine:adenine (T:A) transversions, which are often associated with smoking. The mutational spectrum is also somewhat different according to histologic type, which may also reflect differences in tobacco use. However, a different pattern of p53 mutations was seen in the radon-associated lung cancers from uranium miners, suggesting a different pathogenesis than smoking-associated lung cancer (92). The mutations in p53 involve the entire coding sequence, but tend to occur in certain hot spots. The pattern of specific p53 gene alteration in primary lung carcinomas is preserved in brain metastases (79). Since the addition of a wild-type (normal) p53 gene to a tumor cell line can inhibit tumor formation in an animal model, p53 may be a candidate for gene therapy in lung cancer patients (59).

Wild-type (normal) p53 protein has a short half-life of about 20 minutes and normally does not accumulate to detectable levels. Missense mutations frequently prolong the half-life so that the protein accumulates to levels detectable by immunohistochemistry (7,94) These mutations account for 85 percent of p53 alterations, and diffuse, intense immunostaining in a lung neoplasm usually correlates with mutation. Deletions and nonsense mutations do not produce p53 protein. Immunohistochemical detection of p53 protein overexpression in nonsmall cell lung cancer correlates with the degree of histologic differentiation (94), lymph node metastases (23), and cigarette smoking (94). In stage I and II nonsmall cell lung cancer, p53 protein detection correlates with a poor prognosis (59). Microdissection and genetic analysis of immunohistochemically positive progenitor lesions have shown that p53 mutations can occur before the onset of invasion in squamous cell lung cancer (fig. 3-2) (34). Immunohistochemical analysis of bronchial resections from 34 patients demonstrated p53 protein accumulation in 30 percent of mild dysplasias and showed that most p53 mutations occurred before the onset of invasion (figs. 3-2, 3-3) (7).

Recently, serum antibodies to p53 have been found in 13 percent of lung cancer patients. In small cell lung carcinoma, these antibodies appear to correlate with prolonged survival and good performance status (59). p53-mediated transactivation can be inhibited by a product of the murine double minute 2 gene (mdm-2), a cellular phosphoprotein that forms a complex with both mutant and wild-type p53 protein (63).

A significantly higher level of p53 expression has been shown by multiparameter flow cytometry in c-*myc*–positive compared to c-*myc*–negative tumors (64). This suggests an association between accumulation of p53 protein and c-*myc* overexpression in nonsmall cell lung carcinoma.

The retinoblastoma gene (*Rb*) is mutated in over 80 percent of small cell lung carcinomas and 20 to 30 percent of nonsmall cell lung carcinomas (59). This gene encodes for a 100-kilodalton nuclear phosphoprotein known to form protein complexes with multiple proteins including transcription factors and cyclins. As a result, the *Rb* protein influences the function of multiple proteins, some of which are thought to be transcription factors or other factors that initiate cell growth. Mutations in the *Rb* gene lead to impaired function of this suppressor protein and allow the development of lung cancer. In cell culture, replacement of a damaged *Rb* gene with a normal copy can restore normal cellular growth (59).

Hereditary/Genetic Factors for Lung Cancer. Several hereditary factors are known to predispose to lung cancer. Many patients with Li-Fraumeni syndrome have germ line p53 mutations and develop multiple primary cancers, including lung cancer (59). First degree relatives of lung cancer patients are also predisposed to lung cancer (59). In addition, a significantly increased risk of lung cancer is found in patients with increased activity of the p450 enzyme debrisoquine hydroxylase (an antihypertensive medication) (9); the gene for this phenotype (CYP2D6) has been cloned. Higher levels of another p450 enzyme, aryl hydrocarbon hydroxylase, have been found in peripheral blood lymphocytes, alveolar macrophages, and lung tissues of lung cancer patients (5).

Growth Factors. Tumor cell proliferation occurs under the influence of a variety of growth factors, which are produced either by tumor cells (autocrine) or normal cells (paracrine) (59). One of the first recognized autocrine growth factors in small cell lung carcinoma was gastrin releasing peptide (GRP), which also has a growth stimulatory effect after binding to GRP receptors on the tumor cells (59). A list of growth factors expressed in lung cancer is found in Table 3-4.

DNA Adducts. Covalent DNA addition products (adducts) are useful markers for studying the genetic epidemiology of lung carcinogenesis (82). DNA adducts result from the covalent binding of carcinogens such as polycyclic aromatic hydrocarbons (PAH) to DNA, resulting in DNA damage. These adducts can be measured in peripheral blood leukocytes or in lung tissue (72), including bronchial biopsies. Detection of these adducts in peripheral blood samples allows evaluation of large numbers of patients for molecular epidemiology studies (47). Several studies have investigated the relationship between DNA adducts and activation of proto-oncogenes in lung carcinogenesis (19).

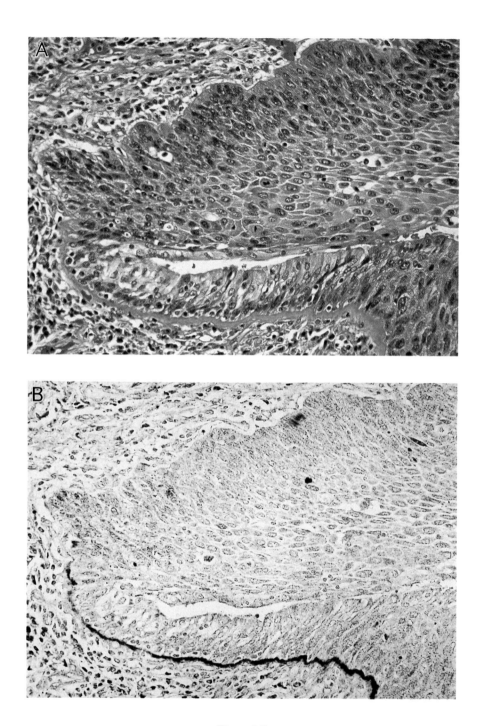

Figure 3-2

p53 PROTEIN ACCUMULATION IN PREINVASIVE BRONCHIAL NEOPLASIA

This case shows a spectrum of squamous neoplasia including mild dysplasia, moderate dysplasia, severe dysplasia, and carcinoma in situ. A,B: Immunohistochemistry of a serial section showed no evidence of p53 accumulation in normal mucosa or mild dysplasia. C,D left: In moderate dysplasia, the basal layers of mucosa contained cells with dark, enlarged, irregularly shaped nuclei; these cells contained detectable levels of nuclear p53 protein. D right: In severe dysplasia and carcinoma in situ, the large, irregularly shaped nuclei were darkly stained by the CM-1 antiserum. There is nuclear immunostaining in the lower layers of moderate dysplasia and in the full thickness of the severe dysplasia. E,F: Severe dysplasia with positive immunostaining in the full thickness of the mucosa. G,H: Carcinoma in situ with intense staining of all mucosal layers. (A,C,E,G are hematoxylin and eosin stained; B,D,F,H are CM-1 immunohistochemistry.) (Courtesy of Drs. William Bennett and Curtis C. Harris, Bethesda, MD.)

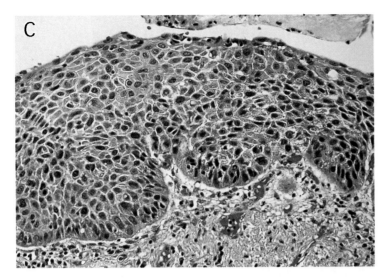

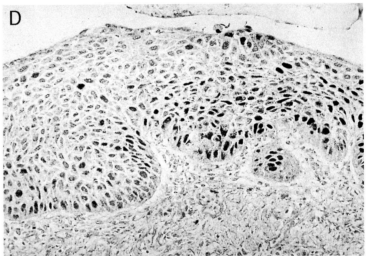

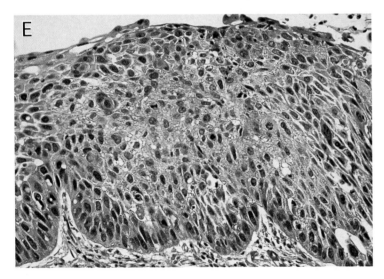

Figure 3-2 (Continued)

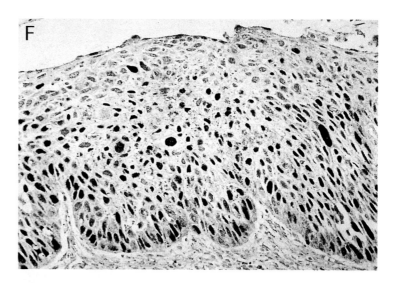

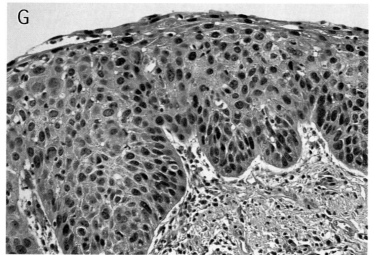

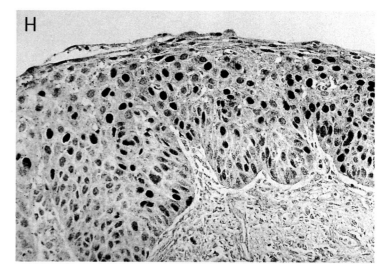

Figure 3-2 (Continued)

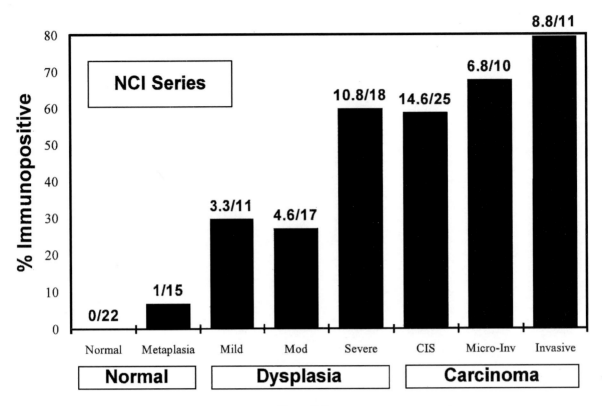

Figure 3-3

FREQUENCY OF p53 ACCUMULATION AT MULTIPLE STAGES OF BRONCHIAL CARCINOGENESIS

These data come from analysis of bronchial resections from 34 patients. The ratios shown at the top of each bar (number positive/total), are the number of immunostained positive lesions divided by the total number of lesions of a specific histologic grade. The numerators are the average interpretations of four observers. (Courtesy of Drs. William Bennett and Curtis C. Harris, Bethesda, MD.)

Invasion and Metastasis. Carcinogenesis is only the initial aspect of the malignant course of lung cancer. After a lung cancer develops the tumor follows a successive series of steps, including invasion, metastasis, and growth of metastases (Table 3-5). Similar to carcinogenesis, each of these steps is associated with specific genetic alterations which result in an imbalance of positive and negative regulation (Table 3-6) (52).

Before metastasis occurs, a cell or group of cells must separate from the primary tumor, penetrate the surrounding tissue, and survive to grow in the host tissue. This requires a complex series of events which includes entry of tumor cells into blood vessels, attachment at the metastatic site, invasion into the organ parenchyma, angiogenesis, and proliferation in the distant tissues. Squamous cell lung carcinoma is the only histologic subtype known to progress

through an in situ phase to invasive carcinoma. This requires interaction with subepithelial basement membrane and involves three steps: 1) attachment to the basement membrane, 2) creation of a defect in the basement membrane, and 3) translocation of the tumor cells across the basement membrane (fig. 3-4). Attachment of the tumor cells involves binding of tumor cell surface proteins to basement membrane glycoproteins such as laminin, type IV collagen, and fibronectin. These binding events are influenced by a variety of adhesion molecules including the integrins, which are a family of transmembrane glycoproteins functioning as adhesion receptors. The tumor cells form a hole in the basement membrane by producing hydrolytic enzymes or by stimulating the host cells to produce proteinases. Examples of proteolytic enzymes include metalloproteinases such as type IV collagenases,

Table 3-5

TUMOR-HOST INTERACTIONS DURING THE METASTATIC CASCADE*

1. Tumor initiation	Carcinogenic insult, oncogene activation or derepression, chromosome rearrangement
2. Promotion and progression	Karyotypic, genetic, and epigenetic instability; gene amplification; promotion associated genes and hormones
3. Uncontrolled proliferation	Autocrine growth factors on their receptors, receptors for host hormones
4. Angiogenesis	Multiple angiogenesis factors including known growth factors
5. Invasion of local tissues, blood and lymphatic vessels	Serum chemoattractants, autocrine motility factors, attachment receptors, degradive enzymes
6. Circulating tumor cell arrest and extravasation	Tumor cell homotypic or heterotypic aggregation
a. Adherence to endothelium	Tumor cell interaction with fibrin, platelets, and clotting factors; adhesion to RGD-type receptors
b. Retraction of endothelium	Platelet factors, tumor cell factors
c. Adhesion to basement membrane	Laminin receptor, thrombospondin receptor
d. Dissolution of basement membrane	Degradive proteases, type IV collagenase, heparinase, cathepsins
e. Locomotion	Autocrine motility factors, chemotaxis factors
7. Colony formation at secondary site	Receptors for local tissue growth factors, angiogenesis factors
8. Evasion of host defenses and resistance to therapy	Resistance to killing by host macrophages, natural killer cells, and activated T cells; failure to express, or blocking of, tumor specific antigens; amplification of drug resistant genes

*Table 4.1 from Liotta LA, Kohn E, Steeg PS, Stetler-Stevenson W. Molecular biology of metastasis. In: Broder S, ed. Molecular foundations of oncology, Vol. 1. Baltimore: Williams & Wilkins, 1991:51–81.

serine proteases such as urokinase, and cysteine proteases such as cathepsins B and L (Table 3-6). Tissue inhibitors of metalloproteinase (TIMP)-1 and -2 are known to negatively regulate collagenases, however, they have not yet been examined in lung cancer. Translocation through the gap in the basement membrane is directed by chemoattractants from the host cells or by motility factors produced by the tumor cells. Angiogenesis is another important factor in allowing tumors to grow, invade, and metastasize; angiogenesis can be inhibited by TIMP. The genes or molecules that participate in tumor invasion and metastasis in either a positive or a negative regulatory fashion in lung cancer are listed in Table 3-6 (52).

Cell Lines from Lung Carcinomas. The study of cell lines provides an extremely valuable tool in the molecular biology of lung carcinoma tumor cells. The development of the cell lines of small cell lung carcinoma characterized the biochemical properties, enzyme or protein products, and cytogenetic changes which led to initial discoveries of genetic alterations in lung cancer (86). One example of the use of cell lines is the transfection of vHa-*ras*, K-*ras*, c-*erb*B-2, or the combination of *myc* and *raf* into BEAS-2B cells, resulting in tumorigenic cell lines (49). Cell lines in lung cancer have also been used to study chemoresistance and cellular factors that modulate tumor growth or invasion (20,32). The ability of a tumor to form a cell line is associated with an adverse prognosis in nonsmall cell lung carcinoma (86).

Transgenic Animal Models. Transgenic animal models enable examination of the genetic events involved in lung carcinogenesis (54). Selected human genes, often with specific mutations, are inserted into the germ line DNA of an animal vector and the animal is then studied for expression of these genes. Lung adenocarcinomas have been found in transgenic mice carrying altered p53 (48) and c-Ha-*ras* genomic sequences (42).

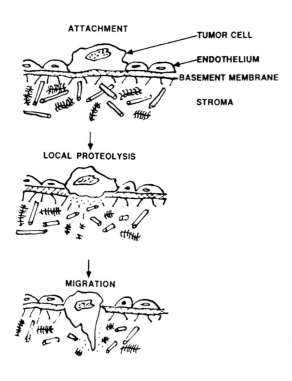

Figure 3-4
THREE-STEP HYPOTHESIS OF INVASION

As depicted for a tumor cell exiting a capillary, the first step is attachment of the tumor cell to the subendothelial basement membrane. This is followed by secretion and activation of proteinases, including metalloproteinases which cleave extracellular matrix components. Proteolytic modification of the matrix barrier is followed by pseudopodial protrusion and locomotion. (Fig. 1 from Aznavoorian S, Murphy AN, Stetler-Stevenson WG, Liotta LA. Molecular aspects of tumor cell invasion and metastasis. Cancer 1993;71:1368–83.)

Table 3-6

MOLECULES INVOLVED IN INVASION AND METASTASIS OF LUNG CANCER

Adhesion
  Positive
    Integrins (family of receptors) (57)
    Laminin (89)
    Fibronectin (20,46)
    Fibrin (96)
    Collagen (26)
    Vitronectin
    von Willebrand factor (83)
  Negative
    RGD (Arg-Gly-Asp) peptides (20)
    YIGSR (Tyr-Ile-Gly-Ser-Arg) peptides* (40)

Proteolysis
  Positive
    Metalloproteinases
      Collagenases: type IV (28,84), type III (43)
    Serine proteases
      Plasminogen activators (31)
        Urokinase (68)
        Tissue plasminogen activator (31)
    Cysteine proteases (13,35)
      Cathepsin B (35)
      Cathepsin L (13)
  Negative
    Tissue inhibitors of metalloproteinase (TIMP-1 and 2) (91)
    Stefins/cystatins (cystine protease inhibitors) (21)
    Serpin (serine protease inhibitor)*

Tumor cell migration
  Positive
    Autocrine motility factor (46)
  Negative
    Metastases suppressor gene nm 23
      (not significant in lung adenocarcinoma) (36)

* Data for lung cancer not available.

The information learned from these special techniques has greatly enhanced our understanding of the mechanisms of lung carcinogenesis, metastasis, and invasion, and is already being used for the development of novel therapeutic approaches for lung cancer such as gene therapy. In the future this technology should lead to new therapies that will hopefully have a greater impact on lung cancer survival than current conventional treatment.

REFERENCES

1. Abe S, Sukoh N, Ogura S, et al. Nucleolar organiser regions as a marker of growth rate in squamous cell carcinoma of the lung. Thorax 1992;47:778–80.

2. American Joint Committee on Cancer. Lung. In: Beahrs OH, Henson DE, Hutter RV, Kennedy BJ, eds. Manual for staging of cancer, Vol. 4. Philadelphia: JB Lippincott, 1992:115–22.

3. Ankrapp DP, Bevan DR. Insulin-like growth factor-I and human lung fibroblast-derived insulin-like growth factor-I stimulate the proliferation of human lung carcinoma cells in vitro. Cancer Res 1993;53:3399–404.

4. Antoniades HN, Galanopoulos T, Neville-Golden J, O'Hara CJ. Malignant epithelial cells in primary human lung carcinomas coexpress in vivo platelet-derived growth factor (PDGF) and PDGF receptor mRNAs and their protein products. Proc Natl Acad Sci U S A 1992;89:3942–6.

5. Anttila S, Vainio H, Hietanen E, et al. Immunohistochemical detection of pulmonary cytochrome P450IA and metabolic activities associated with P450IA1 and P450IA2 isozymes in lung cancer patients. Environ Health Perspect 1992;98:179–82.

6. Aznavoorian S, Murphy AN, Stetler-Stevenson WG, Liotta LA. Molecular aspects of tumor cell invasion and metastasis. Cancer 1993;71:1368–83.

7. Bennett WP, Colby TV, Travis WD, et al. p53 protein accumulates frequently in early bronchial neoplasia. Cancer Res 1993;53:4817–22.

8. Boldy DA, Ayres JG, Crocker J, Waterhouse JA, Gilthorpe M. Interphase nucleolar organiser regions and survival in squamous cell carcinoma of the bronchus: a 10 year follow up study of 138 cases. Thorax 1991;46:871–7.

9. Caporaso NE, Tucker MA, Hoover RN, et al. Lung cancer and the debrisoquine metabolic phenotype. JNCI 1990;82:1264–72.

10. Carey FA, Lamb D, Bird CC. Importance of sampling method in DNA analysis of lung cancer. J Clin Pathol 1990;43:820–3.

11. _____, Prasad US, Walker WS, Cameron EW, Lamb D, Bird CC. Prognostic significance of tumor deoxyribonucleic acid content in surgically resected small-cell carcinoma of lung. J Thorac Cardiovasc Surg 1992;103:1214–7.

12. Carp NZ, Ellison DD, Brophy PF, Watts P, Chang MC, Keller SM. DNA content in correlation with postsurgical stage in non-small cell lung cancer. Ann Thorac Surg 1992;53:680–3.

13. Chauhan SS, Goldstein LJ, Gottesman MM. Expression of cathepsin L in human tumors. Cancer Res 1991;51:1478–81.

14. Churg A, Franklin W, Chan KL, Kopp E, Carrington CB. Pulmonary hemorrhage and immune-complex deposition in the lung. Complications in a patient with systemic lupus erythematosus. Arch Pathol Lab Med 1980;104:388–91.

15. Cibas ES, Melamed MR, Zaman MB, Kimmel M. The effect of tumor size and tumor cell DNA content on the survival of patients with stage I adenocarcinoma of the lung. Cancer 1989;63:1552–6.

16. Dämmrich J, Buchwald J, Papadopoulos T, Müller-Hermelink HK. Special subtypes of pulmonary adenocarcinomas indicated by different tumor cell HLA-ex-pression and stromal infiltrates. A light, electron microscopic and immunohistologic study. Virchows Arch [Cell Pathol] 1991;61:9–18.

17. Dazzi H, Thatcher N, Hasleton PS, Swindell R. DNA analysis by flow cytometry in nonsmall cell lung cancer: relationship to epidermal growth factor receptor, histology, tumour stage and survival. Respir Med 1990;84:217–23.

18. DeLellis RA. Advances in immunohistochemistry. New York: Raven Press, 1988.

19. Devereux TR, Anderson MW, Belinsky SA. Role of ras protooncogene activation in the formation of spontaneous and nitrosamine-induced lung tumors in the resistant C3H mouse. Carcinogenesis 1991;12:299–303.

20. Elices MJ, Urry LA, Hemler ME. Receptor functions for the integrin VLA-3: fibronectin, collagen, and laminin binding are differentially influenced by Arg-Gly-Asp peptide and by divalent cations. J Cell Biol 1991;112:169–81.

21. Erdel M, Spiess E, Trefz G, Boxberger HJ, Ebert W. Cell interactions and motility in human lung tumor cell lines HS-24 and SB-3 under the influence of extracellular matrix components and proteinase inhibitors. Anticancer Res 1992;12:349–59.

22. Filderman AE, Silvestri GA, Gatsonis C, Luthringer DJ, Honig J, Flynn SD. Prognostic significance of tumor proliferative fraction and DNA content in stage I non-small cell lung cancer. Am Rev Respir Dis 1992;146:707–10.

23. Fontanini G, Bigini D, Vignati S, et al. p53 expression in non small cell lung cancer: clinical and biological correlations. Anticancer Res 1993;13:737–42.

24. _____, Macchiarini P, Pepe S, et al. The expression of proliferating cell nuclear antigen in paraffin sections of peripheral, node-negative non-small cell lung cancer. Cancer 1992;70:1520–7.

25. _____, Pingitore R, Bigini D, et al. Growth fraction in non-small cell lung cancer estimated by proliferating cell nuclear antigen and comparison with Ki-67 labeling and DNA flow cytometry data. Am J Pathol 1992;141:1285–90.

26. Gabazza EC, Taguchi O, Yamakami T, et al. Coagulation-fibrinolysis system and markers of collagen metabolism in lung cancer. Cancer 1992;70:2631–6.

27. Gallagher B, Urbanski SJ. The significance of pleural elastica invasion by lung carcinomas. Hum Pathol 1990;21:512–7.

28. Garbisa S, Scagliotti G, Masiero L, et al. Correlation of serum metalloproteinase levels with lung cancer metastasis and response to therapy. Cancer Res 1992;52:4548–9.

29. Gazdar AF. Advances in the biology of lung cancer. Clinical significance of neuroendocrine differentiation. Chest 1989;96:39S–41S.

30. Gibb AR, Seal RM. Examination of lung specimens. J.Clin.Pathol. 1990;43:68–72.

31. Gris JC, Schved JF, Marty-Double C, Mauboussin JM, Balmes P. Immunohistochemical study of tumor cell-associated plasminogen activators and plasminogen activator inhibitors in lung carcinomas. Chest 1993;104:8–13.

32. Hagiya Y, Fukao H, Ueshima S, et al. Urokinase-type plasminogen activator and its specific receptor in high metastatic and non-metastatic cell lines derived from human lung adenocarcinoma. Thromb Res 1992;65:449–56.

33. Haneda H, Miyamoto H, Isobe H, et al. Accuracy of the bronchoscopic DNA content analysis of non-small-cell lung carcinoma. J Surg Oncol 1992;49:182–8.

34. Harris CC, Hollstein M. Clinical implications of the p53 tumor suppressor gene. N Engl J Med 1993;329:1318–27.

35. Higashiyama M, Doi O, Kodama K, Yokouchi H, Tateishi R. Cathepsin B expression in tumour cells and laminin distribution in pulmonary adenocarcinoma. J Clin Pathol 1993;46:18–22.

36. _____, Doi O, Yokouchi H, et al. Immunohistochemical analysis of nm23 gene product/NDP kinase expression in pulmonary adenocarcinoma: lack of prognostic value. Br J Cancer 1992;66:533–6.

37. Ichinose Y, Hara N, Ohta M. Synchronous lung cancers defined by deoxyribonucleic acid flow cytometry. J Thorac Cardiovasc Surg 1991;102:418–24.

38. _____, Hara N, Takamori S, Maeda K, Yano T, Ohta M. DNA ploidy pattern of each carcinomatous component in adenosquamous lung carcinoma. Ann Thorac Surg 1993;55:593–6.

39. Iman DS, Harris CC. Oncogenes and tumor suppressor genes in human lung carcinogenesis. Crit Rev Oncog 1993;2:161–71.

40. Iwamoto Y, Robey FA, Graf J, et al. YIGSR, a synthetic laminin pentapeptide, inhibits experimental metastasis formation. Science 1987;238:1132–4.

41. Kaneko S, Ishida T, Sugio K, Yokoyama H, Sugimachi K. Nucleolar organizer regions as a prognostic indicator for stage I non-small cell lung cancer. Cancer Res 1991;51:4008–11.

42. Katsuki M, Ando K, Saitoh A, et al. Chemically induced tumors in transgenic mice carrying prototype human c-Ha-ras genes. Princess Takamatsu Symp 1991; 22:249–57.

43. Kawamura M, Kato R, Kikuchi K, et al. Assay for type III collagenolytic activity in lung cancer tissue. Clin Chim Acta 1991;203:225–33.

44. Kayser K, Gabius HJ, Ciesiolka T, Ebert W, Bach S. Histopathologic evaluation of application of labeled neoglycoproteins in primary bronchus carcinoma. Hum Pathol 1989;20:352–60.

45. Kempson RL, Association of Directors of Anatomic and Surgical Pathology. Standardization of the surgical pathology report. Am J Surg Pathol 1992;16:84–6.

46. Klominek J, Sundqvist KG, Robèrt KH. Nucleokinesis: distinct pattern of cell translocation in response to an autocrine motility factor-like substance or fibronectin. Proc Natl Acad Sci U S A 1991;88:3902–6.

47. Kriek E, Van Schooten FJ, Hillebrand MJ, et al. DNA adducts as a measure of lung cancer risk in humans exposed to polycyclic aromatic hydrocarbons. Environ Health Perspect 1993;99:71–5.

48. Lavigueur A, Maltby V, Mock D, Rossant J, Pawson T, Bernstein A. High incidence of lung, bone, and lymphoid tumors in transgenic mice overexpressing mutant alleles of the p53 oncogene. Mol Cell Biol 1989; 9:3982–91.

49. Lehman TA, Harris CC. Oncogene and tumor suppressor gene involvement in human lung carcinogenesis. CRC Press 1992;235–59.

50. _____, Reddel R, Peiifer AM, et al. Oncogenes and tumor-suppressor genes. Environ Health Perspect 1991;93:133–4.

51. Liotta LA, Kohn E, Steeg PS, Stetler-Stevenson W. Molecular biology of metastases. In: Broder S, ed. Molecular foundations of oncology, Vol 1. Baltimore: Williams & Wilkins, 1991:57–81.

52. _____, Stetler-Stevenson WG, Steeg PS. Cancer invasion and metastasis: positive and negative regulatory elements. Cancer Invest 1991;9:543–51.

53. Mackay B, Lukeman JM, Ordóñez NG. Technical procedures for lung tumor specimens. In: Bennington JL, ed. Tumors of the lung, Vol 1. Philadelphia: WB Saunders, 1991:381–92.

54. Malkinson AM. Primary lung tumors in mice: an experimentally manipulable model of human adenocarcinoma. Cancer Res 1992;52:2670S–6S.

55. Markman M, Braine HG, Abeloff MD. Histocompatibility antigens in small cell carcinoma of the lung. Cancer 1984;54:2943–5.

56. Matsumoto H, Muramatsu H, Muramatsu T, Shimazu H. Carbohydrate profiles shown by a lectin and a monoclonal antibody correlate with metastatic potential and prognosis of human lung carcinomas. Cancer 1992;69:2084–90.

57. Mette SA, Pilewski J, Buck CA, Albelda SM. Distribution of integrin cell adhesion receptors on normal bronchial epithelial cells and lung cancer cells in vitro and in vivo. Am J Respir Cell Mol Biol 1993;8:562–72.

58. Miller RR, Nelems B. Gross examination of lung resection specimens. In: Thurlbeck WM, ed. Pathology of the lung, Vol 1. New York: Thieme Medical Publishers, 1988:79–94.

59. Minna JD. The molecular biology of lung cancer pathogenesis. Chest 1993;103:449S–56S.

60. Mitsudomi T, Steinberg SM, Oie HK, et al. ras gene mutations in non-small cell lung cancers are associated with shortened survival irrespective of treatment intent. Cancer Res 1991;51:4999–5002.

61. Miyake M, Taki T, Hitomi S, Hakomori S. Correlation of expression of H/Le(y)/Le(b) antigens with survival in patients with carcinoma of the lung. N Engl J Med 1992;327:14–8.

62. Miyamoto H, Harada M, Isobe H, Akita HD, Haneda H, Yamaguchi E, Kuzumaki N, Kawakami Y. Prognostic value of nuclear DNA content and expression of the ras oncogene product in lung cancer. Cancer Res 1991; 51:6346–50.

63. Momand J, Zambetti GP, Olson DC, George D, Levine AJ. The mdm-2 oncogene product forms a complex with the p53 protein and inhibits p53-mediated transactivation. Cell 1992;69:1237–45.

64. Morkve O, Halvorsen OJ, Stangeland L, Gulsvik A, Laerum OD. Quantitation of biological tumor markers (p53, c-myc, Ki-67 and DNA ploidy) by multiparameter flow cytometry in non-small-cell lung cancer. Int J Cancer 1992;52:851–5.

65. _____, Laerum OD. Flow cytometric measurement of p53 protein expression and DNA content in paraffin-embedded tissue from bronchial carcinomas. Cytometry 1991;12:438–44.

66. Nilsson O. Carbohydrate antigens in human lung carcinomas. APMIS Suppl 1992;27:149–61.

67. Ogura S, Abe S, Sukoh N, Kunikane H, Nakajima I, Inoue K, Kawakami Y. Correlation between nucleolar organizer regions visualized by silver staining and the growth rate in lung adenocarcinoma. Cancer 1992; 70:63–8.

68. Oka T, Ishida T, Nishino T, Sugimachi K. Immunohistochemical evidence of urokinase-type plasminogen activator in primary and metastatic tumors of pulmonary adenocarcinoma. Cancer Res 1991;51:3522–5.

69. Oud PS, Pahlplatz MM, Beck JL, Wiersma-Van Tilburg A, Wagenaar SJ, Vooijs GP. Image and flow DNA cytometry of small cell carcinoma of the lung. Cancer 1989;64:1304–9.

70. Perrotti D, Cimino L, Falcioni R, Tibursi G, Gentileschi MP, Sacchi A. Metastatic phenotype: growth factor dependence and integrin expression. Anticancer Res 1990;10:1587–97.

71. Pezzella F, Turley H, Kuzu I, et al. bcl-2 protein in non-small cell lung carcinoma. N Engl J Med 1993; 329:690–4.

72. Randerath E, Miller RH, Mittal D, Avitts TA, Dunsford HA, Randerath K. Covalent DNA damage in tissues of cigarette smokers as determined by 32P-postlabeling assay. JNCI 1989;81:341–7.

73. Redondo M, Ruiz-Cabello F, Concha A, et al. Altered HLA class I expression in non-small cell lung cancer is independent of c-myc activation. Cancer Res 1991; 51:2463–8.

74. Rodenhuis S, Slebos RJ. Clinical significance of ras oncogene activation in human lung cancer. Cancer Res 1992;52:2665S–9S.

75. Rosai J. Guidelines for handling of most common and important surgical specimens. In: Ackerman's surgical pathology, Vol 7. St. Louis: CV Mosby, 1989:1908–11.

76. _____. Standardized reporting of surgical pathology diagnoses for the major tumor types. A proposal. The Department of Pathology, Memorial Sloan-Kettering Cancer Center. Am J Clin Pathol 1993;100:240–55.

77. Rusch V, Baselga J, Cordon-Cardo C, et al. Differential expression of the epidermal growth factor receptor and its ligands in primary non-small cell lung cancers and adjacent benign lung. Cancer Res 1993;53:2379–85.

78. Sara A, el-Naggar AK. Intratumoral DNA content variability. A study of non-small cell lung cancer. Am J Clin Pathol 1991;96:311–7.

79. Schlegel U, Rosenfeld MR, Volkenandt M, Rosenblum M, Dalmau J, Furneaux H. p53 gene mutations in primary lung tumors are conserved in brain metastases. J Neurooncol 1992;14:93–100.

80. Schmidt RA, Rusch VW, Piantadosi S. A flow cytometric study of non-small cell lung cancer classified as T1N0. Cancer 1992;69:78–85.

81. Schmidt WA. The chest. In: Anonymous, ed. Principles and techniques of surgical pathology, Vol 1. Menlo Park, Cal: Addison-Wesley, 1983:389–411.

82. Shields PG, Sugimura H, Caporaso NE, et al. Polycyclic aromatic hydrocarbon-DNA adducts and the CYP1A1 restriction fragment length polymorphism. Environ Health Perspect 1992;98:191–4.

83. Smith JW, Vestal DJ, Irwin SV, Burke TA, Cheresh DA. Purification and functional characterization of integrin alpha v beta 5. An adhesion receptor for vitronectin. J Biol Chem 1990;265:11008–13.

84. Soini Y, Pakk P, Autio-Harmainen H. Genes of laminin B1 chain, alpha 1 (IV) chain of type IV collagen, and 72-kd type IV collagenase are mainly expressed by the stromal cells of lung carcinomas. Am J Pathol 1993; 142:1622–30.

85. Soomro IN, Whimster WF. Growth fraction in lung tumours determined by Ki67 immunostaining and comparison with AgNOR scores. J Pathol 1990; 162:217–22.

86. Stevenson H, Gazdar AF, Phelps R, et al. Tumor cell lines established in vitro: an independent prognostic factor for survival in non-small-cell lung cancer. Ann Intern Med 1990;113:764–70.

87. Stipa S, Danesi DT, Modini C, et al. The importance of heterogeneity and of multiple site sampling in the prospective determination of deoxyribonucleic acid flow cytometry. Surg Gynecol Obstet 1993;176:427–34.

88. Sundaresan V, Reeve JG, Wilson B, Bleehen NM, Watson JV. Flow cytometric and immunohistochemical analysis of p62c-myc oncoprotein in the bronchial epithelium of lung cancer patients. Anticancer Res 1991;11:2111–6.

89. Tagliabue E, Martignone S, Mastroianni A, Mënard S, Pellegrini R, Colnaghi MI. Laminin receptors on SCLC cells. Br J Cancer Suppl 1991;14:83–5.

90. Tungekar MF, Gatter KC, Dunnill MS, Mason DY. Ki-67 immunostaining and survival in operable lung cancer. Histopathology 1991;19:545–50.

91. Urbanski SJ, Edwards DR, Maitland A, Leco KJ, Watson A, Kossakowska AE. Expression of metalloproteinases and their inhibitors in primary pulmonary carcinomas. Br J Cancer 1992;66:1188–94.

92. Vähäkangas KH, Samet JM, et al. Mutations of p53 and ras genes in radon-associated lung cancer from uranium miners. Lancet 1992;339:576–80.

93. Viallet J, Minna JD. Dominant oncogenes and tumor suppressor genes in the pathogenesis of lung cancer. Am J Respir Cell Mol Biol 1990;2:225–32.

94. Westra WH, Offerhaus GJ, Goodman SN, et al. Overexpression of the p53 tumor suppressor gene product in primary lung adenocarcinomas is associated with cigarette smoking. Am J Surg Pathol 1993;17:213–20.

95. Willman CL, Stewart CC. General principles of multiparameter flow cytometric analysis: applications of flow cytometry in the diagnostic pathology laboratory. Semin Diagn Pathol 1989;6:3–12.

96. Wojtukiewicz MZ, Zacharski LR, Memoli VA, et al. Abnormal regulation of coagulation/fibrinolysis in small cell carcinoma of the lung. Cancer 1990;65:481–5.

97. Zimmerman PV, Hawson GA, Bint MH, Parsons PG. Ploidy as a prognostic determinant in surgically treated lung cancer. Lancet 1987;2:530–3.

4
PAPILLARY TUMORS OF THE BRONCHIAL TREE

SQUAMOUS PAPILLOMA AND PAPILLOMATOSIS

Definition. According to the World Health Organization (WHO), squamous papilloma is a benign epithelial neoplasm formed of squamous epithelium (16). The tumor consists of a central fibrovascular core covered by stratified squamous epithelium. It is believed to be caused by human papillomaviruses (10). The occurrence of numerous, recurrent squamous papillomas in the larynx and tracheobronchial tree is termed papillomatosis. Numerous adjectives have been used as modifiers of this name, including *multiple tracheobronchial papillomatosis, tracheobronchial papillomatosis, juvenile laryngobronchial papillomatosis,* and *recurrent respiratory papillomatosis* (9).

Clinical Features. Bronchial papillomas are rare: at one institution, they were only 0.38 percent of all lung tumors (14). Squamous papillomas of the lower respiratory tract most often occur in children or young adults with a history of multiple, recurrent childhood laryngeal papillomas (papillomatosis). It is estimated that 2 to 8 percent of these patients develop tracheal and bronchial papillomas while less than 1 percent eventually have pulmonary parenchymal involvement (1,9,11,12). There is often a history of tracheostomy necessitated by frequent laryngeal and tracheal recurrences, and it has been suggested that electrical or laser fulguration may spread the tumor into the lower respiratory tract by seeding. Pulmonary involvement in the setting of papillomatosis can have a fulminant course and poor prognosis (5).

Solitary squamous papillomas of the tracheobronchial tree without prior laryngeal disease are rare. By 1991, there were only 59 documented cases (3). They most often affect adults from 50 to 70 years of age (5,6,14).

Symptoms vary depending on the number of papillomas and their location. Multiple papillomas of the trachea often produce severe dyspnea, while solitary bronchial papillomas may be asymptomatic or lead to obstruction, recurrent pneumonia, or hemoptysis. When the lung parenchyma is involved, the chest X ray and computerized axial tomograms (CTs) show one or more solid or cystic nodules that grow slowly and may become confluent with time (11). When the lesions are large and extensive, they can cause bronchial obstruction, with the sequelae of atelectasis, pneumonia, sepsis, and a mortality rate as high as 37.5 percent (1,9). Juvenile laryngeal papillomatosis may lead to the development of well-differentiated squamous cell carcinoma of the bronchus (9). The tumor supervenes on average about 15 years after the initial diagnosis of papillomatosis (8). In these cases, there is usually a predisposing factor such as treatment with radiation or cytotoxic drugs, or smoking; rarely, carcinoma supervenes in a patient without such a history (5,8,9,15). By contrast, solitary papillomas have a distinct potential to develop carcinoma without obvious clinical risk factors (6). In general, these cancers are well-differentiated, locally invasive squamous cell carcinomas that can spread to peribronchial lymph nodes, rib, soft tissues, or diaphragm (1,9,15). Most patients die soon after diagnosis of their tumors (8).

Gross Findings. The papillomas appear as one or multiple cauliflower-like excrescences protruding into the bronchial lumens (fig. 4-1). There are often simultaneous papillomas in the trachea. There is distal bronchiectasis with atelectasis or consolidation of the surrounding lung. Intrapulmonary involvement can occur in the form of smooth-walled cavities lined by papillary excrescences or small solid nodules (fig. 4-2).

Microscopic Findings. Papillomas of the bronchi are composed of a loose fibrovascular core covered by cytologically bland, stratified, nonkeratinized or paucikeratinized squamous epithelium (fig. 4-3). The epithelium shows orderly maturation from a basal layer of cuboidal cells to a flattened surface epithelium (fig. 4-4). Intercellular bridges can be found. The squamous cells often show perinuclear clearing (koilocytotic changes) (fig. 4-4). Also, the epithelium sometimes contains admixed vacuolated mucus-secreting cells, intermediate cells, or cells resembling transitional epithelium. Occasionally, a

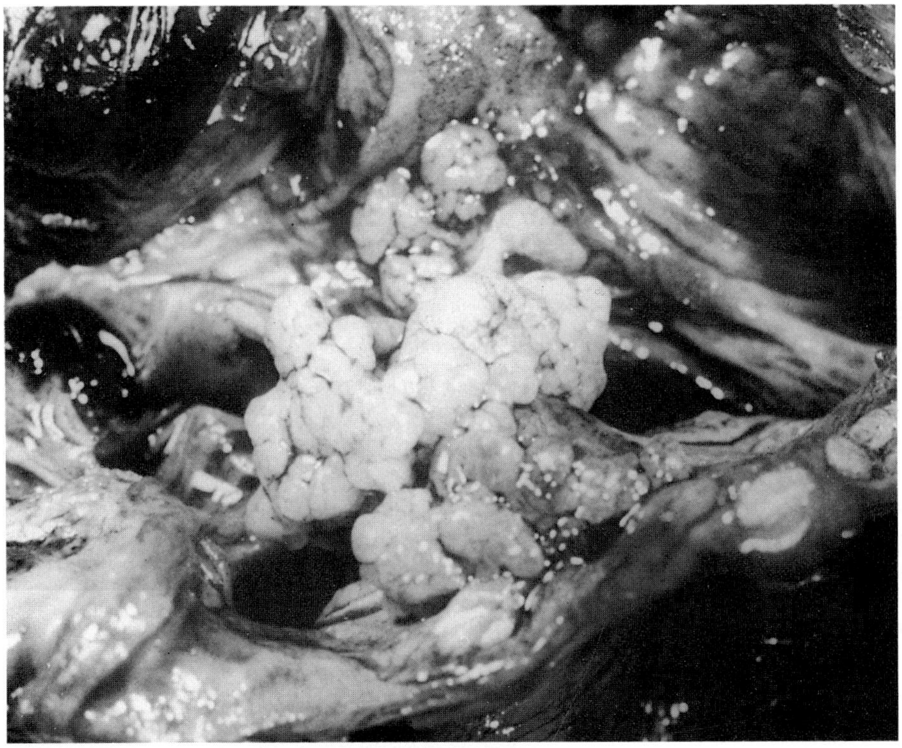

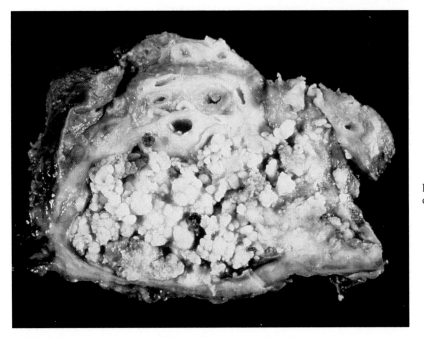

Figure 4-1
GROSS APPEARANCE
OF BRONCHIAL
SQUAMOUS
PAPILLOMA
The lesion, located at
the bifurcation of two bronchi, shows the typical cauliflower-like configuration.

Figure 4-2
CAVITARY PULMONARY
PAPILLOMATOSIS
The inner surface of the cavity is
lined by numerous papillary excrescences.

single layer of ciliated epithelium lines the surface (7). Mitoses are usually infrequent but, occasionally, dyskeratotic atypical cells or mitoses do occur, especially in papillomas of adults (fig. 4-5) (1). Importantly, benign bronchial papillomas typically do not invade subjacent tissues. A single exception in the trachea was termed *invasive tracheal papillomatosis* (7). Squamous papillomas can extend into bronchial surface glands; this should not be regarded as invasion (5).

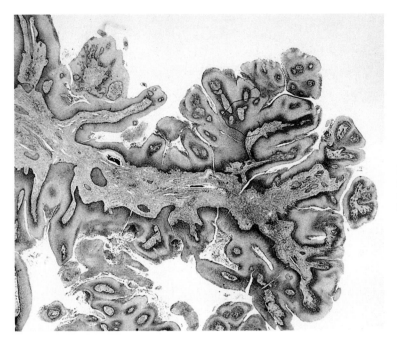

Figure 4-3
SQUAMOUS PAPILLOMA
This bronchial papilloma has a typical low magnification microscopic appearance, namely arborizing fronds composed of fibrovascular cores covered by stratified squamous epithelium.

Figure 4-4
SQUAMOUS PAPILLOMA
The higher magnification view shows nonkeratinized squamous epithelium. There is orderly maturation from the basal layer of cuboidal cells to the flattened surface epithelium. Note the perinuclear clearing (koilocytotic changes) in the squamous cells.

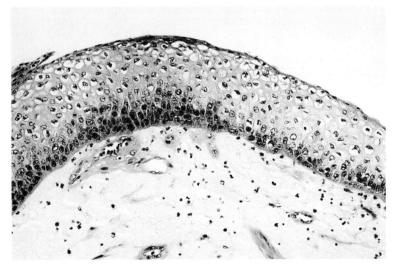

Pulmonary parenchymal papillomatosis occurs as multiple large cavities lined by numerous papillomas (fig. 4-2) (10). Others have described a spectrum of changes from solid clusters of 20 to 30 cytologically bland squamous cells within alveoli to larger cavitary lesions lined by flat, nonkeratinizing squamous epithelium (figs. 4-6, 4-7) (11). When cytologic atypia is present, the distinction from squamous cell carcinoma can be difficult (see chapter 11).

About one third of solitary papillomas show squamous dysplasia, carcinoma in situ, or foci of invasive squamous cell carcinoma (3). Popper and associates (14) suggested a grading system for papillomas. The system is based on that used in cervical neoplasia and grades atypias from mild to severe. Its applicability has not yet been tested.

Squamous cell carcinoma in the setting of papillomas shows prominent cellular pleomorphism, loss of maturation, increased dyskeratosis and

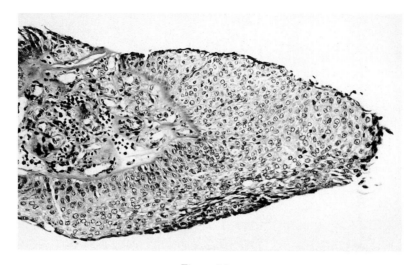

Figure 4-5
SQUAMOUS PAPILLOMA WITH MILD ATYPIA
This frond of a papilloma is covered by squamous epithelium, sectioned tangentially in areas. There is some loss of maturation and mild nuclear atypia.

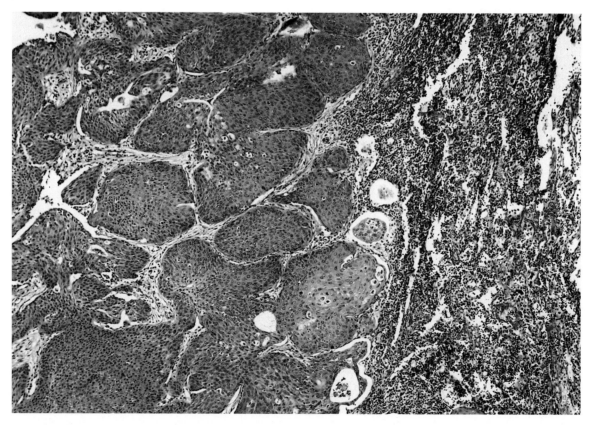

Figure 4-6
INTRAPULMONARY SQUAMOUS PAPILLOMA
This view shows the lining of a cystic nodule consisting of proliferating islands of squamous epithelium surrounded by a delicate fibrous stroma. The nests of squamous cells invade into contiguous alveoli. (Fig. 6c from Kramer SS, Wehunt WD, Stocker JT, Kashima H. Pulmonary manifestations of juvenile laryngotracheal papillomatosis. AJR Am J Roentgenol 1985;144:687–94.)

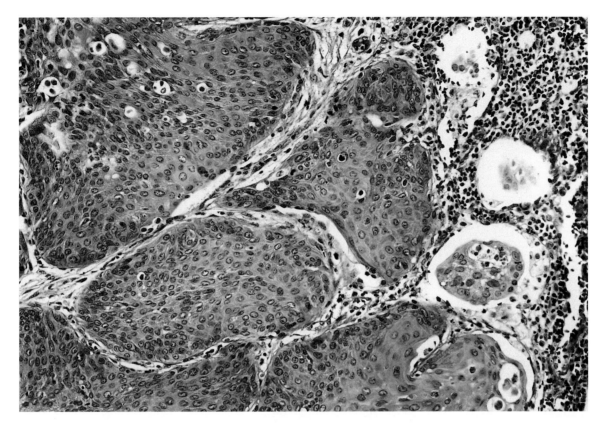

Figure 4-7
INTRAPULMONARY SQUAMOUS PAPILLOMA
Same case as shown in figure 4-6. There are islands of moderately atypical squamous epithelium at the advancing margin of the nodule. The distinction from well-differentiated squamous cell carcinoma can be difficult (see figure 11-6).

hyperkeratosis, and, most importantly, invasion through the bronchial wall into adjacent tissues or lymphatics (fig. 4-8) (1,9). The carcinomas may be keratinizing or nonkeratinizing; some may be papillary. They are all well or moderately differentiated. The malignancy can be focal and easily missed in bronchial biopsies (6).

Ultrastructural Findings. The epithelial cells of papillomas have the typical features of squamous differentiation, including abundant cytoplasmic tonofilaments and desmosomes, but they also have multilobated nuclei, a perinuclear clear zone lacking cytoplasmic organelles, and, on occasion, focal intranuclear virus particles (fig. 4-9) (10).

Molecular Biologic Findings. Papillomaviruses, particularly type 11 and, on occasion, type 6, have been convincingly linked to both laryngeal and lower respiratory tract papillomas (4,8,10,11, 14). Types 16 and 18 and sometimes types 11 and

31/33/35 have been reported in papillomas that precede or are contemporaneous with squamous cell carcinoma of lung or upper respiratory tract in patients without obvious risk factors (see chapter 7) (4,8,14). The virus is also present in at least some of the carcinomas that develop in these cases. Types 16 and 18 may act as promoters in the carcinogenic process (13,14). Popper and associates (14) suggested that human papillomavirus typing might be a useful prognostic tool.

Differential Diagnosis. Bronchial squamous papillomas showing cytologic atypia can be difficult to distinguish from papillary squamous cell carcinoma (see figs. 11-23, 11-24). Their diagnosis has been discussed above. Local invasion into subjacent tissues or lymphatics, marked cellular pleomorphism, loss of maturation, increased dyskeratosis, and hyperkeratosis suggest carcinoma.

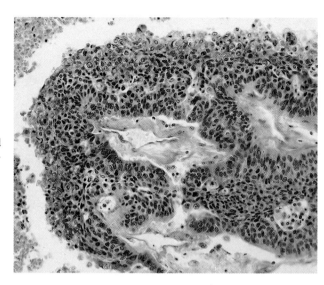

Figure 4-8
PAPILLARY SQUAMOUS CELL CARCINOMA
IN PAPILLOMATOSIS
The loss of maturation of the squamous epithelium and the prominent cytologic atypia are features of carcinoma. Compare with figures 4-4 and 4-5.

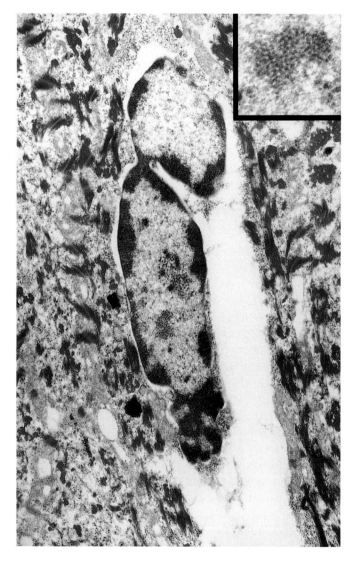

Figure 4-9
ELECTRON MICROSCOPIC APPEARANCE
OF SQUAMOUS PAPILLOMA
Typical surface cell showing squamous differentiation in the form of abundant cytoplasmic tonofilaments and desmosomes, and a perinuclear clear zone (koilocytosis). Inset shows intranuclear papillomavirus particles. (Fig. 3 from Kerley SW, Buchon-Zalles C, Moran J, Fishback JL. Chronic cavitary respiratory papillomatosis. Arch Pathol Lab Med 1989;113:1166–9.)

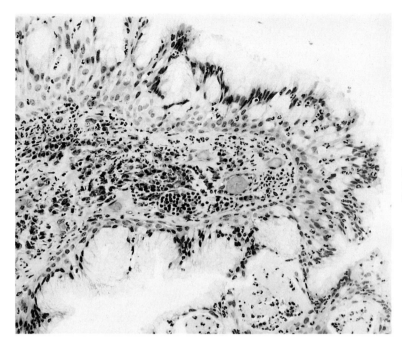

Figure 4-10
COLUMNAR PAPILLOMA
The epithelial surface of the papilloma is lined predominantly by mucus-secreting columnar (goblet) cells, with a few small foci of squamous differentiation.

When squamous papillomas extend into alveoli, the differential diagnosis includes bronchiolar squamous metaplasia of the type seen after viral infection or bleomycin treatment. The presence of diffuse alveolar damage in these diseases as well as the clinical history usually helps in the diagnosis. Well-differentiated squamous cell carcinomas (chapter 11) can be more difficult to exclude in this location. Once again, cellular pleomorphism, loss of maturation, increased dyskeratosis, and hyperkeratosis suggest carcinoma (fig. 4-9) (10).

OTHER BRONCHIAL PAPILLOMAS

Columnar Papillomas

These are rare, benign, solitary papillomas lined largely by columnar cells (3). Patients are usually middle-aged men who present with symptoms of obstruction. The papillary fronds of the tumor consist of a fibrovascular core covered by columnar or cuboidal epithelium that is sometimes mucinous or ciliated (fig. 4-10).

Inverted Papillomas or Polyps

These rare lesions are documented by Dail (5) and Spencer (18). It is unclear whether they are true tumors or result from fibrotic distortion of the submucosa with secondary folding of the overlying epithelium.

Transitional Cell Papillomas

So-called transitional cell papillomas occur in the upper aerodigestive tract (larynx, pharynx), but only a few have been reported in the bronchial tree (2,17,19). There are branching papillary fronds with central fibrovascular cores lined by stratified epithelium. The superficial layers of the epithelium may appear flattened, but keratinization is absent. These lesions resemble transitional cell papillomas of the bladder by light microscopy (hence the name), but electron microscopy shows them to be of squamous phenotype (17); they are therefore a variant of nonkeratinizing squamous papillomas. Like other squamous papillomas, they show a spectrum of cellular atypia, from entirely benign lesions (papillomas) to those with significant cytologic atypia (possibly carcinoma in situ) to those exhibiting microinvasion of the basement membrane (2,17). The natural history of the microinvasive carcinomas cannot be predicted with accuracy at the present time, although some instances of local recurrence have been reported.

Fibroepithelial Polyps

These can occur in the large airways. A typical polyp consists of a fibrovascular core lined by

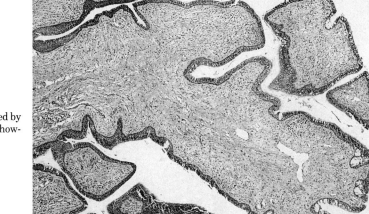

Figure 4-11
FIBROEPITHELIAL POLYP
The polyp shows a fibrovascular core lined by normal bronchial respiratory epithelium showing focal squamous metaplasia.

normal (or metaplastic) bronchial mucosa (fig. 4-11). They are architecturally similar to skin tags. They are probably not neoplasms; some appear to be postinflammatory.

REFERENCES

1. Al-Saleem T, Peale AR, Norris CM. Multiple papillomatosis of the lower respiratory tract. Clinical and pathologic study of eleven cases. Cancer 1968;22:1173–84.
2. Assor D. A papillary transitional cell tumor of the bronchus. Am J Cin Pathol 1971;55:761–4.
3. Basheda S, Gephardt GN, Stoller JK. Columnar papilloma of the bronchus. Case report and literature review. Am Rev Respir Dis 1991;144:1400–2.
4. Byrne PM, Tsao M-S, Fraser RS, Howley PM. Human papillomavirus-11 DNA in a patient with chronic laryngotracheobronchial papillomatosis and metastatic squamous-cell carcinoma of the lung. N Engl J Med 1987;317:873–8.
5. Dail D. Uncommon tumors. In: Dail DH, Hammar SP, eds. Pulmonary pathology. 2nd ed. New York: Springer-Verlag, 1994:1299–300.
6. DiMarco AF, Montenegro H, Payne CB Jr, Kwon KH. Papillomas of the tracheobronchial tree with malignant degeneration. Chest 1978;74:464–5.
7. Fechner RE, Fitz-Hugh GS. Invasive tracheal papillomatosis. Am J Surg Pathol 1980;4:79–86.
8. Guillou L, Sahli R, Chaubert P, Monnier P, Cuttat JF, Costa J. Squamous cell carcinoma of the lung in a nonsmoking, nonirradiated patient with juvenile laryngotracheal papillomatosis. Evidence of human papillomavirus-11 DNA in both carcinoma and papillomas. Am J Surg Pathol 1991;15:891–8.
9. Helmuth RA, Strate RW. Squamous cell carcinoma of the lung in a nonirradiated, nonsmoking patient with juvenile laryngotracheal papillomatosis. Am J Surg Pathol 1987;11:643–50.
10. Kerley SW, Buchon-Zalles C, Moran J, Fishback JL. Chronic cavitary respiratory papillomatosis. Arch Pathol Lab Med 1989;113:1166–9.
11. Kramer SS, Wehunt WD, Stocker JT, Kashima H. Pulmonary manifestations of juvenile laryngotracheal papillomatosis. AJR Am J Roentgenol 1985;144:687–94.
12. Majoros M, Parkhill EM, Devine KD. Papilloma of the larynx in children: a clinicopathological study. Am J Surg 1964;108:470–5.
13. Marshall T, Pater A, Pater MM. Trans-regulation and differential cell specificity of human papillomaviruses types 16, 18, and 11 on acting elements. J Med Virol 1989;29:115–26.
14. Popper HH, Wirnsberger G, Juttner-Smolle FM, Pongratz MG, Sommersgutter M. The predictive value of human papilloma virus (HPV) typing in the prognosis of bronchial squamous cell papillomas. Histopathology 1992;21:323–30.
15. Runckel D, Kessler S. Bronchogenic squamous carcinoma in nonirradiated juvenile laryngotracheal papillomatosis. Am J Surg Pathol 1980;4:293–6.
16. Shanmugaratnam K. Histological typing of tumors of the upper respiratory tract and ear. 2nd ed. International Histological Classification of Tumors. World Health Organization. Berlin: Springer-Verlag, 1991:19.
17. Smith PS, McClure J. A papillary endobronchial tumor with a transitional cell pattern. Arch Pathol Lab Med 1982;106:503–6.
18. Spencer H. Pathology of the lung. 4th ed. Oxford: Pergamon Press, 1985:960.
19. _____, Dail DH, Arneaud J. Non-invasive bronchial epithelial papillary tumors. Cancer 1980;45:1486–97.

5
MISCELLANEOUS BENIGN EPITHELIAL TUMORS

PAPILLARY ADENOMA OF TYPE 2 CELLS

Definition. This rare papillary neoplasm of lung consists of cytologically benign cells of type 2 cell origin. Clara cells may be admixed. Other synonymous terms include *bronchiolar papilloma* (9), *Clara cell adenoma,* and *papillary adenoma of type 2 pneumocytes* (6).

Clinical Features. Patients range in age from 7 to 60 years (2,4-6,9). They are usually asymptomatic. Solitary coin lesions are seen on chest X ray. The tumors may be peripheral or central in location. One tumor was followed radiographically for 10 years prior to resection without evidence of change in size (2). They do not metastasize or recur after resection.

Gross Findings. Papillary adenoma of type 2 cells appears as a well-circumscribed, often peripheral nodule measuring from 1 to 4 cm in diameter. The cut surface is white and spongy or granular. Usually the neoplasm is separate from the airways, but it may involve the wall and protrude into the lumen of small bronchi (4,6,9).

Microscopic Findings. The tumors are well demarcated and compress rather than infiltrate the surrounding lung (fig. 5-1). On occasion, they are associated with a bronchiole or small bronchus (4). The tumor has a branching papillary appearance, sometimes mixed with more solid areas (figs. 5-1, 5-2). The cores of the papillae are fibrous and lined by cytologically bland, cuboidal and columnar cells with oval to round nuclei containing uniformly dispersed fine chromatin (figs. 5-2, 5-3). Occasionally, interspersed ciliated cells may be present (4). The lining cells may show eosinophilic intranuclear inclusions of the type seen in benign and malignant type 2 pneumocytes (fig. 5-3) (4,6). Mitotic figures, necrosis, and intracellular mucin are absent (4,5). The cytoplasm of the tumor cells may show surfactant apoprotein (6) or Clara cell antigen (5), but these findings are inconstant.

Ultrastructurally, there is usually multidirectional differentiation. Most commonly, cells containing cytoplasmic osmiophilic lamellar bodies (similar to those seen in type 2 pneumocytes) are intermixed with cells containing small, apical, electron-dense granules of the type found in Clara cells (2,4-6). In one case, these cell types were joined by ciliated cells, while in another the tumor cells had only laminated osmiophilic inclusions (4).

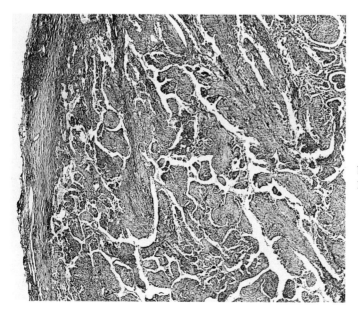

Figure 5-1
PAPILLARY ADENOMA
The lesion shows the typical complex pattern of branching papillae. It is well demarcated and compresses the surrounding lung.

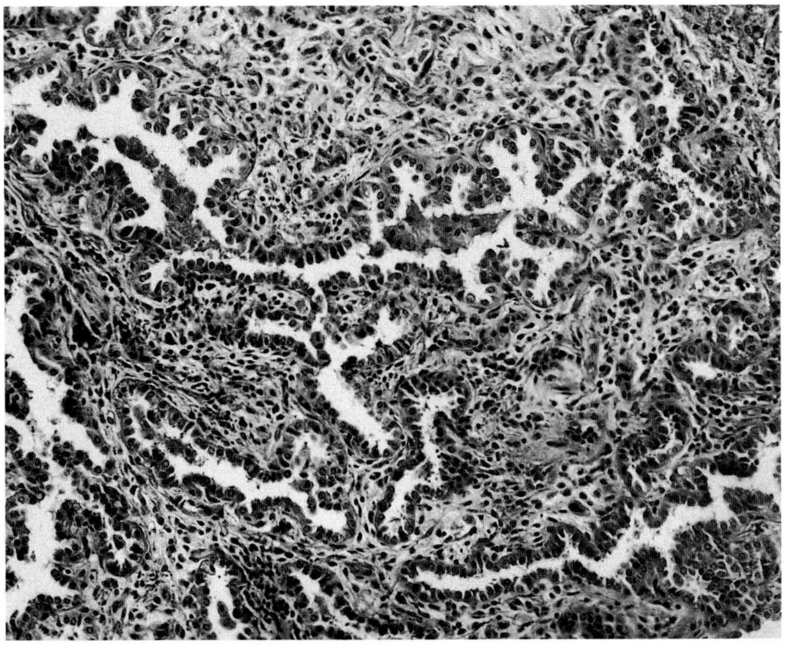

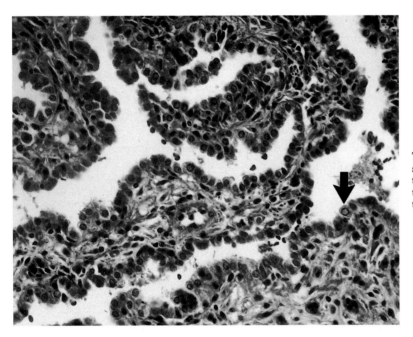

Figure 5-2
PAPILLARY ADENOMA
The fibrous cores of these interanastomosing papillae are lined by cytologically bland cuboidal cells.

Figure 5-3
PAPILLARY ADENOMA
Higher magnification of figure 5-2. The cuboidal cells covering the papillae show uniform oval to round nuclei. Note the intranuclear inclusions (arrow) of the type seen in benign and malignant type 2 pneumocytes.

Differential Diagnosis. The differential diagnosis of papillary adenomas includes other adenomas and papillary tumors of lung. Alveolar adenomas consist of multiple cystic spaces of varying size containing proteinaceous material. They most closely resemble a lymphangioma (which some of the initial cases were believed to be). They do not have the papillary features of papillary adenoma.

Popper and associates (7a) described microscopic (less than 1 mm) nodules composed of benign proliferating type 2 pneumocytes in a patient with tuberous sclerosis. We have also encountered similar micronodules in a patient with tuberous sclerosis and lymphangioleiomyomatosis. These nodules lack the broad papillary appearance and fibrous cores of papillary adenoma.

Papillary bronchioloalveolar carcinomas (chapter 13) have the histologic and cytologic features of malignancy, such as necrosis, mitoses, and nuclear and cellular pleomorphism. Further, papillary bronchioloalveolar carcinomas usually have irregular borders and a lepidic pattern of growth, whereas adenomas are well circumscribed and usually compress the surrounding lung. Similarly, atypical alveolar hyperplasia (acinar atypical proliferation) or "adenomas" resembling incipient bronchioloalveolar carcinomas show greater cytologic atypia than papillary adenomas and they also have a lepidic growth pattern (10). Still, some papillary tumors may be difficult to classify precisely (3).

Papillary adenomas are usually easily distinguished from pulmonary metastases from primaries such as ovary, kidney, pancreas, colon, thyroid, or breast. The presence of multiple lesions, a history of a known primary tumor, and the histologic features of malignancy, such as mitoses, cytologic atypia, and necrosis in these metastatic papillary adenocarcinomas all aid in the differential diagnosis.

Sclerosing hemangiomas (chapter 23) may demonstrate a papillary pattern of growth. Also, the papillae are lined by type 2 pneumocytes. Still, sclerosing hemangiomas show a greater diversity of histologic patterns, including solid areas, blood-filled cysts, and areas of scarring, than do papillary adenomas. In addition, there are bland oval, round, or polygonal tumor cells in the interstitium of sclerosing hemangiomas, a feature not seen in papillary adenoma.

Rarely, a papillary variant of carcinoid tumor may occur in lung (chapter 17). The cells of these tumors have the slightly granular cytoplasm and punctate nucleoplasm typical of carcinoid tumors. Immunohistochemical stains for chromogranin or electron microscopy readily distinguish it.

Comparative Tumors in Animals. So-called bronchioloalveolar adenomas (pulmonary adenomas) can occur as spontaneous or experimentally-induced neoplasms in mice and rats (1,7,8). They are usually solitary peripheral nodules less than 4 mm in diameter. Microscopically, they consist of relatively uniform cuboidal or columnar cells growing in papillary, glandular, solid, or mixed configurations, with little pleomorphism and few mitoses. Their microscopic

appearance can therefore be relatively similar to that of human papillary adenomas. By electron microscopy, the cells show cytoplasmic inclusions suggestive of type 2 pneumocytes and, on occasion, Clara cells, warranting the descriptive term "bronchioloalveolar" (1).

ALVEOLAR ADENOMA

Definition. Alveolar adenoma is a benign multicystic neoplasm that microscopically recapitulates alveolar epithelium and mesenchyme (13).

Clinical Features. Only a small number of cases have been reported, some as lymphangiomas (11,12). The lesion typically presents in older, asymptomatic women who have a solitary nodule. Excision is curative.

Gross Findings. The tumor is usually a solitary, circumscribed, easily shelled out, gray-white or tan peripheral nodule measuring 1 to 2 cm in diameter (fig. 5-4).

Microscopic Findings. At low magnification, alveolar adenoma is well circumscribed and multicystic (fig. 5-5). Delicate septa of variable thickness separate ectatic spaces that tend to be larger in the center of the lesion than at its margin (figs. 5-5, 5-6). The spaces contain eosinophilic and periodic acid-Schiff–positive granular material, sometimes in association with scattered foamy macrophages (fig. 5-6). The spaces are lined by cells that vary from hobnail or cuboidal to flattened. When the lining cells are flat, alveolar adenomas distinctly resemble dilated lymphatic spaces (fig. 5-6). However, these cells are stained by antibodies to keratin and, focally, to carcinoembryonic antigen, supporting an epithelial phenotype (13).

The interstitium between the cysts varies in thickness and consists of a myxoid collagenous matrix containing spindled cells, probably fibroblasts or myofibroblasts. These cells fail to stain for desmin.

By electron microscopy, the cuboidal cells lining the cystic spaces contain lamellar bodies, have blunt surface microvilli, show cell junctions of zonula adherens type, and have an underlying thin basement membrane, features compatible with type 2 pneumocytes (13).

Differential Diagnosis. The ectatic spaces containing proteinaceous material and at times lined by flattened cells may suggest lymphangioma

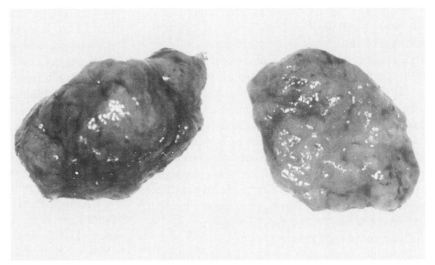

Figure 5-4
GROSS APPEARANCE
OF ALVEOLAR ADENOMA
Left: The excised lesion is tan, with a bulging, glistening external surface.
Right: The cut surface shows a suggestion of multinodularity. (Fig. 1 from Yousem SA, Hochholzer L. Alveolar adenoma. Hum Pathol 1986;17:1066–71.)

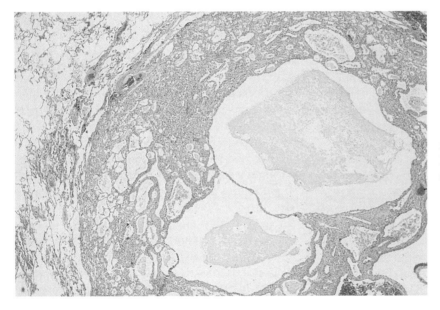

Figure 5-5
ALVEOLAR ADENOMA
Low magnification view shows a well-circumscribed, multicystic lesion. Ectatic spaces are larger in the center of the lesion than at its margin.

(11,12). Staining for keratin and carcinoembryonic antigen easily excludes this possibility.

Sclerosing hemangiomas (chapter 23) may show dilated spaces lined by cuboidal cells, but they are usually not as ectatic as those seen in alveolar adenoma, and when dilated, often contain hemorrhage. They also have greater histologic diversity, encompassing solid or papillary patterns in the same lesion in most cases. Finally, the relevant tumor cells in sclerosing hemangiomas are interstitial, characteristically round or oval with pale cytoplasm, and regularly stain for epithelial membrane antigen in paraffin sections.

Papillary adenomas consistently show type 2 or Clara cell phenotype. They are easily distinguished from alveolar adenomas by their papillary, frond-like architecture, which differs markedly from the multicystic appearance of alveolar adenoma.

Adenoma or atypical alveolar hyperplasia (chapter 7) may occur in lung, particularly in the setting of lung cancer. Like alveolar adenomas, these are proliferations of cuboidal cells, but rather than a multicystic pattern, they show lepidic growth along alveolar septa, and in addition, often demonstrate cytologic atypia.

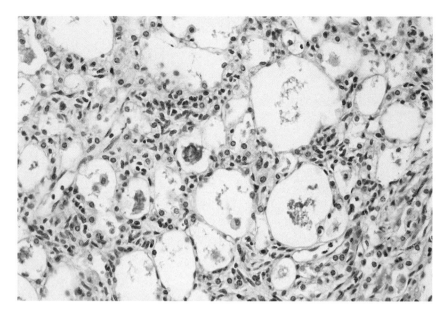

Figure 5-6
ALVEOLAR ADENOMA
The numerous cysts are separated by a delicate stroma, lined by flattened cells, and contain eosinophilic granular material.

MUCINOUS CYSTADENOMA AND PULMONARY MUCINOUS TUMORS OF BORDERLINE MALIGNANCY

Rarely, mucinous cystic tumors of low malignant potential occur in lung. There is debate over whether these tumors, like their counterparts in pancreas and ovary, exist in a morphologic spectrum from benign (cystadenoma) to uncertain or low malignant potential, to well-differentiated mucinous adenocarcinomas, or whether they are all best classified as adenocarcinomas (bronchioloalveolar carcinomas) of low malignant potential (see figs. 13-20–13-22).

Mucinous Cystadenoma

This is a unilocular cystic lesion whose fibrous wall is lined by well-differentiated, presumably benign, columnar mucinous epithelium (18). The few cases that have been reported occur in adult smokers. Chest X ray reveals a solitary nodule. The treatment is complete resection.

Grossly, the lesions are mucus-filled cysts that are less than 2 cm in diameter and unattached to bronchi (18). The walls of the cysts are thin (0.1 cm), without evidence of thickened areas or satellite nodules.

Microscopically, a typical cyst contains abundant mucus, while its wall consists of fibrous connective tissue and is sometimes discontinuous (fig. 5-7). The wall is lined by columnar, mucin-

secreting epithelium with hyperchromatic nuclei (figs. 5-8, 5-9). Invasion of subjacent alveolar tissue and solid areas of adenocarcinoma are not seen. Marked chronic inflammation in the wall or foreign body granulomatous reaction to the mucin may be present (fig. 5-8).

Mucinous Cystic Tumor of Borderline Malignancy

Mucinous cystic tumors can show more advanced cytologic atypia or even foci of frank carcinoma. Graeme-Cook and associates (16) offered the above term to denote this morphologic spectrum. In addition to the mucinous cystadenomas described above, cysts may demonstrate cellular atypia in the form of stratified nuclei with nuclear pleomorphism and hyperchromatism, or even show foci of frank adenocarcinoma in the form of columnar epithelial cells with prominent nucleoli, solid growth pattern, and invasion into subjacent lung. Even when areas suggestive of adenocarcinoma are present, the prognosis is good (14–16).

Distinguishing between these tumors and well-differentiated adenocarcinoma or bronchioloalveolar carcinoma can at times be difficult. In particular, some mucinous bronchioloalveolar carcinomas ("colloid carcinomas") of the lung may show sparse numbers of goblet cells and abundant pools of mucin that fill and distend alveolar lumens (17,20). These mucinous cancers may

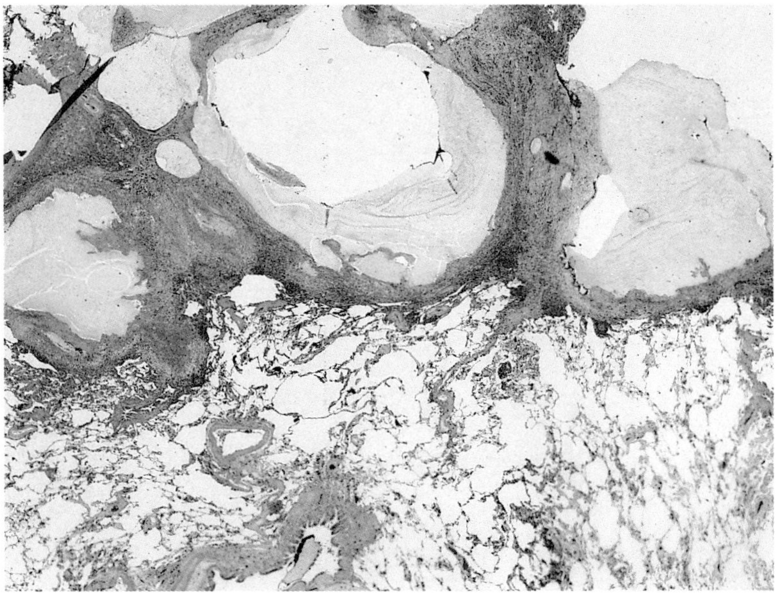

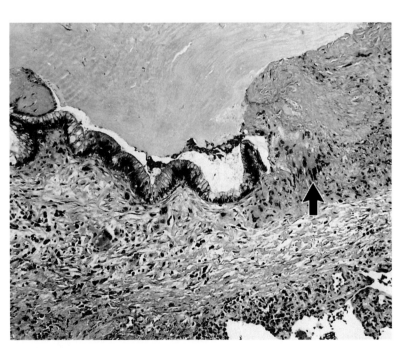

Figure 5-7
MUCINOUS CYSTADENOMA
At low magnification, the cyst shows a fibrous wall that separates its mucinous contents from the surrounding lung. (Figures 5-7–5-9 are from the same lesion.)

Figure 5-8
MUCINOUS CYSTADENOMA
Higher magnification of the fibrous wall shows a discontinuous layer of mucin-secreting cells lining the lumen. The tumor cells do not invade into the capsule or involve the surrounding lung. The epithelial lining is replaced in part by granulomatous reaction, including multinucleated giant cells (arrow), presumably in response to the mucus.

even be multicystic. Still, they usually lack fibrous capsules of the type seen in cystadenomas. One suggestion for classifying mucinous cystic tumors is that those in which the epithelium is cytologically bland and limited to the fibrous wall be termed mucinous cystadenomas; those in which the lining cells show cytologic atypia be termed cystic tumors of borderline malignancy; and those in which mucin-secreting epithelium invades beyond the fibrous cyst wall into adjacent lung or shows foci of frankly anaplastic cells be designated mucinous adenocarcinoma (15,19).

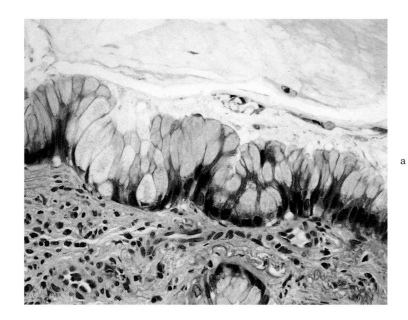

Figure 5-9
MUCINOUS CYSTADENOMA
The epithelial lining of the cyst consists of a single layer of goblet cells.

REFERENCES

Papillary Adenoma of Type 2 Cells

1. Dixon D, Horton J, Haseman JK, et al. Histomorphology and ultrastructure of spontaneous pulmonary neoplasms in strain A mice. Exp Lung Res 1991;17:131–55.
2. Fantone JC, Geisinger KR, Appelman HD. Papillary adenoma of the lung with lamellar and electron dense granules. An ultrastructural study. Cancer 1982;50:2839–44.
3. Fine G, Chang CH. Adenoma of type 2 pneumocytes with oncocytic features. Arch Pathol Lab Med 1991; 115:797–801.
4. Fukuda T, Ohnishi Y, Kanai I, et al. Papillary adenoma of the lung. Histological and ultrastructural findings in two cases. Acta Pathol Jpn 1992;42:56–61.
5. Hegg CA, Flint A, Singh G. Papillary adenoma of the lung. Am J Clin Pathol 1992;97:393–7.
6. Noguchi M, Kodama T, Shimosato Y, et al. Papillary adenoma of type 2 pneumocytes. Am J Surg Pathol 1986;10:134–9.
7. Palmer KC. Clara cell adenomas of the mouse lung. Interaction with alveolar type 2 cells. Am J Pathol 1985;120:455–63.
7a. Popper HH, Juettner-Smolle FM, Pongratz MG. Micronodular hyperplasia of type II pneumocytes—a new lung lesion associated with tuberous sclerosis. Histopathology 1991;18:347–54.
8. Schwartz LW, Hahn FR, Keenan KP, Keenan CM, Brown HR, Mann PC. Proliferative lesions of the rat respiratory tract. In: Guides for toxologic pathology. Washington, D.C.: Society of Toxicologic Pathologists, 1991.
9. Spencer H, Dail DH, Arneaud J. Non-invasive bronchial epithelial papillary tumors. Cancer 1980;45:1486–97.
10. Travis WD, Linnoila RI, Horowitz M, et al. Pulmonary nodules resembling bronchioloalveolar carcinoma in adolescent cancer patients. Mod Pathol 1988;1:372–7.

Alveolar Adenoma

11. Al-Hilli F. Lymphangioma (or alveolar adenoma?) of the lung. Histopathology 1987;11:979–80.
12. Wada A, Tateishi R, Terazawa T, Matsuda M, Hattori S. Case report. Lymphangioma of the lung. Arch Pathol 1974;98:211–3.
13. Yousem SA, Hochholzer L. Alveolar adenoma. Hum Pathol 1986;17:1066–71.

Mucinous Cystadenoma and Pulmonary Mucinous Tumors of Borderline Malignancy

14. Davison AM, Lowe JW, Da Costa P. Adenocarcinoma arising in a mucinous cystadenoma of the lung. Thorax 1992;47:129–30.
15. Dixon AY, Moran JF, Wesselius LJ, McGregor DH. Pulmonary mucinous cystic tumor. Case report with review of the literature. Am J Surg Pathol 1993;17:722–8.
16. Graeme-Cook F, Mark EJ. Pulmonary mucinous cystic tumors of borderline malignancy. Hum Pathol 1991; 22:185–90.
17. Higashiyama M, Doi O, Kodama K, Yokouchi H, Tateishi R. Cystic mucinous adenocarcinoma of the lung: two cases of cystic variant of mucus-producing lung adenocarcinoma. Chest 1992;101:763–6.
18. Kragel PJ, Devaney KO, Meth BM, Linnoila I, Frierson HF, Travis WD. Mucinous cystadenoma of the lung. A report of two cases with immunohistochemical and ultrastructural analysis. Arch Pathol Lab Med 1990;114:1053–6.
19. _____, Devaney KO, Travis WD. In reply to letters of the editor. Arch Pathol Lab Med 1991;115:740–1.
20. Moran C, Hochholzer L, Fishback N, Travis W, Koss M. Mucinous (so-called colloid) carcinoma of lung. Mod Pathol 1992;5:634–8.

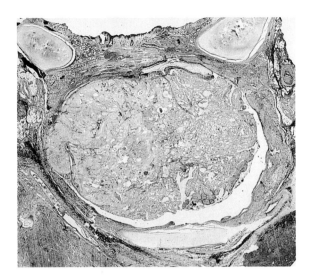

Figure 6-3
MUCOEPIDERMOID CARCINOMA
OF BRONCHUS, LOW GRADE

This scanning microscopic view shows the typical low magnification appearance of the tumor: a polypoid and microcystic nodule protruding into the bronchial lumen. (Fig. 1 from Yousem SA, Hochholzer L. Mucoepidermoid tumors of the lung. Cancer 1987;60:1346–52.)

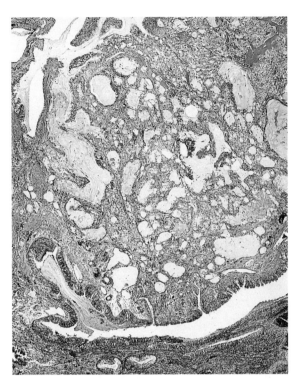

Figure 6-4
MUCOEPIDERMOID CARCINOMA
OF BRONCHUS, LOW GRADE

Note the numerous anastomosing glands and irregularly shaped, mucin-filled cysts that are typical findings.

The overwhelming majority (75 to 80 percent) of mucoepidermoid carcinomas are of low histologic grade (6,25). There is debate over the definition of high-grade tumors and their distinction from adenosquamous carcinoma (6,25). High-grade mucoepidermoid carcinomas have a central endobronchial location. They usually consist largely of sheets or nests of intermediate and squamoid cells intermixed with a smaller population of mucin-secreting cells; however, occasionally, an equal or even dominant glandular component is reported (25). The squamoid cells typically do not show individual cell keratinization or keratin pearl formation. Mitoses are increased, averaging 4 per 10 high-power fields, and there is nuclear pleomorphism, hyperchromasia, and cellular necrosis (figs. 6-13, 6-14) (6,8,25). The stroma frequently has admixed chronic inflammatory cells and can be hyalinized. The tumor invades the pulmonary parenchyma in nearly 50 percent of cases.

Cytology. There are only a few reports of the cytologic diagnosis of bronchial mucoepidermoid carcinoma (15,23). Although sputum cytology is generally not useful, transthoracic and transbronchial fine needle aspiration is occasionally of diagnostic value. The diagnosis is suggested by the finding of clusters of atypical squamous cells with prominent nucleoli dispersed among vacuolated, mucus-secreting polygonal cells; cyst-like spaces; and abundant background mucus.

Ultrastructural Findings. Mucoepidermoid carcinomas of the bronchus are similar in their ultrastructural appearance to those arising in the salivary glands. Undifferentiated cells, glandular cells, and squamous cells with prominent desmosomes and cytoplasmic tonofibrils are typical (8,13,16,22). Intermediate cells have only scattered desmosomes, with occasional small cytoplasmic tonofibril bundles (13). Oncocytes with abundant cytoplasmic mitochondria can occur (22).

Differential Diagnosis. Low-grade mucoepidermoid carcinoma needs to be distinguished from bronchial mucous gland adenoma (Table 6-1). The latter shows numerous mucus-filled cysts or tubules lined by a single row of columnar globlet cells, but it does not have the sheets or clusters of intermediate or squamous cells typical

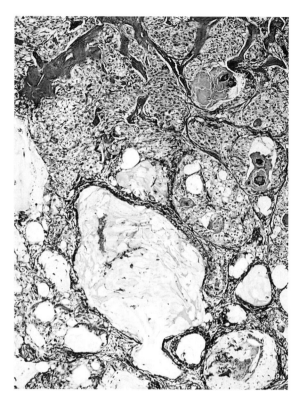

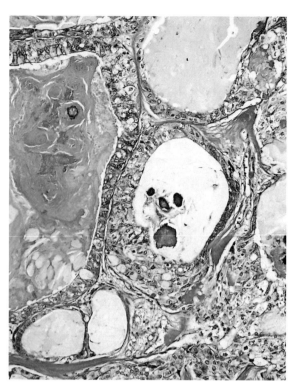

Figure 6-5

MUCOEPIDERMOID CARCINOMA
OF BRONCHUS, LOW GRADE

This view shows glands, mucus-filled cysts lined by flattened cells, and solid nests of cells. Scattered dark, calcific
concretions are present within the intraglandular mucin of
this tumor. (Figures 6-5 and 6-6 are from the same tumor.)

Figure 6-6

GLANDULAR COMPONENT OF MUCOEPIDERMOID
CARCINOMA OF BRONCHUS, LOW GRADE

There are numerous glands lined by columnar, cuboidal,
and flattened mucinous cells, some with clear or bubbly
cytoplasm. The glandular lumens are filled with mucin,
some of which is inspissated and shows calcific concretions.

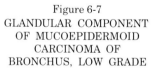

Figure 6-7

GLANDULAR COMPONENT
OF MUCOEPIDERMOID
CARCINOMA OF
BRONCHUS, LOW GRADE

In this area, the tumor consists
largely of glands and tubules streaming through a fibrous stroma.

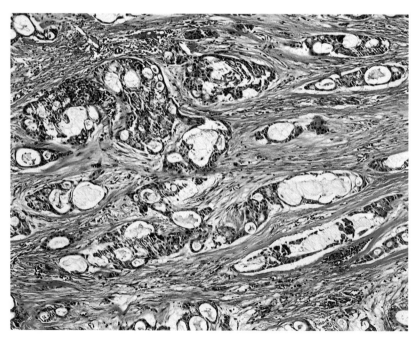

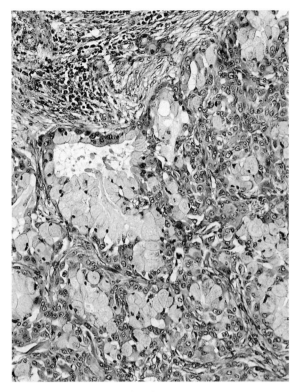

Figure 6-8
GLANDULAR COMPONENT OF MUCOEPIDERMOID
CARCINOMA OF BRONCHUS, LOW GRADE

Glands intermixed with intermediate cells. Note the
presence of goblet cells lining some of the glands and appearing in nests. (Fig. 3 from Yousem SA, Hochholzer L. Mucoepidermoid tumors of the lung. Cancer 1987;60:1346–52.)

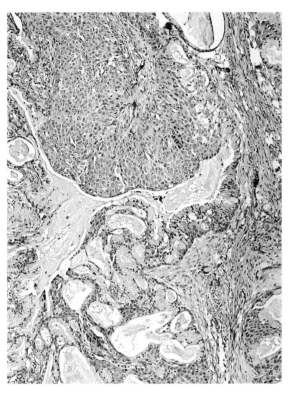

Figure 6-9
MUCOEPIDERMOID CARCINOMA, LOW GRADE

The tumor shows solid nests of intermediate cells in addition to glands. (Fig. 2 from Yousem SA, Hochholzer L. Mucoepidermoid tumors of the lung. Cancer 1987;60:1346–52.)

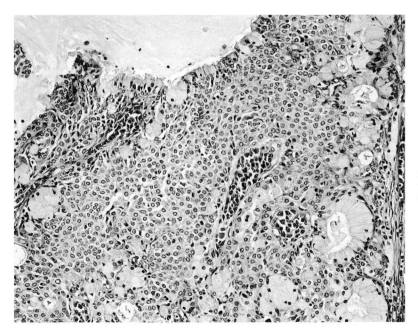

Figure 6-10
INTERMEDIATE CELLS
IN MUCOEPIDERMOID
CARCINOMA, LOW GRADE

Sheets of intermediate cells with central, uniform nuclei and amphophilic or
mildly eosinophilic cytoplasm are intermixed with glands lined by goblet cells.

Table 6-1

COMPARATIVE FEATURES OF SELECTED SALIVARY GLAND TYPE TUMORS OF LUNG

	Adenoid Cystic Carcinoma	Mucoepidermoid Carcinoma	Pleomorphic Adenoma	Mucous Gland Adenoma
Location	Trachea/main stem or lobar bronchi	Main stem/lobar> segmental bronchi	Lobar, segmental bronchi, peripheral	Lobar, segmental bronchi
Gross	Villous, heaped-up margins	Polypoid, well circumscribed, mucus covered, cystic	Polypoid or occlusive, well or poorly circumscribed	Polypoid, spherical, well circumscribed, noninvasive
Histology	Cylinders, glands, tubules, cribriform arrays; nerves and margins often invaded; myxoid stroma without spindle cells	Cysts, glands, squamous cells, intermediate cells	Biphasic pattern; cords, occasional ductules, solid sheets; myxoid stroma with spindle/ stellate cells	Cysts, glands, tubules
Positive Immuno-reactants	Actin, focal S-100, keratin	Keratin	Actin, S-100, GFAP, keratin	Keratin, CEA, EMA

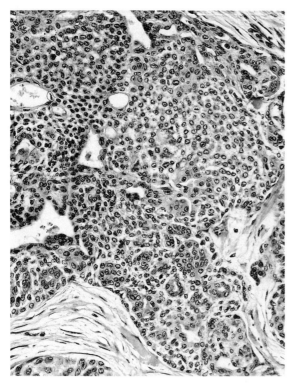

Figure 6-11
INTERMEDIATE CELLS IN MUCOEPIDERMOID CARCINOMA, LOW GRADE

High magnification view shows sheets of intermediate cells with central, uniform nuclei and relatively scant cytoplasm. Small glands are intermixed.

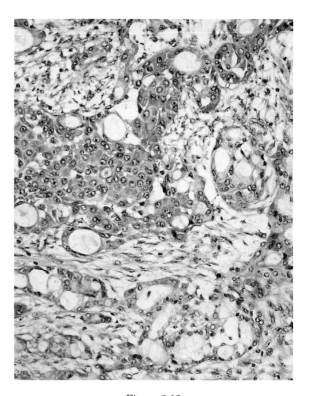

Figure 6-12
SQUAMOUS CELLS IN MUCOEPIDERMOID CARCINOMA, LOW GRADE

The squamous cells in this case have relatively abundant eosinophilic cytoplasm, well-defined cytoplasmic borders, and focal intercellular bridges. However, keratin whorls or pearls are not seen.

70

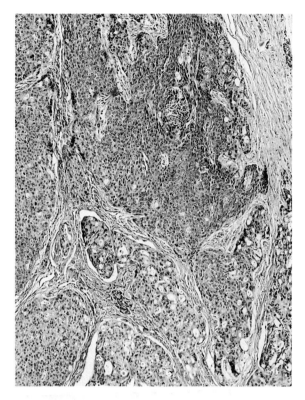

Figure 6-13
MUCOEPIDERMOID CARCINOMA, HIGH GRADE

Solid sheets and nests of intermediate and squamous cells without keratin pearl formation and with intermixed mucin-secreting cells are present. Glands are conspicuously absent. (Fig. 7 from Yousem SA, Hochholzer L. Mucoepidermoid tumors of the lung. Cancer 1987;60:1346–52.)

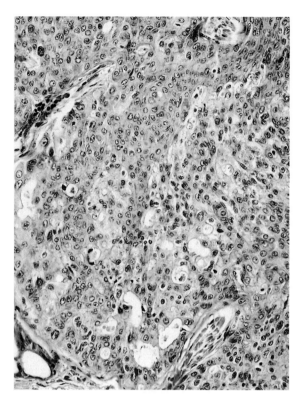

Figure 6-14
MUCOEPIDERMOID CARCINOMA, HIGH GRADE

Note the solid sheet of intermediate/squamous cells without keratin whorls or pearls and with minimal gland formation. Cytologic atypia in the form of nuclear pleomorphism and hyperchromasia is present.

of mucoepidermoid tumors. It is also significantly less frequent than mucoepidermoid carcinoma, in our experience. Still, this distinction can be difficult on occasion, since low-grade mucoepidermoid tumors may have few intermediate cells.

The comparative features of low-grade mucoepidermoid carcinomas and other salivary gland-like tumors are shown in Table 6-1.

The numerous glands or, on occasion, tubules of low-grade tumors may suggest adenocarcinoma, especially in small samples. A similar problem is seen with adenocarcinomas that are thought to arise from bronchial gland epithelium (7). The relative lack of cytologic atypia is helpful, as is the bronchoscopist's report of a smooth-surfaced polypoid endobronchial lesion. The presence of other cellular elements (intermediate cells, squamoid cells) allows definitive distinction.

Carcinosarcomas occasionally have malignant glands and may present as an endobronch-

ial mass. They are easily distinguishable by their greater cytologic atypia, and when present in the biopsy, malignant stroma.

Metastases to the bronchus may cause problems (2). Often, there is a preexisting history of a malignant tumor. Most metastatic neoplasms can be readily excluded on histologic grounds or on the basis of multiple nodules in lung.

As mentioned above, high-grade mucoepidermoid carcinomas are difficult to separate from adenosquamous cell carcinomas of lung (see chapter 16) (4,14). In fact, there are those who view them as histologically indistinguishable tumors that differ only in location within lung (6). Those who advocate separating the tumors note that mucoepidermoid tumors are usually central, have a polypoid endobronchial component, usually lack in situ changes in the bronchial epithelium, and fail to show squamous pearls or whorls, while adenosquamous carcinomas tend to be more peripheral in location, may show in situ bronchial epithelial atypia, and often demonstrate frank keratinization (8,25). Still, there are tumors not easily classified into one or the other category (9).

Treatment and Prognosis. Histologic grade appears to be of great prognostic significance (12). Low-grade tumors are infrequently locally invasive, and metastasis to regional lymph nodes or other sites (such as skin) is rare (1,3,6, 11,25). In one study, only 2 percent of tumors metastasized to the regional lymph nodes (25). In general, conservative, lung-sparing therapy (such as sleeve resection) is appropriate if a clear margin of tissue can be obtained. Completely resectable low-grade tumors generally have an excellent prognosis (6,25). Nearly all mucoepidermoid carcinomas in children or young adults are low grade (9,13).

The usual treatment for high-grade lesions is surgical resection, followed in some instances by postoperative radiation therapy (25). The prognosis of these tumors is guarded. In two studies, the average and median survival of patients was only 5.3 and 5.0 months, respectively, but this very poor prognosis may result from inclusion of individuals with adenosquamous carcinomas (12,18, 24). A different appraisal is offered by a series of 13 patients, only 3 of whom died of disease (including 2 patients with regional lymph node metastases) (25). Intracranial and skin metastases have also been reported.

ADENOID CYSTIC CARCINOMA

Definition. This is an infiltrative, malignant epithelial neoplasm with a distinctive histologic pattern of growth consisting of cribriform or glandular arrays, tubules surrounding central spaces filled with epithelial mucin, and solid foci (42). Two types of tumor cells are present: those lining ducts and myoepithelial cells. Older terms include *cylindroma* and *adenocystic carcinoma*.

Clinical Features. Adenoid cystic carcinomas are the most common salivary gland-like tumor to occur in the lower respiratory tract; however, they are nevertheless infrequent, comprising only about 6 percent of bronchial adenomas and less than 0.2 percent of all primary pulmonary tumors (31,36). They usually arise in the lower trachea, main stem bronchi, or lobar bronchi (26,29,43). An origin in peripheral or subsegmental bronchi is uncommon, occurring in only about 10 percent of cases (36). Patients range from 18 to 79 years of age. Symptoms and chest X-ray abnormalities are usually due to chronic bronchial obstruction or irritation, averaging 2 years' duration before diagnosis (29,40, 43). The tumors may be difficult to localize by chest X ray because of their endobronchial and central location, but they are usually readily found at bronchoscopy (32,35).

Gross Findings. Adenoid cystic carcinomas are usually central in location and occur in association with large cartilage-bearing bronchi; they infrequently arise in secondary bronchi or peripheral lung (30,35,36). The tumors intrude into the bronchial lumens as gray-white or tan, soft, sessile, polypoid, annular, or diffusely infiltrative nodules ranging from 0.9 to 4.0 cm in diameter (fig. 6-15) (43). They may appear well circumscribed but they have a distinct tendency to extend through the bronchial wall and along the bronchial submucosa, producing heaped-up margins (29,33). Centripetal spread along the airways can at times reach exaggerated levels: one tumor arising in the main stem bronchus diffusely invaded the entire trachea, while a second occurring in the lung periphery infiltrated along airways to the level of proximal bronchi (36). In a few cases, adenoid cystic carcinomas grossly infiltrate the pleura or mediastinum, creating large masses, and involve the regional lymph nodes by metastasis (43).

Microscopic Findings. The tumor is microscopically similar to its counterpart in the salivary glands. At low magnification, it is usually a submucosal mass that narrows the bronchial lumen, spreads proximally and distally from the main tumor mass, invades circumferentially around the airway, and penetrates radially between and through the bronchial cartilage plates (figs. 6-16, 6-17). The bronchial epithelium overlying the neoplasm is typically intact (figs. 6-17, 6-18), but it may be ulcerated or show squamous metaplasia.

At higher magnification, small cells with darkly stained nuclei are arranged in cylinders or cribriform arrays (cylindromatous pattern), in trabeculae, glands or tubules, and, least often, in solid or cystic cords. The cylindromatous pattern is the one usually encountered (figs. 6-18, 6-19). Many of the cylindrical spaces are pseudocysts

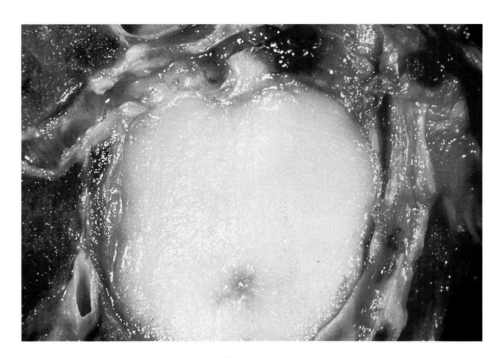

Figure 6-15
ADENOID CYSTIC CARCINOMA OF BRONCHUS: GROSS APPEARANCE
This tumor presented in an iceberg fashion, with deep invasion through and beneath the bronchial cartilage.

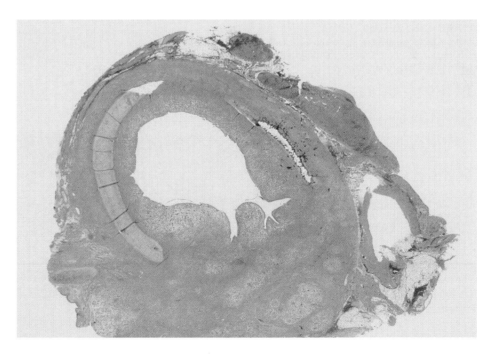

Figure 6-16
ADENOID CYSTIC CARCINOMA OF BRONCHUS
This whole mount section shows tumor extending radially around and away from the bronchus wall, a feature that often leads to local recurrence if an adequate surgical margin is not obtained. (Fig. 3-92 from Colby TV, Lombard C, Yousem SA, Kitaichi M. Atlas of pulmonary surgical pathology. Philadelphia: WB Saunders, 1992.)

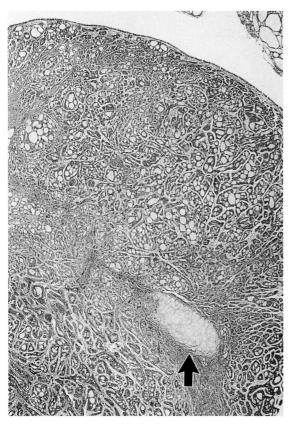

Figure 6-17
ADENOID CYSTIC CARCINOMA

In this view, the tumor penetrates the bronchial wall, destroying the cartilage. A residual island of cartilage is still present (arrow). Bronchial lumen is above.

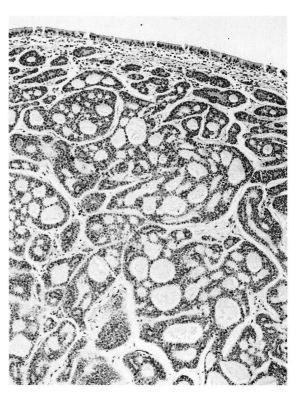

Figure 6-18
ADENOID CYSTIC CARCINOMA:
CYLINDROMATOUS GROWTH PATTERN

Note the cribriform appearance of the tumor cells. The spaces present are pseudocysts rather than true glands. Note intact bronchial epithelium overlying the tumor.

Figure 6-19
ADENOID CYSTIC CARCINOMA:
CYLINDROMATOUS
GROWTH PATTERN

Higher magnification of lesion in previous figure. A delicate cribriform pattern is present in which tumor cells are arrayed about pseudocysts.

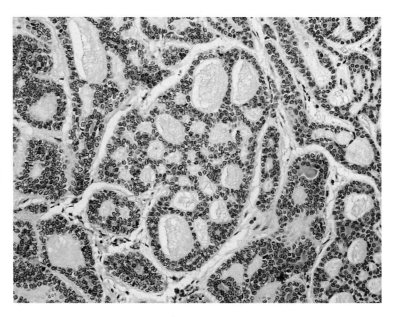

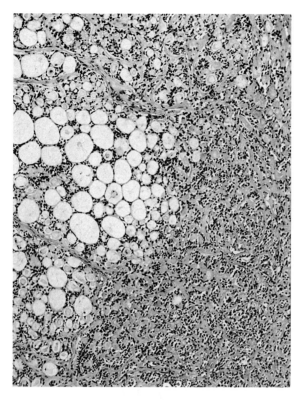

Figure 6-20
ADENOID CYSTIC CARCINOMA
Sclerotic stroma compresses the tumor cells into thin cords that merge with ectatic pseudocysts lined by flattened cells.

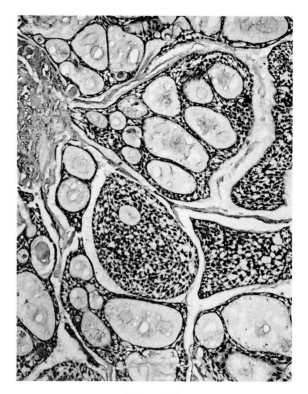

Figure 6-21
ADENOID CYSTIC CARCINOMA
Nests of tumor cells showing ectatic pseudocysts containing myxoid and mucinous material.

or pseudolumens, rather than true glandular lumens, formed by compressed cords of cells coursing through a sclerotic or myxoid stroma (figs. 6-20, 6-21). Pseudocysts often vary greatly in size (some may be markedly ectatic) and contain mucinous or eosinophilic, hyaline basal lamina-like material (see Ultrastructural Findings) (fig. 6-21). This basal lamina-like material is rich in proteoglycans and it, as well as the surrounding stroma, stains consistently and strongly with Alcian blue but only weakly with periodic acid–Schiff (PAS) (38). Alcian blue staining is abolished by hyaluronidase predigestion.

True glands or tubules can occur (fig. 6-22) (35). They are lined by a luminal layer of ductular epithelium and one or more layers of myoepithelial cells. They too may contain mucinous material, but the mucin stains as well with diastase-predigested PAS as with mucicarmine.

Sometimes, there is an abundant hyaline stroma that compresses the epithelial cords into thin ribbons (fig. 6-23). Tangential cutting of tubular structures can create the appearance of longitudinal cords or trabeculae of cells.

The solid growth pattern is characterized by sheets or solid nests of cells largely lacking luminal structures (fig. 6-24). Occasionally, the solid nests have peripheral cell palisades, producing a basaloid pattern. Still, necrosis, cytologic atypia, and increased mitoses are unusual.

It is common for adenoid cystic carcinomas to have foci of scattered glands embedded in a myxoid stroma, resembling pleomorphic adenoma. In addition to myxoid changes, the stroma may be hyalinized (fig. 6-23). Another peculiar growth pattern is one in which clusters of small glands are lined by oval to spindle, myoepithelial-like cells.

Perineural invasion is a striking finding, occurring in 38 percent of cases in the AFIP series (38a) (fig. 6-25). The tumor commonly invades surrounding lung and may involve regional

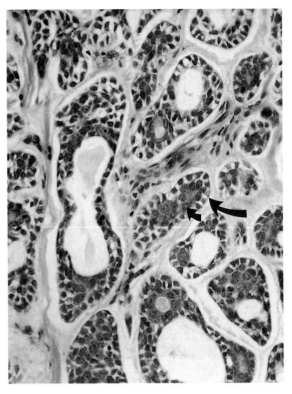

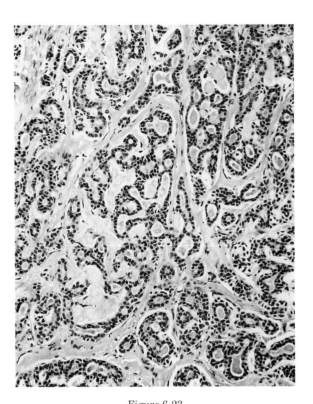

Figure 6-22
ADENOID CYSTIC CARCINOMA
Both pseudocysts and compressed glands are present. The latter are lined by a luminal layer of ductular epithelium (short arrow) and a prominent underlying layer of myoepithelial cells with relatively clear cytoplasm (long arrow). Some of the glandular lumens are obliterated, but one contains a small amount of mucin.

Figure 6-23
ADENOID CYSTIC CARCINOMA
WITH HYALINE STROMA
The stroma compresses the tumor into cords and ribbons.

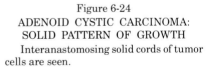

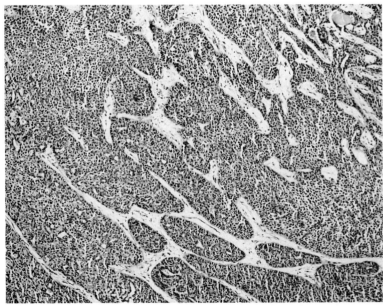

Figure 6-24
ADENOID CYSTIC CARCINOMA:
SOLID PATTERN OF GROWTH
Interanastomosing solid cords of tumor cells are seen.

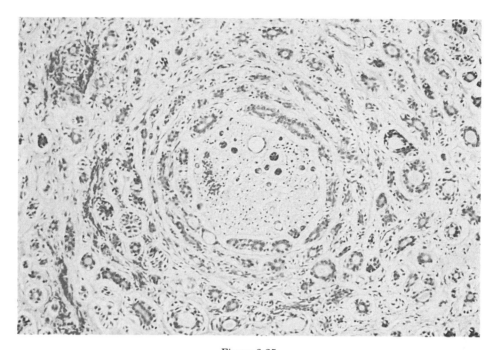

Figure 6-25
ADENOID CYSTIC CARCINOMA: PERINEURAL INVASION
In this view, the nerve is cut in cross section with the tumor circumferentially arrayed about it.

lymph nodes. Most extra-pulmonary metastases histologically resemble the primary tumor and usually have a cribriform growth pattern.

Immunohistochemical Findings. The immunohistochemical staining pattern for adenoid cystic carcinoma of lung and salivary gland is similar. There is strong epithelial reactivity for low molecular weight keratins, vimentin, and actin. Staining for S-100 protein may also be present, but it is more focal. The tumor cells may not express glial fibrillary acidic protein (GFAP), an antigen present in the myoepithelial elements of salivary gland mixed tumors. Antibodies to type IV collagen, laminin, heparin sulfate proteoglycan, and entactin decorate the matrix of the pseudocysts, particularly the outer borders (27).

Ultrastructural Findings. The electron microscopic appearance of adenoid cystic carcinoma is distinctive (38). Pseudocysts consist of entrapped matrix surrounded by cords of infiltrating tumor cells (fig. 6-26). The cells are sometimes lined by highly replicated basal lamina (fig. 6-27). The tumor cells may also form true glands containing microvilli, junctional complexes, and desmosomes. Myoepithelial cells are present and contain cytoplasmic aggregates of

6-nm filaments compatible with myofilaments. The stroma is rich in basal lamina as well as flocculent and fibrillar material.

Differential Diagnosis. The differential diagnosis of salivary gland type tumors originating in lung is shown in Table 6-1. As noted above, adenoid cystic carcinomas may have foci of small glands embedded in a myxoid stroma, suggesting pleomorphic adenoma. This can create particular difficulty in small biopsies. The finding of characteristic cribriform or cylindromatous areas should lead to the diagnosis of adenoid cystic carcinoma.

Mucoepidermoid tumors of the bronchus usually have glandular spaces containing mucin. The gross appearance of the two tumors is different: adenoid cystic carcinomas have a more villous appearance with heaped-up margins, while mucoepidermoid carcinomas present as smooth, well-circumscribed, polypoid endobronchial nodules. Mucoepidermoid tumors are more likely to appear in segmental bronchi. Microscopically, mucoepidermoid tumors have sheet-like arrays of squamous or intermediate cells, a finding not observed in adenoid cystic carcinomas.

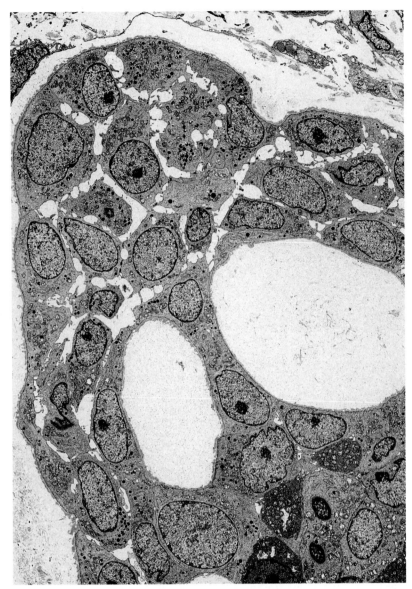

Figure 6-26
ADENOID CYSTIC
CARCINOMA:
ULTRASTRUCTURAL
APPEARANCE
Two pseudocysts are formed within a nest of tumor cells. They contain scant amounts of amorphous material in this view.

Sometimes, adenocarcinomas of lung have cribriform or tubular foci resembling adenoid cystic carcinoma. Still, this pattern is focal and other patterns are seen within adenocarcinomas. Further, adenocarcinomas have greater cytologic atypia, as well as necrosis and increased mitoses.

In crushed tissue obtained by forceps biopsy, the small darkly stained cells of adenoid cystic carcinoma can be readily confused with small cell carcinoma or lymphoma. The presence of a double layer of tumor cells lining ductules favors adenoid cystic carcinoma while punctate nuclear chromatin and nuclear molding suggests small cell carcinoma.

Adenoid cystic carcinoma from extrapulmonary primary sites may metastasize to lung up to 18 years after initial diagnosis (39). History of a previous primary and the presence of multiple or bilateral nodules suggests metastasis.

Prognosis. Adenoid cystic carcinomas, because they tend to infiltrate along the airways, are likely to be incompletely excised and are prone to recur locally, sometimes many years after initial resection (29,43). Spread occurs by direct invasion to mediastinum and by metastasis to regional lymph nodes. Distant metastasis is less common but spread to liver, spleen, kidney,

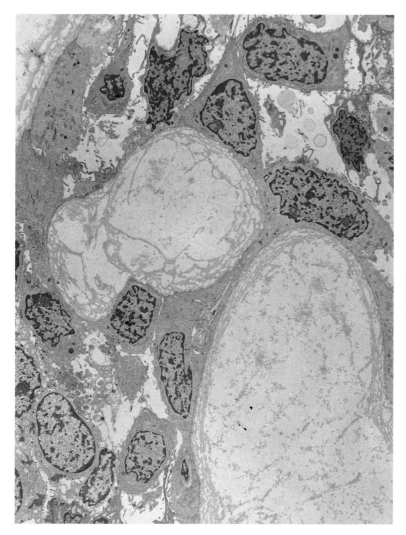

Figure 6-27
ADENOID CYSTIC CARCINOMA:
ULTRASTRUCTURAL
APPEARANCE
Two pseudocysts formed by infiltrating tumor cells contain laminated basal lamina, a feature, which when marked, creates the hyaline appearance seen within some pseudocysts by light microscopy.

bone, and adrenal glands have all been reported (43). In the AFIP series, 2 of 11 patients died of tumor within a year of diagnosis, while in 3 others disease recurred up to 15 years after initial diagnosis (38a). In a series compiled from the Mayo Clinic, only 55 percent of patients resected for cure were alive at 10 years (29).

The prognosis is affected by stage of disease at presentation. In particular, patients with distant metastasis at diagnosis have a poor prognosis, with death due to widespread metastases, while patients with well-circumscribed endobronchial tumors have a relatively good prognosis. However, some patients with regional lymph node involvement still survive long term (29). A relationship between a solid pattern of growth and a poor prognosis, which has been suggested for adenoid

cystic carcinomas of salivary gland origin, has also been raised in lung (37,41). Evaluation of bronchial tumor margins by frozen section is mandatory for successful surgical resection (29).

MUCOUS GLAND ADENOMA

Definition. Mucous gland adenoma is a benign tumor arising from and histologically mimicking bronchial mucous glands. Synonymous terms include *mucous gland cystadenoma, adenomatous polyp,* and *adenomas of mucous gland type.*

Clinical Features. The tumor is rare (44). It occurs in both children and adults. In the largest series of adults, women outnumbered men by 2.5 to 1 (45a). Because of the bronchial location of these neoplasms, patients often have symptoms secondary to airway obstruction or hemorrhage.

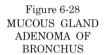

Figure 6-28
MUCOUS GLAND
ADENOMA OF
BRONCHUS
The whole mount sec-
tion shows the numerous
dilated cysts that are often
a prominent feature of
these benign tumors.

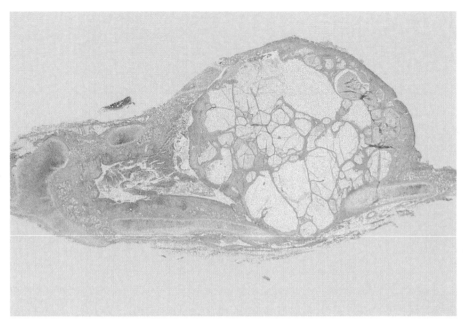

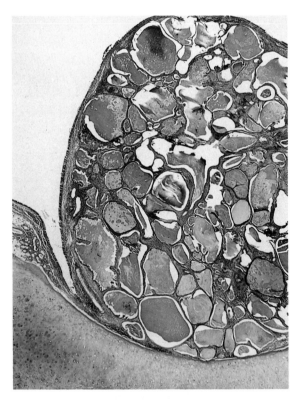

Figure 6-29
MUCOUS GLAND ADENOMA
In this low magnification view, the tumor protrudes into the
bronchial lumen. Note the numerous cystic spaces of varying
sizes produced by the dilated mucin-filled glands of the tumor.

Gross Findings. The tumors are soft, spherical, polypoid endobronchial nodules that are
usually less than 2 cm in diameter but may range
up to 6.8 cm (44-47). They arise in lobar or
segmental bronchi, most often of the lower or
middle lobes (45a). They are well circumscribed
and noninvasive. The mucosa overlying the
tumor is typically intact. The lung distal to the
neoplasm shows the consequences of bronchial
obstruction, with dilated bronchi containing inspissated mucus and cholesterol pneumonia.

Microscopic Findings. The most striking
feature is the presence of cystic, mucus-filled
glands protruding into the bronchial lumen (figs.
6-28–6-30). The glands are lined by cytologically
bland columnar, cuboidal, or flattened mucus-secreting cells (fig. 6-31). In areas, they may show
oncocytic metaplasia (a phenomenon also seen in
aging normal bronchial glands) or focally clear
cytoplasm. The cyst contents often have a colloid-like appearance. Sometimes, small concretions are present in the mucus. Other
morphologic patterns can occur, including small
tubular glands lined by columnar cells and a
mixture of papillary and cystic glandular structures (fig. 6-31). A form of mucous gland adenoma composed of small glands lined by goblet
cells with a focal admixture of intermediate cells
is also reported, but this seems more likely a

variant of mucoepidermoid tumor with a dominant glandular component. The stroma can be fibrous, giving the tumor an adenofibromatous appearance, or it may be chronically inflamed. The tumors stain for neutral and acid mucins and react with immunohistochemical stains for carcinoembryonic antigen, keratin, and epithelial membrane antigen (45a).

Differential Diagnosis. Low-grade mucoepidermoid tumor often is largely glandular and may have dilated cysts (Table 6-1). Distinguishing it from mucous gland adenoma can be difficult, particularly in small biopsies. Although some suggest that mucous gland adenomas may contain small numbers of intermediate cells, in our opinion, the finding of intermediate cells, even in small numbers, suggests mucoepidermoid tumor.

The lack of cytologic atypia, mitoses, and necrosis aids in differentiating the tumor from adenocarcinoma.

Treatment and Prognosis. The treatment of this tumor is conservative surgical excision with sparing of lung parenchyma. Occasionally, lobectomy is required when more limited surgery is not technically feasible or when the lung distal to the tumor is extensively damaged. As their name indicates, mucous gland adenomas are benign and hence truly warrant the name adenoma.

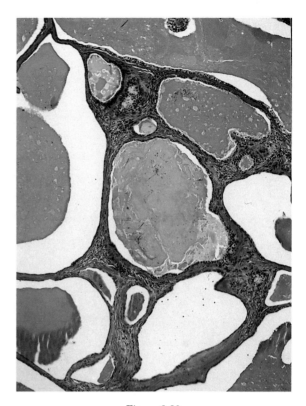

Figure 6-30
MUCOUS GLAND ADENOMA
Cystically dilated, mucin-filled glands are lined by a flattened epithelium that is barely discernible. A fibrous stroma separates the glands.

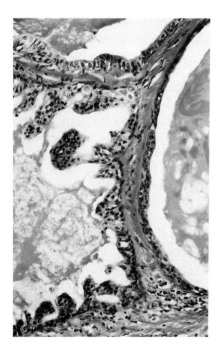 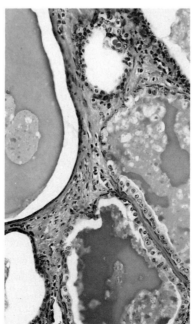

Figure 6-31
MUCOUS GLAND ADENOMA
The two panels show the variety of epithelial linings of the glands, ranging from a flattened, almost inapparent epithelium to cuboidal cells to low papillary structures.

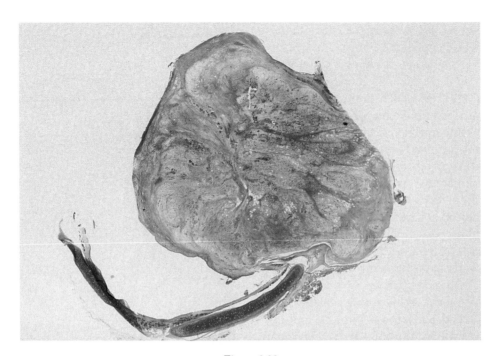

Figure 6-32
PLEOMORPHIC ADENOMA
The tumor presents as a polypoid intrabronchial lesion covered by squamous epithelium.

PLEOMORPHIC ADENOMA

Definition. The WHO classification of salivary gland tumors defines pleomorphic adenoma as a neoplasm of pleomorphic histologic appearance produced by a mixture of luminal-type ductal epithelial cells, myoepithelial tissues, and tissues of myxochondroid, mucoid, or chondroid appearance (54,55). The epithelial and myoepithelial components form ducts, strands, or sheets. An older term is *benign mixed tumor.*

Clinical Features. Pleomorphic adenoma is the most common form of major salivary gland tumor, but it is exceedingly rare in lung (48–53, 56,57). Patients range from 35 to 74 years of age. Most have symptoms and signs of chronic bronchial obstruction. Still, some are asymptomatic, presenting with an incidental finding on chest X ray (51). The neoplasm can occur adjacent to or within bronchi, and it may even appear as a polypoid endobronchial lesion, but it may also be present in the lung periphery without apparent involvement of a bronchus (51,53). Occasionally, the tumor occupies a whole lobe. Pleomorphic adenomas are slow growing, with a potential for aggressive behavior in the form of local recurrence and distant metastasis (52,53,56).

Gross Findings. Pleomorphic adenomas of lung range from 1.5 to 16 cm in diameter (50,56). Most are associated with a major or secondary bronchus where they appear as polypoid and occlusive intraluminal tumors (51,52), but one third to nearly half are peripheral (50,53). They are gray-white, and soft, rubbery, or myxoid on cut surface. They are typically well circumscribed but unencapsulated. The regional lymph nodes are usually free of metastases at thoracotomy.

Microscopic Findings. Most tumors appear sharply circumscribed from the surrounding lung. Polypoid intrabronchial lesions are covered by a thin layer of squamous epithelium (fig. 6-32). When the tumor is peripheral or subpleural, a cartilage-bearing bronchus may not be seen.

Pleomorphic adenomas have a biphasic histology. The epithelial component consists of sheets, compressed anastomosing cords, trabeculae or small islands of round to oval cells that usually have vesicular nuclei and a pale rim of eosinophilic cytoplasm (fig. 6-33). Pleomorphic adenomas of lung, unlike those in the salivary gland, either lack or have few ducts (50,53,56). When present, the ductules are usually small and branching (fig. 6-34). They are lined by a double

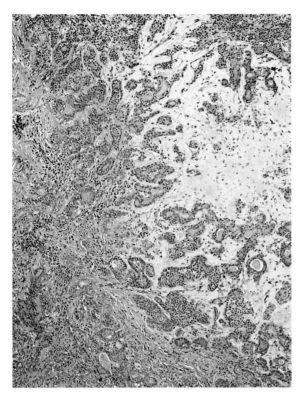

Figure 6-33
PLEOMORPHIC ADENOMA OF LUNG
The tumor shows a biphasic histology. Compressed cords, trabeculae, islands, and small ductules merge with a pale area of hyaline-like stroma.

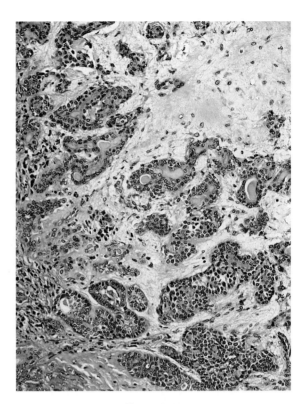

Figure 6-34
PLEOMORPHIC ADENOMA OF LUNG
Small ductules and solid epithelial islands merge with oval and spindle cells in a hyaline stroma. The ductular lumens contain small amounts of mucinous material.

layer of cells: an inner epithelial and an outer myoepithelial layer. Their lumens may contain small amounts of PAS-positive material.

The epithelial component merges with stellate and spindle cells in a myxoid, myxochondroid, or hyaline stroma (fig. 6-34). This stroma is rich in hyaluronic acid, as demonstrated by acid mucopolysaccharide stains with and without hyaluronidase predigestion. In about 25 percent of cases, a chondroid matrix can be seen (50,52,53,56,57).

The epithelial component of pleomorphic adenoma of the lung shows strong cytoplasmic reactivity for low molecular weight keratins. When ductules are present, the basal layer of cells as well as many of the spindle and stellate cells lying in the myxoid matrix are decorated by antibodies to vimentin, actin, S-100 protein, and GFAP (50,53). This pattern of staining is typical of myoepithelial cells and similar to pleomorphic adenomas of salivary gland origin.

Differential Diagnosis. The differential diagnosis includes metastasis from a primary salivary gland tumor. A solitary tumor presenting in the lung, related to a cartilage-bearing bronchus, and appearing as a polypoid intrabronchial mass suggests a pulmonary origin. Histologically, lung primaries also tend to have few duct-like structures in the epithelial component and typically do not have well-developed chondroid components.

Biphasic pulmonary blastomas have a stromal component that can be myxoid, but the stroma is frankly sarcomatous and the epithelial component has the characteristic clear cytoplasm, abundant glycogen, and endometrioid appearance of fetal lung tubules (see chapter 21). By definition, other carcinosarcomas of lung consist of a mixture of malignant epithelium and sarcomas of the type seen in tumors of adults. The presence of a frankly sarcomatous stroma excludes pleomorphic adenoma. Still, there is a variant of malignant mixed

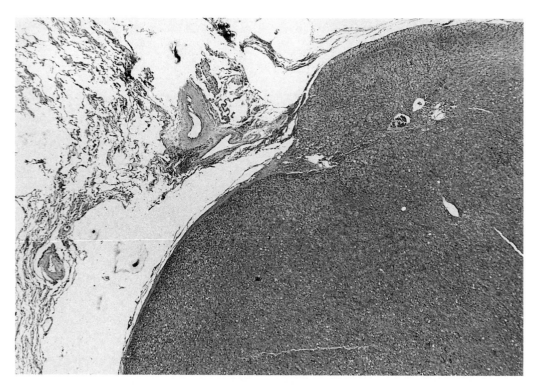

Figure 6-35
ACINIC CELL CARCINOMA OF LUNG
The tumor presents as a solid, sharply defined, parenchymal nodule. (Fig. 1 from Moran CA, Suster S, Koss MN. Acinic cell carcinoma of the lung ("Fechner tumor"). A clinicopathologic, immunohistochemical, and ultrastructural study of five cases. Am J Surg Pathol 1992;16:1039–50.)

tumor in salivary gland characterized by both a carcinosarcomatous pattern and residual pleomorphic adenoma (54); one similar case has been reported in lung (49).

The differential diagnosis with other salivary gland type tumors such as adenoid cystic carcinoma and mucoepidermoid carcinoma is shown in Table 6-1.

ACINIC CELL CARCINOMA

Definition. This tumor was originally described in the salivary glands and consists of epithelial cells morphologically resembling serous cells (62). Serous type secretory granules are seen on electron microscopic examination. This pulmonary tumor has also been termed *Fechner tumor* after its discoverer (58,61), *acinic cell adenocarcinoma,* and *acinic cell tumor*.

Clinical Features. Acinic cell carcinoma of lung is rare: less than 10 cases have been re-

ported as of 1993 (58,59,61,63). The age range of patients is wide, varying from 12 to 75 years, but most patients are adults. The tumor can be endobronchial and polypoid, producing symptoms of bronchial irritation and obstruction, or parenchymal and asymptomatic. Still, even in the latter instance, there is usually contiguity to bronchi. In the cases reported to date, there has been neither recurrence nor metastasis after surgical resection.

Gross Findings. Acinic cell carcinomas are well-circumscribed, unencapsulated, tan to yellow neoplasms (fig. 6-35). When they are intrabronchial, they present as polypoid masses.

Microscopic Findings. Cytologically, the tumor cells are uniform, round to polygonal, with abundant granular, eosinophilic, or basophilic cytoplasm (fig. 6-36). The nuclei are usually small, round to oval, and central, but sometimes larger vesicular nuclei with prominent nucleoli are seen. The characteristic tumor cells are arranged in

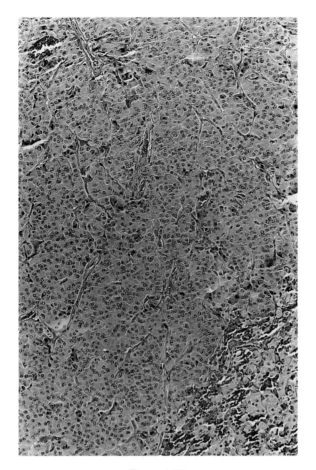

Figure 6-36
ACINIC CELL CARCINOMA OF LUNG

Delicate fibrovascular strands separate the tumor into cords and nests. The tumor cells have abundant cytoplasm and a monotonous appearance. (Fig. 2b from Moran CA, Suster S, Koss MN. Acinic cell carcinoma of the lung ("Fechner tumor"). A clinicopathologic, immunohistochemical, and ultrastructural study of five cases. Am J Surg Pathol 1992;16:1039–50.)

sheets, nests, acini, small glands, or tubulo-papillary formations (fig. 6-36). The nests can be separated by thin or broad bands of fibrous connective tissue, sometimes containing an abundant lymphoid or lymphoplasmacytic infiltrate, or a vascular stroma.

Acinic cell carcinomas of the salivary gland characteristically contain PAS-positive diastase-resistant cytoplasmic granules that express amylase and alpha-1-antichymotrypsin. However, these features are not constant (61). Electron microscopy reveals the characteristic zymogen-type granules: cytoplasmic membrane-bound bodies averaging 600 to 800 nm in diameter (61).

Differential Diagnosis. The first consideration must be to exclude metastatic acinic cell carcinoma of salivary gland origin. A solitary lesion adjacent to a bronchus suggests origin in lung, but clinical evaluation is always in order to exclude metastasis.

Oncocytic carcinoid tumors, like acinic cell carcinomas, can have a sheet-like or acinar pattern of growth as well as cytologically uniform cells with abundant eosinophilic granular cytoplasm. Immunoreactivity for chromogranin, synaptophysin, or Leu-7 and the finding of numerous mitochondria with typical small dense core granules support this diagnosis.

Granular cell tumors of the bronchus have abundant eosinophilic and granular cytoplasm. Still, they have the characteristic ultrastructural feature of abundant autophagic lysosomes not seen in acinic cell carcinomas.

There is a rare form of xanthoma (histiocytoma) that consists of sheets of uniform cells with gray, finely vacuolated cytoplasm set amid gaping staghorn-shaped vessels (60). The presence of intracytoplasmic keratin supports acinic cell carcinoma and excludes this diagnosis.

OTHER RARE SALIVARY GLAND TUMORS

Carcinoma ex Pleomorphic Adenoma (Malignant Mixed Tumor)

This is defined as a tumor showing definitive evidence of malignancy, such as cytologic and histologic characteristics of anaplasia, abnormal mitoses, progressive course, and infiltrative growth and in which evidence of pleomorphic adenoma can still be found (72). These neoplasms occur in only 3 to 4 percent of salivary gland pleomorphic adenomas (72) and they are understandably rare in lung as well.

Grossly, the tumors are less well defined than pleomorphic adenomas, often presenting as masses with peripheral satellite nodules or tumors occupying nearly an entire lobe (69). Microscopically, they show foci of carcinoma characterized by cytologic anaplasia, increased mitoses (5 or more per 10 high-power fields), necrosis, poor circumscription, and lymphatic invasion (fig. 6-37). At the same time, areas resembling pleomorphic adenoma are present.

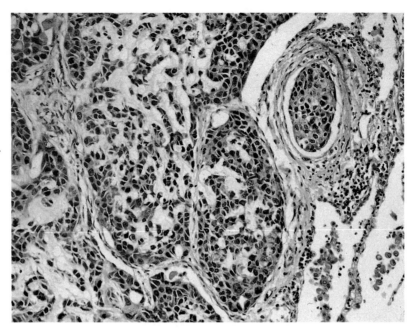

Figure 6-37
CARCINOMA ARISING IN
PLEOMORPHIC ADENOMA
Compressed cords and islands of
tumor cells are embedded in a hyaline
stroma. The tumor shows not only cytologic atypia but also invasion into an
adjacent artery.

Pulmonary Oncocytoma

This rare and controversial tumor is composed of columnar or polyhedral cells with centrally placed vesicular or hyperchromatic nuclei and abundant granular eosinophilic cytoplasm. The cytoplasmic features result from an accumulation of mitochondria. It is interesting to note that oncocytic metaplasia of bronchial glands is a common incidental finding in older individuals.

There are less than 10 reported pulmonary neoplasms designated as oncocytomas based on light and electron microscopic studies (65-68,70). The tumors tend to occur in male smokers. Grossly, they are usually solitary intrabronchial nodules that are 1.0 to 3.5 cm in diameter. Microscopically, they consist of sheets of cells with abundant granular eosinophilic cytoplasm, uniform round central nuclei, and prominent nucleoli. Mitoses and necrosis are rare or absent. Fibrous septa may be present, dividing the tumor into nests.

The controversy over the existence of oncocytomas in lung arises because certain pulmonary neoplasms, notably bronchial carcinoids (71,74), mucoepidermoid carcinomas, and mucous gland adenomas, may have prominent oncocytic changes. In fact, it is possible that many or all of the pulmonary oncocytomas reported to date are oncocytic carcinoids. Not only have

some of the published cases of oncocytomas shown a few cytoplasmic electron-dense granules (66-68), but none has had a complete immunohistochemical evaluation for a neuroendocrine immunophenotype. Nevertheless, the consensus favors retaining oncocytoma as a separate classification at least until the issue of immunophenotype is settled.

Myoepithelioma

This rare tumor is composed of myoepithelial cells without a ductal epithelial component. It may be a morphologic variant of pleomorphic adenoma (64,73). Myoepithelioma is typically found in salivary glands and breast; only one case in lung has been reported (75).

In this single report, the neoplasm was a well-circumscribed, tan, parenchymal pulmonary nodule that had been present for several years in an adult man. Microscopically, it consisted of sheets, nodules, and interdigitating fascicles of spindle and oval cells (figs. 6-38, 6-39). No epithelial elements were found. The tumor cells contained glycogen but not mucin; they reacted with antibodies to S-100 protein and actin but not keratin. A myxoid or chondroid matrix containing stellate cells was present in areas.

The diagnosis was supported by finding numerous fine, parallel, 6-nm cytoplasmic filaments by

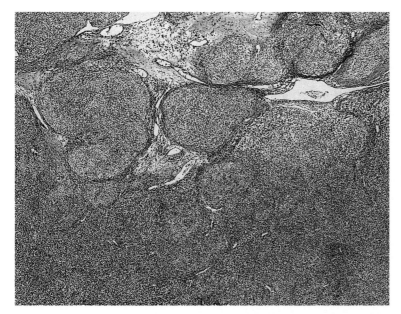

Figure 6-38
PULMONARY MYOEPITHELIOMA
In this section, the tumor appears as a multinodular cellular neoplasm. (Courtesy of Dr. J. Strickler, Minneapolis, MN.)

Figure 6-39
PULMONARY MYOEPITHELIOMA
The tumor is composed of interdigitating fascicles of spindle and oval cells without definite epithelial elements. (Courtesy of Dr. J. Strickler, Minneapolis, MN.)

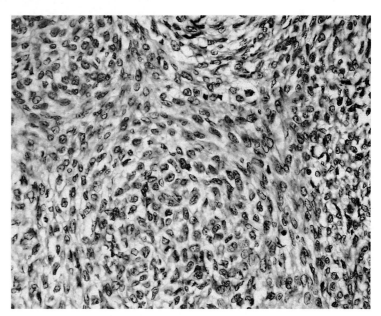

electron microscopy consistent with myofilaments. There were also desmosomes, macula adherens, and a discontinuous basal lamina, as well as cytoplasmic glycogen. These ultrastructural features were consistent with a myoepithelial phenotype.

The differential diagnosis of myoepithelioma includes spindle cell carcinoma and a smooth muscle tumor. The absence of keratin and presence of diffuse staining for S-100 protein separates these tumors.

Adenosquamous Carcinoma with Amyloid-like Stroma

Yousem (76) reported two cases which are described in more detail in chapter 16. A salient feature of these rare neoplasms is the hyaline-like or amyloid-like material surrounding tumor cells. The material consists of basement membrane-like structures rather than amyloid. Despite the histologic resemblance to adenosquamous carcinoma, these tumors are thought to be more closely aligned to salivary gland tumors.

REFERENCES

Mucoepidermoid Carcinoma

1. Barsky SH, Martin SE, Matthews M, Gazdar A, Costa JC. Low grade mucoepidermoid carcinoma of the bronchus with "high grade" biological behavior. Cancer 1983;51:1505–9.
2. Baumgartner WA, Mark JB. Metastatic malignancies from distant sites to the tracheobronchial tree. J Thorac Cardiovasc Surg 1980;79:499–503.
3. Conlan AA, Payne WS, Woolner LB, Sanderson DR. Adenoid cystic carcinoma (cylindroma) and mucoepidermoid carcinoma of the bronchus. Factors affecting survival. J Thorac Cardiovasc Surg 1978;76:369–77.
4. Fitzgibbons PL, Kern WH. Adenosquamous carcinoma of the lung: a clinical and pathologic study of seven cases. Hum Pathol 1985;16:463–6.
5. Green LK, Gallion TL, Gyorkey F. Peripheral mucoepidermoid tumour of the lung. Thorax 1991;46:65–6.
6. Heitmiller RF, Mathisen DJ, Ferry JA, Mark EJ, Grillo HC. Mucoepidermoid lung tumors. Ann Thorac Surg 1989;47:394–9.
7. Hirata H, Noguchi M, Shimosato Y, Uei Y, Goya T. Clinicopathologic and immunohistochemical characteristics of the bronchial gland cell type adenocarcinoma of the lung. Am J Clin Pathol 1990;93:20–5.
8. Klacsmann PG, Olson JL, Eggleston JC. Mucoepidermoid carcinoma of the bronchus: an electron microscopic study of the low grade and the high grade variants. Cancer 1979;43:1720–33.
9. Lack EE, Harris GB, Eraklis AJ, Vawter GF. Primary bronchial tumors in childhood. A clinicopathologic study of six cases. Cancer 1983;51:492–7.
10. Leonardi HK, Jung-Legg Y, Legg MA, Neptune WB. Tracheobronchial mucoepidermoid carcinoma: clinicopathological features and results of treatment. J Thorac Cardiovasc Surg 1978;76:431–8.
11. Metcalf JS, Maize JC, Shaw EB. Bronchial mucoepidermoid carcinoma metastatic to skin. Report of a case and review of the literature. Cancer 1986;58:2556–9.
12. Miller DL, Allen MS. Rare pulmonary neoplasms. Mayo Clin Proc 1993;68:492–8.
13. Mullins JD, Barnes RP. Childhood bronchial mucoepidermoid tumors: a case report and review of the literature. Cancer 1979;44:315–22.
14. Naunheim KS, Taylor JR, Skoskey C, et al. Adenosquamous lung carcinoma: clinical characteristics, treatment and prognosis. Ann Thorac Surg 1987;44:462–6.
15. Nguyen GK. Cytology of bronchial gland carcinoma. Acta Cytol 1988;32:235–9.
16. Perrone TL, Dickersin GR. Ultrastructure of a bronchial mucoepidermoid carcinoma [Letter]. Hum Pathol 1983;14:1011.
17. Reichle FA, Rosemond GP. Mucoepidermoid tumors of the bronchus. J Thorac Cardiovasc Surg 1966;51:443–8.
18. Seo IS, Warren J, Mirkin LD, Weisman SJ, Grosfeld JL. Mucoepidermoid carcinoma of the bronchus in a 4-year-old child. A high-grade variant with lymph node metastasis. Cancer 1984;53:1600–4.
19. Shanmugaratnam K. Histological typing of tumors of the upper respiratory tract and ear. 2nd ed. International Histological Classification of Tumors. Berlin: World Health Organization, 1991:35–6.
20. Sniffen RC, Soutter L, Robbins LL. Mucoepidermoid tumors of bronchus arising from surface epithelium. Am J Pathol 1958;34:671–83.
21. Spencer H. Bronchial mucous gland tumors. Virchows Arch [A] 1979;383:101–15.
22. Stafford JR, Pollock WJ, Wenzel BC. Oncocytic mucoepidermoid tumor of the bronchus. Cancer 1984;54:94–9.
23. Tao LC, Robertson DI. Cytologic diagnosis of bronchial mucoepidermoid carcinoma by fine needle aspiration biopsy. Acta Cytol 1978;22:221–4.
24. Turnbull AD, Huvos AG, Goodner JT, Foote FW Jr. Mucoepidermoid tumors of bronchial glands. Cancer 1971;28:539–44.
25. Yousem SA, Hochholzer L. Mucoepidermoid tumors of the lung. Cancer 1987;60:1346–52.

Adenoid Cystic Carcinoma

26. Attar S, Miller JE, Hankins J, et al. Bronchial adenoma: a review of 51 patients. Ann Thorac Surg 1985;40:126–32.
27. Cheng J, Saku T, Okabe H, Furthmayr H. Basement membranes in adenoid cystic carcinoma. An immunohistochemical study. Cancer 1992;69:2631–40.
28. Colby TV, Lombard C, Yousem SA, Kitaichi M. Atlas of pulmonary surgical pathology. Philadelphia: WB Saunders, 1992:92.
29. Conlan AA, Payne WS, Woolner LB, Sanderson DR. Adenoid cystic carcinoma (cylindroma) and mucoepidermoid carcinoma of the bronchus. Factors affecting survival. J Thorac Cardiovasc Surg 1978;76:369–77.
30. Dalton ML, Gatling RR. Peripheral adenoid cystic carcinoma of the lung. South Med J 1990;83:577–9.
31. de Lima R. Bronchial adenoma. Clinicopathologic study and results of treatment. Chest 1980;77:81–4.
32. Gallagher CG, Stark R, Teskey J, Kryger M. Atypical manifestation of pulmonary adenoid cystic carcinoma. Br J Dis Chest 1986;80:396–9.
33. Goldstraw P, Lamb D, McCormack RJ, Walbaum PR. The malignancy of bronchial adenoma. J Thorac Cardiovasc Surg 1976;72:309–14.
34. Green LK, Gallion TL, Gyorkey F. Peripheral mucoepidermoid tumour of the lung. Thorax 1991;46:65–6.
35. Heilbrunn A, Crosby JK. Adenocystic carcinoma and mucoepidermoid carcinoma of the tracheobronchial tree. Chest 1972;61:145–9.
36. Inoue H, Iwashita A, Kanegae H, Higuchi K, Fujinaga Y, Matsumoto I. Peripheral pulmonary adenoid cystic carcinoma with substantial extension to the proximal bronchus. Thorax 1991;46:147–8.
37. Ishida T, Yano T, Sugimachi K. Clinical applications of the pathological properties of small cell carcinoma, large cell carcinoma, and acinic cell carcinoma of the lung. Semin Surg Oncol 1990;6:53–63.
38. Lawrence JB, Mazur MT. Adenoid cystic carcinoma: a comparative pathologic study of tumors in salivary gland, breast, lung, and cervix. Hum Pathol 1982;13:916–24.
38a. Moran CA, Suster S, Koss MN. Primary adenoid cystic carcinoma of the lung. A clinicopathologic and immunohistochemical study of 16 cases. Cancer 1994;73:1390–7.
39. Pappo O, Gez E, Craciun I, Zajicek G, Okon E. Growth rate analysis of lung metastases appearing 18 years after resection of cutaneous adenoid cystic carcinoma. Arch Pathol Lab Med 1992;116:76–9.
40. Payne WS, Ellis FH, Woolner LB, Moersch HJ. The surgical treatment of cylindroma (adenoid cystic carcinoma) and mucoepidermoid tumors of the bronchus. J Thorac Cardiovasc Surg 1959;38:709–26.

41. Perzin KH, Gullane P, Clairmont AC. Adenoid cystic carcinomas arising in salivary glands: a correlation of histological features and clinical course. Cancer 1978;42:265–82.

42. Seifert G. Histological typing of salivary gland tumours. International Histological Classification of Tumours. 2nd ed. Berlin: World Health Organization, 1991:21.

43. Spencer H. Bronchial mucous gland tumors. Virchows Arch [A] 1979;383:101–15.

Mucous Gland Adenoma

44. Edwards CW, Matthews HR. Mucous gland adenoma of the bronchus. Thorax 1981;36:147–8.

45. Emory WB, Mitchell WT Jr, Hatch HB Jr. Mucous gland adenoma of the bronchus. Am Rev Respir Dis 1973;108:1407–10.

45a. England DM, Hochholzer L. The truly benign "bronchial adenoma": report of 14 cases of mucous gland adenoma with immunohistochemical and ultrastructural findings. Am J Surg Pathol 1995 (in press).

46. Heard BE, Corrin B, Dewar A. Pathology of seven mucous cell adenomas of the bronchial glands with particular reference to ultrastructure. Histopathology 1985;9:687–701.

47. Spencer H. Bronchial mucous gland tumors. Virchows Arch [A] 1979:383;101–15.

Pleomorphic Adenoma

48. Davis PW, Briggs JC, Seal RM, Storring FK. Benign and malignant mixed tumours of the lung. Thorax 1972;27:657–73.

49. Hayes MM, van der Westhuizen NG, Forgie R. Malignant mixed tumor of the bronchus: a biphasic neoplasm of epithelial and myoepithelial cells. Mod Pathol 1993;6:85–8.

50. Moran CA, Suster S, Askin FB, Koss MN. Benign and malignant salivary gland-type mixed tumors of the lung. Clinicopathologic and immunohistochemical study of eight cases. Cancer 1994;73:2481–90.

51. Mori M, Furuya K, Kimura T, Kitade M, Ueda N. Mixed tumor of salivary gland type arising in the bronchus. Ann Thorac Surg 1991;52:1322–4.

52. Payne WS, Scier J, Woolner LB. Mixed tumors of the bronchus (salivary gland type). J Thorac Cardiovasc Surg 1965;49:663–8.

53. Sakamoto H, Uda H, Tanaka T, Oda T, Morino H, Kikui M. Pleomorphic adenoma in the periphery of the lung. Report of a case and review of the literature. Arch Pathol Lab Med 1991;115:393–6.

54. Seifert G. Histological typing of salivary gland tumours. International Histological Classification of Tumours. 2nd ed. Berlin: World Health Organization, 1991:11.

55. Shanmugaratnam K. Histological typing of tumors of the upper respiratory tract and ear. 2nd ed. International Histological Classification of Tumors. Berlin: World Health Organization, 1991:22.

56. Spencer H. Bronchial mucous gland tumors. Virchows Arch [A] 1979;383:101–15.

57. Wright ES, Pike E, Couves CM. Unusual tumors of the lung. J Surg Oncol 1983;24:23–9.

Acinic Cell Carcinoma

58. Fechner RE, Bentinck BR, Askew JB Jr. Acinic cell tumor of the lung. A histologic and ultrastructural study. Cancer 1972;29:501–8.

59. Gharpure KJ, Deshpande RK, Vishweshvara RN, Raghu CR, Bhargava MK. Acinic cell carcinoma of the bronchus (a case report). Indian J Cancer 1985;22:152–6.

60. Katzenstein AA, Maurer JJ. Benign histiocytic tumor of lung: a light and electron-microscopic study. Am J Surg Pathol 1979;3:61–8.

61. Moran CA, Suster S, Koss MN. Acinic cell carcinoma of the lung ("Fechner tumor"). A clinicopathologic, immunohistochemical, and ultrastructural study of five cases. Am J Surg Pathol 1992;16:1039–50.

62. Shanmugaratnam K. Histological typing of tumors of the upper respiratory tract and ear. 2nd ed. International Histological Classification of Tumors. Berlin: World Health Organization, 1991:35.

63. Yoshida K, Koyama I, Matsui T, Tsukiyama M, Mizushima M. Acinic cell tumor of the bronchial gland. Nippon Geka Gakkai Zasshi 1989;90:1810–3.

Other Rare Salivary Gland Tumors

64. Barnes L, Appel BN, Perez H, El-Attar AM. Myoepitheliomas of the head and neck: case report and review. J Surg Oncol 1985;28:21–8.

65. Cwierzyk TA, Glasberg SS, Virshup MA, Cranmer JC. Pulmonary oncocytoma. Report of a case with cytologic, histologic and electron microscopic study. Acta Cytol 1985;29:620–3.

66. De Jesus MG, Poon T, Chung KY. Pulmonary oncocytoma. NY State J Med 1989;89:477–80.

67. Fechner RE, Bentinck BR. Ultrastructure of bronchial oncocytoma. Cancer 1973;31:1451–7.

68. Fernandez MA, Nyssen J. Oncocytoma of the lung. Can J Surg 1982;25:332–3.

69. Moran CA, Suster S, Askin FB, Koss MN. Benign and malignant salivary gland-type mixed tumors of the lung. Clinicopathologic and immunohistochemical study of eight cases. Cancer 1994;73:2481–90.

70. Santos-Briz A, Terron J, Sastre R, Romero L, Valle A. Oncocytoma of the lung. Cancer 1977;40:1330–6.

71. Scharifker D, Marchevsky A. Oncocytic carcinoid of lung. Cancer 1981;47:530–2.

72. Seifert G. Histological typing of salivary gland tumours. International Histological Classification of Tumours. 2nd ed. Berlin: World Health Organization, 1991:29.

73. Shanmugaratnam K. Histological typing of tumors of the upper respiratory tract and ear. 2nd ed. International Histological Classification of Tumors. Berlin: World Health Organization, 1991:22–3.

74. Sklar JL, Churg A, Bensch KG. Oncocytic carcinoid tumor of the lung. Am J Surg Pathol 1980;4:287–92.

75. Strickler JG, Hegstrom J, Thomas MJ, Yousem SA. Myoepithelioma of the lung. Arch Pathol Lab Med 1987;111:1082–5.

76. Yousem SA. Pulmonary adenosquamous carcinomas with amyloid-like stroma. Mod Pathol 1989;2:420–6.

7

CARCINOMA OF THE LUNG:
OVERVIEW, INCIDENCE, ETIOLOGY, AND SCREENING

OVERVIEW

The common tumors generally included under the heading of carcinoma of the lung are squamous cell carcinoma, adenocarcinoma, small cell carcinoma, and large cell carcinoma. These tumors share many clinical, etiologic, and demographic features. Bronchioloalveolar carcinoma is included as a subset of adenocarcinoma, although it has distinctive features of its own.

The incidence of the major subtypes of lung carcinoma from several large studies is shown in Table 7-1. Most recent series suggest that adenocarcinoma is now more frequent than squamous cell carcinoma (fig. 7-1) (4,12); in fact, adenocarcinoma represented 56 percent of the lung carcinomas seen at Johns Hopkins Hospital from 1984 to 1987 (7). Adenocarcinoma is the most frequent subtype seen in women. A relative decrease in the incidence of squamous cell carcinoma has accompanied the increased incidence of adenocarcinoma from the 1960s through the 1980s (1,3,6, 12,13). Although not as dramatic as the change

Table 7-1

FREQUENCY OF SUBTYPES OF LUNG CARCINOMA

Cell Type	Percent of Cases
A. Series prior to 1985 (21,139 cases)*	
Squamous cell carcinoma	37.7
Adenocarcinoma	24.9
(Bronchioloalveolar carcinoma: 2-2.8%)**	
Small cell carcinoma	18.7
Large cell carcinoma	18.7
B. SEER data 1983-1987 (59,260 cases)†	
Squamous cell carcinoma	30.0
Adenocarcinoma	32.2
(Bronchioloalveolar carcinoma: 0.7%)	
Small cell carcinoma	18.2
Large cell carcinoma	9.7
Other/unspecified	9.9

*From references 3,6,11,13 primarily reflecting data from prior to 1985.
**From references 10,13.
†From reference 12.

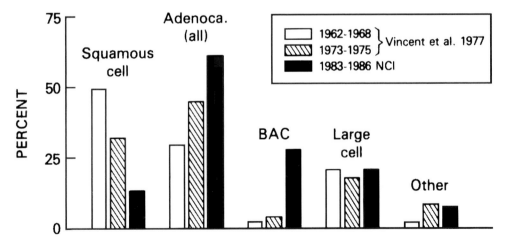

Figure 7-1
INCIDENCE OF LUNG CARCINOMA

The changing incidence of squamous cell carcinoma, adenocarcinoma, bronchioloalveolar carcinoma, and large cell carcinoma is shown for three time periods between 1962 and 1986. The period from 1983 to 1986 is represented by 100 consecutive cases seen by the National Cancer Institute, whereas data for the two earlier periods are from the literature. (Fig. 1 from Gazdar AF, Linnoila RI. The pathology of lung cancer—changing concepts and newer diagnostic techniques. Semin Oncol 1988;15:215–25.)

in the incidence of adenocarcinoma, the incidence of small cell carcinoma has also increased in recent years (12).

A relative decrease in the percent of central tumors compared to peripheral tumors has accompanied the change in histologic subtypes. Auerbach and Garfinkel (1) found a decrease in central tumors from 69.3 to 57.3 percent when comparing tumors seen prior to 1978 to those seen between 1986 and 1989.

The change in incidence in lung carcinoma subtypes may, in part, be related to changing histologic criteria in addition to a real change in incidence (4). Another complicating factor is the histologic heterogeneity of lung carcinomas, discussed in chapter 9.

Multiple separate primary carcinomas of the lung are well recognized; the incidence ranges from 0.2 to 2.0 percent of patients with lung carcinoma (2,9). Synchronous lung carcinomas are seen in about 2 percent of surgical resections (2). Of 50 cases reported by Martini and Melamed (8), 18 were synchronous and 32 were metachronous, with the time to diagnosis of the second tumor varying from 4 months to 16 years. The criteria for the diagnosis of two (or more) separate primary lung carcinomas used by Martini and Melamed are shown in Table 7-2. Squamous cell carcinoma is the most common subtype associated with multiple primary carcinomas of the lung, but many combinations occur (Table 7-3).

While gross and histologic features can be used to recognize synchronous primary lung carcinomas, other techniques may also be useful. Ichinose et al. (5) have shown that DNA flow cytometric patterns can separate synchronous primaries from intrapulmonary metastases.

Table 7-2

CRITERIA FOR DIAGNOSIS OF MULTIPLE PRIMARY LUNG CARCINOMAS*

Metachronous tumors
1. Histologically different**
2. Similar histology, but
   a. free interval between tumors of at least 2 years
   b. origin from carcinoma in situ
   c. second tumor in different lobe, but
      (1) no carcinoma in lymphatics common to both tumors
      (2) no extrapulmonary metastases at time of diagnosis

Synchronous tumors
1. Tumors physically distinct and separate
2. Histology
   a. different**
   b. same, but in different segments if
      (1) origin from carcinoma in situ
      (2) no carcinoma in lymphatics common to both
      (3) no extrapulmonary metastases at time of diagnosis

*Modified from reference 8.
**Adequate sampling mandatory.

Table 7-3

HISTOLOGY OF MULTIPLE PRIMARY LUNG CARCINOMAS*

Cell Type		Synchronous	Metachronous	Total
Tumor #1	Tumor #2			
Squamous	Squamous	31	59	90
Squamous	Adenocarcinoma	21	10	31
Squamous	Small cell	22	13	35
Squamous	Large cell**	5	6	11
Adenocarcinoma	Adenocarcinoma	4	9	13
Adenocarcinoma	Small cell	5	1	6
Adenocarcinoma	Large cell**	1	2	3
Small cell	Large cell**	1	0	1
Large cell**	Large cell**	4	1	5
		94	101	195

*Modified from reference 8 (195 cases).
**Includes some unspecified "anaplastic carcinomas."

INCIDENCE

Data from the American Cancer Society show that in 1989 carcinoma of the lung was the most common cause of cancer death in both men (34.1 percent) and women (19.9 percent) (14). It was estimated that 170,000 new cases of lung carcinoma would occur in the United States in 1993. Based on data from the United States for the year 1989, 23.1 percent of all deaths were due to cancer, and 27.6 percent of the cancer deaths were due to carcinoma of the lung. Thus, approximately 6.4 percent of all deaths in the United States in 1989 were due to carcinoma of the lung. The age-adjusted cancer death rate for 1989 was close to 30 per 100,000 for women and 75 per 100,000 for men.

Death rates from lung carcinoma have risen steadily in both men and women since 1930, with the rise occurring earlier and being steeper in men. However, since 1970 there has been a sharp increase in the death rate in women (14). Evidence suggests that the rate may be leveling off or decreasing in men as a result of public health efforts to curb cigarette smoking (15).

ETIOLOGY AND PATHOGENESIS

Cigarette smoking is the major cause of lung carcinoma in the United States and around the world (38). The lung carcinoma rate parallels smoking prevalence. There is a dose-response association between the number of cigarettes smoked and the risk of carcinoma of the lung, although changes in the composition of cigarettes and the introduction of filter tips in the 1950s and 1960s have lowered the risk of lung carcinoma 20 to 50 percent compared to earlier "high yield" cigarettes (30). The risk of lung carcinoma is also increased in individuals who are pipe or cigar smokers. The increased risk in smokers is seen for all types of lung carcinoma and decreases exponentially over time after cessation of cigarette smoking (38).

There are some variations in the histologic subtypes among smokers and nonsmokers (Table 7-4), with squamous cell carcinoma and small cell carcinoma showing the highest association with smoking. It is possible that the recent decrease in the frequency of squamous cell carcinoma is in part attributable to changing smoking habits (1).

Table 7-4

HISTOLOGIC SUBTYPES OF CARCINOMA IN SMOKERS AND NONSMOKERS*

Histologic Subtype	Smokers** (percent)	Non-smokers† (percent)
Squamous cell carcinoma	98.0	2.0
Adenocarcinoma	81.6	18.4
Bronchioloalveolar carcinoma	70.6	29.4
Small cell carcinoma	98.9	1.1
Large cell carcinoma	93.3	6.7

*Modified from reference 9.
**No. = 2708.
†No. = 218.

Some 80 percent of lung cancer deaths in men and 75 percent of lung cancer deaths in women can be attributed to cigarette smoking (38,45). In addition, it has been estimated that up to 25 percent of cases of carcinoma of the lung occurring in nonsmokers are the result of passive exposure to cigarette smoke (38), but this is controversial. In one study, 17 percent of the cases of lung carcinoma in nonsmokers were ascribed to childhood or adolescent exposure to cigarette smoke (31).

Asbestos is thought to be responsible for 4,000 to 6,000 deaths per year from carcinoma of the lung, less than 5 percent of all lung carcinoma deaths (38). A strong dose-response effect has been shown between asbestos exposure and the development of lung carcinoma; all histologic subtypes can be seen. There is a synergistic and multiplicative effect of smoking and asbestos exposure, with a 50-fold increased risk in the development of lung carcinoma (25). Although there is considerable debate, several studies suggest that the increased risk of lung carcinoma from asbestos exposure is only seen in those individuals with concomitant asbestosis (50).

Radiation is known to cause lung carcinoma (38). The association has been most extensively studied in uranium miners exposed to radon daughters. All types of lung carcinoma are seen, and a dose effect has been shown. An increased incidence of lung carcinoma has also been found in atom bomb survivors (35). Recently, considerable

Table 7-5

AGENTS OR EXPOSURES WITH PROVEN, PUTATIVE, OR POSSIBLE ASSOCIATION WITH LUNG CARCINOMA*

Ionizing radiation	Tobacco smoke
Asbestos	Shipyard workers
Chloromethyl ether	Truck drivers
Cadmium	Plumbers
Arsenic	Rubber workers
Chromate	Coke oven workers
Hexavalent chromium	Petroleum workers
Formaldehyde	Mustard gas workers
Terpenes	Coal tar workers
Vinyl chloride	Roofers
Soots and tars	Pottery workers
Nickel	Printers
Isopropyl oils	Female cosmetologists
Antimony	Leather industry workers
Beryllium	Building laborers
Cobalt	Construction workers
Iron and iron oxides	Cooks, bakers, and pastry cooks
N-nitrosamines	Asbestos insulation workers
Polycyclic aromatic hydrocarbons	Uranium miners
Fibrous zeolites	
Manmade mineral fibers	Other factors:
Fiberglass	Lung scarring
Glass wool	Alveolar epithelial hyperplasia/
Rock wool	bronchioloalveolar cell adenoma
Ceramics	Previous bronchogenic carcinoma
Alumina	Hereditary carcinomas (chapter 3)
Lead	

*From references 17,25,28,35,38,39,42,43.

interest has centered on nonoccupational exposure to radon daughters in houses. Some studies have suggested that 5 to 15 percent of lung carcinomas are due to nonoccupational radon daughter exposure and that these cases account for 25 percent of the lung carcinomas occurring in nonsmokers and for 5 percent of the carcinomas in smokers (38). These figures have not been universally accepted (21), and further confirmatory studies are needed.

There has been some evidence that diet may have an impact on the risk of carcinoma of the lung. In a review by Colditz et al. (26), it was concluded that vitamin C might offer slight protection from lung carcinoma, but there was little evidence that vitamin C or vitamin E had any major influence. Data on a protective effect from selenium was limited but thought to warrant further study.

There are a number of other potential or proven agents or exposures associated with an increased risk of lung carcinoma, as shown in Table 7-5. In some instances, an occupation is associated with an increased incidence of carcinoma of the lung, but the specific causative agent or agents have not been identified. Some of the exposures listed in Table 7-5 are controversial and not universally accepted as proven or putative causes of lung carcinoma.

The concept of *scar carcinoma*, namely carcinoma of the lung arising in the vicinity of fibrosis (fig. 7-2), has been accepted for decades since first being studied in 1930s (17,36). In early studies, most of the scars were attributed to old tuberculosis; however, infarcts, pneumoconioses, and other chronic inflammatory scarring of the lung have all been implicated in individual

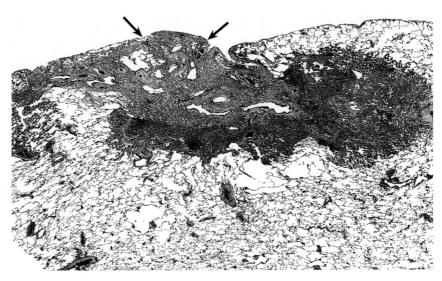

Figure 7-2
SCAR CANCER

Small peripheral adenocarcinoma, bronchioloalveolar type, arising in association with a scar. There is a scar associated with some pleural puckering (arrows) around and from which the darker-appearing neoplasm extends. The surrounding lung tissue shows no significant fibrosis and only slight emphysema. In the majority of such cases, including this, the scar is probably the result of, rather than a precursor to, the carcinoma.

cases. In some studies, nearly half of all peripheral lung carcinomas were associated with a scar (36). The concept of scar carcinoma suggests that progressively atypical epithelial changes develop in the vicinity of the scar and ultimately lead to the development of a carcinoma. Meyer and Liebow (36) and subsequently others (27,51) described lung carcinomas arising in association with diffuse interstitial fibrosis and drew an analogy with carcinomas associated with focal scarring.

Tumors that have been labeled scar carcinomas are typically subpleural adenocarcinomas associated with retraction or puckering of the overlying pleura (17,22). Cut sections grossly show a central sclerotic zone ("scar") which may have anthracotic pigment and necrosis. Larger tumors (greater than 3 cm) tend to have more extensive scarring (22). In 1980, Shimosato (49) and subsequently others (22,32–34) suggested that the fibrosis in most scar carcinomas is a secondary phenomenon rather than a precursor to the carcinoma. Studies showed that the scar had abundant type III collagen and an extracellular matrix, suggesting an ongoing fibrosing process supporting a host response to the neoplasm (19,34), i.e., these tumors were desmoplastic carcinomas rather than carcinomas arising in scars.

Nevertheless, there are well-documented cases (52) showing carcinomas arising adjacent to old granulomas (fig. 7-3). It seems likely, however, that most scars are a secondary reaction rather than a preexisting lesion. This phenomenon is easily appreciated in sclerosing bronchioloalveolar carcinomas (chapter 13) in which only the alveolar walls involved by carcinoma are inflamed, thickened, and fibrosed.

While the pathogenesis of many scar carcinomas has been questioned, the concept of *atypical type 2 cell hyperplasia (atypical adenomatous hyperplasia)* as a precursor of adenocarcinoma has been reemphasized in several recent studies (23,40,41). Nakanishi (40) studied 15 cases of alveolar epithelial hyperplasia coexistent with lung carcinoma in a series of 70 patients. A histogenetic relationship between atypical alveolar epithelial hyperplasia (fig. 7-4) and pulmonary adenocarcinoma was suggested. Nakayama et al. (41) showed that atypical adenomatous hyperplasia (probably synonymous with *atypical alveolar epithelial hyperplasia*) was a clonal cellular proliferation closely related to well-differentiated adenocarcinoma.

In a series of 247 consecutive resections for carcinoma of the lung, Miller (37) found 23 (9.3

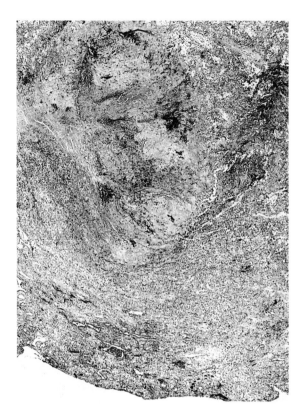
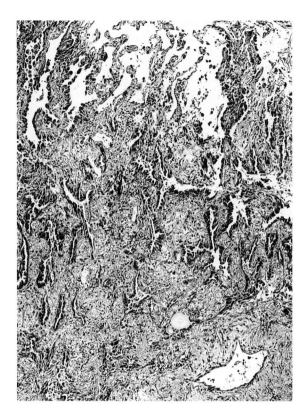

Figure 7-3
SCAR CANCER

Adenocarcinoma arising in association with a scar. These sections are from a physician's wife who had been followed for several decades with a stable lesion on her chest radiograph following a documented bout of tuberculosis. When the radiographic lesion started to enlarge, it was resected. Evidence of old healed granulomatous disease with increased anthracotic pigmentation can be seen at the left; in the surrounding fibrotic tissue, there is a proliferation of atypical epithelium (lower left and right) which was continuous with an obvious bronchioloalveolar carcinoma extending from the edge of the fibrotic region. This case probably represents a bona fide scar carcinoma.

percent) with incidental 1- to 7-mm nodules separate from the main tumor mass. These nodules were composed of localized proliferations of type 2 cells and were termed *bronchioloalveolar cell adenomas* (chapter 13). Miller concluded that these adenomas might be an early or premalignant phase of glandular neoplasia with the potential for progression to carcinoma. She also suggested that the finding might explain some examples of multicentricity among lung carcinomas. In individual cases, atypical type 2 cell hyperplasia and bronchioloalveolar cell adenoma may be difficult to distinguish and part of a disease spectrum.

Patients with a history of a resected lung carcinoma have an appreciable risk of a second lung carcinoma. The risk is in the range of 2 percent per year for patients with long-term survival (over 5 years) (44). Long-term survivors of small cell carcinoma have a particularly high risk, estimated at 5.6 percent per person year (29).

Bejui-Thivolet et al. (20) have used in situ hybridization to show the presence of human papilloma virus (HPV) DNA in well-differentiated squamous cell carcinomas of the lung. They studied 33 carcinomas and 10 bronchial squamous metaplasias with probes for HPV subtypes 6, 11, 16, and 18. Of the 43 cases studied, 7 showed the presence of HPV DNA, including 1 case of squamous cell metaplasia and 6 cases of squamous cell carcinoma. Fourteen of the 43 lesions studied showed condylomatous changes, and 6 of the 7 cases in which HPV was detected by in situ hybridization came from among these cases. The authors suggested that HPV infection might be potentially oncogenic in the lung as it

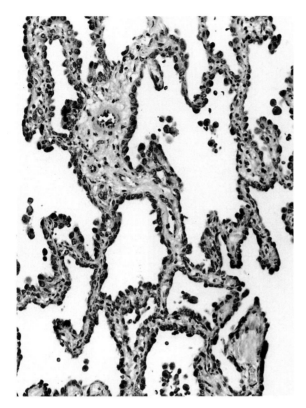

Figure 7-4
ATYPICAL ADENOMATOUS HYPERPLASIA
There is a relatively uniform proliferation of low cuboidal cells lining alveolar walls. Obvious cytologic features of malignancy are not present. Such atypical adenomatous hyperplasia is thought by some to represent a precursor to the development of adenocarcinoma of the lung, and such proliferations are relatively common in lungs resected for bronchioloalveolar carcinoma, as was this case.

is in the genital tract, but that its exact role needs to be clarified.

The morphogenesis of squamous cell carcinoma has been studied for several decades and is illustrated cytologically in figures 7-5 and 7-6. Since cigarette smoking increases squamous metaplasia (46), most studies have used serial sputum cytology specimens from cigarette smokers (16,18) or uranium miners. There is loss of normal ciliated lining cells with basal cell hyperplasia, low columnar nonciliated epithelium or squamous metaplasia, and increasing degrees of atypical squamous metaplasia (dysplasia), ultimately followed by squamous cell carcinoma in situ (CIS) and invasive squamous carcinoma. Not all cases of CIS of the bronchial tree are progressive, and some cases regress (24).

In practice, CIS is not found in all patients with squamous cell carcinoma and rarely in other histologic subtypes of lung carcinoma. In meticulous studies of serial sections of the bronchial tree taken at autopsy, Auerbach (18) found CIS in 26 of 34 patients with carcinoma of the lung. It is much less frequently seen in surgical specimens, as shown in the data of Rilke et al. (47): CIS at the bronchial margin was seen in only 3 of 67 cases (4.5 percent).

The molecular biology of carcinogenesis in the lung is discussed in chapter 3.

SCREENING FOR CARCINOMA OF THE LUNG

In 1971, the National Cancer Institute organized the Cooperative Early Lung Cancer Group to develop a screening program for the early detection of lung cancer in high-risk patients (male smokers) (53–59). Over 30,000 men older than 45 years of age enrolled in the study; at the time of entry into the study, none were suspected of having a lung carcinoma. Sputum cytologic examinations, chest radiographic examination, or both, along with a medical questionnaire were the screening tests used.

At the initial screening, a number of unsuspected lung carcinomas were identified, and these comprised the prevalence cancers in the study. The proportion of cases in each histologic subtype was roughly similar to that for all cases of lung carcinoma. Fifty-nine percent of the tumors were resectable, a figure more than double that seen in routine practice.

The carcinomas that were detected during the study period represented the incidence cancers. A number of both the prevalence cancers and the incidence cancers represented early or occult lung carcinomas, which are described and illustrated in chapter 10.

The study showed that with screening there was increased cancer detection, resectability, and survival. Regarding the incidence cancers: less than half were actually detected by the screening studies despite rescreening every 4 months; cancers detected on the basis of clinical symptoms were rarely resectable; and the proportion that could be completely resected was 46 percent for the screened group and 32 percent for the control group (58).

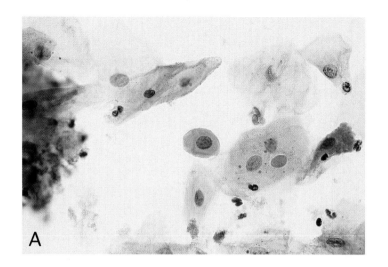

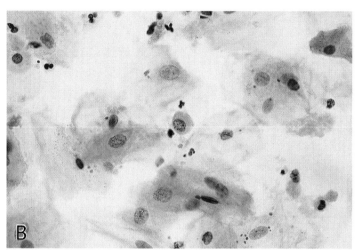

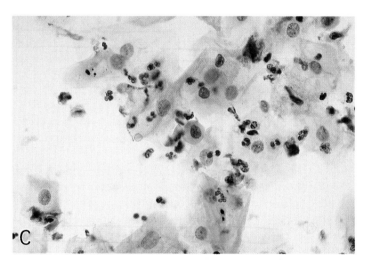

Figure 7-5
MORPHOGENESIS OF CARCINOMA OF THE LUNG
Mild (A–C), moderate (D–F), and severe (G–I) squamous atypia (dysplasia) developing in uranium miners followed with sputum cytology examinations. (Courtesy of Drs. G. Saccomanno and M. Turner, Grand Junction, CO.)

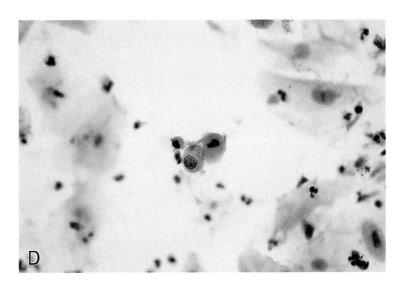

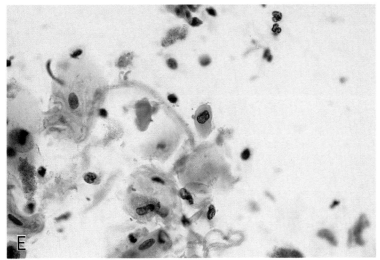

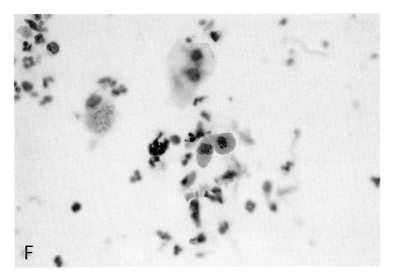

Figure 7-5 (Continued)

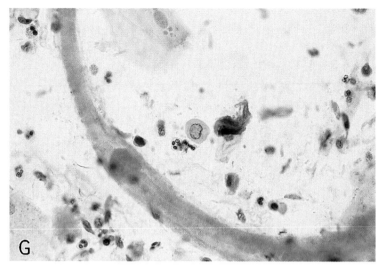

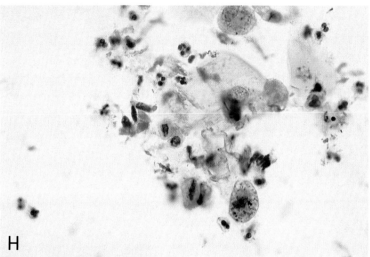

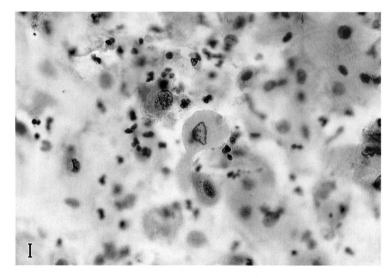

Figure 7-5 (Continued)

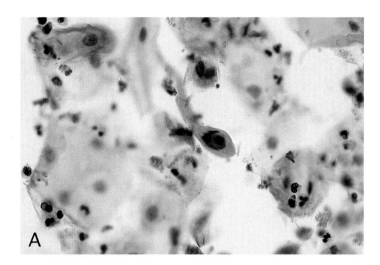

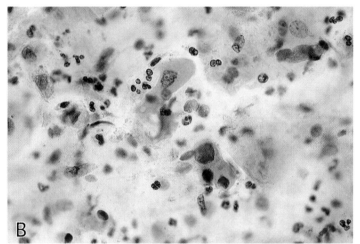

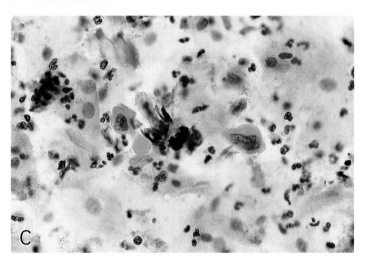

Figure 7-6
MORPHOGENESIS OF BRONCHOGENIC CARCINOMA
Even though degrees of squamous atypia (dysplasia) may progress to squamous cell carcinoma (A–C), squamous atypia may also precede small cell carcinoma (D–F) or adenocarcinoma (G–I) in uranium miners. (Courtesy of Drs. G. Saccomanno and M. Turner, Grand Junction, CO.)

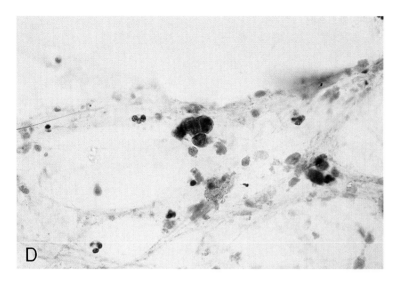

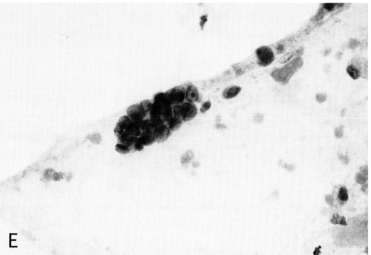

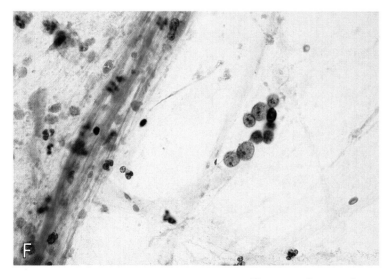

Figure 7-6 (Continued)

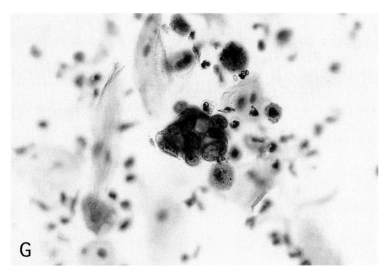

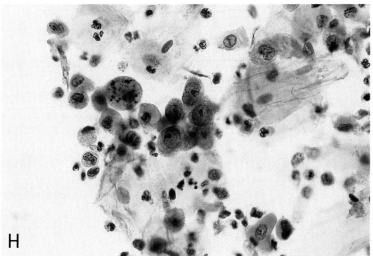

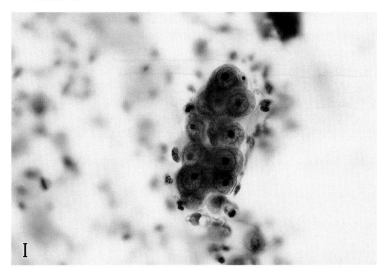

Figure 7-6 (Continued

Table 7-6

**DETECTION OF LUNG CARCINOMA
BY SCREENING METHODS***

| | % Detected By: | | |
	X Ray Only	Cytology Only	X Ray & Cytology
Squamous cell (no. = 81)	38	43	19
Adenocarcinoma (no. = 43)	81	0	19
Small cell (no. = 15)	73	0	27
Large cell (no. = 20)	75	10	15

*From reference 54.

The screening methods showed considerable variability in effectiveness for identifying histologic subtypes of lung carcinoma (Table 7-6). Over 60 percent of the squamous cell carcinomas had a positive cytology, and in data not shown, it was found that 95 percent of all cancers detected by cytology alone were squamous cell carcinomas (54). For the other histologic subtypes, the chest radiograph was the primary means of detection.

The 5-year survival data from the Mayo Lung Project revealed the following (56): cases identified cytologically, about 80 percent; cases identified roentgenographically, about 35 percent; symptomatic cases, about 10 percent; every 4-month screened group, about 35 percent; and control group, less than 15 percent.

Despite these findings, there was no statistically significant difference in the mortality rate for lung carcinoma between the study groups and the control groups, either in the Mayo Lung Project or in the other two institutions taking part in the study (56). For the Mayo Lung Project there were 122 lung cancer deaths in the study group (3.2 per 1000 man years) and 115 lung cancer deaths in the control group (3.0 per 1000 man years). Although tumors were detected in the study group and overall there was a better 5-year survival, the fact that the mortality rates were similar between the study group and the control group suggests that some of the tumors identified in the study group may have been relatively indolent and slower growing and might not have manifested for a number of years or been fatal. It is possible that these tumors had inherent biologic differences from the more highly aggressive tumors that accounted for the mortality in both groups and characterize most lung carcinomas.

Other general conclusions from the Cooperative Early Lung Cancer Group study were (54): 1) the chest roentgenogram is the most sensitive method available for detecting lung carcinoma, and 2) sputum cytology is the most effective method for detecting early squamous cell carcinoma of the lung.

These studies suggest that mass screening does not have a significant impact on mortality, and thus question the usefulness of mass screening for carcinoma of the lung. This conclusion has recently been challenged by Strauss et al. (61) who concluded, after reworking the original data, that there was insufficient evidence to firmly recommend against lung cancer screening.

While mass screening may not have a significant impact on mortality, screening of select populations may yet prove to be of value. Saccomanno et al. (60) described the results of periodic cytologic examinations of sputum in a group of uranium miners, a subset now known to be at high risk for the development of lung carcinoma. In this group, abnormalities progressed in degree over time and changes were readily detectable in sputum cytology specimens (figs. 7-5, 7-6); there was an average of 4 to 5 years during which individuals would exfoliate abnormal cells prior to the development of an invasive carcinoma. The authors concluded that this 4- to 5-year period represented a window of opportunity for early detection and treatment.

REFERENCES

Overview

1. Auerbach O, Garfinkel L. The changing pattern of lung carcinoma. Cancer 1991;68:1973–7.
2. Carey FA, Donnelly SC, Walker WS, Cameron EW, Lamb D. Synchronous primary lung cancers: prevalence in surgical material and clinical implications. Thorax 1993;48:344–6.
3. el-Torky M, el-Zeky F, Hall JC. Significant changes in the distribution of histologic types of lung cancer. A review of 4928 cases. Cancer 1990;65:2361–7.
4. Gazdar AF, Linnoila RI. The pathology of lung cancer—changing concepts and newer diagnostic techniques. Semin Oncol 1988;15:215–25.
5. Ichinose Y, Hara N, Ohta M. Synchronous lung cancers defined by deoxyribonucleic acid flow cytometry. J Thorac Cardiovasc Surg 1991;102:418–24.
6. Johnston WW. Histologic and cytologic patterns of lung cancer in 2580 men and women over a 15-year period. Acta Cytol 1988;32:163–8.
7. Linnoila I. Pathology of non-small cell lung cancer. New diagnostic approaches. Hematol Oncol Clin North Am 1990;4:1027–51.
8. Martini N, Melamed MR. Multiple primary lung cancers. J Thorac Cardiovasc Surg 1975;70:606–12.
9. Rohwedder JJ, Weatherbee L. Multiple primary bronchogenic carcinoma with a review of the literature. Am Rev Respir Dis 1974;109:435–45.
10. Rosenow EC, Carr DT. Bronchogenic carcinoma. Cancer J Clin 1979;29:233–45.
11. Teeter SM, Holmes FF, McFarlane MJ. Lung carcinoma in the elderly population. Influence of histology on the inverse relationship of stage to age. Cancer 1987;60:1331–6.
12. Travis WD, Travis LB, Percy C, Devesa SS. Lung cancer incidence and survival by histologic type. Cancer. In press.
13. Vincent RG, Pickren JW, Lane WW, et al. The changing histopathology of lung cancer: a review of 1682 cases. Cancer 1977;39:1647–55.

Incidence

14. Boring CC, Squires TS, Tong T. Cancer statistics, 1993. CA Cancer J Clin 1993;43:7–26.
15. Garfinkel L, Silverberg E. Lung cancer and smoking trends in the United States over the past 25 years. CA Cancer J Clin 1991;41:137–45.

Etiology

17. Auerbach O, Garfinkel L, Parks VR. Histologic type of lung cancer in relation to smoking habits, year of diagnosis, and sites of metastases. Chest 1975;67:382–7.
18. _____, Garfinkel L, Parks VR. Scar cancer of the lung: increase over a 21-year period. Cancer 1979;43:636–42.
16. _____, Gere JB, Forman JB, et al. Changes in the bronchial epithelium in relation to smoking and cancer of the lung. N Engl J Med 1957;256:97–104.
19. Barsky SH, Huang SJ, Bhuta S. The extracellular matrix of pulmonary scar carcinomas is suggestive of a desmoplastic origin. Am J Pathol 1986;124:412–9.
20. Bejui-Thivolet F, Liagre N, Chignol MC, Chardonnet Y, Patricot LM. Detection of human papilloma virus DNA in squamous bronchial metaplasia and squamous cell carcinomas of the lung by in situ hybridization using biotinylated probes in paraffin-embedded specimens. Hum Pathol 1990;12:111–6.
21. Bowie C, Bowie SH. Radon and health. Lancet 1991;337:409–13.
22. Cagle PT, Cohle SD, Greenberg SD. Natural history of pulmonary scar cancers. Clinical and pathologic implications. Cancer 1985;56:2031–5.
23. Carey FA, Wallace WA, Fergusson RJ, Kerr KM, Lamb D. Alveolar atypical adenomatous hyperplasia in association with primary pulmonary adenocarcinoma: a clinicopathologic study of ten cases. Thorax 1992;47:1041–3.
24. Carter D. Squamous cell carcinoma of the lung: an update. Semin Diagn Pathol 1985;2:226–34.
25. Churg A, Greene FH. Pathology of occupational lung disease. New York: Igaku-Shoin, 1988:50.
26. Colditz GA, Stampfer MJ, Willett WC. Diet and lung cancer. A review of the epidemiologic evidence in humans. Arch Intern Med 1987;147:157–60.
27. Fraire AE, Greenberg SD. Carcinoma and diffuse interstitial fibrosis of lung. Cancer 1973;31:1078–86.
28. Frank AL. The epidemiology and etiology of lung cancer. Clin Chest Med 1982;3:219–28.
29. Heyne KH, Lippman SM, Lee JJ, Lee JS, Hong WK. The incidence of second primary tumors in long-term survivors of small-cell lung cancer. J Clin Oncol 1992;10:1519–24.
30. Hoffmann D, Hoffmann I, Wynder EL. Lung cancer and the changing cigarette. IARC Sci Publ 1991;105:449–59.
31. Janerich DT, Thompson WD, Varela LR, et al. Lung cancer and exposure to tobacco smoke in the household. N Engl J Med 1990;323:632–6.
32. Kolin A, Koutoulakis T. Role of arterial occlusion in pulmonary scar cancers. Hum Pathol 1988;19:1161–7.
33. Kung IT, Lui IO, Loke SL, et al. Pulmonary scar cancer. The pathologic reappraisal. Am J Surg Pathol 1985;9:391–400.
34. Madri JA, Carter D. Scar cancers of the lung: origin and significance. Hum Pathol 1984;15:625–31.
35. Marchevsky AM. Pathogenesis and experimental models of lung cancer. Lung Biol Health Dis 1990;44:7–27.
36. Meyer EC, Liebow AA. Relationship of interstitial pneumonia honeycombing and atypical epithelial proliferation to cancer of the lung. Cancer 1965;18:322–51.
37. Miller RR. Bronchioloalveolar cell adenomas. Am J Surg Pathol 1990;14:904–12.
38. Minna JD, Pass H, Glatstein E, Ihde DC. Cancer of the lung. In: DeVita VT, Hellman S, Rosenberg SA, eds. Cancer: principles and practice of oncology. Philadelphia: JB Lippincott, 1988:591–705.
39. Mohsenifar Z. Epidemiology of lung cancer. Lung Biol Health Dis 1990;44:1–5.

40. Nakanishi K. Alveolar epithelial hyperplasia and adenocarcinoma of the lung. Arch Pathol Lab Med 1990;114:363–8.

41. Nakayama H, Noguchi M, Tsuchiya R, Kodama T, Shimosato Y. Clonal growth of atypical adenomatous hyperplasia of the lung: cytofluorometric analysis of nuclear DNA content. Mod Pathol 1990;3:314–20.

42. Nemery B. Metal toxicity in the respiratory tract. Eur Respir J 1990;3:202–19.

43. Owens AH, Abeloff MD. Neoplasms of the lung. In: Calabresi P, Schein PS, Rosenberg SA, eds. Medical oncology: basic principles and clinical management of cancer. New York: MacMillan, 1985:715–57.

44. Pairolero PC, Williams DE, Bergstralh EJ, Piehler JM, Bernatz PE, Payne WS. Postsurgical stage I bronchogenic carcinoma: morbid implications of recurrent disease. Ann Thorac Surg 1984;38:331–8.

45. Parkin DM, Sasco AJ. Lung cancer: worldwide variation in occurrence and proportion attributable to tobacco use. Lung Cancer (Elsevier) 1993;9:1–16.

46. Peters EJ, Morice R, Benner SE, et al. Squamous metaplasia of the bronchial mucosa and its relationship to smoking. Chest 1993;103:1429–32.

47. Rilke F, Carbone A, Clemente C, Pilotti S. Surgical pathology of resectable lung cancer. In: Muggia F, Rozencweig M, eds. Lung cancer: progress in therapeutic research. New York: Raven Press, 1979:129–42.

48. Saccomanno G, Archer VE, Auerbach O, Saunders RP, Brennan LM. Development of carcinoma of the lung as reflected in exfoliated cells. Cancer 1974;33:256–70.

49. Shimosato Y, Suzuki A, Hashimoto T, et al. Prognostic implications of fibrotic focus (scar) in small peripheral lung cancers. Am J Surg Pathol 1980;4:365–73.

50. Sluis-Cremer GK, Bezuidenhout BN. Relation between asbestosis and bronchial cancer in amphibole asbestos miners. Br J Ind Med 1989;46:537–40.

51. Turner-Warwick M, Lebowitz M, Burrows B, Johnson A. Cryptogenic fibrosing alveolitis and lung cancer. Thorax 1980;35:496–9.

52. Yoneda K. Scar carcinomas of the lung in a histoplasmosis endemic area. Cancer 1990;65:164–8.

Screening

53. Berlin NI, Buncher CR, Fontana RS, Frost JK, Melamed MR. The National Cancer Institute Cooperative Early Lung Cancer Detection Program. Results of the initial screen (prevalence). Early lung cancer detection: introduction. Am Rev Respir Dis 1984;130:545–9.

54. Early lung cancer detection: summary and conclusions. Am Rev Respir Dis 1984;130:565–70.

55. Flehinger BJ, Melamed MR, Zaman MB, Heelan RT, Perchick WB, Martini N. Early lung cancer detection: results of the initial (prevalence) radiologic and cytologic screening in the Memorial Sloan-Kettering study. Am Rev Respir Dis 1984;130:555–60.

56. Fontana RS. Screening for lung cancer. Recent experience in the United States. In: Hansen HH, ed. Lung cancer: basic and clinical aspects. Boston: Martinus Nijhoff, 1986:91–111.

57. _____, Sanderson DR, Taylor WF, et al. Early lung cancer detection. Results of the initial (prevalence) radiologic and cytologic screening in the Mayo Clinic study. Am Rev Respir Dis 1984;130:561–5.

58. _____, Sanderson DR, Woolner LB, et al. Screening for lung cancer. A critique of the Mayo Lung Project. Cancer 1991;67:1155–64.

59. Frost JK, Ball WC Jr, Levin ML, et al. Early lung cancer detection: results of the initial (prevalence) radiologic and cytologic screening the Johns Hopkins study. Am Rev Respir Dis 1984;130:549–54.

60. Saccomanno G, Archer VE, Auerbach O, Saunders RP, Brennan LM. Development of carcinoma of the lung as reflected in exfoliated cells. Cancer 1974;33:256–70.

61. Strauss GM, Gleason RE, Sugarbaker DJ. Screening for lung cancer re-examined. A reinterpretation of the Mayo Lung Project randomized trial on lung cancer screening. Chest 1993;103:337S–41S.

◇◇◇

8
CARCINOMA OF THE LUNG: CLINICAL AND RADIOGRAPHIC ASPECTS, SPREAD, STAGING, MANAGEMENT, AND PROGNOSIS

DEMOGRAPHICS

Carcinoma of the lung primarily affects adults over the age of 45. The number of men affected exceeds that of women, although the sex difference is decreasing. Estimated new cancer cases for 1993 predict that only 58.8 percent of new cases will occur in men, and 41.2 percent will occur in women, reflecting the dramatic increase in lung carcinoma among women in the past two decades (1).

Most patients with carcinoma of the lung are between 50 and 80 years of age. Figure 8-1 shows the age-specific rate by histologic subtype from the SEER data for 1978 to 1986 (74). Patients under 40 years of age are rare: 2.3 percent in one series (5). Eight percent of cases occur after 80 years of age (25). There is some evidence that the incidence of squamous cell carcinoma increases with age while that of adenocarcinoma and small cell carcinoma decreases (25). Increasing age may also correlate with a greater likelihood of low-stage disease, especially among men (25).

SIGNS AND SYMPTOMS

The signs and symptoms associated with lung carcinoma may be related to the direct or indirect effects of the tumor. Most patients (over 80 percent) are symptomatic (3); the clinical manifestations

AGE SPECIFIC RATE BY HISTOLOGIC TYPE (1983-1987)

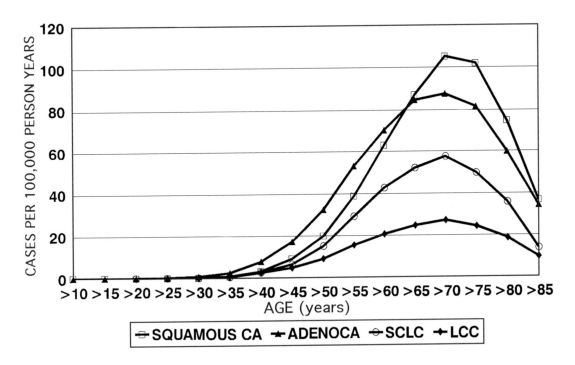

Figure 8-1
AGE-SPECIFIC RATE OF LUNG CANCER
The age-specific rate of lung cancer by histologic type is shown from the SEER data for 1983-1987 (74).

Table 8-1

CAUSES OF CLINICAL MANIFESTATIONS OF LUNG CARCINOMAS*

Tumor	Effects of Primary Tumor	Intrathoracic Spread	Distant Metastases	Paraneo-plastic Syndromes	Endocrine Syndromes
Squamous cell carcinoma	>50%	10-25%	<10%	10-25%	<10%
Adenocarcinoma	10-25%	<10%	10-25%	10-25%	<10%
Small cell carcinoma	>50%	up to 50%	up to 50%	10-25%	10-25%
Large cell carcinoma	up to 50%	10-25%	10-25%	10-25%	<10%

*Modified from reference 4.

vary with the histologic subtype (Table 8-1). Squamous cell carcinoma tends to be associated with direct tumor effects while small cell carcinoma is the subtype most often associated with secondary endocrine and paraneoplastic syndromes.

Table 8-2 is a compilation of signs and symptoms associated with lung carcinoma. In one series, the symptoms in decreasing order of incidence were: cough (64 percent), weight loss (53 percent), pain (53 percent), increased sputum production (45 percent), hemoptysis (28 percent), malaise (27 percent), fever (21 percent), and neuromyopathy (10 percent)(5). Twelve percent of the patients in that series were asymptomatic. In another series, 27 percent of the patients presented with symptoms from the primary tumor; 32 percent with symptoms from metastatic disease; and 34 percent with systemic complaints, particularly anorexia, weight loss, and fatigue (17). Only 6 percent of the patients were asymptomatic.

As shown in Table 8-1, only a minority of patients with lung carcinoma actually have an identifiable endocrine syndrome, even though a large number of different syndromes are associated with lung carcinoma (Table 8-2). Most endocrine syndromes are found in patients with small cell carcinoma; the syndrome of inappropriate antidiuretic hormone (ADH) secretion (SIADH) is one of the best known, but Cushing syndrome and somatostatinoma syndrome are also recognized. Hyperparathyroidism due to secretion of a parathormone-like substance is an exception, since it is most common in patients with squamous cell carcinoma (17,22).

In some cases, the identification of a serum marker correlates with the clinically recognized endocrine or paraneoplastic syndrome, but there are many more serum markers associated with lung carcinoma than there are syndromes ascribed to them (Table 8-3). One can expect the number of serum markers associated with lung carcinoma to increase along with the sensitivity of the techniques identifying them. In general, serum levels of tumor markers are higher in disseminated disease; the levels may decrease with therapy-induced remission, although there are many exceptions (10,22).

Peptide hormones can be demonstrated in the tumor cells by immunoperoxidase techniques and the results of Gropp (9) are shown in Table 8-4. This is a rapidly evolving area, and these data will undoubtedly be updated.

Neuromyopathies are the most frequent paraneoplastic syndromes associated with lung carcinoma. They most commonly are associated with small cell carcinoma (56 percent) followed by squamous cell carcinoma (22 percent), large cell carcinoma (16 percent), and adenocarcinoma (5 percent) (22).

One of the most distinctive paraneoplastic syndromes is the Lambert-Eaton syndrome, a myasthenic syndrome associated with small cell carcinoma. Studies have shown the presence of anticalcium channel antibodies in the serum of many patients with small cell carcinoma and antibodies may be found in patients with small cell carcinoma who do not have the syndrome (21). Serum antineuronal nuclear antibodies are found with peripheral neuropathies and encephalomyeloradiculopathies associated with small cell carcinoma (12).

Table 8-2

SIGNS AND SYMPTOMS OF LUNG CARCINOMA*

None: Clinically occult (5-20% of cases)
General/systemic: Weakness, anorexia, cachexia, malaise, fever, orthostatic hypotension
Local/direct effects (from endobronchial growth and/or invasion of adjacent structures including chest wall and
    vertebral column):
    Cough, dyspnea, wheeze, stridor, hemoptysis
    Chest pain/back pain
    Obstructive pneumonia (+/- cavitation)
    Pleural effusion
Extension to mediastinal structures:
    Nerve entrapment syndromes: recurrent laryngeal nerve (hoarseness), phrenic nerve (diaphragmatic
        paralysis), sympathetic system (Horner syndrome), brachial plexus (brachial plexopathy from "superior
        sulcus" tumors)
    Vena cava obstruction: superior vena cava syndrome
    Pericardium: effusion, tamponade
    Myocardium: arrythmia, heart failure
    Esophagus: dysphagia, bronchoesophageal fistula
    Mediastinal lymph nodes: pleural effusion
Metastatic disease: Direct effects related to the organ(s) involved (for example, seizures, abnormal
    liver function tests)
Paraneoplastic syndromes:
    Acanthosis nigricans
    Dermatomyositis/polymyositis
    Autonomic overactivity
    Clubbing
    Hypertrophic pulmonary osteoarthropathy
    Tylosis
    Encephalopathy/cortical degeneration
    Subacute cerebellar degeneration
    Peripheral neuropathies
    Myasthenic syndromes (including Lambert-Eaton)
    Transverse myelitis
    Progressive multifocal leukoencephalopathy
    Retinal blindness
Endocrine syndromes:
    Parathormone-like substance: hypercalcemia
    Inappropriate antidiuretic hormone: hyponatremia
    ACTH: Cushing syndrome, hyperpigmentation
    Serotonin: carcinoid syndrome
    Gonadotropins: gynecomastia
    Melanocyte-stimulating hormone: increased pigmentation
    Hypoglycemia, hyperglycemia
    Hypercalcitonemia
    Elevated growth hormone
    Prolactinemia
    Hypersecretion of vasoactive intestinal polypeptide (VIP): diarrhea
Hematologic/coagulation defects:
    Disseminated intravascular coagulation
    Recurrent venous thromboses
    Nonbacterial thrombotic (marantic) endocarditis
    Anemia
    Dysproteinemia
    Granulocytosis
    Eosinophilia
    Hypoalbuminemia
    Leukoerythroblastosis
    Marrow plasmacytosis
    Thrombocytopenia
Miscellaneous:
    Henoch-Schönlein purpura
    Glomerulonephritis
    Nephrotic syndrome
    Hypouricemia
    Hyperamylasemia
    Amyloidosis
    Lactic acidosis
    Systemic lupus erythematosus

*Compiled from references 3,4,11,17,19,20,22.

Table 8-3

TUMOR MARKERS FOUND IN THE SERUM OF PATIENTS WITH LUNG CARCINOMA*

Hormones	Adrenocorticotropic hormone (ACTH)
	Melanocyte-stimulating hormone (MSH)
	Human chorionic gonadotropin (hCG)
	Human placental lactogen (HPL)
	Human growth hormone (HGH)
	Parathyroid hormone (PTH)
	Calcitonin
	Antidiuretic hormone (ADH)
	Prolactin
	Bombesin (gastrin-releasing peptide)
	5-Hydroxytryptophan (serotonin)
	Estradiol
	Hypoglycemic factor
	Renin
	Erythropoietin
	Glucagon
	Vasoactive intestinal polypeptide (VIP)
	Neuron-specific enolase (NSE)
	β-Endorphin
	Lipotropin
	Oxytocin
	Gastrin
	Secretin
	Insulin
Other	Alpha fetoprotein (AFP)
	Carcinoembryonic antigen (CEA)
	Placental alkaline phosphatase (PAP)
	Histaminase
	L-dopa decarboxylase
	Anti-Purkinje cell antibodies
	Antineuronal nuclear antibodies (ANNA)
	Ferritin

*From references 2,10,22.

RADIOGRAPHIC FEATURES

The radiographic evaluation of the chest and extrathoracic structures plays a critical role in the diagnosis, staging, and determination of resectability of lung carcinoma. An overview of the various imaging techniques used in the staging of lung cancer is presented in Table 8-5. The chest radiographic findings according to the histologic subtype are summarized in Table 8-6.

The radiographic criteria supporting a diagnosis of malignancy for a solitary pulmonary nodule were developed over a number of years and include a size greater than 3 cm, a spiculated border, and absence of benign-pattern calcification (14). Computed tomography (CT) has added considerably to the radiographic evaluation of the solitary pulmonary nodule by improving the accuracy rate in separating benign from malignant lesions (24,28). Despite advances in chest radiology, the final diagnosis of malignancy is ultimately based on microscopic examination of either histologic or cytologic specimens.

In some cases, the secondary effects of a lung carcinoma are the most prominent radiographic features, particularly obstructive pneumonia, atelectasis, and pleural effusion (22).

CT studies of the chest are useful for the staging of lung cancers. The improved accuracy of CT compared to conventional tomography and chest roentgenograms has been documented (6, 8,18). CT is particularly useful for noninvasive evaluation of mediastinal lymph nodes. In normal subjects, 85 to 95 percent of the mediastinal lymph nodes are less than 10 mm in diameter; node size of greater than 10 mm is considered abnormal.

Table 8-4

IDENTIFICATION OF PEPTIDE HORMONES IN PARAFFIN SECTIONS OF LUNG CARCINOMA BY THE IMMUNOPEROXIDASE TECHNIQUE*

Tumor	ACTH	β-Lipotropin	β-Endorphin	α-MSH	Calcitonin	β–hCG
Small cell carcinoma	18/36	9/36	3/36	3/19	3/36	7/36
Squamous cell carcinoma	12/21	7/21	4/21	4/13	2/21	10/21
Large cell carcinoma	10/19	6/19	1/19	3/10	3/19	9/19
Adenocarcinoma	3/5	1/4	0/4	1/3	1/4	1/4
Total	43/81	23/80	8/80	11/45	9/80	27/80

*From reference 9.

Table 8-5

IMAGING TECHNIQUES IN LUNG CANCER STAGING*

Modality	Uses
Conventional radiographs	Primary detection/characterization of parenchymal tumor Assessment of main bronchi/tracheal involvement Detection of chest wall invasion Assessment of hilar and mediastinal invasion/adenopathy Detection of obstructive atelectasis/pneumonitis Detection of pleural effusion
CT	Assessment of main bronchi/tracheal involvement Detection of chest wall invasion Assessment of hilar and mediastinal invasion/adenopathy Detection of liver, adrenal, brain metastases
MRI	Detection of chest wall invasion (particularly superior sulcus [tumors]) Detection of mediastinal or spinal canal invasion Assessment of hilar and mediastinal adenopathy in patients with equivocal CT examinations or contraindications to intravenous contrast media Characterization of isolated adrenal masses
Ultrasound	Detection of pleural effusion/guidance for thoracentesis Guidance for biopsy of peripheral lung or mediastinal mass
Gallium-67 scan	Detection of hilar and mediastinal adenopathy Detection of distal metastases
Pulmonary angiography	Evaluation of central pulmonary artery invasion

*Modified from reference 13.

Table 8-6

CHEST RADIOGRAPHIC FINDINGS AT PRESENTATION ACCORDING TO HISTOLOGIC TYPE OF LUNG CARCINOMA*

Radiographic Feature	Squamous Cell Carcinoma	Adeno-carcinoma	Small Cell Carcinoma	Large Cell Carcinoma
Nodule ≤4 cm	14%	46%	21%	18%
Peripheral location	29%	65%	26%	61%
Central location	64%	5%	74%	42%
Hilar/perihilar mass	40%	17%	78%	32%
Cavitation	5%	3%	0%	4%
Pleural/chest wall involvement	3%	14%	5%	2%
Hilar adenopathy	38%	19%	61%	32%
Mediastinal adenopathy	5%	9%	14%	10%

*Modified from references 4,16.

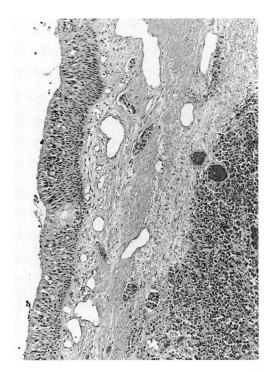 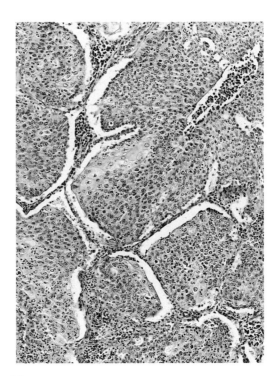

Figure 8-2
SPREAD OF LUNG CARCINOMA

Left: Direct bronchial submucosal infiltration by small cell carcinoma is seen as direct interstitial infiltration (lower right) and as nests of carcinoma within dilated lymphatics.
Right: Direct extension into intact alveolar spaces is seen at the periphery of a moderately differentiated squamous cell carcinoma.

Increasing lymph node size increases the likelihood of metastases, but CT cannot entirely replace formal node sampling at surgery (15).

There is not a significant difference in the accuracy of CT and magnetic resonance imaging (MRI) in the assessment of mediastinal nodes; they are also comparable for differentiating T0 to T2 versus T3 to T4 tumors (18,27). MRI, however, may be superior for identification of direct invasion of mediastinal structures (27).

The gold standard for the staging of lung carcinoma remains microscopic evaluation of cytologic or histologic specimens since not all nodes harboring metastases are enlarged and not all enlarged nodes are metastatically involved. Reactive follicular hyperplasia causing lymph node enlargement is common in patients with chronic bronchitis or obstructive pneumonia, both of which are frequent concomitant findings in patients with lung carcinoma. In McLoud's study (15), 7 of 19 (37 percent) nodes measuring 2 to 4 cm were found to be hyperplastic.

PATTERNS OF SPREAD

The patterns of spread of lung carcinoma are extensively reviewed by Spencer (38). They can be grouped as: direct extension to adjacent structures; aerogenous spread; lymphatic spread; hematogenous dissemination; and pleural seeding.

Direct extension of lung carcinoma includes involvement of the immediately adjacent lung parenchyma and bronchovascular bundles (figs. 8-2, 8-3) as well as structures in the chest wall, mediastinum, and vertebral column. Within the lung parenchyma, tumor cells spread by direct extension into contiguous airspaces, along interstitial or submucosal planes, or intraluminally in airways. Tumors cells are commonly seen lying free within architecturally intact airspaces at the periphery of many lung carcinomas. A study by Pääkkö et al. (37) provided immunohistochemical evidence that most bronchogenic carcinomas, regardless of histologic type, grow along intact alveolar basement membranes at

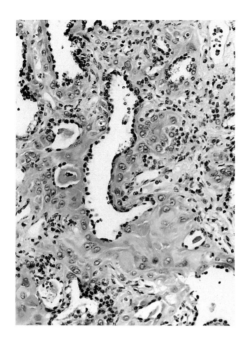
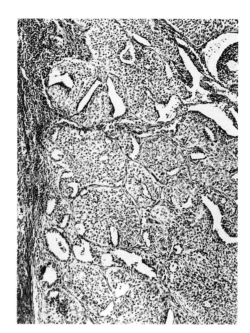

Figure 8-3
SPREAD OF LUNG CARCINOMA

Left: Transbronchial lung biopsy showing interstitial extension by squamous cell carcinoma. There is widening of the alveolar septa by carcinoma cells with distorted alveolar spaces lined by type 2 cells.

Right: Similarly, a resected poorly differentiated adenocarcinoma shows tumor spread under type 2 cells, which are left as small acini surrounded by carcinoma within intact alveoli.

their periphery. Maintenance of preexisting pulmonary architectural framework throughout the entire tumor is characteristic of, and one of the defining features of, bronchioloalveolar carcinoma. Growth within intact airspaces may also lead to replacement or elevation of the alveolar lining cells; the latter produce a small central acinus of reactive type 2 cells surrounded by neoplastic cells which abut the intact basement membrane of the alveolus (fig. 8-3).

Aerogenous dissemination implies spread of tumor cells through the air passages with the development of secondary deposits at some distance from the main mass (fig. 8-4), even in different lobes. This occurs commonly with bronchioloalveolar carcinoma, and as a result, large numbers of tumor cells may be shed in the sputum. In routine sections of bronchioloalveolar carcinoma, multiple, discrete, and widely separated nodules of carcinoma, unassociated with interstitial or lymphangitic spread, are often seen. Radiographically, a solitary nodule of bronchioloalveolar carcinoma may eventually spread aerogenously to involve multiple lobes and lead to death by progressive consolidation of

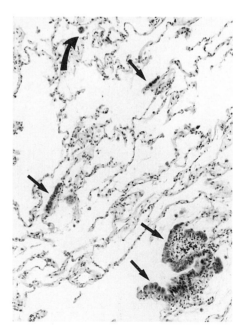

Figure 8-4
SPREAD OF LUNG CARCINOMA

Aerogenous dissemination from a case of bronchioloalveolar carcinoma. Away from the main mass there are multiple discrete and separate foci of involvement on intact alveolar walls (arrows), and a tiny cluster of carcinoma cells floating free within an alveolus (curved arrow).

113

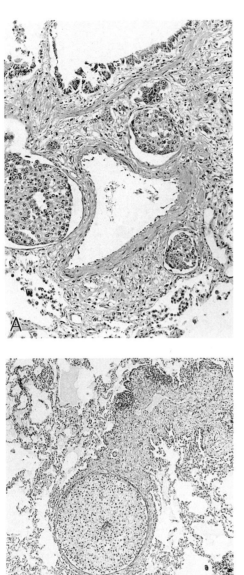

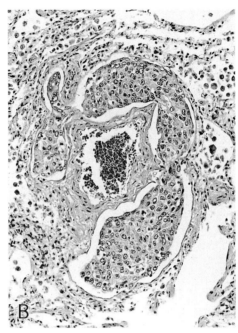

Figure 8-5
SPREAD OF LUNG CARCINOMA
Lymphangitic spread of carcinoma. Tumor cell nests are in dilated lymphatic spaces around bronchovascular structures (A), pulmonary veins (B), and filling a septal lymphatic (C).

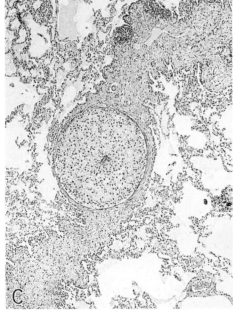

intact lung parenchyma without any evidence of extrapulmonary disease.

Lymphatic invasion and spread is extremely common in lung carcinoma (fig. 8-5), and the anatomy of the lymphatic drainage of the lung is one of the foundations of the staging of lung carcinoma. Lymph node groups outside the chest are commonly affected late in the natural history of the disease. In autopsy series, Spencer (38) found involvement of the tracheobronchial lymph nodes in 70 percent of patients, intra-abdominal lymph nodes in 20 percent, cervical lymph nodes in 17 percent, retroperitoneal lymph nodes in 8 percent, axillary lymph nodes in 7 percent, pancreatic lymph nodes in 7 percent, and supraclavicular lymph nodes in 7 percent.

Table 8-7
LYMPHATIC AND HEMATOGENOUS SPREAD OF LUNG CARCINOMA*

Site	Total (%)	Squamous Cell Carcinoma (%)	Adeno- carcinoma (%)	Small Cell Carcinoma (%)	Large Cell Carcinoma (%)
Any metastasis	96	94	94	99	97
Regional nodes	89	83	91	96	89
Pleura	24	24	30	23	18
Chest wall	16	16	18	12	14
Pericardium	18	15	19	20	17
Esophagus	13	14	10	18	9
Distant nodes	45	29	48	62	45
Brain	45	36	47	50	49
Liver	44	37	42	62	33
Adrenal	34	20	41	44	36
Bone	30	26	44	35	25
Kidney	24	23	26	25	19
Heart	18	20	16	20	16

*Modified from reference 29.

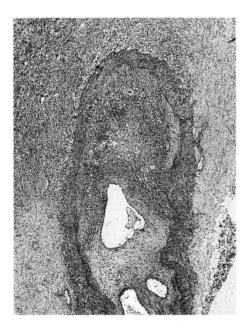 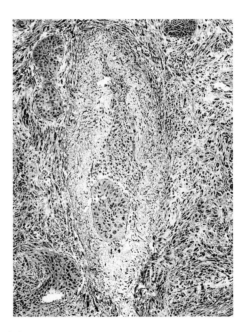

Figure 8-6
SPREAD OF LUNG CARCINOMA
Vascular invasion by lung carcinoma into a large artery (left) and a medium-sized vein (right). The lesion depicted on the right is a spindled squamous cell carcinoma, and both the epithelial and spindled components are present in the vessel lumen.

Hematogenous dissemination is extremely common in lung carcinoma (Table 8-7), and there are few carcinomas that spread more widely. While invasion of large vessels is occasionally seen in routine lung carcinoma sections (fig. 8-6), evalua-tion with elastic tissue stains shows that this is actually very common. In a study of 59 resection specimens, Ballantyne et al. (30) found vascular invasion in 52 (88 percent) and pulmonary arte-rial invasion in 10 (17 percent). Collier et al. (31)

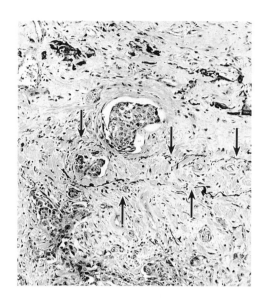 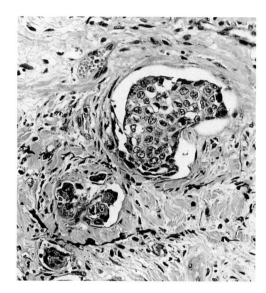

Figure 8-7
SPREAD OF LUNG CARCINOMA
Pleural invasion by lung carcinoma with nests of tumor cells traversing the pleural elastica (left, arrows) in the dilated lymphatics (right).

showed vascular invasion in 161 of 215 (74 percent) carcinomas. In a recent study of small (3 cm or less) resected peripheral carcinomas by Kolin and Koutoulakis (33), arterial invasion or occlusion was very common (90 percent).

Venous invasion allows widespread dissemination of tumor cells to extrathoracic organs, whereas pulmonary arterial invasion is associated with infarction and scarring, the effects of which may overshadow the tumor itself. Kolin and Koutoulakis (33) implicated arterial invasion in the pathogenesis of many "scar cancers."

Pleural seeding may be the result of direct invasion of the pleura by a peripheral tumor or spread to the pleura by hematogenous or lymphatic routes (fig. 8-7). Invasion of the pleural elastica can be subtle and obscured by reactive fibroblastic proliferation, and accurate assessment of whether the pleural elastica has been breached is best made with elastic tissue stains (32). Once the pleura is breached, tumor cells can seed the entire pleural space and mimic a diffuse malignant mesothelioma (pseudomesotheliomatous carcinoma).

Pleural effusions are a common finding in patients with bronchogenic carcinoma, and they carry a poor prognosis regardless of whether or not carcinoma cells are identified in them cytologically (36). Pleural effusions associated with bronchogenic carcinomas have several etiologies: lymphatic obstruction, pulmonary venous obstruction, pleural seeding by neoplastic cells, or inflammatory reactions caused by the tumor.

The sites affected by all methods of spread for the major subtypes of lung carcinoma are summarized from the data of Auerbach et al. (29) in Table 8-7. Almost any site can be affected.

The high frequency of occult metastatic disease at the time of presentation in patients with lung carcinoma is illustrated by data from Matthews et al. (35). She showed that of 202 patients who underwent curative surgical resection for lung cancer (i.e., there was no clinical evidence of residual carcinoma) and died (of unrelated causes) within 1 month of surgery, 73 (35 percent) had persistent carcinoma identified at autopsy (Table 8-8). Current staging techniques might have identified some, but probably not all, of the metastatic deposits in these patients.

The sites of clinical relapse after curative resection of nonsmall cell carcinoma parallel the data of Matthews. Relapse tends to be at distant sites, even in patients with regional lymph node metastases at the time of resection. Follow-up data on 111 patients who relapsed after undergoing curative resection for N2 disease with involvement of ipsilateral mediastinal or subcarinal lymph nodes is shown in Table 8-9 (34).

Table 8-8

**PERSISTENT LUNG CARCINOMA AT AUTOPSY
IN 202 PATIENTS DYING WITHIN 30 DAYS OF CURATIVE SURGERY***

Histologic Subtype	Number of Patients	Residual Local Disease	Distant Metastases	Total with Residual Disease no. (%)
Squamous cell	131	22	22	44 (33)
Adenocarcinoma	30	1	12	13 (43)
Small cell	19	1	12	13 (14)
Large cell	22	—	3	3 (14)
Totals	202	24	49	73 (35)

*Modified from reference 35.

Table 8-9

**RELAPSE SITES IN 111 OF 149 PATIENTS UNDERGOING
CURATIVE RESECTION FOR N2 NONSMALL CELL LUNG CARCINOMA***

	Squamous Cell	Adenocarcinoma	Large Cell	Total
No. of patients	46	92	11	149
Relapses	30 (65%)	71 (77%)	10 (91%)	111 (75%)
Local	2 (7%)	4 (6%)	1 (10%)	7 (6%)
Regional	4 (13%)	10 (14%)	3 (30%)	17 (15%)
Distant	24 (80%)	57 (80%)	6 (60%)	87 (79%)
Brain	8	20	8	36
Bone	6	7	6	19
Liver	1	5	1	7
Lung	4	9	4	17
Multiple	1	7	—	8
Others	2	5	—	7
Unknown	2	4	—	6

*Modified from reference 34.

STAGING, MANAGEMENT, AND PROGNOSIS

Surgical resection offers the only reasonable chance of cure in cases of carcinoma of the lung. Surgery is possible in approximately 20 percent of nonsmall cell carcinomas (squamous cell carcinoma, adenocarcinoma, large cell carcinoma) and in less than 5 percent of small cell carcinomas (17, 36,54). For patients with relapses following surgery and for those who are not surgical candidates, a number of radiation and chemotherapy protocols are available, depending on histologic subtype, extent of disease, and sites of involvement (52,69). Small cell carcinoma is responsive to chemotherapy in at least three fourths of the cases (51); fewer patients with nonsmall cell carcinoma respond to chemotherapy. Whether or not a patient can be considered a candidate for surgical resection depends on stage and identification of localized disease.

Staging represents a determination of the anatomic extent of disease based on clinical, radiographic, pathologic, and other evidence (17,65). Staging is important in the evaluation and management of lung carcinoma and is the most important prognostic parameter, far outweighing histologic subtype in importance among cases of nonsmall cell carcinoma. Staging of lung carcinoma can be performed at various points in patient management and can be grouped as follows (17): 1) pretreatment clinical diagnostic staging including information from endoscopy, mediastinoscopy, and other studies; 2) surgical evaluative staging taking into account findings at exploratory thoracotomy; 3) postsurgical pathologic staging combining the results of histologic evaluation of resection specimens and accompanying biopsies; 4) retreatment staging representing restaging of the disease at the time of relapse; and 5) autopsy staging representing the final analysis of anatomic disease extent on the basis of autopsy studies.

The currently accepted staging system for lung carcinoma is that proposed by Mountain in 1986 (36,62,63,71). It is a TNM-based system, where T refers to the size and extent of the primary tumor; N, to the presence and extent of regional lymph node involvement; and M, to the presence or absence of distant metastases. The system is modified for each organ system and provides a carefully defined framework for reporting the anatomic extent of disease in a common and reproducible format; it facilitates comparison of studies from different centers and has proven to be of value (42).

The defining features of the TNM system for lung carcinoma are shown in Table 8-10. This system can be applied to findings from radiographic as well as pathologic examinations and in any given case, the data used in staging may vary considerably. In some cases, staging is based entirely on radiographic data (when there are findings of inoperability), whereas in others, staging is primarily based on pathologic information derived from tissues taken at mediastinoscopy or thoracotomy. Table 8-11 illustrates the prognostic value of staging.

A diagram of regional lymph node groups in the chest and their locations on a chest radiograph are shown in figures 8-8 and 8-9. Figures 8-10 and 8-11 illustrate examples of TNM staging of lung carcinomas.

Once the TNM status is determined, a clinical stage is assigned. It is on the basis of clinical stage that operability is assessed and on which considerable prognostic information rests. Clinical staging and resectability based on TNM staging are shown in Table 8-12. Individuals with clinical stage IIIA or lower tumor may be candidates for resection whereas those with clinical stage IIIB and IV are not. The role of surgery

in stage IIIA lung carcinoma is controversial and not unanimously advocated.

The staging system and assessment of operability as shown in Table 8-12 apply primarily to nonsmall cell carcinomas. Mountain (36) has shown the value of TNM staging for nonsmall cell carcinomas; survival according to stage for squamous cell carcinoma and adenocarcinoma of the lung are shown in figures 8-12 and 8-13.

TNM staging does not apply well to small cell carcinomas as shown in fig. 8-14; resection is reserved for a small number of peripheral small cell carcinomas that are clinical stage I (54). Small cell carcinoma is considered primarily a systemic disease and therefore treated chemotherapeutically. This is why the pathologic distinction between nonsmall cell carcinoma and small cell carcinoma is so important (17,44).

A two-stage system is favored in the management of small cell carcinoma (Table 8-13) (44, 51,66,72). Limited disease refers to involvement confined to one hemithorax, with or without lymph node involvement (including ipsilateral and contralateral mediastinal and supraclavicular nodes) and pleural effusion independent of cytology. Extensive disease is defined as any disease more advanced than limited disease, usually including involvement of distant lymph nodes, brain, liver, bone marrow, bone, and intraabdominal or soft tissue sites. The key factor in this system is that the anatomic extent of limited disease can be included within an irradiation field (66). The 5-year survival for limited disease is about 10 percent, and for extensive disease 0 to 2 percent (44,51,72).

Pleural effusion associated with lung carcinoma carries a poor prognosis regardless of histologic subtype or pleural fluid cytology (fig. 8-15).

While there are differences in staging and survival for the histologic subtypes, lung carcinoma overall remains a disease with a poor prognosis and high stage at presentation. Recent statistics from the National Cancer Institute reveal a 13 percent 5-year survival for whites and 11 percent for blacks for all stages of lung carcinoma (Table 8-14A) (41). Some differences based on sex, race, and histology are also apparent in the SEER data (Table 8-14B). There has been a slight improvement in overall 5-year survival for all stages in both blacks and whites since 1960: from 8 to 13 percent for whites and

Table 8-10

DEFINING FEATURES OF TNM SYSTEM FOR LUNG CARCINOMA

ANATOMIC FEATURES OF THE PRIMARY TUMOR (T)*

TX — Tumor proven by the presence of malignant cells in bronchopulmonary secretions but not visualized roentgenographically or bronchoscopically, or any tumor that cannot be assessed in treatment staging.

T0 — No evidence of primary tumor.

TIS — Carcinoma in situ.

T1 — A tumor that is 3.0 cm or less in greatest dimension, surrounded by lung or visceral pleura, and without evidence of invasion proximal to a lobar bronchus at bronchoscopy.

(Note: The uncommon superficial tumor of any size with its invasive component limited to the bronchial wall which may extend proximal to the main bronchus is also classified as T1.)

T2 — A tumor more than 3.0 cm in greatest dimension or a tumor of any size that either invades the visceral pleura or has associated atelectasis or obstructive pneumonitis extending to the hilar region. At bronchoscopy, the proximal extent of demonstrable tumor must be within a lobar bronchus or at least 2.0 cm distal to the carina. Any associated atelectasis or obstructive pneumonitis must involve less than an entire lung.

T3 — A tumor of any size with direct extension into the chest wall (including superior sulcus tumors), diaphragm, or the mediastinal pleura or pericardium without involving the heart, great vessels, trachea, esophagus, or vertebral body, or a tumor in the main bronchus within 2.0 cm of the carina without involving the carina.

T4 — A tumor of any size with invasion of the mediastinum or involving heart, great vessels, trachea, esophagus, vertebral body, or carina or presence of malignant pleural effusion.

(Note: Most pleural effusions associated with lung cancer are due to tumor. There are, however, a few patients in whom cytopathologic examination of pleural fluid (on more than one specimen) is negative for tumor, the fluid is not bloody, and is not an exudate. In such cases where these elements and clinical judgment dictate that the effusion is not related to the tumor, the patient should be staged T1, T2, or T3, excluding effusion as a staging element.)

STATUS AND EXTENT OF INVOLVEMENT OF REGIONAL LYMPH NODES (N)*

NX — Regional lymph nodes cannot be assessed.

N0 — No demonstrable metastasis to regional lymph nodes.

N1 — Metastasis to lymph nodes in the peribronchial or ipsilateral hilar region, or both, including direct extension.

N2 — Metastasis to ipsilateral mediastinal lymph nodes or subcarinal lymph nodes.

N3 — Metastasis to contralateral mediastinal lymph nodes, contralateral hilar nodes, ipsilateral or contralateral scalene, or supraclavicular lymph nodes.

DISTANT METASTASES (M)*

MX — Presence of distant metastases cannot be assessed.

M0 — No (known) distant metastasis.

M1 — Distant metastasis present—specify site(s).

*From references 40,62.

Table 8-11

LUNG CANCER PROGNOSIS ACCORDING TO TNM FACTORS IN 1479 PATIENTS*

TNM Stage	Number	5-Year Survival (%)
T1N0M0	245	75.5
T2N0M0	291	57.0
T1N1M0	66	52.5
T2N1M0	153	38.4
T3N0M0	106	33.3
T3N1M0	85	39.0
T1-3N2M0	368	15.1
T1-3N3M0	55	0
T4 any N	104	8.2

*From reference 40.

from 5 to 11 percent for blacks (41). The overall poor prognosis of lung carcinoma is due to the fact that few patients present with localized disease (Table 8-15).

Staging remains the best prognostic indicator for lung carcinoma, especially for nonsmall cell subtypes. Small cell carcinoma appears to be a biologically more aggressive histologic subtype, and its distinction from the nonsmall cell subtype is important. Among the nonsmall cell carcinomas of the lung, including squamous cell carcinoma, adenocarcinoma, and large cell carcinoma, there are minor differences in prognosis stage for stage in some, but not all, studies (63,67). The survival figures from the SEER data for a huge number of patients (approximately 50,000) stratified by histologic subtype is shown in figure 8-16 (74).

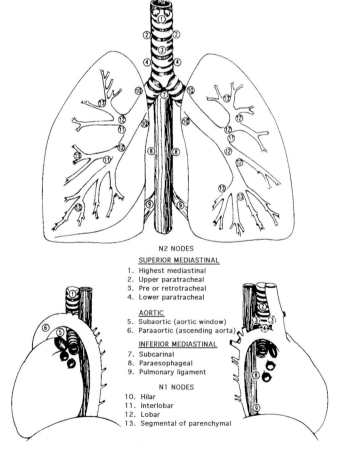

Figure 8-8
LYMPH NODE STATIONS
Lymph node stations within the mediastinum and lung are shown with their associated numerical designations. (Fig. 3 from Bains MS. Surgical treatment of lung cancer. Chest 1991;100:826–37.)

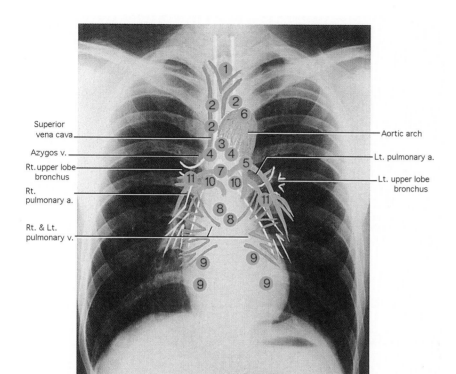

Superior vena cava
Azygos v.
Rt. upper lobe bronchus
Rt. pulmonary a.
Rt. & Lt. pulmonary v.

Aortic arch
Lt. pulmonary a.
Lt. upper lobe bronchus

Figure 8-9
LYMPH NODE STATIONS
Lymph node stations are shown projected onto a chest roentgenogram. (Fig. 11 from Okada Y. Lymphatic system of the human lung. Kinpodo, Kyoto, Japan 1989.)

Table 8-12

STAGE GROUPING OF TNM SUBSETS AND POTENTIAL OPERABILITY*

Stage	Cases** (%)	T Factor	N Factor	M Factor	Consider Surgery?
Occult		TX	N0	M0	Yes
0		TIS	N0	M0	Yes
I	13	T1	N0	M0	Yes
		T2	N0	M0	Yes
II	10	T1	N1	M0	Yes
		T2	N1	M0	Yes
IIIA	22	T3	N0	M0	Yes
		T3	N1	M0	Yes
		T1-T3	N2	M0	Yes
IIIB	22	Any T	N3	M0	No
		T4	Any N	M0	No
IV	32	Any T	Any N	M1	No

* Modified from references 39,62.
**From reference 42 (No. = 3823).

Table 8-13

TWO-STAGE CLASSIFICATION FOR SMALL CELL CARCINOMA*

Limited disease (30 percent of cases)

Primary tumor confined to hemithorax

Ipsilateral hilar nodes

Ipsilateral and contralateral supraclavicular nodes

Ipsilateral and contralateral mediastinal nodes

Pleural effusion

Extensive disease (70 percent of cases)

More advanced than limited disease

Metastases to contralateral lung

Distant metastases

*Modified from reference 51.

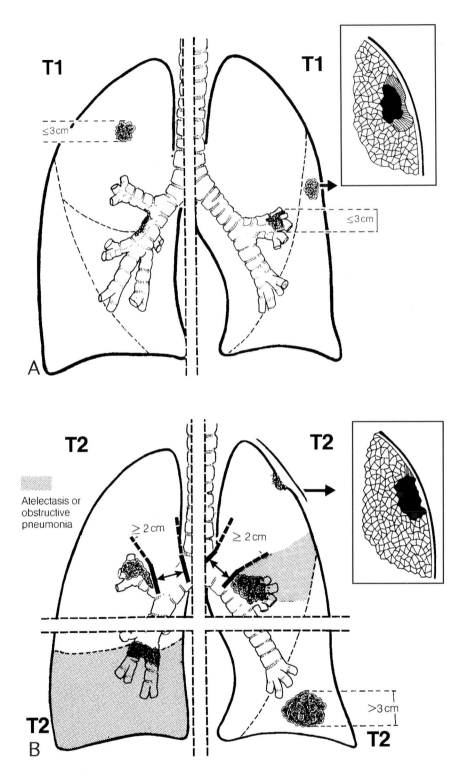

Figure 8-10
TNM STAGING

Diagrammatic representations of features of the primary tumor (T) in the TNM staging system for T1 tumors (A), T2 tumors (B), T3 tumors (C), and T4 tumors (D–K). See Table 8-12 for details. (From Spiessl B, ed. International Union Against Cancer. TNM atlas: illustrated guide to the TNM/pTNM-classification of malignant tumours. 3rd ed. New York: Springer-Verlag, 1989.)

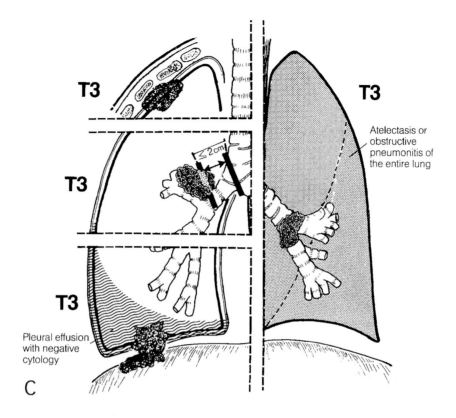

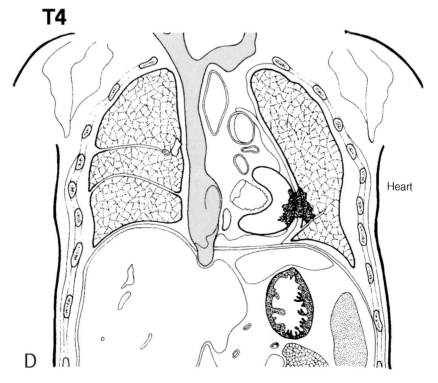

Figure 8-10 (Continued)

T4

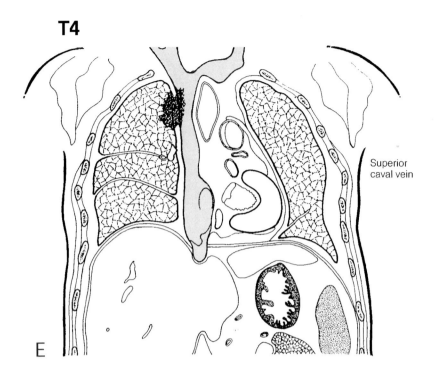

Superior
caval vein

E

T4

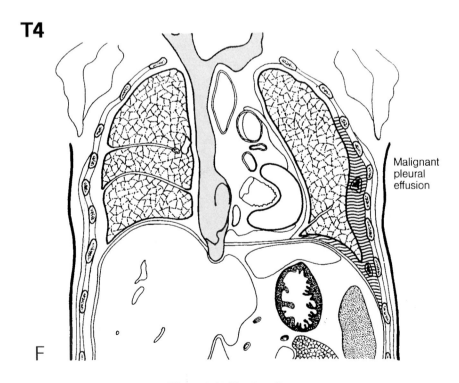

Malignant
pleural
effusion

F

Figure 8-10 (Continued)

T4

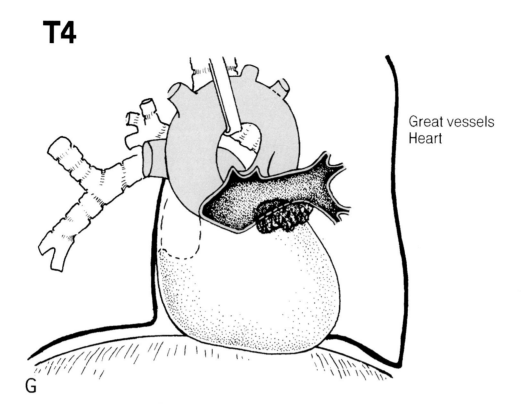

Great vessels
Heart

G

T4

Malignant
pleural
effusion

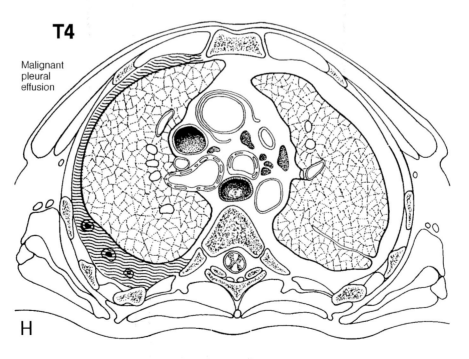

H

Figure 8-10 (Continued)

T4

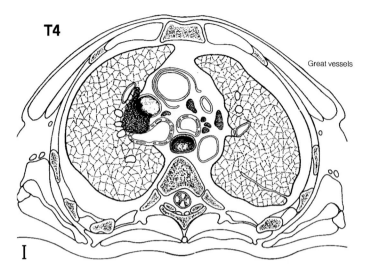

Great vessels

I

T4

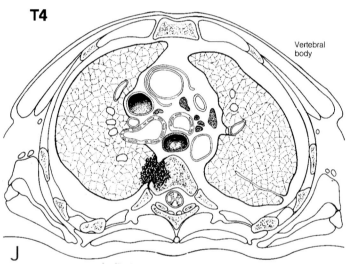

Vertebral body

J

T4

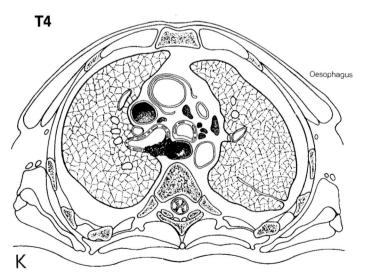

Oesophagus

K

Figure 8-10 (Continued)

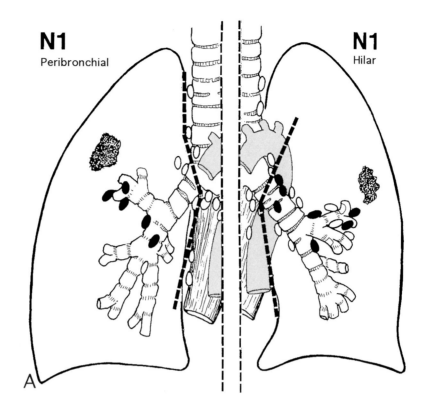

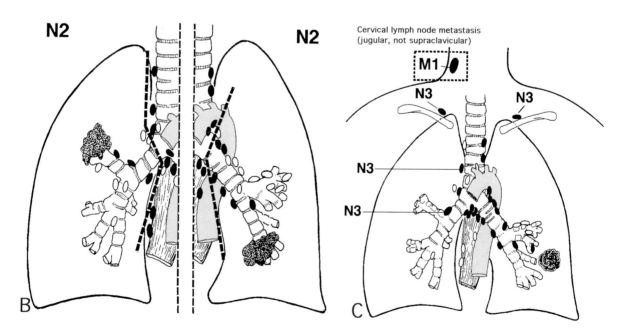

Figure 8-11

TNM STAGING

Patterns of lymph node involvement (N) for TNM staging of lung carcinoma are depicted for N1 tumors (A), N2 tumors (B), and N3 tumors (C). Metastatic disease (M1) is also shown in C. See Tables 8-13 and 8-14 for details. (From Spiessl B, ed. International Union Against Cancer. TNM atlas: illustrated guide to the TNM/pTNM-classification of malignant tumours. 3rd ed. New York: Springer-Verlag, 1989.)

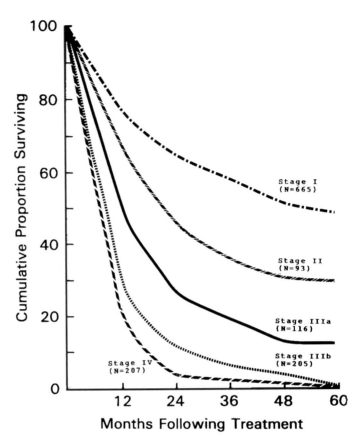

Figure 8-12
SQUAMOUS CELL
CARCINOMA SURVIVAL
Survival by stage for squamous cell carcinoma
of the lung. (Fig. 9 from Mountain CF. Prognostic
implications of the International Staging System
for Lung Cancer. Semin Oncol 1988;15:236–45.)

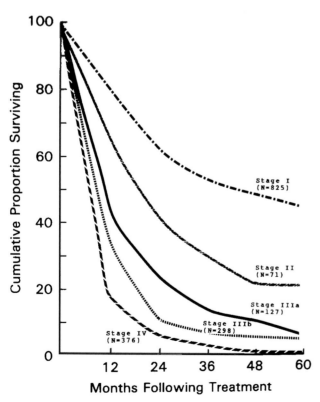

Figure 8-13
ADENOCARCINOMA SURVIVAL
Survival by stage for adenocarcinoma of the lung.
(Fig. 10 from Mountain CF. Prognostic implications of
the International Staging System for Lung Cancer.
Semin Oncol 1988;15:236–45.)

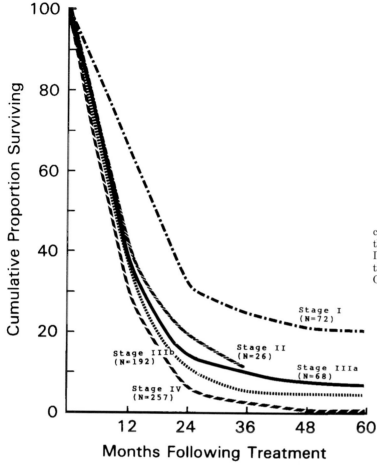

Figure 8-14
SMALL CELL
CARCINOMA SURVIVAL
Although patients with stage I disease do significantly better than those with the other three stages, there is little separation between stages II, III, and IV. (Fig. 11 from Mountain CF. Prognostic implications of the International Staging System for Lung Cancer. Semin Oncol 1988;15:236–45.)

Figure 8-15
PLEURAL EFFUSION AND SURVIVAL
Survival for patients with lung carcinoma and an associated pleural effusion. No difference is seen between those with positive versus those with negative pleural fluid cytology examinations. (Fig.1 from Mountain CF. Prognostic implications of the International Staging System for Lung Cancer. Semin Oncol 1988;15:236–45.)

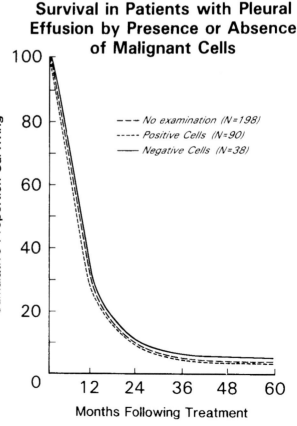

Survival in Patients with Pleural Effusion by Presence or Absence of Malignant Cells

--- No examination (N=198)
····· Positive Cells (N=90)
—— Negative Cells (N=38)

Table 8-14

LUNG CARCINOMA—FIVE-YEAR SURVIVAL

A. Overall by stage 1981-1987*

Disease at Presentation	Whites	Blacks
Localized	41%	35%
Regional	14%	10%
Distant metastases	2%	2%
All stages	13%	11%

B. By stage, race, sex, and histology 1978-1986**

	Local	Regional	Distant	Unstaged	All Stages
			Patients Alive at 5 Years (%)		
Squamous cell carcinoma					
White men	33.4	14.6	1.4	6.5	15.0
White women	40.5	17.8	1.5	12.2	18.8
Black men	26.7	11.3	1.5	5.2	11.3
Black women	32.7	14.9	4.8	0	15.8
Adenocarcinoma					
White men	48.6	16.1	1.4	8.9	16.7
White women	59.9	21.1	2.4	14.9	23.9
Black men	40.3	12.0	1.4	4.4	12.9
Black women	54.7	19.0	0.7	16.3	20.3
Small cell carcinoma					
White men	8.8	6.8	1.3	3.8	3.7
White women	18.5	9.0	1.8	8.0	6.3
Black men	4.7	4.9	1.1	2.3	2.6
Black women	17.2	13.1	1.7	0	6.5
Large cell carcinoma					
White men	32.7	12.5	1.6	8.1	10.7
White women	36.0	15.0	1.4	6.7	12.5
Black men	43.1	9.9	0.7	0 [†]	10.6
Black women	51.5	19.6	5.9	—	18.4

* From reference 41.
**From reference 74.
[†]Less than 25 cases for calculation of relative survival.

Table 8-15

STAGE OF LUNG CARCINOMA AT PRESENTATION

A. Cancer statistics 1981-1987*

Localized	18%
Regional lymph node involvement	31%
Distant metastases	39%
Unknown	12%

B. SEER data 1983-1987; stage at presentation by histologic subtype**

	Squamous	Adeno-carcinoma	Small cell	Large cell
Localized	21.5%	22.2%	8.2%	15.2%
Regional	38.5%	33.1%	26.1%	31.5%
Distant	25.2%	35.9%	52.8%	40.3%
Unstaged	14.8%	8.8%	12.8%	12.9%

* From reference 41.
**Modified from reference 74.

5-YEAR RELATIVE SURVIVAL RATE

BY HISTOLOGIC TYPE OF LUNG CANCER

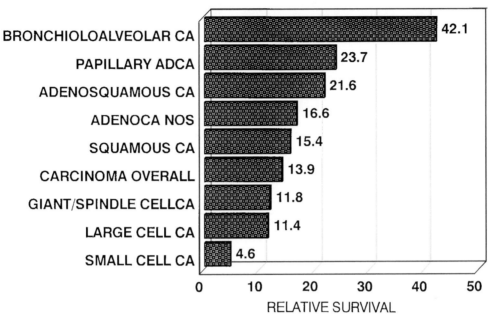

SEER (TABLE 7, 1978-86)

Figure 8-16
FIVE-YEAR SURVIVAL
The 5-year relative survival rate by histologic subtype is shown from the SEER data 1978–1986 (74).

Many specific histologic parameters have been assessed as possible prognostic indicators among lung carcinomas with variable results. Most of these have been based on surgically resected (generally nonsmall cell) tumors, so that clear differences in outcome may be apparent at follow-up. Some of these studies, which have not always agreed with one another, are summarized in Table 8-16. The application and prognostic implications of newer techniques of study, including flow cytometry and molecular genetics, are discussed in chapter 3 (56).

REFERENCES

Demographic, Clinical, and Radiographic Features

1. Boring CC, Squires TS, Tong T. Cancer statistics, 1993. CA Cancer J Clin 1993;43:7–26.
2. Broder LE, Primack A. Marker substances in bronchogenic carcinoma: a review. In: Strauss MJ, ed. Lung cancer: clinical diagnosis and treatment. 2nd ed. New York: Grune and Stratton, 1983:37–63.
3. Carter D, Eggleston JC. Tumors of the lower respiratory tract. Atlas of Tumor Pathology, Second Series, Fascicle 17. Washington, D.C.: Armed Forces Institute of Pathology, 1980.
4. Cohen MH. Signs and symptoms of bronchogenic carcinoma. In: Strauss MJ, ed. Lung cancer: clinical diagnosis and treatment. 2nd ed. New York: Grune and Stratton, 1983:97–112.
5. Cromartie RS III, Parker EF, May JE, Metcalf JS, Bartles DM. Carcinoma of the lung: a clinical review. Ann Thorac Surg 1980;30:30–5.
6. Dales RE, Stark RM, Raman S. Computed tomography to stage lung cancer. Approaching a controversy using meta-analysis. Am Rev Respir Dis 1990;141(5 Pt 1):1096–101.

Table 8-16
SELECTED PROGNOSTIC PARAMETERS IN LUNG CARCINOMA*

Favorable	Unfavorable
Lymphocytes predominant and germinal center predominance in regional nodes (53)	Lymphocyte depleted or unstimulated regional nodes (53)
Regional nodes with sinus histiocytosis or paracortical hyperplasia (64,73)	Follicular hyperplasia in regional nodes (73)
Peritumor lymphoplasmacytic infiltrates (45,55,58)	Tumor necrosis, venous invasion (45,68)
Peritumor infiltrates of Langerhans and related cells (47)	High mitotic index (43)
Increased numbers of cellular junctions between tumor cells as seen ultrastructurally (59)	K-*ras* mutations in adenocarcinomas (70)
Immunohistochemical identification of neuroendocrine features (48) or expression of certain peripheral airway markers: surfactant-associated protein and Clara cell protein (57).	*Ras* p21 expression in nonsmall cell carcinoma (50,61)
	Ras mutations in nonsmall cell carcinoma (60)
	C-*erb* B1 oncogene expression in squamous cell carcinoma (75)

*See also chapter 3.

7. el-Torky M, el-Zeky F, Hall JC. Significant changes in the distribution of histologic types of lung cancer. A review of 4928 cases. Cancer 1990;65:2361–7.
8. Ferguson MK, MacMahon H, Little AG, Golomb HM, Hoffman PC, Skinner DB. Original accuracy of computed tomography of the mediastinum in staging of lung cancer. J Thorac Cardiovasc Surg 1986;91:498–504.
9. Gropp C. Peptide hormones in lung cancer. In: McVie JG, Bakker W, Wagenaar SJ, Curney D, eds. Clinical and experimental pathology of lung cancer. Boston: Martinus-Nijhoff, 1986:123–30.
10. Havemann K, Gropp C, Holle R. Peptide in hormones and small cell lung cancer: the usefulness for diagnosis, staging, and monitoring of treatment. In: Hansen HH, ed. Lung cancer: basic and clinical aspects. Boston: Martinus-Nijhoff, 1986:113–28.
11. Jett JR, Cortese DA, Fontana RS. Lung cancer: current concepts and prospects. CA Cancer J Clin 1983;33:74–86.
12. Kiers L, Altermatt HJ, Lennon VA. Paraneoplastic anti-neuronal nuclear IgG autoantibodies (type I) to localized antigen in small cell lung carcinoma. Mayo Clin Proc 1991;66:1209–16.
13. Klein JS, Webb WR. The radiologic staging of lung cancer. J Thorac Imaging 1991;7:29–47.
14. Lyubsky S, Jacobson MJ. Lung cancer. Making the diagnosis. Chest 1991;100:511–20.
15. McLoud TC, Bourgouin PM, Greenberg RW, et al. Bronchogenic carcinomas: analysis of staging in the mediastinum with CT by correlative lymph node mapping sampling. Radiology 1992;182:319–23.
16. Miller WE. Roentgenographic manifestations of lung cancer. In: Strauss MJ, ed. Lung cancer: clinical diagnosis and treatments. 2nd ed. New York: Grune and Stratton, 1983:175–84.
17. Minna JD, Pass H, Glatstein E, Ihde DC. Cancer of the lung. In: DeVita VT, Hellman S, Rosenberg SA, eds. Cancer: principles and practice of oncology. 3rd ed. Philadelphia: JB Lippincott, 1989:591–705.
18. Naidich DP. CT/MR correlation in the evaluation of tracheobronchial neoplasia. Radiol Clin North Am 1990;28:555–71.
19. Owens AH, Abeloff MD. Neoplasms of the lung. In: Calabresi P, Schein PS, Rosenberg SA, eds. Medical oncology: basic principles and clinical management of cancer. New York: MacMillan, 1985:715–57.
20. Patel AM, Davila DG, Peter SG. Paraneoplastic syndromes associated with lung cancer. Mayo Clin Proc 1993;68:278–87.
21. Pelucchi A, Ciceri E, Clementi F, Marazzini L, Foresi A, Sher E. Calcium channel antibodies in myasthenic syndrome and small cell lung cancer. Am Rev Respir Dis 1993;147:1229–32.
22. Richards F, Choplin RH. Diagnostic workup. In: Scarantino CW, ed. Lung cancer: diagnostic procedures and therapeutic management with special reference to radiotherapy. New York: Springer-Verlag, 1985:55–75.
23. Rosenow EC, Carr DT. Bronchogenic carcinoma. CA Cancer J Clin 1979;29:233–45.
24. Swensen SJ, Jett JR, Payne WS, Viggiano RW, Pairolero PC, Trastek VF. An integrated approach to evaluation of the solitary pulmonary nodule. Mayo Clin Proc 1990;65:173–86.
25. Teeter SM, Holmes FF, McFarlane MJ. Lung carcinoma in the elderly population. Influence of histology on the inverse relationship of stage to age. Cancer 1987;60:1331–6.
25a. Travis WD, Travis LB, Percy C, Devesa SS. Lung cancer incidence and survival by histologic type. Cancer. In press.
26. Vincent RG, Pickren JW, Lane WW, et al. The changing histopathology of lung cancer: a review of 1682 cases. Cancer 1977;39:1647–55.

27. Webb WR, Gatsonis C, Zerhouni EA, et al. CT and MR imaging in staging non-small cell bronchogenic carcinoma: report of the Radiologic Diagnostic Oncology Group. Radiology 1991;178:705–13.

28. Zerhouni EA, Stitik FP, Siegelmann SS, et al. CT of the pulmonary nodule: a cooperative study. Radiology 1986;160:319–27.

Spread of Lung Carcinoma

29. Auerbach O, Garfinkel L, Parks VR. Histologic type of lung cancer in relation to smoking habits, year of diagnosis and sites of metastases. Chest 1975;67:382–7.

30. Ballantyne AJ, Clagett OT, McDonald JR. Vascular invasion in bronchogenic carcinoma. Thorax 1957;12:294–9.

31. Collier FC, Enterline HT, Kyle RH, Tristan TT, Greening R. The prognostic implications of vascular invasion in primary carcinomas of the lung. Arch Pathol 1958;66:594–603.

32. Gallagher B, Urbanski SJ. The significance of pleural elastica invasion by lung carcinomas. Hum Pathol 1990;21:512–7.

33. Kolin A, Koutoulakis T. Invasion of pulmonary arteries by bronchial carcinomas. Hum Pathol 1987;18:1165–71.

34. Martini N, Flehinger BJ. The role of surgery in N2 lung cancer. Surg Clin North Am 1987;65:1037–49.

35. Matthews MJ, Kanhouwa S, Pickren J, Robinette D. Frequency of residual and metastatic tumor in patients undergoing curative surgical resection for lung cancer. Cancer Chemother Rep 1973;4:63–7.

36. Mountain CF. Prognostic implications of the International Staging System for Lung Cancer. Semin Oncol 1988;15:236–45.

37. Pääkkö P, Risteli J, Risteli L, Autio-Harmainen H. Immunohistochemical evidence that lung carcinomas grow on alveolar basement membranes. Am J Surg Pathol 1990;14:464–73.

38. Spencer H. Pathology of the lung. 4th ed. New York: Pergamon Press, 1985:915–25.

Staging, Management, and Prognosis

39. Bains MS. Surgical treatment of lung cancer. Chest 1991;100:826–37.

40. Beahrs OH. Manual for staging of cancer. 4th ed. American Joint Committee on Cancer (AJCC). Philadelphia: JB Lippincott, 1992:115–22.

41. Boring CC, Squires TS, Tong T. Cancer statistics, 1992. CA Cancer J Clin 1992;42:19–38.

42. Bülzebruck H, Bopp R, Drings P, et al. New aspects in the staging of lung cancer. Prospective validation of the International Union Against Cancer TNM classification. Cancer 1992;70:1102–10.

43. Carbajo M, Ondiviela R, Garijo F, Val-Bernal F, Buelta L, Blanco C. The mitotic index in the prognosis of non-small cell lung cancer. Surg Pathol 1993;5:35–46.

44. Diggs CH, Engeler JE Jr, Prendergast EJ, Kramer K. Small cell carcinoma of the lung. Treatment in the community. Cancer 1992;69:2075–83.

45. Elson CE, Roggli VL, Vollmer RT, et al. Prognostic indicators for survival in stage 1 carcinoma of the lung: a histologic study of 47 surgically resected cases. Mod Pathol 1988;4:288–91.

46. Funa K, Steinholtz L, Nou E, Bergh J. Increased expression of N-myc in human small cell lung cancer biopsies predicts lack of response to chemotherapy and poor prognosis. Am J Clin Pathol 1987;88:216–20.

47. Furukawa T, Watanabe S, Kodama T, Sato Y, Shimosato Y, Suemasu K. T-zone histiocytes in adenocarcinoma of the lung in relation to postoperative prognosis. Cancer 1985;56:2651–6.

48. Graziano SL, Mazid R, Newmann N, et al. The use of neuroendocrine immunoperoxidase markers to predict chemotherapy response in patients with non-small cell lung cancer. J Clin Oncol 1989;7:1398–406.

49. Greenberg SD, Fraire AE, Kinner BM, Johnson EH. Tumor cell type versus staging in the prognosis of carcinoma of the lung. Pathol Annu 1987;22(Pt 2):387–405.

50. Harada M, Dosaka-Akita H, Miyamoto H, Kuzumaki N, Kawakami Y. Prognostic significance of the expression of ras oncogene product in non-small cell lung cancer. Cancer 1992;69:72–7.

51. Iannuzzi MC, Scoggin CH. Small cell lung cancer. Am Rev Respir Dis 1986;134:593–608.

52. Jett JR. Current treatment of unresectable lung cancer. Mayo Clin Proc 1993;68:603–11.

53. Kitaichi M, Asamoto H, Izumi T, Furuta M. Histological classification of regional lymph nodes in relation to postoperative survival in primary lung cancer. Hum Pathol 1981;12:1000–5.

54. Kreisman H, Wolkove N, Quoix E. Small cell lung cancer presenting as a solitary pulmonary nodule. Chest 1992;101:225–31.

55. Lee TK, Horner RD, Silverman JF, Chen YH, Jenny C, Scarantino CW. Morphometric and morphologic evaluations in stage III non-small cell lung cancers. Prognostic significance of quantitative assessment of infiltrating lymphoid cells. Cancer 1989;63:309–16.

56. Linnoila I. Pathology of non-small cell lung cancer. New diagnostic approaches. Hematol Oncol Clin North Am 1990;4:1027–51.

57. Linnoila RI, Jensen SM, Steinberg SM, Mulshine JL, Eggleston JC, Gazdar AF. Peripheral airway cell marker expression in non-small cell lung carcinoma. Association with distinct clinicopathologic features. Am J Clin Pathol 1992;97:233–43.

58. Lipford EH, Eggleston JC, Lillemoe KD, Sears DL, Moore GW, Baker RR. Prognostic factors in surgically resected limited stage non-small cell carcinoma of the lung. Am J Surg Pathol 1984;8:357–65.

59. McDonagh D, Vollmer RT, Shelburne JD. Intercellular junctions and tumor behavior in lung cancer. Mod Pathol 1991;4:436–40.

59a. Minna JD, Pass H, Glatstein E, Ihde DC. Cancer of the lung. In: DeVita VT, Hellman S, Rosenberg SA, eds. Cancer: principles and practice of oncology. 3rd ed. Philadelphia: JB Lippincott, 1989:591–705.

60. Mitsudomi T, Steinberg SM, Oie HK, et al. ras gene mutations in non-small cell lung cancers are associated with shortened survival irrespective of treatment intent. Cancer Res 1991;51:4999–5002.

61. Miyamoto H, Harada M, Isobe H, et al. Prognostic value of nuclear DNA content and expression of the ras oncogene product in lung cancer. Cancer Res 1991;51(23 Pt 1):6346–50.

62. Mountain CF. A new international staging system for lung cancer. Chest 1986;89:225S–33S.

62a. Mountain CF. Prognostic implications of the International Staging System for Lung Cancer. Semin Oncol 1988;15:236–45.

63. _____, Lukeman JM, Hammar SP, et al. Lung cancer case classification: the relationship of disease extent and cell type to survival in a clinical trials population. J Surg Oncol 1987;35:147–56.

64. Ogawa J, Iwazaki M, Tsurumi T, Inoue H, Shohtsu A. Prognostic implications of DNA histogram, DNA content, and histologic changes of regional lymph nodes in patients with lung cancer. Cancer 1991;67:1370–6.

65. Patel AM, Dunn WF, Trastek VF. Staging systems of lung cancer. Mayo Clin Proc 1993;68:475–82.

66. Pignon JP, Arriagada R, Ihde DC, et al. A meta-analysis of thoracic radiotherapy for small-cell lung cancer. N Engl J Med 1992;327:1618–24.

67. Rosenthal SA, Curran WJ. The significance of histology in non-small cell lung cancer. Cancer Treat Rev 1990;17:409–25.

68. Shahab I, Fraire AE, Greenberg SD, Johnson EH, Langston C, Roggli VL. Morphometric quantitation of tumor necrosis in stage I non-small cell carcinoma of the lung: prognostic implications. Mod Pathol 1992;5:521–4.

69. Shaw EG, Bonner JA, Foote RL, et al. Role of radiation therapy in the management of lung cancer. Mayo Clin Proc 1993;68:593–602.

70. Slebos RJ, Kibbelaar RE, Dalesio O, et al. K-ras oncogene activation as a prognostic marker in adenocarcinoma of the lung. N Engl J Med 1990;323:561–5.

71. Speissl B, Behrs OH, Hermanek P, et al International Union Against Cancer TNM atlas. New York: Springer-Verlag, 1989:134–44.

72. Stahel RA. Diagnosis, staging, and prognostic factors of small cell lung cancer. Cur Opin Oncol 1991;3:306–11.

73. Tosi P, Luzi P, Leoncini L, Miracco C, Gambacorta M, Grossi A. Bronchogenic carcinoma: survival after surgical treatment according to stage, histologic type and immunomorphologic changes in regional lymph nodes. Cancer 1981;48:2288–95.

74. Travis WD, Travis LB, Percy C, Devesa SS. Lung cancer incidence and survival by histologic type. Cancer. In press.

75. Volm M, Efferth T, Mattern J. Oncoprotein (c-myc, c-erbB1, c-erbB2, c-fos) and suppressor gene product (p53) expression in squamous cell carcinomas of the lung. Clinical and biological correlations. Anticancer Res 1992;12:11–20.

❖❖❖

9
MORPHOLOGIC DIAGNOSIS AND
HETEROGENEITY OF CARCINOMA OF THE LUNG

DIAGNOSIS

The diagnosis of lung carcinoma is based either on histologic or cytologic evaluation of specimens from the lung (see Table 3-1), direct extension sites, or metastases. About three fourths of cases of lung carcinoma are diagnosed cytologically. Some specimens, especially bronchial biopsies and cytologic preparations, include scant material, and a definitive diagnosis should be made with caution, particularly when further confirmatory or supportive material is usually readily available (for example, with sputum specimens). Since lung carcinoma is fatal in over 85 percent of cases, the diagnosis carries considerable implications and an overall conservative approach is warranted, especially for patients who have clinical evidence of a concurrent acute inflammatory process in the lungs or bronchi.

In making a histologic diagnosis of carcinoma of the lung, the following factors should be taken into account: 1) Are the clinical setting and ra-diographic findings consistent with lung carcinoma?; 2) Could a reactive or non-neoplastic process explain the changes?; 3) Have other lung tumors, such as sarcoma or lymphoma, been excluded?; 4) Is metastasis a consideration? Is there a past history of malignancy?; 5) Have sufficient criteria been met for confident subclassification according to the World Health Organization (WHO) criteria? In the case of small cell carcinoma, for example, there are a number of mimics, and one must be certain that histologic standards for diagnosis are maintained.

Pitfalls in the diagnosis of lung carcinoma are grouped broadly into those seen in histologic specimens (Table 9-1) and those seen in cytologic specimens (Table 9-2), although there is considerable overlap (figs. 9-1–9-8) (6,13,15). Awareness of a clinical history of an inflammatory process and knowledge of the spectrum of changes seen with reactive pneumocytes helps one avoid such misinterpretations.

Table 9-1

HISTOLOGIC PITFALLS IN THE DIAGNOSIS OF LUNG CARCINOMA

Poor fixation, processing, or staining

Overinterpretation of reactive bronchiolar or alveolar cell atypia associated with inflammation, radiation, viral cytopathic effect, reparative changes, chemotherapy, and so forth

Florid squamous metaplasia associated with organizing diffuse alveolar damage and around healing infarcts

Florid bronchiolar metaplasia in severely scarred lungs (honeycomb lung) and around fibrotic small airways

Interpretation of crush artifact as indicative of small cell carcinoma in chronic inflammatory lesions, lymphomas, carcinoid tumors, atypical carcinoid tumors, and metastases (particularly prostate carcinoma and breast carcinoma)

Overinterpretation of detached strips of bronchiolar mucosa as neoplastic

Interpretation of a sarcoma with epithelioid features (such as leiomyosarcoma, epithelioid sarcoma, etc.) or a melanoma as a lung carcinoma

Metastatic carcinoma (especially breast, kidney, prostate, colon), melanoma, or sarcoma mimicking a primary carcinoma

Pleural involvement by lung carcinoma misinterpreted as mesothelioma (and vice versa)

Table 9-2

CYTOLOGIC PITFALLS IN THE DIAGNOSIS OF BRONCHOGENIC CARCINOMA*

Granulomatous inflammation: infectious and noninfectious

Lung abscess

Pneumonias: bacterial and viral

Exogenous lipoid pneumonia

Bronchial asthma (creola bodies)

Pulmonary infarction

Radiation therapy

Chemotherapeutic agents

Emphysema and chronic bronchitis

Bronchiectasis

Autoimmune diseases (especially rheumatoid disease and pemphigus)

Chemical pneumonitis

---

*Modified from reference 9. These conditions may be associated with marked cytologic atypia.

HISTOLOGIC HETEROGENEITY

While the WHO classification for lung carcinomas appears relatively straightforward, it may prove difficult to apply in individual cases. A major reason for this is the histologic heterogeneity of lung carcinomas, a phenomenon recognized for many years (11). In 1967, Ashley and Davies (1) evaluated 666 cases of lung carcinoma and showed that even with a classification system that recognized only five categories (well and poorly differentiated squamous cell carcinoma, well and poorly differentiated adenocarcinoma, and undifferentiated carcinoma), 107 (16 percent) showed two or more patterns. In a recent study of 100 lung carcinomas (65 resections and 35 autopsies) that were extensively sampled and classified by five pathologists using WHO criteria, Roggli et al. (12) found that only 34 percent of the tumors were homogeneous, as agreed upon by a majority of the reviewers. Forty-five percent showed a major discrepancy (i.e., a major heterogeneity) in the WHO histologic subtypes present in at least one slide. Similarly, Dunnill and Gatter (5) found that only 18 of 66

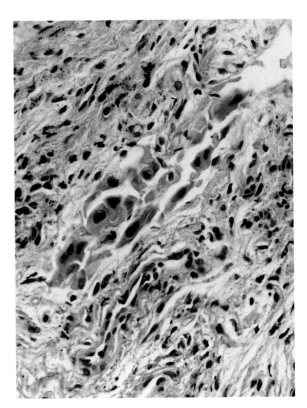

Figure 9-1
REACTIVE TYPE 2 CELLS
Atypical reactive type 2 alveolar lining cells interpreted as adenocarcinoma on a transbronchial biopsy specimen. The patient had signs and symptoms compatible with pneumonitis. The patient was well and without evidence of lung disease 1 year later. Clues to a diagnosis of reactive changes: the cells are in a single layer and vary in size and shape (in contrast to bronchioloalveolar carcinoma); the adjacent alveolar walls show a reactive fibroblastic proliferation (not shown); and the clinical history was of an inflammatory process.

carcinomas examined by light microscopy, electron microscopy, and immunohistochemical techniques comprised only one cell type; in the remaining cases, two or three cell types were present.

Most cases of large cell carcinoma show some evidence of differentiation when studied ultrastructurally or immunohistochemically (2–4,7, 10,16). Churg (3) examined eight cases of large cell carcinoma ultrastructurally and ultimately reclassified all eight as either adenocarcinoma or squamous cell carcinoma. Mooi et al. (10) examined 44 resected lung carcinomas ultrastructurally and found that 26 showed more than one type of differentiation in at least one sample examined.

Cellular heterogeneity, whether found by routine light microscopy (figs. 9-9, 9-10), histochemistry,

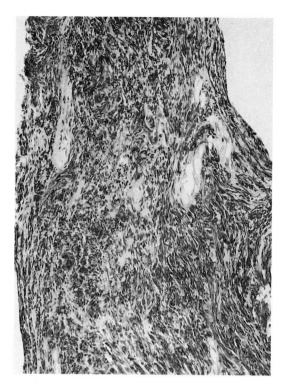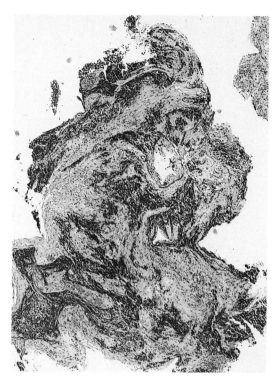

Figure 9-2
CRUSH ARTIFACT

Left: Biopsy of a small cell carcinoma without any recognizable cells in a generous biopsy. The diagnosis was confirmed on cytology specimens taken at the time of the biopsy.

Right: Biopsy from a nonsmall cell carcinoma showing crush artifact. The diagnosis of nonsmall cell carcinoma was made on concurrent cytology specimens and the rare foci showing cytologic preservation in the biopsy.

immunohistochemistry, or electron microscopy is present in most cases of lung carcinoma. This is probably because lung carcinomas are derived from pluripotential cells (8). At present, it is not clear how this should impact on routine practice and diagnosis of lung carcinomas. It is important to emphasize that the WHO classification of lung tumors is based on light microscopic criteria, and when using this system of classification, it is not appropriate to change an interpretation based solely on findings from electron microscopy or immunohistochemistry. This is not meant to minimize the usefulness of these techniques but to emphasize the necessity of uniform histologic criteria for clinical studies. Immunohistochemistry will undoubtedly take on a much greater role in future classification, and even at present is used to help define neuroendocrine lung tumors.

As has been pointed out by Sobin (14), the "accuracy" of histologic subclassification of lung carcinomas is technique-dependent, and while more precise characterization may be possible with special techniques, such as electron microscopy, it is not always clear that such studies are necessary for clinical management. For example, Sobin quotes three studies that showed a 17 to 46 percent variation in the incidence of adenosquamous carcinoma (as identified by ultrastructural features).

Since clinical management currently depends primarily on distinguishing small cell carcinomas from nonsmall cell carcinomas, the fact that this latter group shows considerable heterogeneity is not a practical problem at present. Studies have shown that the separation of small cell from nonsmall cell carcinomas is usually readily accomplished (17).

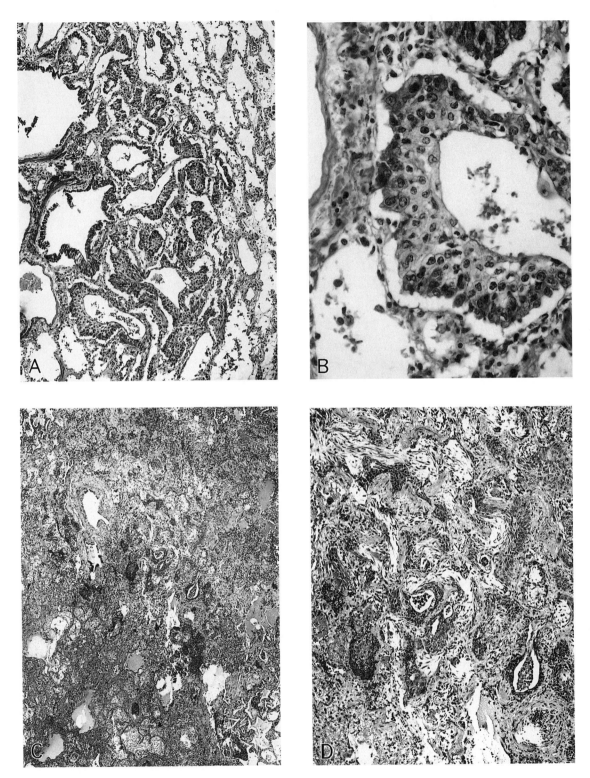

Figure 9-3
SQUAMOUS METAPLASIA
Florid peribronchiolar squamous metaplasia associated with organizing diffuse alveolar damage (A,B) and adjacent to an infarct (C,D). The case depicted in A was from a young women who died of acute diffuse pulmonary disease, and the sections were initially suspected as showing bronchioloalveolar carcinoma. In C a portion of the infarct can be seen at the lower left.

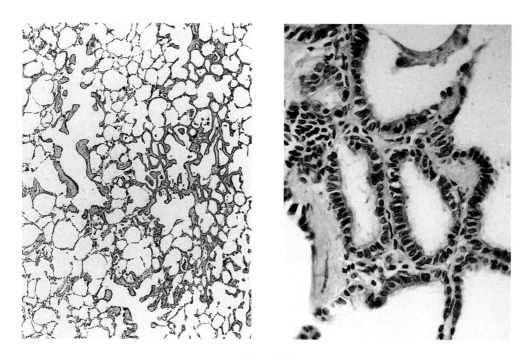

Figure 9-4
BRONCHIOLAR METAPLASIA

Bronchiolar metaplasia simulating bronchioloalveolar carcinoma.

Left: Centered on a bronchiole is a metaplastic proliferation of bronchiolar mucosa with associated peribronchiolar and interstitial scarring.

Right: Cytologically, the cells are bland and cilia can be identified.

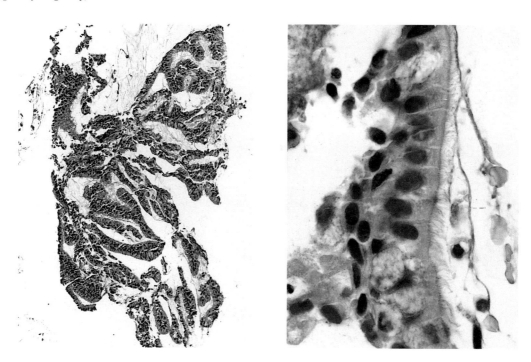

Figure 9-5
STRIPPED BRONCHIAL MUCOSA

Left: The stripped and heaped-up bronchial mucosa in this bronchial biopsy mimics a papillary carcinoma.
Right: Cilia are seen at high power.

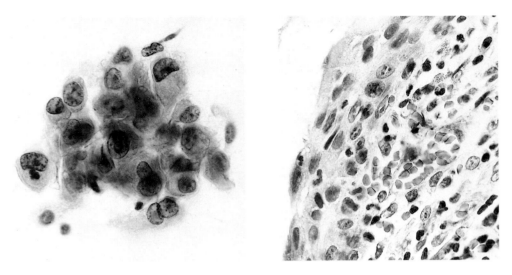

Figure 9-6
REACTIVE BRONCHIAL CELLS
Bronchial mucosal reactive changes associated with blastomycosis were overinterpreted as adenocarcinoma.
Left: The cells from a bronchial brush cytology specimen (and others like them) were interpreted as adenocarcinoma.
Right: The resected mass showed blastomycosis with atypical and reparative changes in the bronchiolar mucosa.

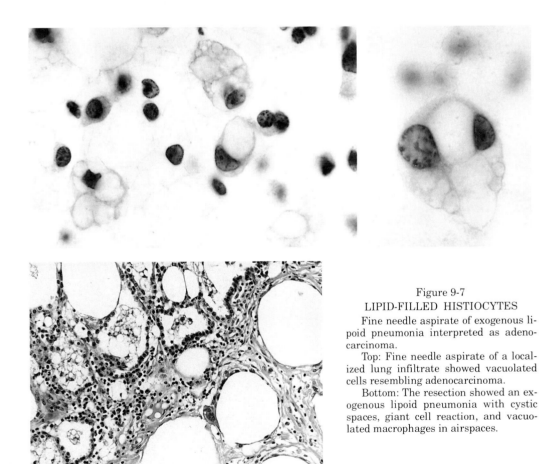

Figure 9-7
LIPID-FILLED HISTIOCYTES
Fine needle aspirate of exogenous lipoid pneumonia interpreted as adenocarcinoma.
Top: Fine needle aspirate of a localized lung infiltrate showed vacuolated cells resembling adenocarcinoma.
Bottom: The resection showed an exogenous lipoid pneumonia with cystic spaces, giant cell reaction, and vacuolated macrophages in airspaces.

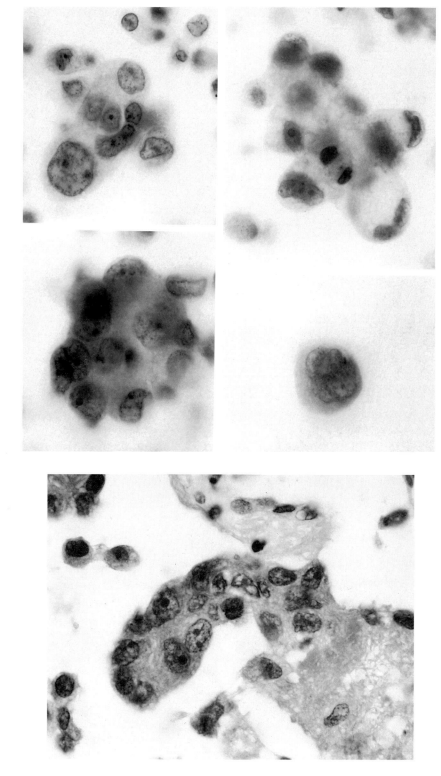

Figure 9-8
REACTIVE TYPE 2 CELLS
Top: Acute lung injury (*Klebsiella* pneumonia) mimicking bronchioloalveolar carcinoma in a bronchoalveolar lavage specimen.
Bottom: Histologic section from a biopsy of organizing pneumonia showing similar cells lying free in an alveolar space.

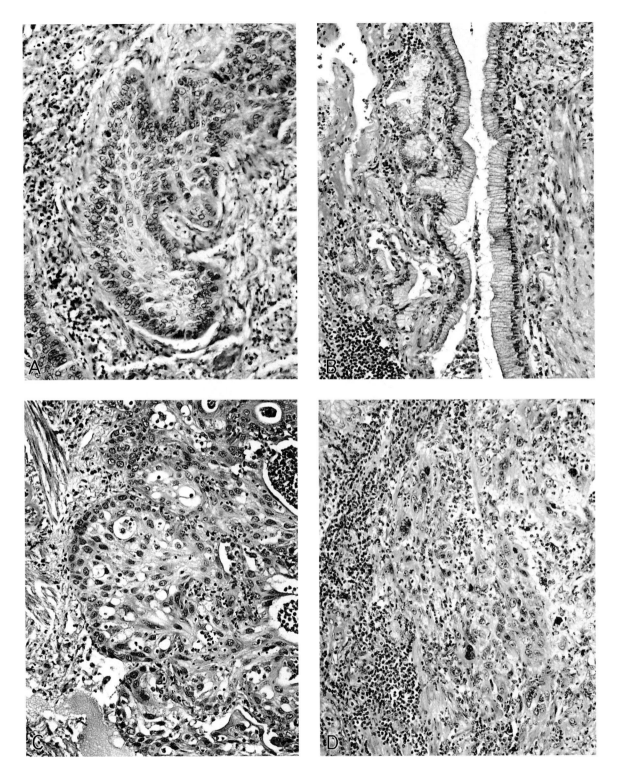

Figure 9-9
HETEROGENEITY OF BRONCHOGENIC CARCINOMA

All the fields depicted (A–E) come from two tissue blocks of a patient with a resected peripheral lung carcinoma. Foci of well-differentiated squamous cell carcinoma (A), well-differentiated mucinous adenocarcinoma (B), poorly differentiated adenocarcinoma with a somewhat mucoepidermoid appearance (C), poorly differentiated squamous cell carcinoma (D), and peculiar adenoid foci with hyalinized nodules (E) were all found.

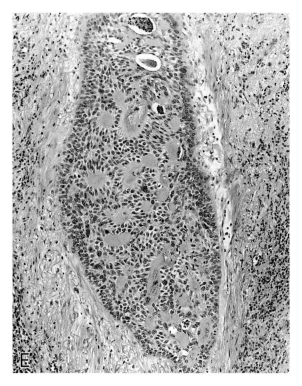

Figure 9-9 (continued)

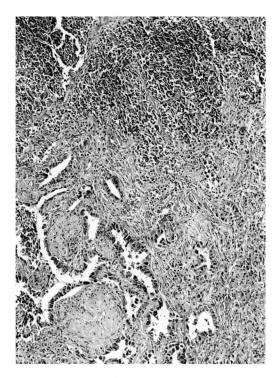

Figure 9-10
HETEROGENEITY OF
BRONCHOGENIC CARCINOMA
This mixed carcinoma shows adenocarcinoma (bottom)
and small cell carcinoma (top) in the same field.

REFERENCES

1. Ashley DJ, Davies HD. Cancer of the lung: histology and biological behavior. Cancer 1967;20:165–74.
2. Auerbach O, Frasca JM, Parks BR, Carter HW. A comparison of World Health Organization (WHO) classification of lung tumors by light and electron microscopy. Cancer 1982;50:2079–88.
3. Churg A. Fine structure of large cell undifferentiated carcinoma of the lung. Evidenced for its relation to squamous cell carcinomas and adenocarcinomas. Hum Pathol 1978;9:143–56.
4. Delmonte VC, Alberti O, Saldiva PH. Large cell carcinoma of the lung. Ultrastructural and immunohistochemical features. Chest 1986;90:524–7.
5. Dunnill MS, Gatter KC. Cellular heterogeneity in lung cancer. Histopathology 1986;10:461–75.
6. Johnston WW. Type II pneumocytes in cytologic specimens. A diagnostic dilemma [Editorial]. Am J Clin Pathol 1992;97:608–9.
7. Leong AS. The relevance of ultrastructural examination and the classification of primary lung tumors. Pathology 1982;14:37–46.
8. Linnoila I. Pathology of non-small cell lung cancer. New diagnostic approaches. Hematol Oncol Clin North Am 1990;4:1027–51.
9. Mackay B, Lukeman JM, Ordonez NG. Tumors of the lung. Philadelphia: WB Saunders, 1991:55–89.
10. Mooi WJ, Dingemans KP, Wagenaar SS, Hart AA, Wagenvoort CA. Ultrastructural heterogeneity of lung carcinomas: representativity of samples for electron microscopy in tumor classification. Hum Pathol 1990;21:1227–34.
11. Olcott CT. Cell types and histologic patterns in carcinoma of the lungs: observations on the significance of tumors containing more than one type of cell. Am J Pathol 1955;31:975–96.
12. Roggli VL, Vollmer RT, Greenberg SD, McGavran MH, Spjut HJ, Yesner R. Lung cancer heterogeneity: a blinded and randomized study of 100 consecutive cases. Hum Pathol 1985;16:569–79.
13. Saito Y, Imai T, Sato M, et al. Cytologic study of tissue repair in human bronchial epithelium. Acta Cytol 1988;32:622–8.
14. Sobin LH. The histologic classification of lung tumors: the need for a double standard. Hum Pathol 1983;14:1020–1.
15. Stanley MW, Henry-Stanley MJ, Gajl-Peczalska KJ, Bitterman PB. Hyperplasia of type II pneumocytes in acute lung injury. Cytologic findings of sequential bronchoalveolar lavage. Am J Clin Pathol 1992;97:669–77.
16. Yesner R. Large cell carcinoma of the lung. Semin Diagn Pathol 1985;2:255–69.
17. _____, Seydel GH, Asbell SO, et al. Biopsies of non-small lung cancer: central review and cooperative studies of the Radiation Therapy Oncology Group. Mod Pathol 1991;4:432–5.

10

IN SITU AND EARLY INVASIVE (OCCULT) SQUAMOUS CELL CARCINOMA

Definition. Most early squamous cell carcinomas are identified cytologically at a stage when chest roentgenograms are negative, hence the term "occult" squamous cell carcinomas (5,7,9,11,13). Many of the reported cases were found during the screening studies described in chapter 7 (7–9,11,13). Virtually all involve large airways, and about half are in situ and half are invasive (13). Most can be localized bronchoscopically either with cytologic studies (bronchial brushings and washings) or by direct visualization and bronchial biopsy (11). In the series by Cortese et al. (5), three fourths of the cases were localized within 6 months after the first positive sputum cytology, but in a small number the interval to localization was as long as 34 months.

Clinical Features. By definition, chest roentgenograms are negative. A small percentage of these cases may have lesions identifiable by computerized tomography (CT).

Some series include only asymptomatic patients (other than cough) (8,9) whereas other series include patients with a history of hemoptysis or pneumonia (7,11). All patients are smokers over the age of 40 years; the mean age in one series was 64.5 years (10). Most cases occur in men, owing largely to the fact most series are derived from screening studies of male smokers.

Gross Findings. In situ squamous cell carcinomas of the large airways are grossly visible in about half the cases (13): slight irregularities in the bronchial mucosa are seen with granularity, papillation, and loss of rugae; in the remainder, the involved regions of the bronchial mucosa cannot be distinguished from normal tissue (fig. 10-1A). In early invasive squamous cell carcinomas, the former features are more pronounced, with nodular thickening but without extensive exophytic growth (fig. 10-2).

Occult squamous cell carcinomas are typically situated in a segmental bronchus, and invasion occurs in the setting of associated carcinoma in situ. The distribution and associated mucosal changes of seven lesions described by Melamed et al. (9) are shown in figure 10-3. The distribu-

tion of 20 early squamous cell carcinomas described by Carter (2) is shown in Table 10-1.

Microscopic Findings. Atypical mucosal changes that fall short of carcinoma in situ may or may not be seen in association with occult squamous cell carcinoma (2–4,8). These changes include squamous metaplasia, degrees of mucosal atypia (dysplasia/dyskaryosis), basal cell hyperplasia, and basal cell atypia (fig. 10-4). The exact distinction and grading of these findings is somewhat arbitrary, but the criteria of Saccomanno (see figs. 7-5 and 7-6) (12) are generally accepted for sputum cytology. Figure 10-4 shows the histologic spectrum of these changes. These changes are not always seen, and in some cases carcinoma in situ directly abuts normal bronchial mucosa (fig. 10-5) (2,3,9).

The microscopic criteria for squamous cell carcinoma in situ of the lung are similar to those applied elsewhere in the body and include an intact basement membrane with a full-thickness abnormality in the mucosa (1,2–4,9,13). The nuclei show abnormalities in size and shape, chromatin pattern with hyperchromasia, increased and often abnormal mitotic figures, and an increased nuclear-cytoplasmic ratio (figs. 10-1, 10-5–10-8). Since some squamous maturation may be seen at the surface, the criteria for full-thickness involvement may be difficult to apply, and the distinction between severe atypia and carcinoma in situ may be arbitrary. In invasive carcinoma, surface changes that do not fulfill the criteria of carcinoma in situ may be seen in

Table 10-1

FEATURES OF 20 EARLY SQUAMOUS CELL CARCINOMAS

	Airways Affected		
	Segmental	Lobar	Main Stem
Invasive carcinoma	9	1	2
Carcinoma in situ	15	16	6

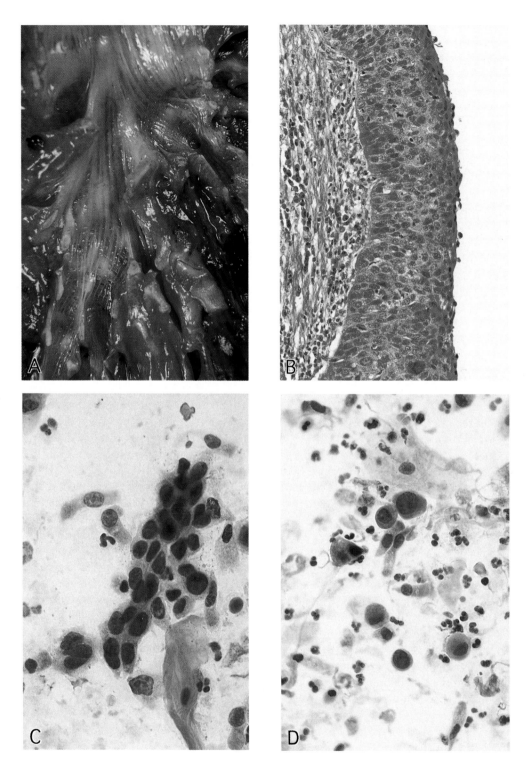

Figure 10-1
CARCINOMA IN SITU

There are no gross mucosal abnormalities (A) in this case of squamous cell carcinoma in situ (B). Preoperative bronchoscopic evaluation in this case showed carcinoma cells in the bronchial brush (C) and bronchial wash (D) specimens. In C there is a cluster of hyperchromatic cells with a high nuclear-cytoplasmic ratio. Adjacent bland-appearing keratinized squamous cells are also present. The bronchial wash specimen (D) shows isolated keratinized cells with deeply orangophilic cytoplasm, hyperchromatic nuclei, and a high nuclear-cytoplasmic ratio.

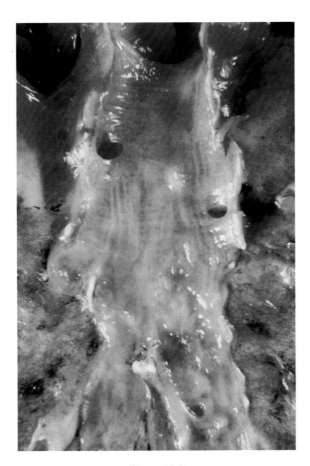

Figure 10-2
EARLY INVASIVE SQUAMOUS CELL
CARCINOMA: GROSS FINDINGS
This case showed carcinoma in situ with foci of early invasion. The latter foci can be seen grossly as areas of nodular thickening (lower right) in subsegmental bronchi adjacent to a bronchial bifurcation.

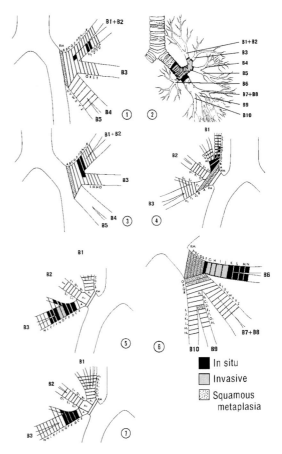

Figure 10-3
CARCINOMA IN SITU
Diagram of the mucosal changes in seven cases of radiologically occult squamous cell carcinoma of the lung. (Figs. 1-7 from Melamed MR, Zaman MB, Flehinger BJ, Martini N. Radiologically occult in situ and incipient epidermoid lung cancer: detection by sputum cytology in a survey of asymptomatic cigarette smokers. Am J Surg Pathol 1977;1:5–16.)

continuity with the underlying invasive lesion (fig. 10-9). In such cases, invasion is the most important finding, but for lesions that are entirely in situ, maintenance of strict criteria is appropriate.

Histologically, carcinoma in situ is usually associated with thickening of the mucosa; bulbous masses of cells may replace the mucosa. Carcinoma in situ often extends down the ducts of submucosal glands (fig. 10-8), and invasion may start at this site (3). However, unless the cells cross the basement membrane and invade the adjacent stroma, the tumor is still considered in situ even if there is extensive submucosal gland

involvement. Carcinoma in situ involving the ducts may be difficult to distinguish from broad-based submucosal invasive nests that have minimal stromal reaction (fig. 10-8). Chronic inflammation may be seen with both, but stromal desmoplasia is often a feature of invasion.

Most early invasive carcinomas are moderate to well-differentiated tumors (13). The criteria for early invasion in squamous carcinomas of the lung are similar to other sites, with the same attendant problems. Invasion is readily identified if there are single cells (fig. 10-9) or irregular jagged nests of cells with an associated stromal

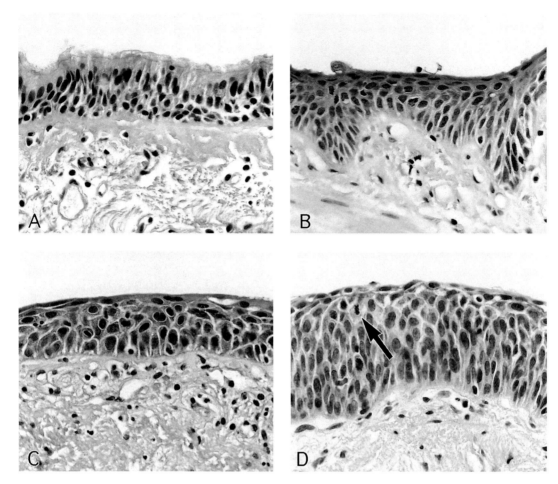

Figure 10-4
MUCOSAL ATYPIA

The spectrum of associated atypical mucosal changes is illustrated in a case of carcinoma in situ. There is mild basal cell hyperplasia in mucosa that maintains its ciliary border (A), squamous metaplasia with mild to moderate atypia (B), squamous metaplasia with moderate atypia (C), and marked squamous atypia with mitotic figures (arrow) extending close to the surface (D).

Table 10-2

CLASSIFICATION OF 68 OCCULT SQUAMOUS CELL CARCINOMAS*

Category	Depth of Invasion	No. of Cases (%)
Carcinoma in situ	0	23 (34)
Intramucosal invasion	<0.1 cm	12 (18)
Invasion to bronchial cartilage	0.11-0.30 cm	11 (16)
Deep invasion to full thickness of bronchial wall	0.31-0.5 cm	10 (14)
Extrabronchial invasion	> 0.5 cm	12 (18)

*From reference 13.

reaction and vascular invasion (fig. 10-10). Cases that show invasion as broad nests with little stromal reaction may be extremely difficult to separate from carcinoma in situ (fig. 10-8). In a series of 68 cases, Woolner et al. (13) recognized five categories of occult squamous cell carcinoma based on absence or presence of invasion and depth of invasion (Table 10-2). The term intramucosal was used to signify early stromal (submucosal) invasion that did not extend to the bronchial cartilage. As shown in Table 10-2, occult squamous cell carcinomas may be deeply invasive, but in the absence of luminal occlusion or sufficient size for roentgenographic recognition, they remain occult.

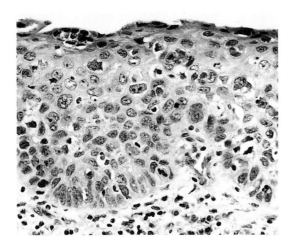
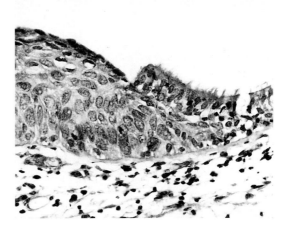

Figure 10-5
CARCINOMA IN SITU
Squamous carcinoma in situ showing full thickness cytologic atypia with some cytoplasmic keratinization near the surface.
Left: Despite the maturation, there is complete cellular disarray, and atypical nuclei extend all the way to the surface.
Right: In another case, there is an abrupt transition between squamous carcinoma in situ and normal mucosa.

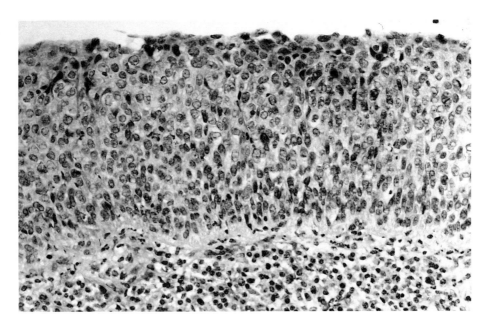

Figure 10-6
CARCINOMA IN SITU
Squamous carcinoma in situ with full thickness mucosal replacement by atypical small cells with little squamous differentiation. There is prominent submucosal chronic inflammation.

Nagamoto et al. (10) studied 92 occult squamous cell carcinomas in 83 resection specimens. Based on serial studies comparing depth of invasion and superficial extent (length of airway affected) of the carcinoma in situ, two groups were delineated. The "creeping type" of carcinoma was the more common of the two. These tumors were slow growing, with a greater propensity for longitudinal growth within the mucosa rather than deep invasion. The "penetrating type" was much less common. These tumors were rapidly evolving, with a greater propensity for deep penetration.

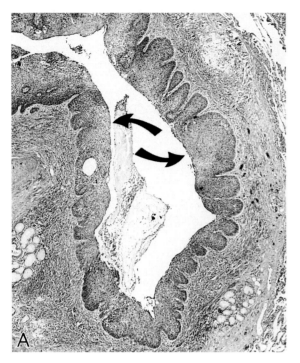

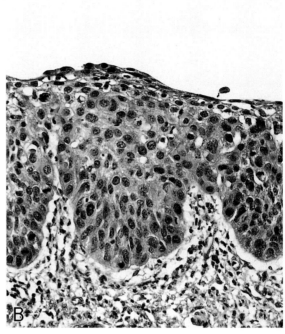

Figure 10-7
CARCINOMA IN SITU

Squamous carcinoma in situ entirely replacing the mucosa of a small bronchus (A,B). In some foci (B), the features of carcinoma in situ are obvious, with full thickness replacement in the mucosa, whereas in other foci (arrows), definite maturation is apparent. The preresection bronchial brush cytology specimen from this case shows neoplastic squamous cells (C). The nuclei are cytologically malignant and there is relatively abundant cytoplasm showing the irregular shape and increased density typical of squamous differentiation.

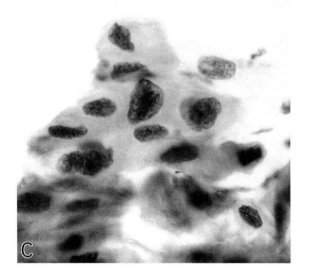

The cytologic features of occult squamous cell carcinoma (see figs. 7-5, 7-6 and 10-1, 10-7, 10-8, 10-11, 10-12) are similar to those of ordinary squamous cell carcinoma and are outlined in Table 10-2. Briefly, cytologic preparations show malignant squamous cells in a relatively clean background due to the lack of necrosis. Degrees of squamous atypia usually accompany the malignant cells (see fig. 7-5).

Differential Diagnosis. The differential diagnosis of squamous cell carcinoma in situ and lesser degrees of dysplasia in the bronchial mucosa includes two broad groups of lesions: reactive mucosal atypias and invasive squamous carcinoma. As in the cervix, reactive changes in the bronchial mucosa may be difficult to distinguish from dysplasia and carcinoma in situ. A history of radiation therapy, pneumonia, or bronchitis;

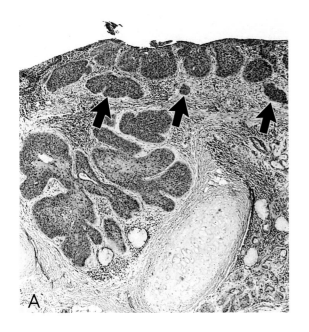

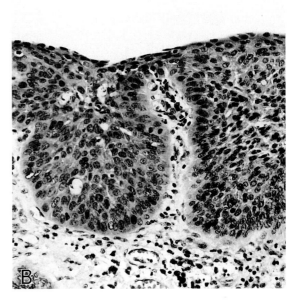

Figure 10-8
CARCINOMA IN SITU

Squamous carcinoma in situ (A,B) with prominent involvement of submucosal glands (A). This case probably has early submucosal invasion (arrows), but it is extremely difficult to separate from involvement of submucosal glands and their ducts. Markedly atypical cells had been identified in sputum cytology specimens (C) 2 years before this lesion could be localized and resected.

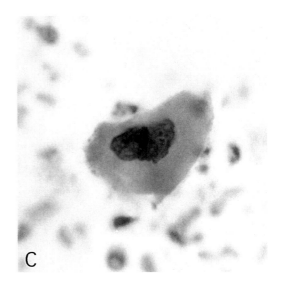

inflammatory changes seen at bronchoscopy; acute inflammatory cells infiltrating the mucosa; and foci of ulceration point to reactive bronchial mucosal changes. Reactive epithelium may overlie invasive carcinoma. Reactive lesions generally have a tendency to mature, and the cells often have relatively abundant cytoplasm and large vesicular nuclei with prominent nucleoli. The nuclei are more uniform and lack the hyperchromasia and nuclear membrane irregularities seen in carcinoma in situ. In difficult cases, follow-up sputum cytology specimens and

sometimes even repeat bronchoscopy are necessary for accurate diagnosis.

Invasive squamous carcinoma enters the differential diagnosis when a sample is insufficient to confirm definite evidence of invasion and small detached fragments raise the possibility of carcinoma in situ. The radiographic and bronchoscopic findings are extremely helpful in such cases. Carcinoma in situ is not associated with a mass on the chest radiograph, and the mucosa may appear grossly normal or show only minor abnormalities to the bronchoscopist; invasive carcinomas are

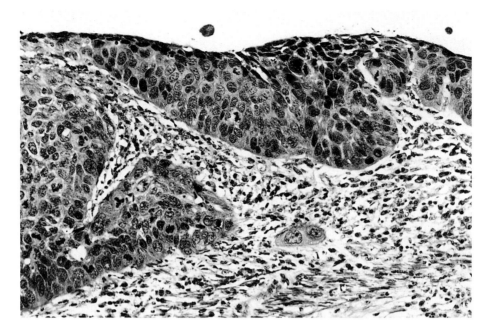

Figure 10-9
EARLY INVASIVE SQUAMOUS CARCINOMA
Early submucosal invasion is seen as a detached pair of squamous cells (right center) in the submucosa. The overlying mucosa shows features of carcinoma in situ.

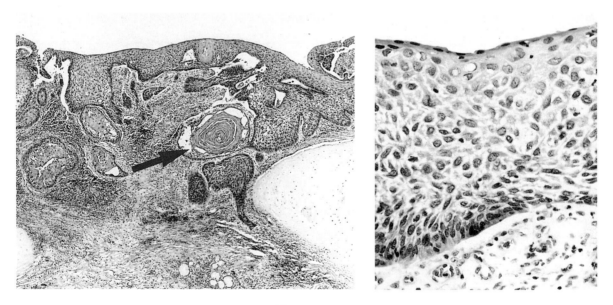

Figure 10-10
EARLY INVASIVE SQUAMOUS CARCINOMA
Left: Invasive well-differentiated keratinizing squamous carcinoma with extension to the bronchial cartilage. A large nest of keratinized cells are apparent (arrow), and tongues of carcinoma extend below and around a bronchial cartilage.
Right: The overlying mucosa does not show classic full thickness cytologic features of carcinoma in situ.

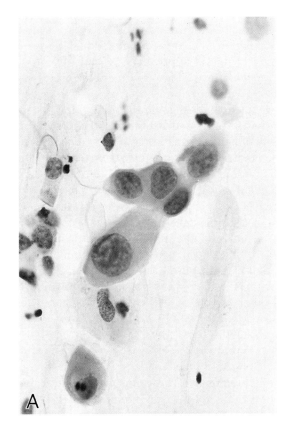

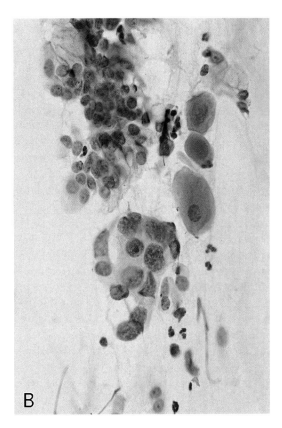

Figure 10-11
CARCINOMA IN SITU

Neoplastic squamous cells (A,B) from a bronchial brush specimen of the case illustrated in figure 10-4. Not all the cells show orangeophilic cytoplasm; however, the marked hyperchromasia of the nuclei, lack of nucleoli, and a dense cytoplasm all favor squamous differentiation. In B, keratinized cells lacking features of carcinoma can be seen adjacent to a cluster of carcinoma cells. Such metaplastic squamous cells are commonly seen in this setting; they can be compared with the normal bronchial mucosal cells adjacent to them.

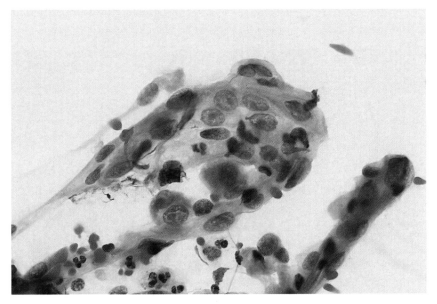

Figure 10-12
CARCINOMA IN SITU

A bronchial brush specimen shows orangophilia of the cytoplasm which is not as dense as is typically seen in squamous carcinoma. In addition, some of the cells have nucleoli. Nevertheless, the cells have malignant nuclei that are hyperchromatic and have an irregular nuclear border and an elongated cytoplasm which is in keeping with squamous differentiation.

usually readily visible to the bronchoscopist and are often visible on the chest radiograph.

Spread. The majority of occult squamous cell carcinomas are indolent tumors with a relatively favorable prognosis (see below), and as such, may be biologically different from ordinary squamous cell carcinomas. The data of Nagomoto et al. (10) support this: the less common but much more aggressive penetrating type of early squamous cell carcinoma may simply represent very early squamous cell carcinoma of the ordinary type which has been fortuitously identified.

In Woolner's series (13) only 3 of 68 cases showed vascular (capillary) invasion. This contrasts with the over 80 percent incidence of vascular invasion seen in ordinary lung carcinomas (chapter 8). Lymph node metastases from occult squamous cell carcinomas were seen in 9 of 62 resections in Woolner's series; in all 9 a single peribronchial lymph node was involved.

Multicentricity and the Risk of Subsequent Primary Carcinomas. The frequency of epithelial atypia at some distance from an invasive lesion (fig. 10-1) suggests that multicentricity should be expected. Similarly, the classic study by Auerbach et al. (1) showed that carcinoma in situ was relatively widespread in the bronchial tree of smokers, particularly in those with lung carcinoma. Data summarized by Carter (3), showed that 22 percent of patients with occult squamous cell carcinoma develop a second primary carcinoma at a later date. Woolner et al. (13) found 4 concurrent second primary carcinomas among 54 cases (7 percent) and showed that the risk for sequential second carcinoma was 10 times the risk

of lung carcinoma generally seen in high-risk populations; all second carcinomas were squamous cell, and approximately half were in situ.

Treatment. The treatment of occult squamous cell carcinoma of the lung is resection provided the lesion can be adequately localized prior to surgery (3,13). Frozen section confirmation of a negative bronchial margin is important since direct visualization at bronchoscopy or at the time of resection is not reliable for identifying normal mucosa.

Recently, photodynamic therapy with hematoporphyrin derivatives has been used as an alternative in the management of biopsy-proven early superficial squamous cell carcinoma (6). Edell et al. (6) used this therapy on 13 patients (with 14 lesions) who were otherwise surgical candidates. Thirteen lesions showed a complete response after one (10 lesions) or two (3 lesions) treatments. Ten of the 13 (77 percent) lesions did not recur during a follow-up period of 49 months.

Prognosis. The prognosis for occult squamous cell carcinoma of the lung is very favorable in comparison to lung carcinoma in general (3). The resectability rate is 60 to 95 percent, with a 5-year survival of 57 to 87 percent (3). The favorable prognosis may reflect the fact that most occult squamous cell carcinomas are biologically different from their clinically apparent counterparts, being inherently indolent and more slowly growing, i.e., the creeping type of Nagamoto et al. (10).

For patients who develop a second primary after resection of occult squamous cell carcinoma, the prognosis is poor due to insufficient pulmonary reserve for a second resection (3).

REFERENCES

1. Auerbach O, Gere JB, Pawlowski JM, Muehsam GE, Smolin HJ, Stout AP. Carcinoma in situ and early invasive carcinoma occurring in the tracheal bronchial trees in cases of bronchial carcinoma. J Thorac Surg 1957;34:298–309.
2. Carter D. Pathology of early squamous cell carcinoma of the lung. Pathol Annu 1978;13(Pt 1):131–47.
3. _____. Squamous cell carcinoma of the lung: an update. Semin Diagn Pathol 1985;2:226–34.
4. _____, Marsh BR, Baker R, Erozan YS, Frost JK. Relationships of morphology to clinical presentation in ten cases of early squamous cell carcinoma of the lung. Cancer 1976;37:1389–96.
5. Cortese DA, Pairolero PC, Bergstralh EJ, et al. Roentgenographically occult lung cancer. J Thorac Cardiovasc Surg 1983;86:373–80.
6. Edell ES, Cortese DA. Photodynamic therapy in the management of early superficial squamous cell carcinoma as an alternative to surgical resection. Chest 1992;102:1319–22.
7. Martini N, Beattie EJ Jr, Cliffton EE, Melamed MR. Radiologically occult lung cancer. Report of 26 cases. Surg Clin North Am 1974;54:811–23.
8. Melamed MR, Flehinger BJ, Zaman MB, Heelan RT, Hallerman ET, Martini N. Detection of true pathologic stage I lung cancer in a screening program and the effect on survival. Cancer 1981;47:1182–7.

9. _____, Zaman MB, Flehinger BJ, Martini N. Radiologically occult in situ and incipient invasive epidermoid lung cancer: detection by sputum cytology in a survey of asymptomatic cigarette smokers. Am J Surg Pathol 1977;1:5–16.

10. Nagamoto N, Saito Y, Suda H, et al. Relationship between length of longitudinal extension and maximal depth of transmural invasion and roentgenographically occult squamous cell carcinoma of the bronchus (nonpolypoid type). Am J Surg Pathol 1989;13:11–20.

11. Pearson FG, Thompson DW, Delarue NC. Experience with the cytologic detection, localization, and treatment of radiologically undemonstrable bronchial carcinoma. J Thorac Cardiovasc Surg 1967;54:371–82.

12. Saccomanno G, Archer VE, Auerbach O, Saunders RP, Brennan LM: Development of carcinoma of the lung as reflected in exfoliated cells. Cancer 1974;33:256–70.

13. Woolner LB, Fontana RS, Cortese DA, et al. Roentgenographically occult lung cancer: pathologic findings and frequency of multicentricity during a ten-year period. Mayo Clin Proc 1984;59:453–66.

11
SQUAMOUS CELL CARCINOMA AND VARIANTS

Definition. Squamous cell carcinoma (*epidermoid carcinoma*) of the lung is a malignant epithelial tumor with the differentiating features of squamous epithelium: keratinization, intercellular bridges, or both (25). The extent to which an individual tumor has these features varies with the degree of differentiation: well-differentiated squamous cell carcinomas often are abundantly keratinized and intercellular bridges are usually easy to find; these features are less prominent in moderately differentiated tumors and focal in poorly differentiated squamous carcinomas where much of the tumor resembles large cell carcinoma. When well-defined components of adenocarcinoma or small cell carcinoma are present, a diagnosis of mixed carcinoma is appropriate, and each component present should be designated. An occasional mucin droplet on mucin stains, or an occasional lumen ultrastructurally, is not uncommon in otherwise typical squamous cell carcinoma of the lung and is a reminder of the histologic heterogeneity so frequently seen in lung carcinomas.

The tumors discussed in this section are clinically manifest squamous cell carcinomas in contrast to the occult tumors discussed in chapter 10.

Clinical Features. The clinical features of lung carcinoma in general are discussed in chapters 7 and 8. Squamous cell carcinoma has recently been surpassed in frequency by adenocarcinoma in many series (11). Squamous cell carcinomas tend to be central (two thirds of cases) rather than peripheral, and because of the frequent involvement of large airways, exfoliated cells are more commonly identified in sputum cytology specimens than in other types of lung carcinoma; symptoms related to the local effects of the tumor are also more frequent (11, 17,18,20). Ninety-eight percent of patients with squamous cell carcinoma of the lung have a history of cigarette smoking, and the majority are men (see Table 7-4). Human papillomavirus has been found in an appreciable percentage of squamous cell carcinomas (18 percent) and bronchial squamous metaplasias (10 percent), partic-ularly when condylomatous changes are seen histologically (1).

Gross Findings. Clinically manifest squamous cell carcinomas vary from small endobronchial obstructive tumors to large cavitated masses that can replace an entire lung (figs. 11-1–11-3) (11,17,18,20,24). Even small tumors may cavitate. The masses are gray-white or yellowish, often with a dry, flaky appearance that reflects the keratinization. Necrosis and hemorrhage are common; cavitation is seen in one third of cases. Secondary infections in cavitated masses may occur. Some tumors are firm and white due to prominent stromal desmoplasia.

Most tumors involve the segmental and subsegmental bronchi (18); an in situ carcinomatous component or mucosal atypia of varying degree may be identified in the adjacent bronchial mucosa (proximal or distal). These features should be specifically sought in sections of the bronchial resection margin, particularly in frozen sections taken at the time of resection (20). Squamous cell carcinomas are smaller than other lung carcinomas because they tend to manifest earlier with symptoms of obstruction (20). Endobronchial exophytic polypoid masses may or may not be associated with invasion into the surrounding parenchyma. Gross and histologic evidence of obstruction is commonly present in the parenchyma distal to the tumor mass and includes atelectasis, mucostasis, organization, secondary infection, or abscess formation; their presence should be noted.

Microscopic Findings. Squamous cell carcinoma of the lung may be divided into well-differentiated, moderately differentiated, and poorly differentiated subtypes, depending on the degree of squamous differentiation present (figs. 11-4–11-11) (25). Intercellular bridges and keratinization are most marked in well-differentiated tumors. Some tumors have an oncocytoid appearance correlating with prominent mitochondria seen ultrastructurally (12,13). Many nonsquamous lung tumors may be squamoid and should not be interpreted as squamous cell carcinoma unless definite keratinization or intercellular bridges can be identified.

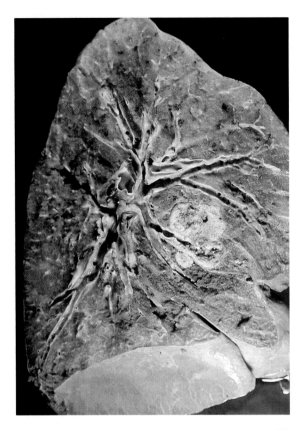
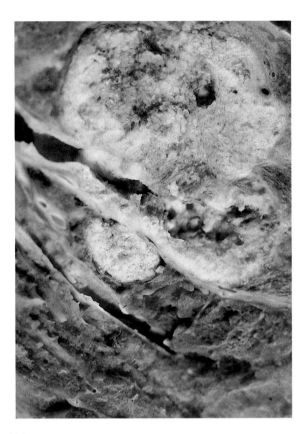

Figure 11-1
SQUAMOUS CELL CARCINOMA

This squamous cell carcinoma involves a segmental bronchus (left, right), which is eroded and destroyed by the cavitating mass. The tumor has a somewhat granular or flaky appearance due to the keratinization. The high frequency of positive exfoliative cytology specimens from such cases results from the degree of bronchial involvement.

Figure 11-2
SQUAMOUS
CELL CARCINOMA

Squamous cell carcinoma involving a subsegmental bronchus with distal chronic obstructive pneumonia. The tumor is seen as a rounded nodule, approximately 2 cm in diameter, proximal to a more irregular focus of chronic obstructive pneumonia with fibrosis.

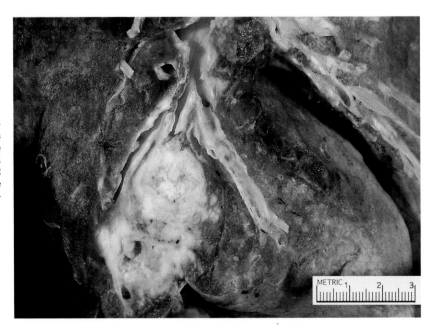

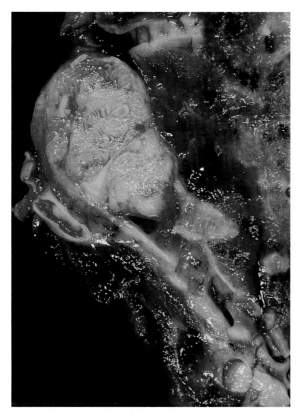

Figure 11-3
ENDOBRONCHIAL SQUAMOUS CELL CARCINOMA
Endobronchial, polypoid, moderately differentiated squamous cell carcinoma filling a segmental bronchus. Only minimal extension outside the bronchial cartilage is present. This is the same case as illustrated in figure 11-8.

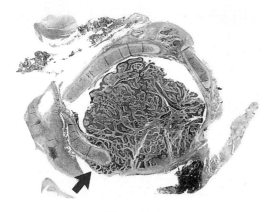

Figure 11-4
SQUAMOUS CELL CARCINOMA
Endobronchial growth by the moderately differentiated squamous cell carcinoma illustrated in figure 11-3. Only minimal extension of the carcinoma around the outside of the bronchial cartilage can be seen (arrow).

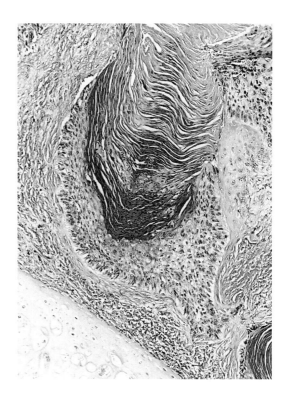

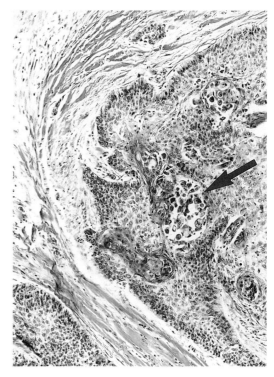

Figure 11-5
SQUAMOUS CELL CARCINOMA
Well-differentiated squamous cell carcinoma showing layered keratin formation (top) and central dyscohesion (arrow) by keratinized cells (bottom).

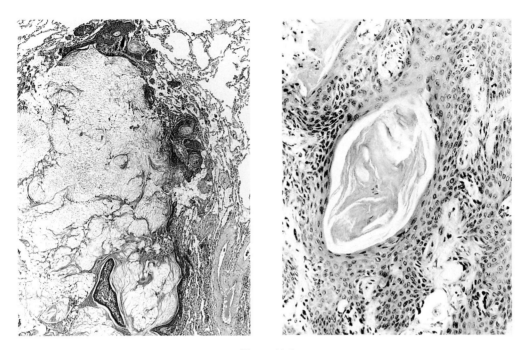

Figure 11-6
EXTREMELY WELL-DIFFERENTIATED KERATINIZING SQUAMOUS CELL CARCINOMA
This elderly woman, with no history of prior laryngeal or large airway disease, had a solitary pulmonary mass resected.
Left: Histologically, this is an extremely well-differentiated keratinizing squamous cell carcinoma with a large central mass of keratin.
Right: The infiltrative edges are composed of well-differentiated cells lacking overt cytologic features of malignancy.

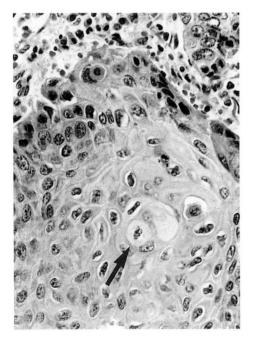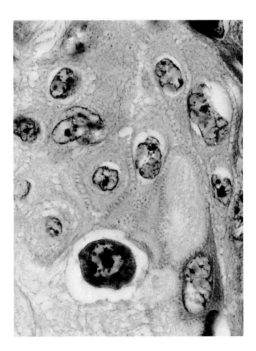

Figure 11-7
SQUAMOUS CELL CARCINOMA
Left: Moderately differentiated squamous cell carcinoma showing well-defined cell nests with central squamous maturation and increased cytoplasm. Individual cell keratinization and keratin pearl formation (arrow) can be identified.
Right: Intercellular bridges are best seen with the condenser diaphragm partially closed.

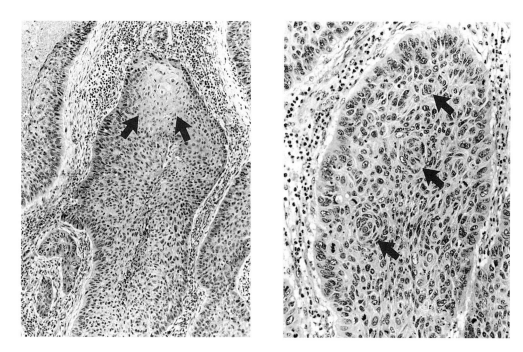

Figure 11-8
SQUAMOUS CELL CARCINOMA

Moderately differentiated squamous cell carcinoma showing central squamous differentiation with large cells with voluminous cytoplasm (left, arrows) and squamous pearl formation (right, arrows).

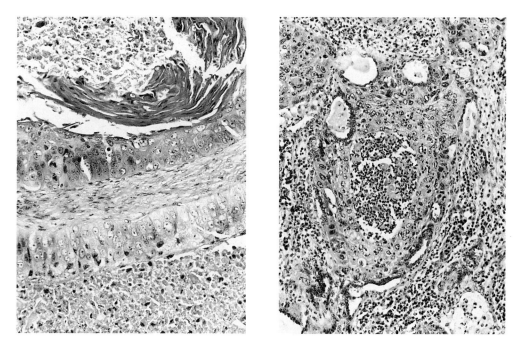

Figure 11-9
SQUAMOUS CELL CARCINOMA

Left: Poorly differentiated squamous cell carcinoma showing keratinization directly from poorly differentiated cells (top) and amorphous necrotic debris associated with similar cells (bottom).

Right: In another poorly differentiated squamous cell carcinoma, the cell nests show necrosis and accumulation of acute inflammatory cells (center). Growth of the tumor nests around the alveolar spaces has left behind small acinar structures (the residual alveoli) lined by reactive type 2 cells.

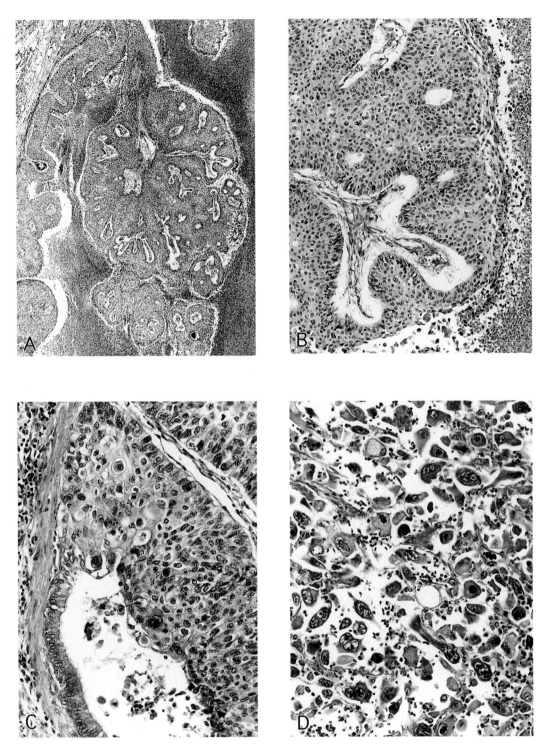

Figure 11-10
SQUAMOUS CELL CARCINOMA
Moderately differentiated squamous cell carcinoma with a variable histologic picture. The endobronchial component of this tumor has replaced the bronchial mucosa (A) and grown as an endobronchial papillary mass with surrounding necrotic debris (A,B). A sharp transition between normal bronchial mucosa and endobronchial growth is present (C). The extrabronchial component of this tumor is represented by a mass composed of pleomorphic malignant cells (D) lacking any squamous differentiation and most closely resembling a bizarre sarcoma. Transitions were seen between the histologic components of this carcinoma.

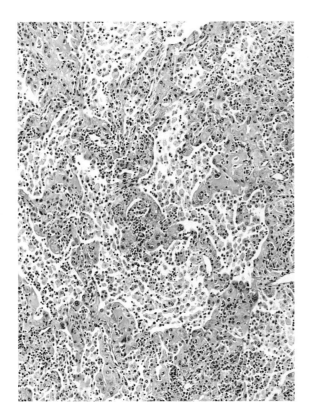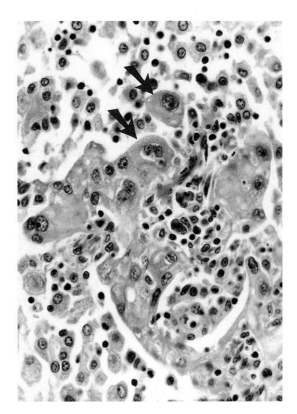

Figure 11-11
SQUAMOUS CELL CARCINOMA
Left: Poorly differentiated squamous carcinoma manifesting as an endobronchial dyscohesive mass with numerous inflammatory cells.
Right: The neoplastic squamous cells are seen as small clusters and individual cells showing dense eosinophilic cytoplasm characteristic of squamous differentiation (arrows).

Squamous cell carcinomas tend to grow as nests of cells, with surrounding stroma that may be desmoplastic and infiltrated by acute or chronic inflammatory cells. The nests typically show zonation, with increasing amounts of cytoplasm centrally where keratinization and intercellular bridges are most prominent. Acute inflammation and foreign body giant cell reaction are often seen among the keratinous debris; central cavitation of cell nests is common. Some poorly differentiated squamous cell carcinomas show marked cellular dyscohesion with extensive infiltration by inflammatory cells and they may be difficult to distinguish from the inflammatory variant of malignant fibrous histiocytoma or Hodgkin disease. The dyscohesive component may have features of giant cell carcinoma (chapter 15).

At the periphery of the nodules, tumor cell nests often grow in intact airspaces (see fig. 8-2). The neoplastic cells may replace or elevate the alveolar lining cells, producing small acini among the large pleomorphic carcinoma cells (see figs. 8-3, 11-9).

Rare mucin vacuoles may be found in otherwise typical squamous cell carcinomas of the lung (fig. 11-12) and do not necessarily indicate a component of adenocarcinoma. A distinct glandular component (over 5 percent) should be present before a diagnosis of adenosquamous carcinoma is considered (chapter 16). In a study by Gatter et al. (8), approximately half the squamous cell carcinomas showed intracellular Alcian blue–positive mucinous material and one fourth showed at least focal staining with the argyrophil (Grimelius) stain.

The nuclei are hyperchromatic, sometimes with prominent nucleoli and thick chromatin condensation along the nuclear membrane. Nuclei vary from cell to cell (except in very well-differentiated carcinomas), and the cytologic diagnosis

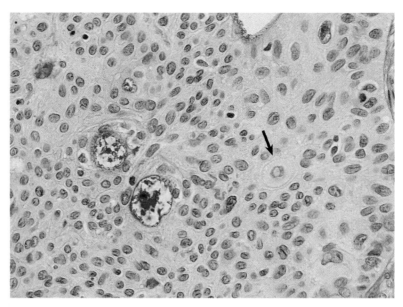

Figure 11-12
SQUAMOUS
CELL CARCINOMA
Mucin production in a moderately differentiated squamous carcinoma. Digested PAS stain shows mucin droplets of varying sizes. Squamous cells with intercellular bridges are present (arrow).

of malignancy is usually straightforward. In foci of keratinization, the nuclei become progressively more dense, lose their nuclear structure, and appear as hyperchromatic, densely hematoxyphilic blobs in bizarre-shaped keratinized cells.

There is a subset of squamous cell carcinoma that is extremely well-differentiated and lacks obvious cytologic features of malignancy (see fig. 11-6); these carcinomas are recognized as malignant by their invasion of the surrounding lung parenchyma. They produce large amounts of keratin and are thus similar to the well-differentiated squamous cell carcinomas developing in chronic draining sinus tracts. These carcinomas are difficult to distinguish from laryngeal papillomatosis that has descended into the bronchial tree. The few cases we have seen have not shown condylomatous features cytologically. In addition, marked keratinization in a squamous cell carcinoma of the lung should lead to consideration of a metastasis, particularly from the head and neck.

Like other lung carcinomas, squamous cell carcinoma may show diverse morphologic patterns: spindling, tumor giant cells, osteoclastic giant cells (16,19), and clear cells (15).

Inflammatory changes commonly occur in the surrounding lung tissue. Squamous cell carcinomas are associated with airway obstruction and distal inflammatory changes in the lung parenchyma. These include accumulations of foamy macrophages in the airspaces, interstitial inflam-

matory infiltrates, type 2 cells, and varying degrees of organization and fibrosis. If there is secondary infection, acute inflammation may be present. A non-necrotizing granulomatous reaction is sometimes seen and may involve hilar lymph nodes; distinguishing such a reaction from sarcoidosis is difficult and somewhat arbitrary. Obstruction of airways may be associated with a necrotizing granulomatous reaction resembling bronchocentric granulomatosis; granulomatous infections should also be carefully excluded.

Histologic grading is difficult in lung carcinomas that show a variation in pattern and differentiation from one tumor block to the next (20). In addition, it is not clear whether grade has any prognostic significance at present. Nevertheless, provided the lesion has been adequately sampled, tumors should be graded by the most predominant component, using three categories: well, moderately, and poorly differentiated. Specific comments about any other components present should be included.

The cytologic features of squamous cell carcinoma (figs. 11-13–11-15) vary with the degree of differentiation and whether or not the cells are keratinized (14,17,18). Most tumors show some cellular dyscohesion, especially in exfoliated cells. Nonkeratinized tumor cells have a high nuclear-cytoplasmic ratio; large hyperchromatic nuclei, sometimes with prominent nucleoli, especially in bronchial brush and aspiration material;

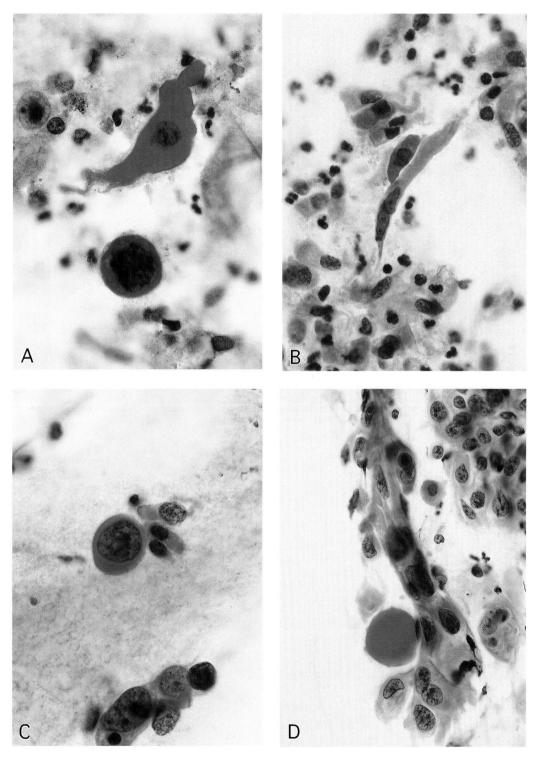

Figure 11-13
CYTOLOGIC FEATURES OF SQUAMOUS CELL CARCINOMA
There are large bizarre-shaped keratinized cells with hyperchromatic nuclei, some of which show cytoplasmic orangophilia (A). Keratinized carcinoma cells can be compared with normal ciliated bronchial lining cells (B). Some cells lack keratinization (C). A strip of nonkeratinized carcinoma cells has an adjacent anucleate squamous cell (D). All these illustrations are from bronchial wash cytology specimens.

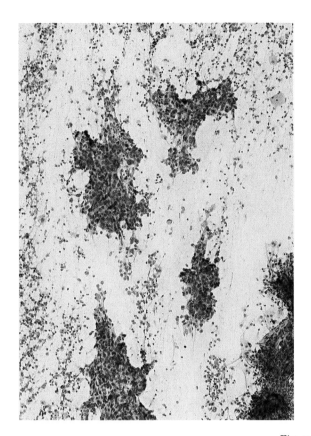
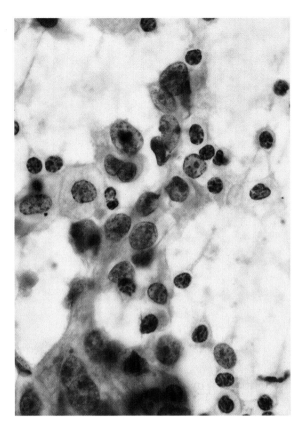

Figure 11-14
SQUAMOUS CELL CARCINOMA
Fine needle aspirate of poorly differentiated squamous cell carcinoma reveals a cellular specimen with irregular-shaped cell groups (left) and cytologically malignant cells (right) lacking definitive squamous differentiation. The surgical resection showed focal squamous differentiation.

Figure 11-15
SQUAMOUS
CELL CARCINOMA
Poorly differentiated squamous carcinoma in a bronchial wash specimen. The cells show cytologic features of malignancy, but no evidence of squamous differentiation, and the diagnosis of squamous cell carcinoma was based on other cell groups.

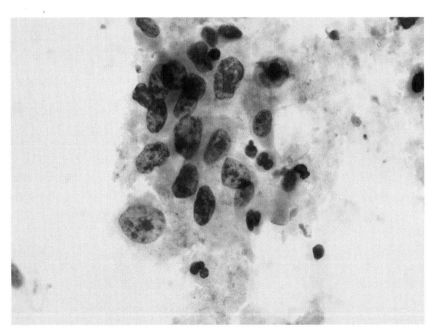

and dense chromatin. Evidence of early keratinization can be seen as a deeply staining, somewhat dense-appearing cytoplasmic fibrillar change oriented in a perinuclear fashion. This feature, which corresponds to tonofilaments ultrastructurally, is recognized as squamous differentiation cytologically.

Fully keratinized cells from squamous cell carcinoma tend to be orangophilic in Papanicolaou-stained material and to show marked cellular pleomorphism: cells have bizarre sizes and shapes, with dense, hyperchromatic nuclei. The cytoplasm has a refractile character that can be appreciated by lowering the condenser on the microscope. The nuclei often lack a recognizable internal nuclear structure, although they are large, hyperchromatic, and bizarre in shape with indentations and angulations. Nucleoli are usually not present. In well-differentiated, heavily keratinized tumors, the nuclear-cytoplasmic ratio may be quite low. Some observers have noted that it may be easier to identify squamous differentiation in cytologic specimens than in histologic specimens from the same tumor (18).

Atypical squamous cells that lack features of malignancy often accompany squamous carcinoma cells but are also seen in many nonmalignant conditions such as infections and following radiation.

The morphogenesis of squamous cell carcinoma can be appreciated in cytologic specimens as shown in figures 7-5 and 7-6.

Immunohistochemical Findings. Immunohistochemistry is not necessary for a diagnosis of squamous cell carcinoma of the lung. The diagnosis is readily made histologically, and the problems encountered in routine light microscopic evaluation (such as lung cancer heterogeneity) may actually be compounded with immunohistochemical studies.

Squamous cell carcinomas typically stain for both high and low molecular weight keratins; the staining for high molecular weight keratins is usually in regions of keratinization (2,8–10,12, 17,22,23). Other intermediate filaments may also be present including vimentin, neurofilaments, synaptophysin, and even desmin (8–10, 22,23,28). Squamous cell carcinomas also may stain positively for epithelial membrane antigen (EMA), human milk fat globule (HMFG-2), S-100 protein, Leu-M1, and carcinoembryonic antigen (CEA) (9,12,13,22,28).

Ultrastructural Findings. Electron microscopy is only rarely necessary in the diagnosis of squamous cell carcinoma of the lung, such as in confirming squamous differentiation ultrastructurally in a spindle cell squamous carcinoma. In squamous cell carcinoma there are true desmosomal attachments with tonofilaments that extend into the cytoplasm as bundles of filaments (figs. 11-16–11-18) (6,12,13,17,18). Well- and moderately differentiated squamous carcinomas may have blunt microvillous surface processes that interdigitate with adjacent cells and connect to them by desmosomes. Mucin and neurosecretory-type granules are occasionally seen. An intact basement membrane is often present around tumor cell nests. Increased cytoplasmic mitochondria are found in cases appearing oncocytoid by light microscopy. Gatter et al. (8) found cytoplasmic secretory vacuoles in 10 of 58 cases (17 percent) and dense core granules in 35 (60 percent). Mackay et al. (17) believe that some of the structures resembling dense core granules may represent lysosomes. In some spindle cell squamous carcinomas (see below) ultrastructural features of squamous differentiation may be focally lost (26).

Histologic Variants of Squamous Cell Carcinoma. *Small Cell Variant.* Some squamous cell carcinomas of the lung are composed of small cells with a high nuclear-cytoplasmic ratio, nuclei that often show nuclear molding, and a resemblance to small cell carcinoma (figs. 11-19– 11-21). Squamous differentiation may be only focal. In general, the small cell variant of squamous cell carcinoma tends to show better defined cell nests, less necrosis, and a more mature fibrous stroma than small cell carcinoma. The nuclei are more vesicular and have definite nucleoli. The possibility of combined small cell carcinoma/squamous cell carcinoma (4) should always be considered in such cases before rendering a diagnosis of small cell squamous cell carcinoma. Hammar (12,13) has shown that the ultrastructural features of small cell squamous carcinoma are similar to those of conventional squamous cell carcinoma of the lung.

Clear Cell Type. Occasional clear cell foci are common in squamous cell carcinomas (fig. 11-22). A small percentage of tumors are composed predominantly or almost entirely of clear cells, yet still show foci of squamous differentiation

Figure 11-16
ULTRASTRUCTURAL
APPEARANCE OF
SQUAMOUS CELL
CARCINOMA

The microvillous border
between cells is well maintained; tonofilaments and
desmosomal attachments
(arrows) are present but not
numerous. There is considerable nuclear pleomorphism
with some cells showing complex nuclear membranes.
Moderate numbers of mito-
chondria can be seen in many
of the cells. (X4400) (Courtesy of Dr. Bruce Mackay,
Houston, TX.)

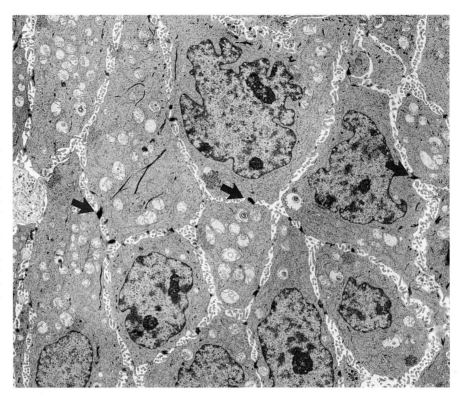

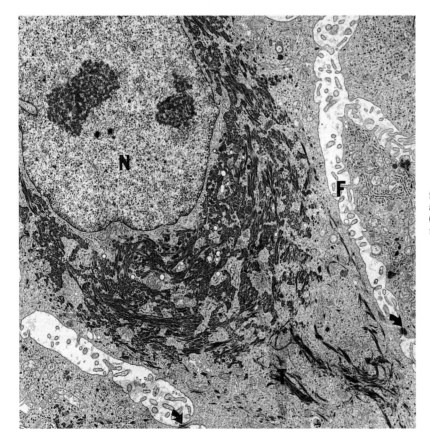

Figure 11-17
ULTRASTRUCTURAL
APPEARANCE OF
SQUAMOUS CELL CARCINOMA

This case shows numerous tonofilaments (T), desmosomes (arrow),
and filopodia (F) of the cell membrane.
(X7000) (Courtesy of Dr. Sam Hammar, Bremerton, WA.)

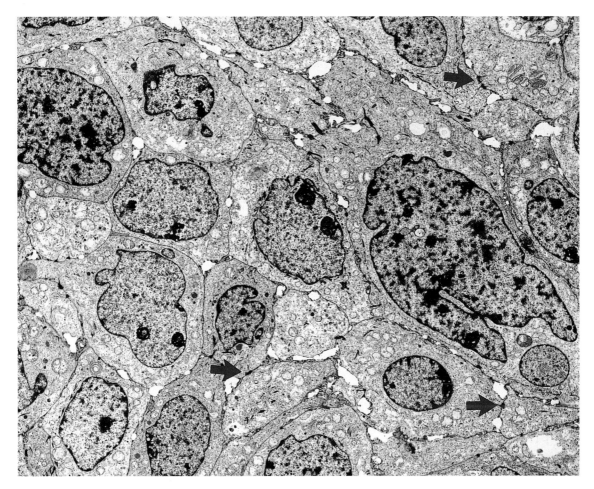

Figure 11-18
ULTRASTRUCTURE OF SQUAMOUS CELL CARCINOMA
This poorly differentiated squamous carcinoma shows only focal tonofilaments and desmosomal attachments between cells (arrows). There is marked nuclear pleomorphism and loss of the blunt microvilli between the cells. Some of the cells are relatively small with a high nuclear-cytoplasmic ratio. (X3000) (Courtesy of Dr. Bruce Mackay, Houston, TX.)

(15). Large cell carcinoma and adenocarcinoma of the lung may also show extensive clear cell change (see chapters 12 and 15). The main differential diagnostic consideration is metastatic clear cell carcinoma from an extrapulmonary site, particularly the kidney.

Well-differentiated Papillary and Verrucous Types. While many endobronchial squamous cell carcinomas are exophytic necrotic masses, there is a subset that are well-differentiated, have little necrosis, and present as delicate intrabronchial papillary lesions restricted to the bronchial lumen (figs. 11-23, 11-24) (7,24). Cellular pleomorphism is not marked, and there is often little or no stromal invasion; i.e., many of these tumors are papillary

in situ carcinomas. Well-differentiated papillary squamous cell carcinomas tend to occur in older individuals and have a favorable prognosis. In a review by Dulmet-Brender (7), there was a male predominance, with most tumors staged as T1N0. There is an excellent 5-year survival of over 60 percent, but this does not differ from other T1N0 lung carcinomas.

Primary lung carcinomas resembling verrucous carcinomas are rare and little is known of their natural history.

Well-differentiated papillary squamous cell carcinoma should be distinguished from pulmonary involvement by papillomatosis (21) and solitary papillomas (27). The clinical history is helpful in

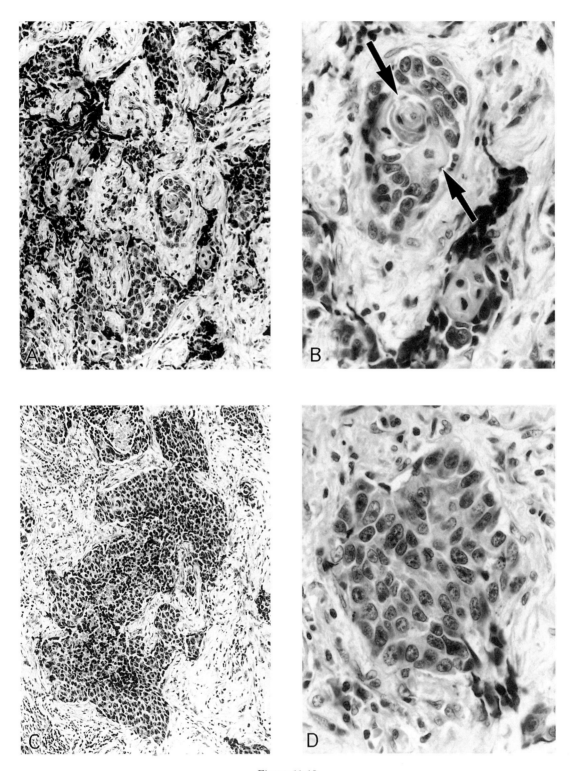

Figure 11-19
SMALL CELL SQUAMOUS CELL CARCINOMA

Small cell squamous cell carcinoma showing nuclear crush artifact (A,B) with focal keratinization (B, arrows). The cell nests (C,D) show sharp demarcation from the well-developed fibrous stroma. Detail of the nuclei (B,D) show discrete chromatin clumping of prominent nuclei. In addition, the cells have modest amounts of cytoplasm and somewhat less nuclear molding than classic small cell carcinoma.

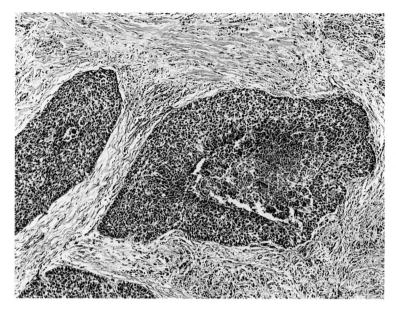

Figure 11-20
SMALL CELL
SQUAMOUS CELL CARCINOMA
Small cell squamous carcinoma showing a discrete cell nest distinct from the fibrous stroma. There is central necrosis.

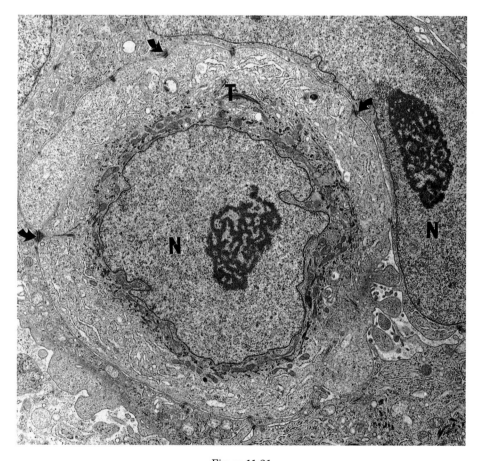

Figure 11-21
SQUAMOUS CELL CARCINOMA
Ultrastructural appearance of this squamous cell carcinoma shows relatively small cells with a high nuclear-cytoplasmic ratio, prominent nuclear molding (N), and tonofilaments (T) with desmosomes (arrows). (X6000) (Courtesy of Dr. Sam Hammar, Bremerton, WA.)

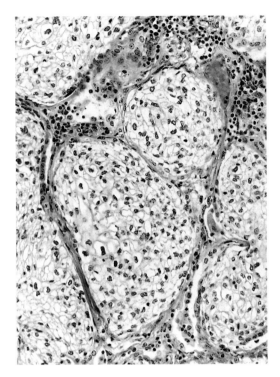

Figure 11-22
CLEAR CELL SQUAMOUS CELL CARCINOMA
This tumor is composed entirely of clear cells with only focal keratinization (not shown).

the former and attention to cytologic detail and lack of invasion in the latter. Some well-differentiated papillary squamous cell carcinomas may have foci that are deceptively benign appearing (fig. 11-24).

Basaloid Type. Primary basaloid lung carcinomas are rare, and have been considered rare variants of squamous cell carcinoma (5). Some tumors closely resemble basal cell carcinoma of the skin or basaloid carcinoma in the upper respiratory tract (fig. 11-25). In a recent series of 38 tumors studied by Brambilla et al. (3), 19 were "pure" and 19 showed associated squamous cell, large cell, or adenocarcinoma components. The authors considered basaloid carcinomas separable from other lung carcinomas, including squamous cell carcinoma, by lack of expression of neuroendocrine markers and ultrastructural evidence of glandular or squamous differentiation. The authors noted a poor prognosis for the group: median survival of only 22 months for stage I and II disease.

Pleomorphic/Giant Cell Type. Some squamous carcinomas show marked cellular pleomorphism with numerous tumor giant cells (fig. 11-14). These tumors often have large zones showing cellular dyscohesion with infiltrates of inflammatory cells, particularly neutrophils. Cohesive cell

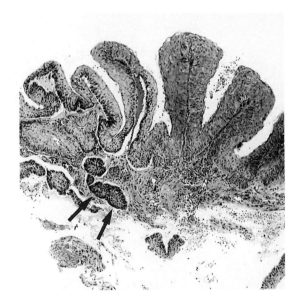

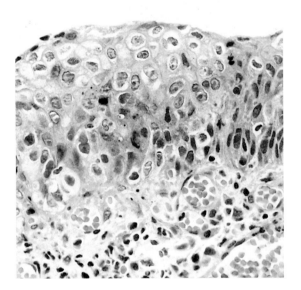

Figure 11-23
PAPILLARY SQUAMOUS CELL CARCINOMA
Well-differentiated papillary squamous cell carcinoma seen in a transbronchial biopsy. Delicate papillae are present, and there is a focus suspicious for submucosal invasion (arrows). Cytologically, the cells comprising the papillae show only modest maturation and moderate nuclear atypia. The cytologic features in the nuclei and lack of orderly maturation are features in favor of a low-grade carcinoma.

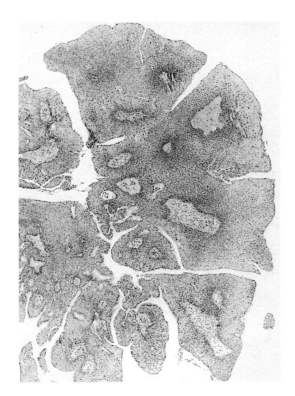 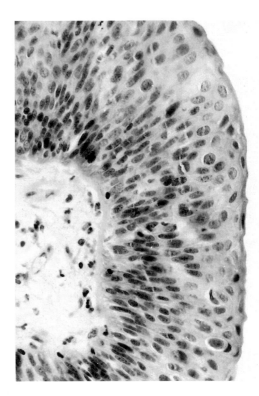

Figure 11-24
PAPILLARY SQUAMOUS CELL CARCINOMA
Well-differentiated papillary squamous cell carcinoma manifesting as blunt papillae in this endobronchial tumor. While the low-power appearance (left) suggests good maturation, detail shows foci of full-thickness cytologic atypia and lack of maturation (right).

nests may be quite focal and evidence of squamous differentiation may only be recognizable in these foci. These carcinomas overlap with pleomorphic carcinomas (chapter 15).

Spindle Cell Type. Some degree of spindling and cellular elongation is frequent in squamous cell carcinoma; a small percentage of tumors show marked spindling, which may be associated with other histologic patterns, including tumor giant cells and even osteoclastic giant cells (figs. 11-26–11-30) (16). These tumors fall into two categories. In the first, the tumor is composed entirely of spindled squamous cells or there is an identifiable transition between squamous cells and spindle cells, with the latter maintaining squamous features at the light microscopic, immunohistochemical, or ultrastructural level (26). In the second, there is a biphasic appearance, with discrete components that do not merge with one another and in which the

malignant spindle cell component has lost its epithelial differentiation by light microscopy. When heterologous elements are present, carcinosarcoma should be considered (chapter 21). Spindle cell squamous carcinomas lacking heterologous elements fall within the spectrum of pleomorphic carcinoma (chapter 15).

Differential Diagnosis. The following should be considered in the differential diagnosis of squamous carcinoma of the lung: florid squamous metaplasia (for example, around an organizing infarct or in organizing diffuse alveolar damage (see fig. 9-3); squamous metaplasia in the bronchial mucosa overlying another tumor (either primary or metastatic); postinflammatory squamous metaplasia (infection, radiation); pseudoepitheliomatous hyperplasia associated with other tumors (granular cell tumor) or inflammatory processes (blastomycosis); squamous papillomas, papillomatosis, and condylomas (27) involving the

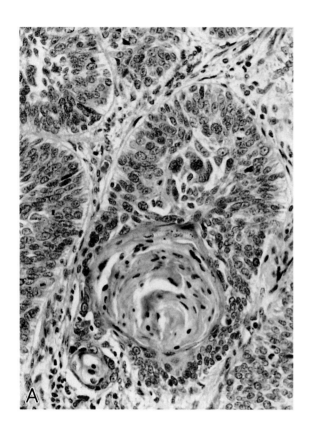

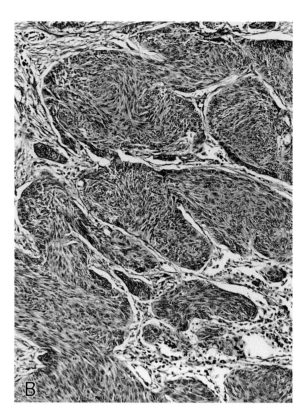

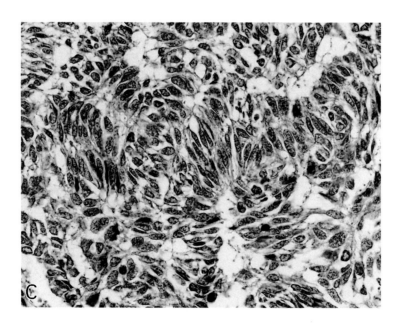

Figure 11-25
BASALOID SQUAMOUS CELL CARCINOMA
Basaloid squamous cell carcinoma of the lung showing marked similarities to basal cell carcinoma of the skin.

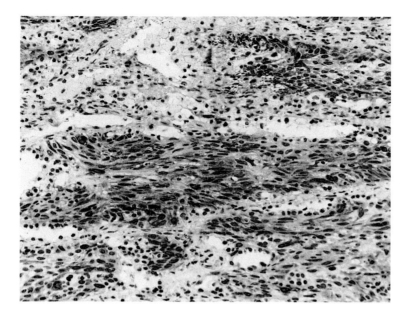

Figure 11-26
SPINDLE CELL
SQUAMOUS CELL CARCINOMA
In this case, all the cell nests show spindling and were recognizably squamous on routine sections. Immunohistochemical stains for keratin are positive and are depicted here; there is diffuse cytoplasmic staining in most, but not all, of the nests. (Courtesy of Dr. Sam Hammar, Bremerton, WA.)

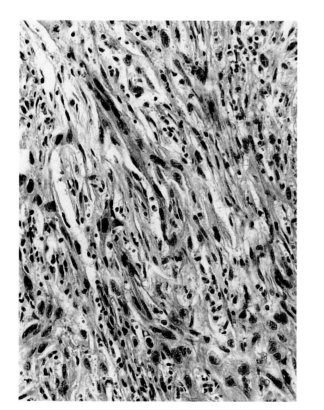
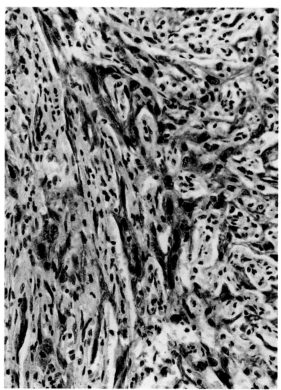

Figure 11-27
SPINDLE CELL SQUAMOUS CELL CARCINOMA
In this case, recognizable poorly differentiated squamous carcinoma was present in another field. It merged with a malignant spindle cell pattern (left) which shows cytoplasmic positivity for cytokeratin (right). (Courtesy of Dr. Sam Hammar, Bremerton, WA.)

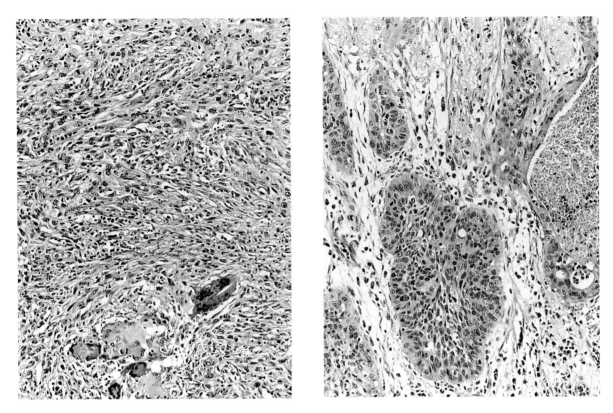

Figure 11-28
SPINDLE CELL SQUAMOUS CELL CARCINOMA
Left: Spindled squamous cell carcinoma showing some zones resembling a pleomorphic spindle cell sarcoma with occasional multinucleate giant cells. The latter may be a reaction to keratin production.
Right: Foci of recognizable squamous cell carcinoma were identified in this case and showed a transition to the spindle cell zones (top).

Figure 11-29
SPINDLE CELL SQUAMOUS CELL
CARCINOMA

Spindled squamous cell carcinoma of the lung showing a pleomorphic spindle cell component (lower left) adjacent to epithelial nests showing squamous differentiation (upper right).

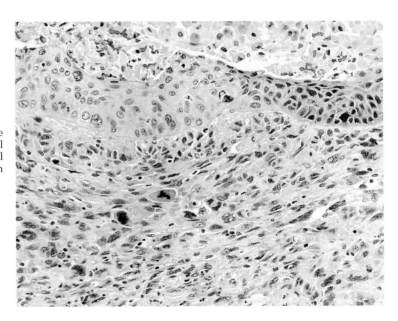

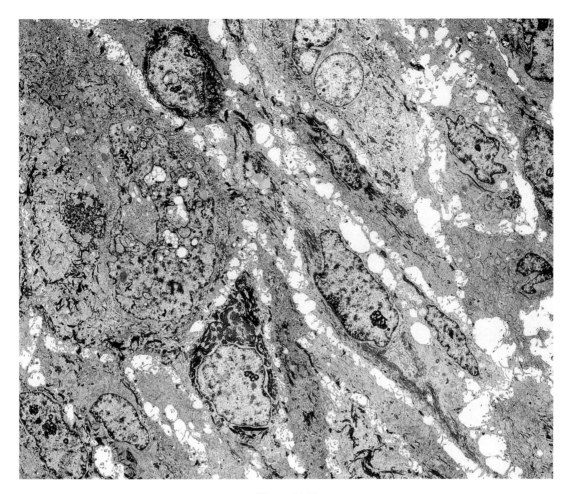

Figure 11-30
SPINDLE CELL SQUAMOUS CELL CARCINOMA
The spindle cells (center) show well-developed tonofilaments and desmosomal attachments with other cells. There is a prominent intercellular space in which blunt microvilli can be seen. (X2000) (Courtesy of Dr. Bruce Mackay, Houston, TX.)

lung and large airways; other primary tumors with a squamous component (mucoepidermoid carcinoma, adenosquamous carcinoma); primary lung tumors with a squamoid or epithelioid appearance; small cell carcinomas (in the case of small cell squamous carcinoma); and metastatic squamous carcinomas and other squamoid tumors (melanoma).

Treatment and Prognosis. The overall 5-year relative survival rate for squamous cell carcinoma cell is 15.4 percent (see fig. 8-16). Surgical resection offers the only reasonable chance of cure. Radiotherapy provides long-term local control for some localized unresectable tumors, such as superior sulcus tumors. A number of chemotherapy and radiation therapy protocols are used in the management of squamous cell carcinoma as part of the therapeutic regimen for nonsmall cell carcinoma of the lung and may result in prolonged survival. For the few of cases that are surgically resectable, the 5-year survival figures of Mountain et al. are representative (see fig. 8-12): stage 1, 50 percent; stage 2, 30 percent; stage 3A, slightly over 10 percent.

REFERENCES

1. Bejui-Thivolet F, Liagre N, Chignol MC, Chardonnet Y, Patricot LM. Detection of human papillomavirus DNA in squamous bronchial metaplasia and squamous cell carcinomas of the lung by in situ hybridization using biotinylated probes in paraffin-embedded specimens. Hum Pathol 1990;21:111–6.

2. Blobel GA, Moll R, Franke WW, Vogt-Moykopf I. Cytokeratins in normal lung and lung carcinomas. I. Adenocarcinomas, squamous cell carcinomas and cultured cell lines. Virchows Arch [Cell Pathol] 1984;45:407–29.

3. Brambilla E, Moro D, Veale D, et al. Basal cell (basaloid) carcinoma of the lung: a new morphologic and phenotypic entity with separate prognostic significance. Hum Pathol 1992;23:993–1003.

4. Churg A, Johnston WH, Stulbarg M. Small cell squamous and mixed small cell squamous—small cell anaplastic carcinomas of the lung. Am J Surg Pathol 1980;4:255–63.

5. Daroca PJ, Robishaux WH. Basaloid carcinoma of the bronchus. Surg Pathol 1989;2:339–44.

6. Dingemans KP, Mooi WJ. Ultrastructure of squamous cell carcinoma of the lung. Pathol Annu 1974;19(Pt 1):249–73.

7. Dulmet-Brender E, Jaubert F, Huchon G. Exophytic endobronchial epidermoid carcinoma. Cancer 1986; 57:1358–64.

8. Gatter KC, Dunnill MS, Heryet A, Mason DY. Human lung tumors: does intermediate filament coexpression correlate with other morphological or immunocytochemical features? Histopathology 1987;11:705–14.

9. _____, Dunnill MS, Pulford KA, Heryet A, Mason DY. Human lung tumors: a correlation of antigenic profile with histologic type. Histopathology 1985;9:805–23.

10. _____, Dunnill MS, Van Muijen GN, Mason DY. Human lung tumours may co-express different classes of intermediate filaments. J Clin Pathol 1986;39:950–4.

11. Gazdar AF, Linnoila RI. The pathology of lung cancer—changing concepts and newer diagnostic techniques. Semin Oncol 1988;15:215–25.

12. Hammar S. The use of electron microscopy and immunohistochemistry in the diagnosis and understanding of lung neoplasms. Clin Lab Med 1987;7:1–30.

13. _____, Bolen JW, Bockus D, Remington F, Friedman S. Ultrastructural and immunohistochemical features of common lung tumors: an overview. Ultrastruct Pathol 1985;9:283–318.

14. Johnston WW, Frable WJ. The cytopathology of the respiratory tract. A review. Am J Pathol 1976;84:372–424.

15. Katzenstein AL, Prioleau PG, Askin FB. The histologic spectrum and significance of clear-cell change in lung carcinoma. Cancer 1980;45:943–7.

16. Love GL, Daroca PJ Jr. Bronchogenic sarcomatoid squamous cell carcinoma with osteoclast-like giant cells. Hum Pathol 1983;14:1004–6.

17. Mackay B, Lukeman JM, Ordonez NG. Tumors of the lung. Philadelphia: WB Saunders, 1991:165–89.

18. Matthews MJ, Mackay B, Lukeman J. Pathology of non-small cell carcinoma of the lung. Semin Oncol 1983;10:34–55.

19. Oyasu R, Battifora HA, Buckingham WB, Hidvegi D. Metaplastic squamous carcinoma of bronchus simulating giant cell tumor of bone. Cancer 1977;39:1119–28.

20. Rilke F, Carbone A, Clemente C, Pilotti S. Surgical pathology of resectable lung cancer. In: Muggia FM, Rozencweig M, eds. Lung cancer: progress in therapeutic research. New York: Raven Press, 1979:129–42.

21. Runckel D, Kessler S. Bronchogenic squamous carcinoma in nonirradiated juvenile laryngotracheal papillomatosis. Am J Surg 1980;4:293–6.

23. Said J. Immunohistochemistry of lung tumors. Lung Biol Health Dis 1990;44:635–51.

23. _____, Nash G, Banks-Schlegel S, Sassoon AF, Murakami S, Shintaku IP. Keratin in human lung tumors: patterns of localization of different-molecular-weight keratin proteins. Am J Pathol 1983;113:27–32.

24. Sherwin RP, LaForet EG, Strieder JW. Exophytic endobronchial carcinoma. J Thorac Cardiovasc Surg 1962;43:716–30.

25. Sobin L, Yesner R. Histological typing of lung tumors. International Histological Classification of Tumors, Vol 1. 2nd ed. Geneva: World Health Organization, 1981.

26. Suster S, Huszar M, Herczeg E. Spindle cell squamous carcinoma of the lung. Immunocytochemical and ultrastructural study of a case. Histopathology 1987;11:871–8.

27. Trillo A, Guha A. Solitary condylomatous papilloma of the bronchus. Arch Pathol Lab Med 1988;112:731–3.

28. Visscher DW, Zarbo RJ, Trojanowski JQ, Sakr W, Crissman JD. Neuroendocrine differentiation in poorly differentiated lung carcinomas: a light microscopic and immunohistologic study. Mod Pathol 1990;3:508–12.

❖❖❖

12

ADENOCARCINOMA OF THE LUNG
(EXCLUDING BRONCHIOLOALVEOLAR CARCINOMA)

Definition. Adenocarcinoma of the lung is a glandular epithelial malignancy manifesting tubular, papillary, or acinar growth patterns or a solid growth pattern with mucin production. In the World Health Organization (WHO) classification of lung tumors (41), adenocarcinomas are grouped as *acinar, papillary, bronchioloalveolar,* and *solid adenocarcinoma with mucin production.*

Although there is considerable overlap among these groups, it is reasonable to segregate bronchioloalveolar carcinomas because of their distinctive clinicopathologic features, and they are discussed in chapter 13. Adenocarcinomas discussed in this chapter include histologically diverse tumors with a variety of patterns and variable degrees of differentiation. Unusual patterns included are: *signet ring adenocarcinoma, spindle cell adenocarcinoma,* and *adenocarcinoma showing hepatoid differentiation.*

Some putative precursor lesions of adenocarcinoma, including lung scarring, atypical adenomatous hyperplasia, and bronchioloalveolar cell adenomas, are discussed in chapter 7.

Clinical Features. The clinical features of adenocarcinoma of the lung are discussed in detail in chapter 8. In many recent studies, adenocarcinoma has become the most common form of lung carcinoma (60 percent in one series) (12,24), particularly among resected tumors (14). Adenocarcinomas are more common in women than men, and there is not as strong a relationship with smoking as with squamous cell, small cell, or large cell carcinoma (28). Small, sometimes occult, primary adenocarcinomas of the lung may be associated with widespread metastases or massive pleural involvement.

Gross Findings. Adenocarcinomas are generally peripheral, well-circumscribed masses, often associated with overlying pleural fibrosis or puckering (12,14,27,29,30,43). The gross and histologic assessment of the exact relationship of the tumor to the pleural elastica is important for staging purposes. Adenocarcinomas may also be central or even endobronchial in location (23).

Adenocarcinomas of the lung vary from lesions under a centimeter in size to tumors that replace an entire lung (figs. 12-1–12-3). On cut section, they are gray-white, sometimes lobulated, and often have central scarring which may contain anthracotic pigment; so-called scar carcinomas are

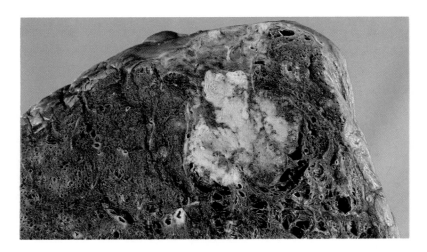

Figure 12-1
ADENOCARCINOMA
There is a small apical mass with some surrounding fibrosis and emphysematous change. Pigmentation within the mass is apparent.

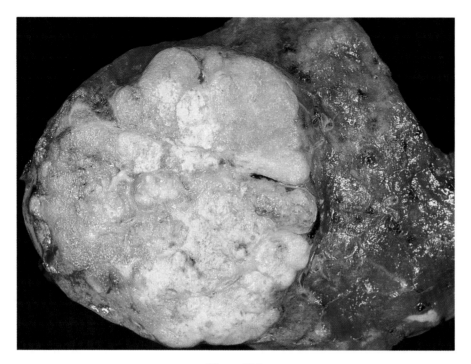

Figure 12-2
ADENOCARCINOMA
This lobectomy specimen shows a lobulated, somewhat glistening mass.

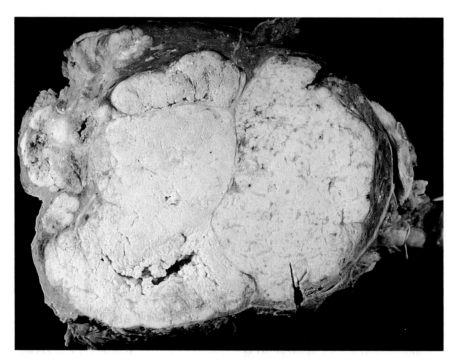

Figure 12-3
ADENOCARCINOMA
The case shows an adenocarcinoma replacing an entire lung at autopsy. There is extensive necrosis seen as somewhat opaque chalky foci and associated pleural thickening.

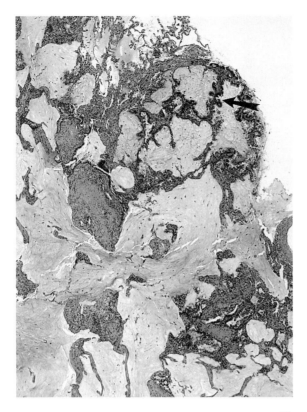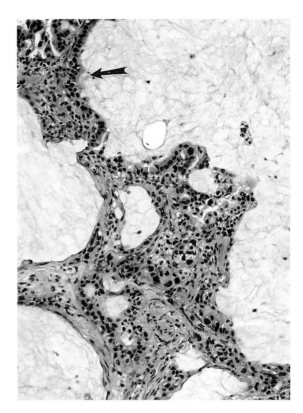

Figure 12-4
WELL-DIFFERENTIATED ADENOCARCINOMA, ACINAR TYPE
At low power this well-differentiated mucin-producing adenocarcinoma resembles a bronchioloalveolar carcinoma. Many of the mucinous spaces lack an epithelial lining, although one can be seen focally (left and right, arrows). At low power stroma production is apparent (left) and invasion is apparent by neoplastic cells that show significant cytologic atypia (right, lower middle).

discussed in chapter 7. Necrosis and hemorrhage are common. Tumors with extensive mucus production have a mucoid appearance on cut section; those with a desmoplastic stroma are quite firm. Adenocarcinomas may be single or multiple (27,31); when multiple, distinction from a single primary with satellite metastases may be difficult or impossible. In one series of 62 consecutive cases, 12 (19 percent) had multiple primary tumors (31).

Pulmonary adenocarcinomas close to the pleura may invade the pleura with extensive pleural seeding that mimics a malignant mesothelioma (pseudomesotheliomatous carcinoma).

Most adenocarcinomas are unrelated to bronchi except by secondary invasion, but central tumors may be associated with large airways and some tumors have a prominent endobronchial component.

Microscopic Findings. Histologically, adenocarcinomas of the lung have tubular, papillary, or acinar growth patterns, or mucin production (figs. 12-4–12-13) (12,14,27, 29,30,43). Variation in differentiation from field to field is common with well-differentiated foci merging with poorly differentiated foci. In poorly differentiated or anaplastic tumors, glandular features may be focal. Solid adenocarcinomas produce intracellular mucin (fig. 12-10). According to Sørensen (42, 43), the frequency of subtypes varies between unresectable (biopsy only) and resectable cases: acinar, 50 versus 57 percent; bronchioloalveolar, 5 versus 18 percent; solid adenocarcinoma, 12 versus 14 percent; and papillary, 9 versus 12 percent. Among the inoperable cases, nearly 24 percent were adenocarcinomas that were difficult to classify based on available material.

Papillary adenocarcinomas are defined by the presence of papillae (fig. 12-9). Many cases represent bronchioloalveolar carcinomas with prominent papillary growth (see chapter 13), but others

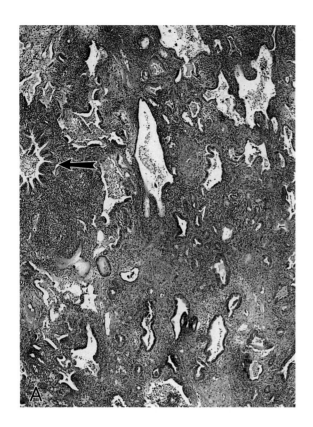

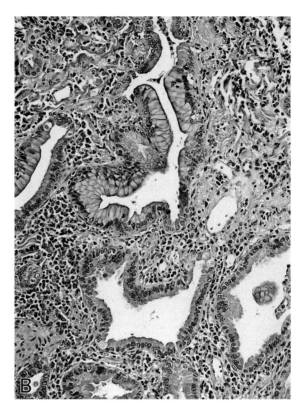

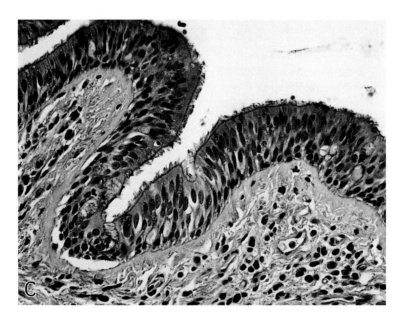

Figure 12-5
WELL-DIFFERENTIATED ADENOCARCINOMA, ACINAR TYPE

The lung parenchyma is replaced by a proliferation of gaping glandular structures (A). A higher magnification view (B) shows well-differentiated adenocarcinoma with tall, columnar, mucin-secreting, glandular epithelium. In C, benign bronchiolar epithelium from the bronchiole in A (arrow) is contrasted with malignant epithelium in B.

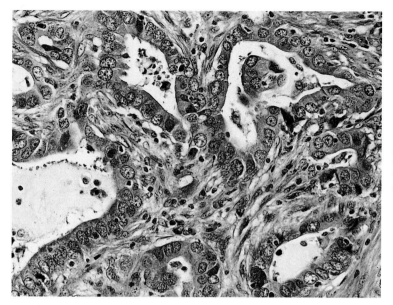

Figure 12-6
MODERATELY DIFFERENTIATED
ADENOCARCINOMA, ACINAR TYPE
This moderately differentiated adenocarcinoma shows well-formed glands lined by cuboidal cells with prominent eosinophilic cytoplasm. The nuclei are moderately atypical, and most of them have prominent nucleoli.

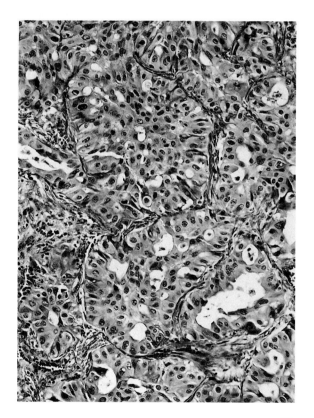
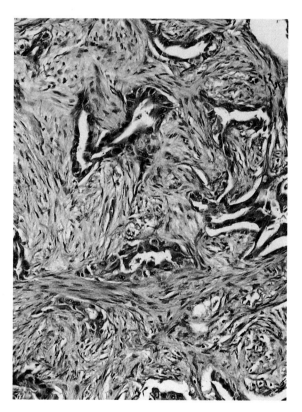

Figure 12-7
MODERATELY DIFFERENTIATED ADENOCARCINOMA
This moderately differentiated adenocarcinoma of the lung shows cellular foci with delicate vascular stroma (left) and other foci with stromal desmoplasia around irregular carcinomatous nests (right). Glandular differentiation is seen in both regions.

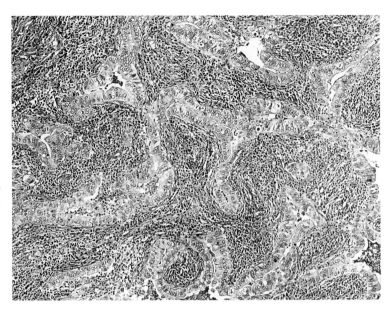

Figure 12-8
MODERATELY DIFFERENTIATED
ADENOCARCINOMA, ACINAR TYPE,
WITH MARKED
LYMPHOID INFILTRATE
This moderately differentiated adeno-
carcinoma has a dense infiltrate of lympho-
cytes and plasma cells. The possibility of
lymphoma or chronic lymphocytic leukemia
has to be considered in such a case.

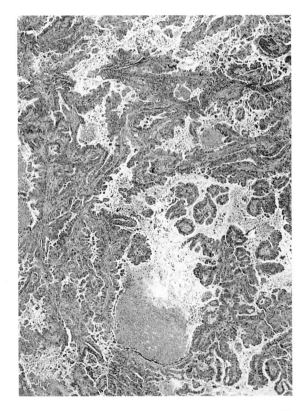
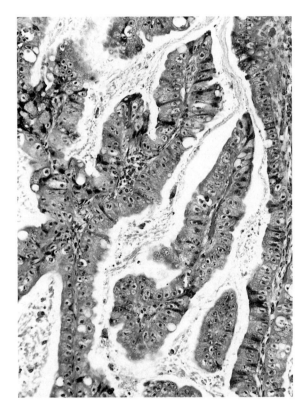

Figure 12-9
PAPILLARY ADENOCARCINOMA
This moderately differentiated adenocarcinoma has numerous papillae with fibrovascular cores (left) lined by cells with
large vesicular nuclei containing very prominent nucleoli (right). This tumor was associated with architectural destruction
and extensive necrosis (which can be seen as the debris between the papillae), and this excluded the possibility of a papillary
variant of bronchioloalveolar carcinoma.

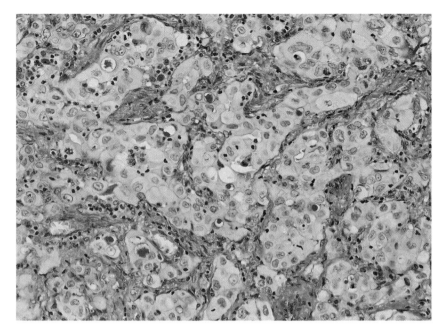

Figure 12-10
SOLID ADENOCARCINOMA
WITH MUCIN PRODUCTION
This poorly differentiated
(solid) adenocarcinoma shows
many cells with mucin vacuoles
stained with digested PAS. The
vacuoles were difficult to see on
routine sections, and the case had
originally been classified as large
cell carcinoma.

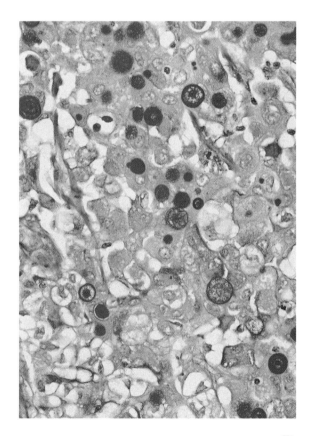
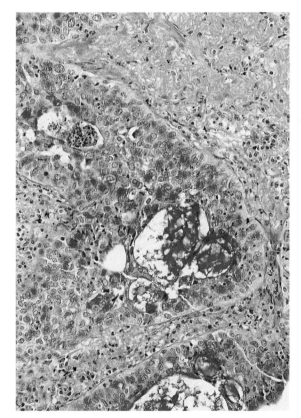

Figure 12-11
MUCIN STAINING IN ADENOCARCINOMA (DIGESTED PAS)
These two cases illustrate variations in mucin stain patterns: cytoplasmic (left) and intraluminal pools (right).

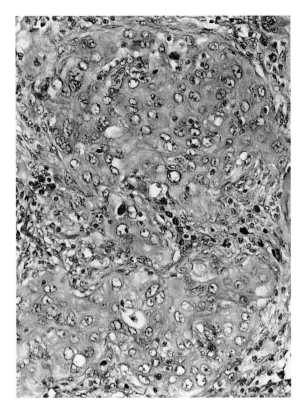

Figure 12-12
POORLY DIFFERENTIATED ADENOCARCINOMA
This poorly differentiated adenocarcinoma shows sheets of neoplastic epithelial cells, which in this field are indistinguishable from large cell carcinoma. Other fields showed acinar differentiation.

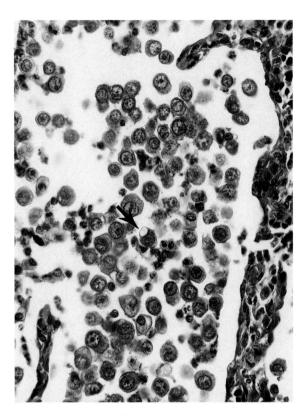

Figure 12-13
POORLY DIFFERENTIATED ADENOCARCINOMA
Dyscohesive adenocarcinoma cells flood alveoli. Other regions showed cohesive nests with acini. Cells within the airspaces were mucin positive, and a cell containing a mucin vacuole is present in the center of the field (arrow).

are associated with architectural destruction and are separable from bronchioloalveolar carcinoma.

Some pulmonary adenocarcinomas have dyscohesive zones with large numbers of single cells that infiltrate the interstitium or flood intact airspaces (fig. 12-13); this last feature can also be seen in some bronchioloalveolar carcinomas. The cells are large and polygonal, with a high nuclear-cytoplasmic ratio. The diagnosis of adenocarcinoma rests on finding mucin production in some of the cells or glandular growth patterns in regions away from the dyscohesive foci.

The cells comprising adenocarcinomas are large, cuboidal, columnar, or polygonal with large vesicular nuclei and prominent nucleoli. The nuclear atypia varies with the degree of differentiation. Solid adenocarcinomas may be virtually indistinguishable from large cell carcinoma except for the mucin production; mucin stains (mucicarmine, pe-

riodic acid–Schiff (PAS) diastase, Alcian blue) are required for diagnostic confirmation.

Cytoplasmic glandular differentiation may be obvious when large mucin vacuoles are present. More often, however, the cytoplasm is eosinophilic without obvious mucin vacuoles, and the cells form glands. Clara cell differentiation includes eosinophilic cytoplasm with knob-like protrusions at the apical surface (2,35). PAS stains show diastase-resistant apical staining corresponding to Clara cell granules; the phosphotungstic acid hematoxylin (PTAH) stain may also be positive (36). Type 2 cell differentiation in adenocarcinoma may be identified by intranuclear PAS-positive eosinophilic inclusions and by positive cytoplasmic staining with the Luxol-fast blue and Sudan black stains (2).

Clear cell change may be seen in adenocarcinoma just as in other lung carcinomas (figs. 12-14,

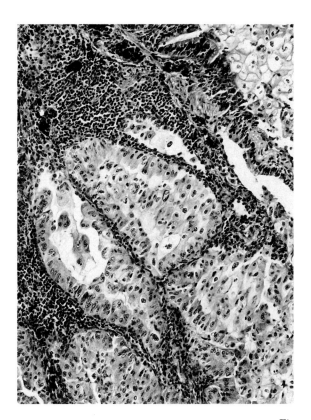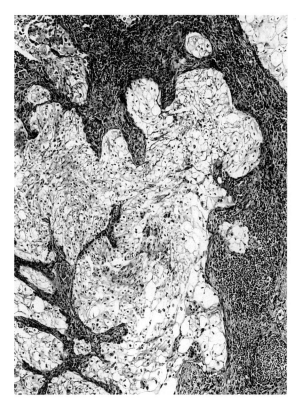

Figure 12-14
ADENOCARCINOMA WITH CLEAR CELLS
This acinar adenocarcinoma shows acini with columnar cells (left) which merged with fields showing clear cell features (right).

12-15). The change may be focal or widespread, and when more than 50 percent of the tumor is involved, a diagnosis of adenocarcinoma with clear cells is appropriate (19). Unless mucin is demonstrated in such cases, metastatic renal cell carcinoma and other clear cell carcinomas should be considered. Katzenstein et al. (19) studied 348 consecutive resected lung carcinomas: 139 were adenocarcinomas and 38 of these (27 percent) showed foci of clear cells.

Scroggs et al. (40) described the presence of eosinophilic intracytoplasmic globules in pulmonary adenocarcinomas. They were similar to the intracytoplasmic eosinophilic globules seen in many other tumors and tended to occur at sites of cell injury.

Mucin production varies from occasional positive cells to large pools containing nests of tumor cells (figs. 12-10, 12-11). When there is extensive mucin production, muciphages are also prominent; there may be an associated giant cell reac-

tion. Mucus may occasionally dissect into the connective tissue and incite a giant cell reaction.

Mucin stains in the following patterns: positive staining of mucinous material within glandular lumens; diffuse cytoplasmic staining of single cells or groups of cells; or intracellular mucin droplets representing mucin secretion into intracellular lumens (figs. 12-10, 12-11). Adenocarcinomas commonly contain abundant glycogen.

The stroma of adenocarcinomas varies from thin, delicate fibrous septa to dense sclerotic zones. Some tumors have a dense lymphoid infiltrate which may be of sufficient intensity to overshadow the carcinoma and suggest the diagnosis of lymphoma (fig. 12-8). A histiocytic reaction, including Langerhans cells (15,16), may also be identified. A secondary granulomatous reaction is sometimes present; if accompanied by necrosis, a coexisting granulomatous infection should be excluded. A reaction resembling bronchocentric granulomatosis may be observed. Inflammatory and obstructive changes in lung tissue surrounding or distal

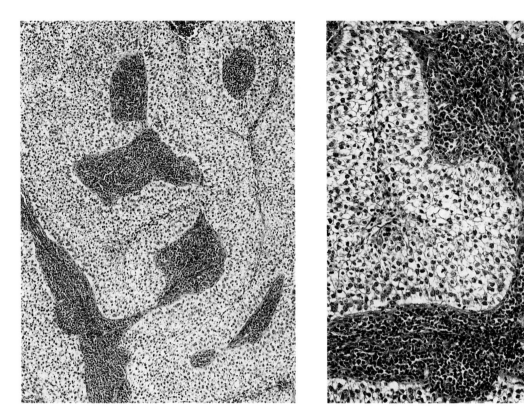

Figure 12-15
ADENOCARCINOMA WITH CLEAR CELLS
This adenocarcinoma has extensive clear cell change and prominent chronic inflammation in the stroma. Acinar differentiation was present focally (not illustrated here).

to the tumor are common. The extent of necrosis varies considerably, but tends to be greater in more poorly differentiated tumors.

Unusual histologic patterns of pulmonary adenocarcinoma are seen either alone or in combination with other patterns. Signet ring cells, identical to those in other tumors, may be a prominent component in a small percentage of pulmonary adenocarcinomas (fig. 12-16). Kish et al. (22) reported five cases (two of which were bronchioloalveolar carcinomas) in which the signet ring cell component varied from 10 to 50 percent. The patients ranged in age from 54 to 74 years; three of the five died of their disease.

Some pleomorphic adenocarcinomas have foci of spindle cells (figs. 12-17–12-19), or giant cells (fig. 12-19) (5,7). These cases may manifest biphasic glandular and spindled patterns in which the spindle cell component is diffusely positive for cytokeratin. Adenocarcinomas with spindle cell foci should be distinguished from

biphasic malignant mesotheliomas, carcinosarcomas, metastatic carcinosarcomas, and primary and metastatic tumors with interstitial growth and metaplasia of alveolar lining cells simulating a glandular component. Pleomorphic carcinoma is discussed in chapter 15.

Hepatoid differentiation was described by Ishikura et al. (17) in seven alpha-fetoprotein–producing tumors of the lung (fig. 12-20). The patients were all men between 40 and 73 years of age, and their serum alpha-fetoprotein levels varied from 1039 to 320,000 ng/mL. Five of the seven tumors had a hepatoid appearance, one resembled an endodermal sinus tumor, and one was a papillary adenocarcinoma. Alpha-fetoprotein was demonstrated immunohistochemically in all but one of the cases.

Cystadenocarcinomas of the lung and related tumors, including cystadenomas and mucinous cystic tumors of borderline malignancy, have recently been reported. We believe most of these

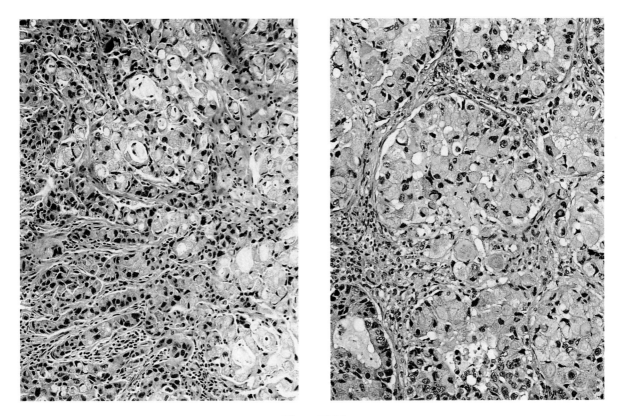

Figure 12-16
ADENOCARCINOMA WITH SIGNET RING CELLS
Two cases of adenocarcinoma with extensive (over 25 percent) signet ring cells are illustrated. In both, acinar foci were identified in addition to the signet ring cells.

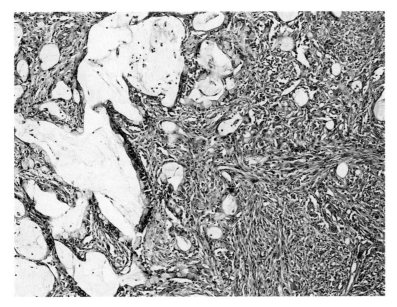

Figure 12-17
ADENOCARCINOMA WITH
GLANDULAR AND
SPINDLE CELL FEATURES
This moderately well-differentiated adeno-carcinoma shows glands with mucin production (left) and spindling of tumor cells (right).

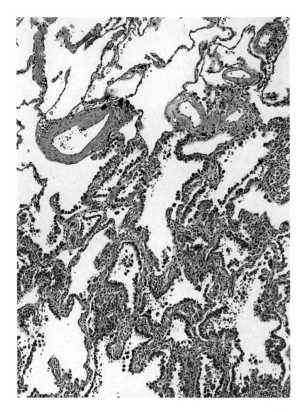 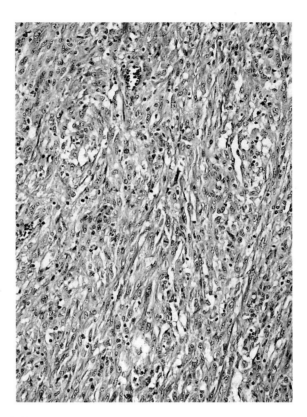

Figure 12-18
ADENOCARCINOMA WITH SPINDLE CELL FOCI
This adenocarcinoma has a bronchioloalveolar pattern (left) and a component of high-grade spindle cell carcinoma (right). The latter component comprised the majority of the tumor and was the sole component seen in pleural implants.

tumors are closely related to, and are probably variants of, bronchioloalveolar carcinoma and they are discussed in chapters 5 and 13.

Enteric differentiation has been reported (fig. 12-21). Tsao and Fraser (45) described a peculiar adenocarcinoma of the lung with cytologic features of differentiated small bowel epithelium. Cells with features of columnar absorptive, goblet, Paneth, and neuroendocrine cell differentiation were all present. A primary tumor in the gastrointestinal tract was not identified in the 4-year follow-up period. The authors thought the occurrence of this tumor in the lung could be explained by common stem cells for the lower respiratory and gastrointestinal tract mucosae.

Paget disease of the bronchus is discussed in chapter 16.

Cytologically, adenocarcinomas of the lung show just as much variation as they do histologically (figs. 12-22–12-25) (18,27,29,30). The cyto-

logic appearance varies with the degree of differentiation and the histologic pattern. The cells are more uniform than those of squamous cell carcinoma and they have a propensity to form three-dimensional clusters, with overlapping of cells and a common cell border. The nuclear appearance varies with the degree of differentiation: the nuclei tend to be vesicular, with prominent eosinophilic nucleoli and relatively fine chromatin that may clump along the nuclear membrane. Cytoplasmic vacuolization, reflecting mucin production, is seen in some cases; in other cases, the cytoplasm has a feathery quality and indistinct cell borders. In poorly preserved specimens, the cytoplasm may be eosinophilic, whereas similar cells in well-prepared specimens have cyanophilic cytoplasm. The nuclear-cytoplasm ratio is increased in poorly differentiated tumors.

Histologic grading is based on a relatively simple three-grade system: poorly differentiated,

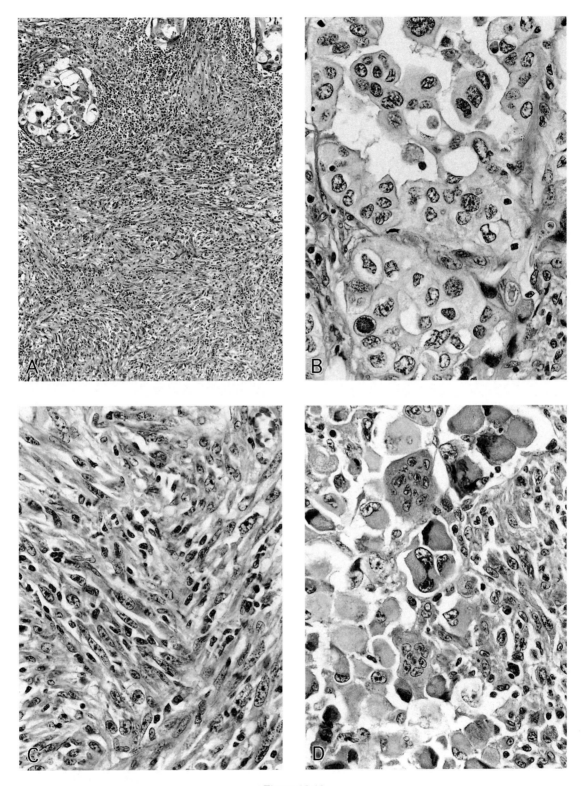

Figure 12-19
ADENOCARCINOMA WITH SPINDLE CELL AND GIANT CELL FOCI
This biphasic neoplasm of the lung shows foci of poorly differentiated adenocarcinoma (A,B) which merged with a neoplastic keratin-positive spindle cell component (A,C) in which foci of giant cell carcinoma were found (D).

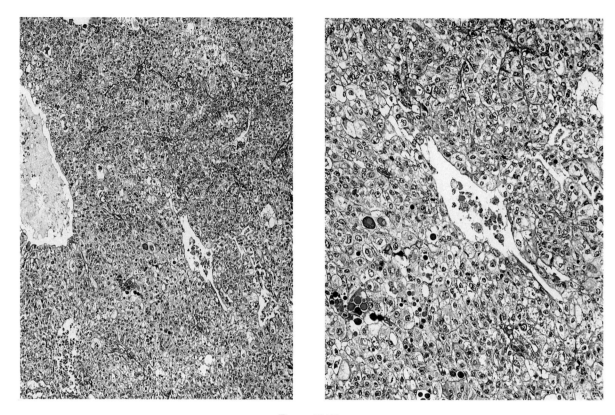

Figure 12-20
HEPATOID ADENOCARCINOMA

This poorly differentiated adenocarcinoma with a hepatoid pattern was associated with alpha-fetoprotein production. Alpha-fetoprotein production can be seen as opaque eosinophilic blobs (right figure, lower left). (Courtesy of Dr. Hiroshi Ishikura, Sapporo, Japan.)

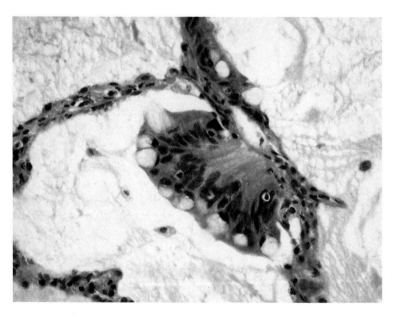

Figure 12-21
ADENOCARCINOMA WITH
ENTERIC DIFFERENTIATION

This adenocarcinoma is associated with extensive mucin production and neoplastic cells lining the alveolar walls. The cells show features of enteric absorptive cells with interspersed goblet cells; focal Paneth cell differentiation was also found. (Courtesy of Dr. Richard Fraser, Montreal, Quebec.)

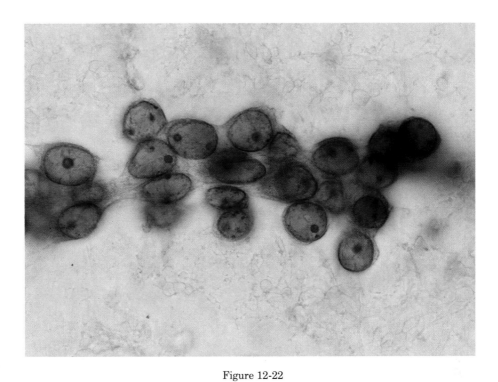

Figure 12-22
ADENOCARCINOMA
This sputum cytology shows a cluster of cells with a high nuclear-cytoplasmic ratio and vesicular nuclei with prominent nucleoli.

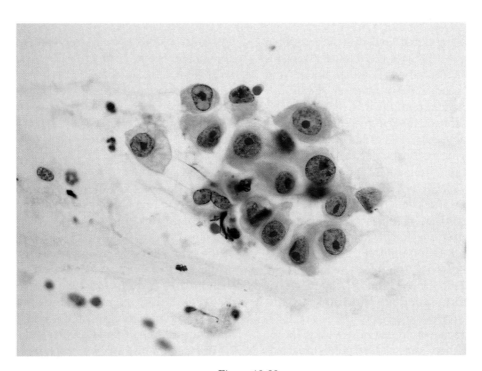

Figure 12-23
ADENOCARCINOMA
Bronchial wash specimen shows cells with vesicular nuclei and prominent nucleoli; the cells are somewhat dyscohesive and have a moderate amount of cyanophilic cytoplasm.

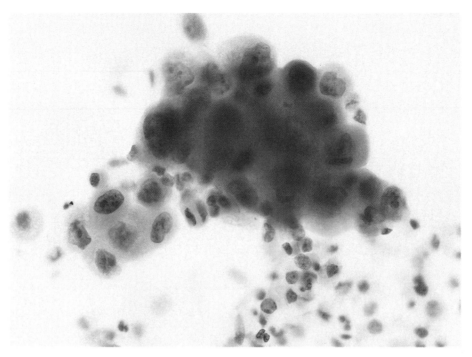

Figure 12-24
ADENOCARCINOMA
Bronchial wash specimen shows cells that overlap and form a three-dimensional group. Atypical features of the nuclei can be seen at the edge of the group. Some of the cells have prominent nucleoli.

moderately differentiated, and well-differentiated (27). Most tumors (70 percent) are moderately differentiated, 5 percent are well- differentiated, and 25 percent are poorly differentiated (27). Even with such a simplified system, the inherent heterogeneity of lung cancer makes grading somewhat difficult and arbitrary. The grade should reflect the predominant histologic pattern. Grading is dependent on sampling and is not accurate with small biopsy specimens. It should reflect the degree of differentiation (tubular, acinar, papillary) and proportion of solid foci, architectural regularity, degree of cytologic atypia, and extent of necrosis. Well-differentiated tumors show architectural regularity, relatively little cytologic atypia, little solid growth, and little necrosis.

Immunohistochemical Findings. Immunohistochemistry is usually not necessary for a diagnosis of adenocarcinoma of the lung except in certain settings, such as distinguishing primary from metastatic adenocarcinoma and malignant mesothelioma from adenocarcinoma. Adenocarcinomas typically, but not invariably, express high and low molecular weight keratins,

epithelial membrane antigen (EMA), HMFG-2, carcinoembryonic antigen (CEA), Leu-M1, and B72.3 (1,3,4,10,11,15,16,38,39).

Pulmonary adenocarcinomas may be positive for a number of neuroendocrine markers: neuron-specific enolase (NSE) (nearly half of adenocarcinomas are positive); Leu-7 (nearly one third are positive); and chromogranin or synaptophysin (10 to 20 percent are positive) (24,26,46). The issue of whether tumors that are positive for neuroendocrine markers should be called large cell neuroendocrine carcinoma is discussed in chapter 14.

Approximately one fourth of adenocarcinomas of the lung stain for vimentin, nearly two thirds are positive for secretory component, and one third to half are positive for surfactant apoprotein (6,20,30). Rarely expressed are bombesin, calcitonin, serotonin, corticotropin (ACTH), vasopressin, neurofilament, and S-100 protein (24,26,46).

The peripheral airway markers, surfactant-associated protein and Clara cell protein, are positive in over 40 percent of adenocarcinomas of the lung and only rarely positive in adenocarcinomas primary in other organs (25).

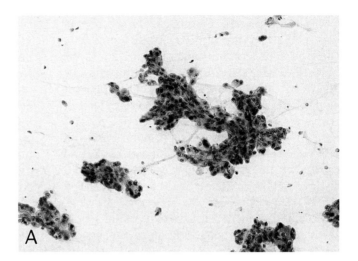

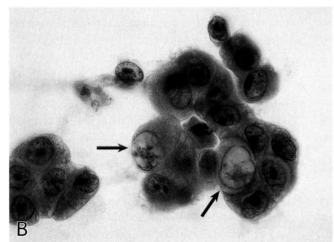

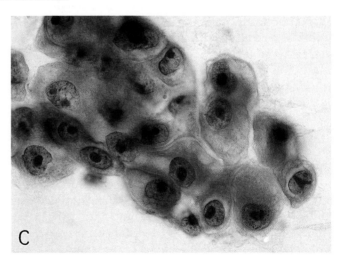

Figure 12-25
ADENOCARCINOMA

This fine needle aspiration specimen shows cohesive three-dimensional cell groups (A) containing cells with vesicular nuclei, thickened nuclear rims, and prominent nucleoli (B,C). The cytoplasm is cyanophilic, and some cells show formation of acini containing mucin vacuoles (arrows) (B). Other cells show some polarity suggesting a columnar shape (C).

Ultrastructural Findings. Adenocarcinomas of the lung are ultrastructurally similar to adenocarcinomas at other sites (figs. 12-26, 12-27) (2,15,16,27,28,30,38). Acinar structures may be identified ultrastructurally when not apparent light microscopically. The most consistent feature is the presence of microvilli, which are present even in poorly differentiated tumors. Microvilli project into an acinar space and have an associated glycocalyx; they may even have terminal webs and distinct rootlets similar to carcinomas of the colon (15,16). According to McGregor et al. (32), microvilli are a more sensitive indicator of adenocarcinoma than the identification of lumens and positive staining for mucin.

The cells are large, cuboidal, or columnar and have large nuclei with prominent nucleoli. Adjacent cells may be joined by junctional complexes. The cells typically have numerous organelles and contain mucin.

Adenocarcinomas usually lack tonofilaments and have fewer desmosomes than squamous cell carcinomas. Tumors that show features of adenocarcinoma by light microscopy may have some evidence of squamous differentiation ultrastructurally, and exactly how such cases are labeled depends on one's criteria. According to WHO criteria, the diagnosis of adenocarcinoma is made at the light microscopic level and such cases are not called adenosquamous carcinomas (43). Similarly, neurosecretory granules may be identified ultrastructurally, just as they may occasionally stain for neuroendocrine markers. The distinction between adenocarcinoma with neuroendocrine differentiation and large cell neuroendocrine carcinoma is discussed in chapter 14.

There are at least three basic cell types comprising pulmonary adenocarcinoma (2,21). The first shows type 2 cell differentiation. These cases have osmiophilic whorls resembling myelin figures and may have intranuclear microtubular arrays corresponding to the eosinophilic intranuclear inclusions seen light microscopically (15,16). The second type shows Clara cell (nonciliated bronchiolar cell) differentiation (35). There are apical knob-like projections of cytoplasm in which osmiophilic Clara cell granules are identifiable. Clara cell differentiation is present in most adenocarcinomas of the lung (21). The third type shows mucinous or goblet cell differentiation and some have recognized

two subtypes in this group (21): cells resembling goblet cells and cells resembling mucus cells of bronchial glands. Mucinous cells are identified by their mucin granules, which may be opaque or flocculent and surrounded by a clear membrane, or by large cytoplasmic accumulations of low-density flocculent mucinous material.

In some poorly differentiated adenocarcinomas, identifying one of these three cell types is difficult. For this reason, some have recognized adenocarcinomas of indeterminate cell type (2).

Differential Diagnosis. The differential diagnosis of adenocarcinoma of the lung includes reactive and metaplastic epithelial changes simulating adenocarcinoma: organizing diffuse alveolar damage, chemotherapy effect, radiation effect, honeycombing, reactive atypia associated with inflammatory processes, and others; benign lesions with glandular features primary in the lung: sclerosing hemangioma, alveolar adenoma, papillary adenoma of type 2 cells, atypical adenomatous hyperplasia, and bronchioloalveolar adenoma; other primary lung malignancies with glandular features: carcinoid, atypical carcinoid, large cell neuroendocrine carcinoma, and pure epithelial blastoma; metastatic adenocarcinoma from extrapulmonary sites: gastrointestinal tract, kidney, breast, prostate, and others; and mesothelioma (in the case of pleural involvement).

The clinical history is extremely helpful in avoiding overinterpretation of reactive epithelial changes and those following chemotherapy or radiation. In general, metaplastic and reactive changes show a heterogeneity of cell types; in bronchiolar metaplasia, ciliated cells are identifiable. Bronchiolar metaplasia lacks significant atypia which is usually identifiable in adenocarcinomas. Metaplastic type 2 alveolar lining cells may be quite bizarre appearing, particularly in cytotoxic-drug lung injury, but they are few in number and lack the monotony typical of neoplasms.

Solitary benign tumors of the lung may resemble adenocarcinomas and these are discussed in chapters 5 and 6. Bronchioloalveolar carcinomas are discussed in chapter 13. Carcinoid tumor and atypical carcinoid tumor are discussed in chapter 17. Large cell neuroendocrine carcinomas may contain glands, produce mucin, and have the same degree of nuclear atypia as seen in adenocarcinoma of the lung. These are discussed in chapter 14. Monophasic

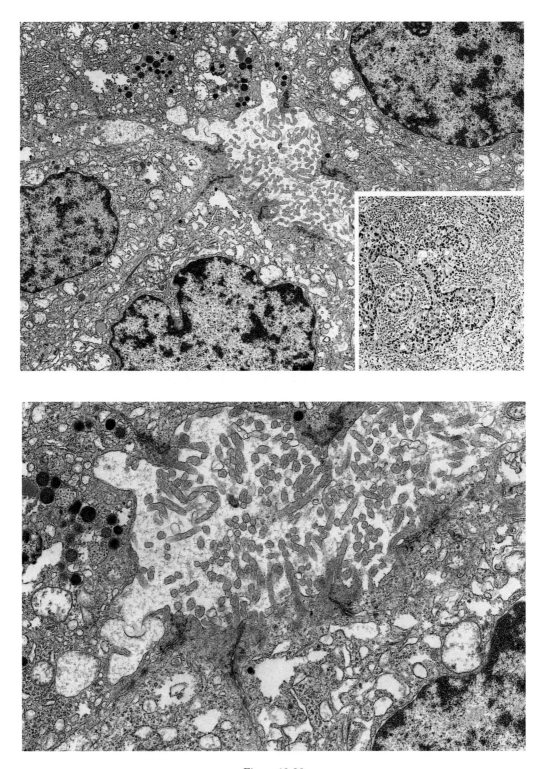

Figure 12-26
ADENOCARCINOMA

Top: The low-power electron micrograph shows lumen formation with a few microvilli protruding into it. The histologic appearance of this tumor is shown in the inset (at lower right). (X1500)

Bottom: Detail of the lumen showing dense apical granules, intercellular attachments, and actin filament cores in the microvilli. (X12,000)

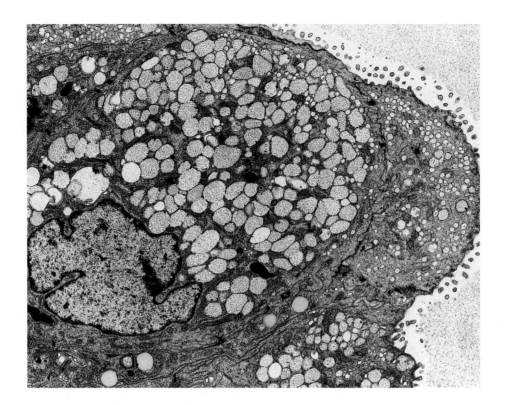

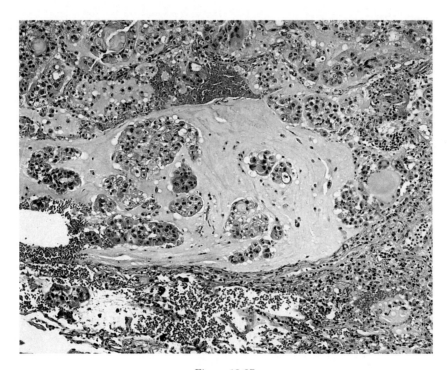

Figure 12-27
MUCIN-PRODUCING ADENOCARCINOMA

Top: An electron micrograph of a mucin-producing adenocarcinoma shows a cell stuffed with flocculent mucin vacuoles. Short surface microvilli are present. (X6500)

Bottom: A histologic section from a similar area in the same tumor.

pulmonary blastomas represent adenocarcinomas in the generic sense, but they have a distinct histology resembling fetal lung. They are discussed in chapter 21.

Some adenocarcinomas metastatic to the lung are impossible to distinguish from a primary adenocarcinoma of the lung. In such cases, sections of the primary tumor, if known, should be compared to the adenocarcinoma. In some cases, immunostaining may be helpful, as shown by the usefulness of anti-CEA antibodies (D-14) in separating metastatic colon carcinoma from lung carcinoma (8,13). Metastatic colon carcinoma is a centrally necrotic tumor with abundant dirty necrosis, better differentiation than most adenocarcinomas of the lung, and lack of the heterogeneity and variation in differentiation from field to field that is so typical of lung adenocarcinoma.

Breast carcinomas may present in the lung or metastasize to the lung and should be considered in any woman, particularly a nonsmoker, who has an unusual clinical presentation for primary carcinoma of the lung or in whom the tumor is composed of intermediate-size cells with relatively little pleomorphism. Raab et al. (37) showed that a panel of immunohistochemical studies could distinguish most primary lung cancers from metastatic breast carcinoma. Lung carcinomas tend to be CEA positive, S-100 negative, estrogen receptor negative, and gross cystic disease fluid protein negative; breast carcinomas tend to show the converse (37).

Renal cell carcinoma may present as single or multiple nodules in the lung or as metastases in a patient with a history of renal cell carcinoma. Histologic patterns are as varied as they are in the kidney, but in most there is clear cell change, prominent vascularity, lack abundant glandular differentiation, and lack of mucin.

It is likely that monoclonal antibodies to antigens primarily restricted to lung carcinomas will become widely available and aid in the differential diagnosis. Antibodies to major surfactant-associated protein and 10-KD Clara cell protein are examples that are often positive in lung carcinomas, both in primary and metastatic sites, and rarely positive in carcinomas primary at other sites (25).

A tumor involving the pleura and showing epithelioid differentiation may be a mesothelioma or an adenocarcinoma. The distinction between these two entities is addressed in the second series Fascicle, Tumors of Serous Membranes (30a).

Although monoclonal antibodies to specific proteins may help in the recognition of various tumors, there is no replacement for careful review of the clinical history, radiographic findings, and routine light microscopy in the differential diagnosis of tumors in the thorax. Most cases can be solved with confidence without resorting to immunohistochemistry or electron microscopy. Current radiographic techniques have allowed for identification of primary tumors in many sites that would previously have been clinically occult, such as the abdomen and retroperitoneum, and these findings, along with knowledge of the usual histologic appearance of tumors (colonic carcinoma, for example, is recognizable in the vast majority of cases regardless of the site of biopsy) have allowed for considerable diagnostic accuracy.

Staging, Spread, and Metastases. See chapter 8.

Treatment and Prognosis. The overall 5-year survival for adenocarcinoma is 19.2 percent (see fig. 8-16). Complete surgical resection is the only hope of cure and is possible in only a minority of cases. As shown in chapter 8, most patients with carcinoma of the lung present with high-stage disease and are not candidates for resection. Nevertheless, of the patients who do undergo resection for cure, between 50 and 80 percent survive 5 years (see fig. 8-13) (43,44). Many studies suggest that the prognosis may be even better with small peripheral bronchiolo-alveolar carcinomas (chapter 13), but this may simply reflect their better differentiation.

REFERENCES

1. Blobel GA, Moll R, Franke WW, Vogt-Moykopf I. Cytokeratins in normal lung and lung carcinomas. I. Adenocarcinomas, squamous cell carcinomas and cultured cell lines. Virchows Arch [Cell Pathol] 1984;45:407–29.

2. Bolen JW, Thorning D. Histogenetic classification of pulmonary carcinomas. Peripheral adenocarcinomas studied by light microscopy, histochemistry, and electron microscopy. Pathol Annu 1982;17(Pt 1):77–100.

3. Brockmann M, Brockmann I, Herberg U, Müller KM. Adenocarcinoma of the lung. Immunohistochemical findings (keratin/CEA). J Cancer Res Clin Oncol 1987;113:379–82.

4. Bruderman I, Cohen R, Leitner O, et al. Immunocytochemical characterization of lung tumors in fine-needle aspiration. The use of cytokeratin monoclonal antibodies for the differential diagnosis of squamous cell carcinoma and adenocarcinoma. Cancer 1990;66:1817–27.

5. Cagle PT, Alpert LC, Carmona PA. Peripheral biphasic adenocarcinoma of the lung: light microscopic and immunohistochemical findings. Hum Pathol 1992;23:197–200.

6. Dempo K, Satoh M, Tsuji S, Mori M, Kuroki Y, Akino T. Immunohistochemical studies on the expression of pulmonary surfactant apoproteins in human lung carcinomas using monoclonal antibodies. Path Res Pract 1987;182:669–75.

7. Fishback N, Travis WD, Moran C, Guinee DG, McCarthy W, Koss M. Pleomorphic (spindle/giant cell) carcinoma of the lung: a clinicopathologic study of 78 cases. Cancer 1994;73:2936–45.

8. Flint A, Lloyd RV. Pulmonary metastases of colon carcinoma: distinction from primary pulmonary adenocarcinoma. Mod Pathol 1991;4:115A.

9. Gatter KC, Dunnill MS, Heryet A, Mason DY. Human lung tumors: does intermediate filament co-expression correlate with other morphologic or immunocytochemical features? Histopathology 1987;11:705–14.

10. _____, Dunnill MS, Pulford KA, Heryet A, Mason DY. Human lung tumors: a correlation of antigenic profile with histologic type. Histopathology 1985;9:805–23.

11. _____, Dunnill MS, Van Muijen GN, Mason DY. Human lung tumours may coexpress different classes of intermediate filaments. J Clin Pathol 1986;39:950–4.

12. Gazdar AF, Linnoila RI. The pathology of lung cancer—changing concepts and newer diagnostic techniques. Semin Oncol 1988;15:215-25.

13. Ghoneim AH, Brisson ML, Fuks A, Mobasher AA, Kreisman H. Monoclonal anti-CEA antibodies in the discrimination between primary pulmonary adenocarcinoma and colon carcinoma metastatic to the lung. Mod Pathol 1990;3:613–8.

14. Greenberg SD, Fraire AE, Kinner BM, Johnson EH. Tumor cell type versus staging in the prognosis of carcinoma of the lung. Pathol Annu 1987;22(Pt 2):387–405.

15. Hammar S. The use of electron microscopy and immunohistochemistry in the diagnosis and understanding of lung neoplasms. Clin Lab Med 1987;7:1-30.

16. Hammar SP, Bolen JW, Bockus D, Remington F, Friedman S. Ultrastructural and immunohistochemical features of common lung tumors: an overview. Ultrastruct Pathol 1985;9:283–318.

17. Ishikura H, Kanda M, Ito M, Nosaka K, Mizuno K. Hepatoid adenocarcinoma: a distinctive histological subtype of alpha-fetoprotein-producing lung carcinoma. Virchows Arch [A] 1990;417:73–80.

18. Johnston WW, Frable WJ. The cytopathology of the respiratory tract. A review. Am J Pathol 1976;84:372–413.

19. Katzenstein AL, Prioleau PG, Askin FB. The histologic spectrum and significance of clear cell change in lung carcinoma. Cancer 1980;45:943–7.

20. Kawai T, Torikata C, Suzuki M. Immunohistochemical study of pulmonary adenocarcinoma. Am J Clin Pathol 1988;89:455–62.

21. Kimula Y. A histochemical and ultrastructural study of adenocarcinoma of the lung. Am J Surg Pathol 1978;2:253–64.

22. Kish JK, Ro JY, Ayala AG, McMurtrey MJ. Primary mucinous adenocarcinoma of the lung with signet-ring cells: a histochemical comparison with signet-ring cell carcinomas of other sites. Hum Pathol 1989;20:1097–102.

23. Kodama T, Shimosato Y, Koide T, Watanabe S, Yoneyama T. Endobronchial polypoid adenocarcinoma of the lung. Histological and ultrastructural studies of five cases. Am J Surg Pathol 1984;8:845–54.

24. Linnoila RI. Pathology of non-small cell lung cancer. New diagnostic approaches. Hematol Oncol Clin North Am 1990;4:1027–51.

25. _____, Jensen SM, Steinberg SM, Mulshing JL, Eggleston JC, Gazdar AF. Peripheral airway cell marker expression in non-small cell lung carcinoma. Am J Clin Pathol 1992;97:233–43.

26. _____, Mulshine JL, Steinberg SM, et al. Neuroendocrine differentiation in endocrine and nonendocrine lung carcinomas. Am J Clin Pathol 1988;90:641–52.

27. Mackay B, Lukeman JM, Ordonez NG. Tumors of the lung. In: Major problems in pathology, Vol 24. Philadelphia: WB Saunders, 1991:100–64.

28. _____, Ordonez NG, Bennington JL, Dugan CC. Ultrastructural and morphometric features of poorly differentiated and undifferentiated lung tumors. Ultrastruct Pathol 1989;13:561–71.

29. Matthews MJ. Morphology of lung cancer. Semin Oncol 1974;1:175–82.

30. _____, Mackay B, Lukeman J. The pathology of non-small cell carcinoma of the lung. Semin Oncol 1983;10:34-55.

30a. McCaughey WT, Kannerstein M, Churg J. Tumors and pseudotumors of the serous membranes. Atlas of Tumor Pathology, 2nd Series, Fascicle 20. Washington, D.C.: Armed Forces Institute of Pathology, 1985.

31. McElvaney G, Miller RR, Müller NL, Nelems B, Evans KG, Ostrow DN. Multicentricity of adenocarcinoma of the lung. Chest 1989;95:151–4.

32. McGregor DH, Dixon AY, McGregor DK. Adenocarcinoma of the lung: a comparative diagnostic study using light and electron microscopy. Hum Pathol 1988;19:910–3.

33. Miller RR, Nelems B, Evans KG, Müller NL, Ostrow DN. Glandular neoplasia of the lung. A proposed analogy of colonic tumors. Cancer 1988;61:1009–14.

34. Mizutani Y, Nakajima T, Morinaga S. Immunohistochemical localization of pulmonary surfactant apoproteins in various lung tumors. Special reference to nonmucus producing lung adenocarcinomas. Cancer 1988;61:532–7.

35. Montes M, Binette JP, Chaudhry AP, Adler RH, Guarino R. Clara cell adenocarcinoma. Light and electron microscope studies. Am J Surg Pathol 1977;1:245–53.

36. Ogata T, Endo K. Clara cell granules of peripheral lung cancers. Cancer 1984;54:1635–44.

37. Raab SS, Berg LC, Swanson PE, Wick MR. Adenocarcinoma in the lung in patients with breast cancer. A prospective analysis of the discriminatory value of immunohistology. Am J Clin Pathol 1993;100:27–35.

38. Saba SR, Espinoza CG, Richman AV, Azar HA. Carcinomas of the lung: an ultrastructural and immunocytochemical study. Am J Clin Pathol 1983;80:6–13.

39. Said JW. Immunohistochemistry of lung tumors. Lung Biol Health Dis 1990;44:635–51.

40. Scroggs MW, Roggli VL, Fraire AE, Sanfilippo F. Eosinophilic intracytoplasmic globules in pulmonary adenocarcinomas: a histochemical, immunohistochemical, and ultrastructural study of six cases. Hum Pathol 1989;20:845–9.

41. Sobin L, Yesner R. Histological typing of lung tumors. International Histological Classification of Tumors, Vol. 1. 2nd ed. Geneva: World Health Organization, 1981.

42. Sørensen JB, Hirsch FR, Olsen J. The prognostic implication of histopathologic subtyping of pulmonary adenocarcinoma according to the classification of the World Health Organization. An analysis of 259 consecutive patients with advanced disease. Cancer 1988;62:361–7.

43. _____, Olsen JE. Prognostic implications of histopathologic subtyping in patients with surgically treated stage I or II adenocarcinoma of the lung. J Thorac Cardiovasc Surg 1989;97:245–51.

44. Takise A, Kodama T, Shimosato Y, Watanabe S, Suemasu K. Histopathologic prognostic factors in adenocarcinomas of the peripheral lung less than 2 cm in diameter. Cancer 1988;61:2083–8.

45. Tsao MS, Fraser RS. Primary pulmonary adenocarcinoma with enteric differentiation. Cancer 1991;68:1754–7.

46. Visscher DW, Zarbo RJ, Trojanowski JQ, Sakr W, Crissman JD. Neuroendocrine differentiation in poorly differentiated lung carcinomas: a light microscopic and immunohistologic study. Mod Pathol 1990;3:508–12.

✧✧✧

13
BRONCHIOLOALVEOLAR CARCINOMA

Definition. Bronchioloalveolar carcinoma (BAC), also called *alveolar cell carcinoma* and *bronchoalveolar tumor* is a subset of pulmonary adenocarcinoma common and distinctive enough to warrant separation from the other subtypes. According to the World Health Organization (WHO) classification, BACs are adenocarcinomas "in which cylindrical tumor cells grow upon the walls of preexisting alveoli" (34). The key feature is preservation of the underlying architecture of the lung. Since many adenocarcinomas of the lung include regions with a BAC pattern, the designation BAC should be restricted to cases that show only this pattern. BACs are composed of two main cell types: mucinous and nonmucinous, with the latter being more common. Sclerosing BACs, which have some alveolar septal fibrosis, are a subset of the nonmucinous type. Many nonmucinous BACs have central scarring and foci of distortion (but not destruction) of architecture which may simulate invasive carcinoma.

Most tumors called mucinous cystadenomas, mucinous cystic tumors of borderline malignancy, and mucinous (colloid) adenocarcinomas of the lung (10,18,21,23,31) are probably closely related to mucinous BAC, although they represent a distinct subgroup (10). Most of the carcinomas complicating lung cysts are BACs (chapter 16).

Clinical Features. In most series, the incidence of BAC varies from 1 to 5 percent of lung carcinomas, although some recent reviews have shown an incidence as high as 15 percent (17). Over 50 percent present as asymptomatic, solitary peripheral nodules, often as incidental findings on chest radiographs taken for some other reason (19). Some solitary peripheral BACs grow slowly for several years without dissemination; others, seen initially as solitary nodules, rapidly develop satellite metastases and then widespread bilateral disease (12,19,28). A few BACs present as lobar consolidation radiographically. Air bronchograms in the affected lung tissue are distinctive, reflecting the nondestructive growth pattern of BAC.

The average patient age at presentation is in the sixth decade, although patients in the second decade have been reported (8,11). Symptomatic patients complain of cough, sputum production, dyspnea, chest pain, or weight loss (8,11). Although a classic sign of BAC, copious mucus in the sputum (bronchorrhea), is seen in less than 10 percent of the cases, and when it is present it is generally late in the course of the disease and associated with a poor prognosis (8,11). Symptoms increase with the extent of disease, and patients with extensive bilateral disease have marked respiratory compromise. Symptoms related to metastases, paraneoplastic syndromes, and hormone production are unusual.

Gross Findings. There are nodules or foci of consolidation without destructive or invasive features (figs. 13-1–13-3) (3,6,7,24,26,29). Most BACs are peripheral, although rare examples are central (6,7).

The nodules of nonmucinous BAC manifest as gray-white foci of parenchymal consolidation, sometimes associated with a central scar, which may be anthracotic, and is probably a secondary phenomenon. In a small number of cases, evidence of old granulomatous disease may be found in the scar. The problem of so-called scar carcinoma is discussed in chapter 7. Hemorrhage and necrosis are lacking, and architectural preservation is apparent. In cases close to the pleural surface, pleural puckering and fibrosis may be evident, although pleural invasion is unusual. The presence or absence of pleural invasion should be addressed for staging purposes.

Mucinous BACs are often larger and more multifocal than nonmucinous variants; mucinous BAC is the usual cause of the lobar pneumonic form of BAC in which an entire lobe is replaced by glistening mucinous consolidation (figs. 13-2, 13-14). There is preservation of the underlying lung architecture, although large pools of mucus may grossly distort airspaces.

In both the mucinous and nonmucinous variants, tumors that may have appeared solitary radiographically may have one or more satellite nodules at the time of gross or microscopic evaluation.

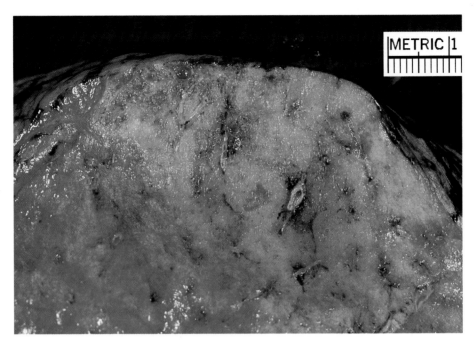

Figure 13-1
BRONCHIOLOALVEOLAR CARCINOMA, NONMUCINOUS TYPE
There is a zone of subpleural consolidation without hemorrhage, necrosis, or loss of lung architecture. Some increased anthracotic pigment is noted. The histology showed nonmucinous BAC.

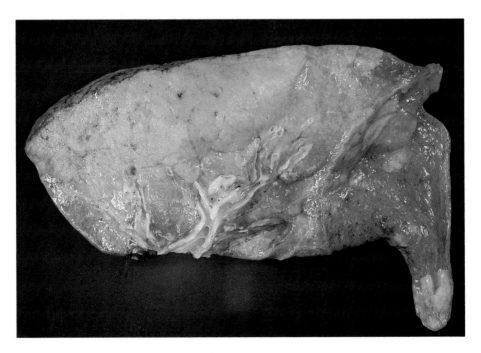

Figure 13-2
BRONCHIOLOALVEOLAR CARCINOMA, MUCINOUS TYPE
The superior portion of this upper lobe (left) is almost entirely consolidated by mucinous BAC. Despite the consolidation, there is an absence of necrosis and hemorrhage, and the architecture is maintained.

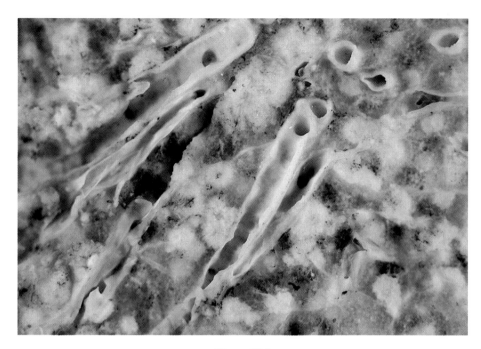

Figure 13-3
BRONCHIOLOALVEOLAR CARCINOMA, NONMUCINOUS TYPE
This gross photograph is from the lungs of a patient who died of widespread bilateral BAC. A cut surface of the formalin-inflated lungs shows multiple, small, gray-white nodules with absence of necrosis, hemorrhage, or architectural distortion. The bronchi course normally through the lung tissue, and the presence of air bronchograms radiographically in such cases is not surprising.

A small BAC (usually nonmucinous) is an occasional incidental finding in a lobectomy for some other problem. Distinction of a small BAC from bronchioloalveolar cell adenoma is discussed below.

Mucinous cystic tumors (colloid carcinomas) (10,31), which, for the most part, are variants of bronchioloalveolar carcinoma, resemble mucinous (colloid or gelatinous) carcinomas at other sites. There is a well-demarcated, though not necessarily circumscribed, pool of glistening mucus, which may be clear, cloudy, or hemorrhagic (see figs. 13-20, 13-21). The masses vary from 0.5 to 10 cm in diameter and generally lack visible cysts. Mucinous cystic tumors of borderline malignancy (19) and mucinous cystadenomas (23) have either partial or complete fibrous walls surrounding the mucin pools.

Microscopic Findings. BACs are separated into two major subtypes: nonmucinous (figs. 13-4–13-13), comprising two thirds to three fourths of the cases, and mucinous (figs. 13-14–13-19), comprising most of the remainder (6–8,16,19,24, 26,27,29). Nonmucinous BACs are composed of

cells with Clara cell or type 2 cell differentiation, or both. Mucinous BACs are composed of goblet or mucin-producing cells and are usually very well-differentiated. A small percentage combine cells of both types, and some of the lesser differentiated cases are difficult to subclassify.

The key feature of BAC is the growth of well-differentiated cuboidal or columnar tumor cells along intact alveolar walls, either as a single layer or, occasionally, as papillae into alveolar spaces. When giant papillae are present and alveolar architecture is no longer discernible, the diagnosis of BAC is no longer appropriate. Tumors resembling BAC but having foci of stromal invasion with irregular nests of tumor cells surrounded by a fibroblastic response should be designated "adenocarcinomas with a prominent bronchioloalveolar growth pattern." These tumors usually also show moderate to marked cytologic atypia, particularly in the foci of stromal invasion.

A characteristic histologic feature of BACs, which probably correlates with aerogenous spread, is the presence of single cells, acinar clusters, and papillary groups lying free in alveolar

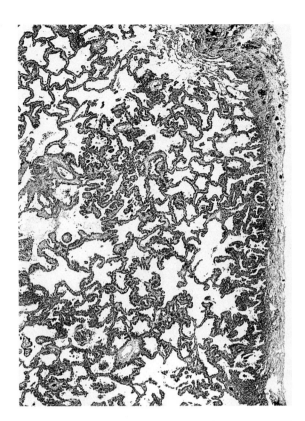
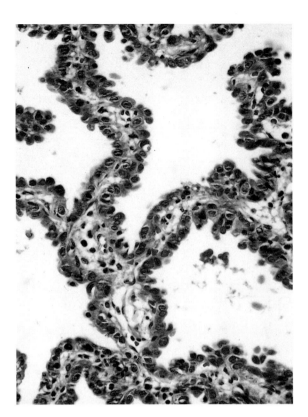

Figure 13-4
NONMUCINOUS BRONCHIOLOALVEOLAR CARCINOMA
There is uniform involvement of the alveolar walls by proliferation of uniform cuboidal cells (left) with moderate nuclear atypia (right).

spaces. Aerogenous spread of these cells probably accounts for some, if not all, of the satellite lesions that are so commonly seen microscopically with BAC. The possibility that some satellite lesions are independent primaries cannot be excluded histologically.

Nonmucinous Bronchioloalveolar Carcinomas. Nonmucinous BAC cells are more cuboidal rather than tall columnar and often have bright eosinophilic cytoplasm. The nuclei are larger, considerably more hyperchromatic and atypical, and have more prominent nucleoli than the mucinous variety. Clara cell differentiation may be seen as apical snouting of the tumor cells. The nucleus may protrude into the snout in a hobnail fashion. Cilia are rarely seen, and when present, are strong evidence of a benign process. While the cell size, shape, and degree of nuclear atypia may vary somewhat, there is an overall uniformity of the cells lining the alveoli. This helps distinguish BAC from reactive and metaplastic

lesions which show a heterogeneity of cell types and include ciliated cells.

Nonmucinous BACs commonly have central scarring (fig. 13-6), which is probably a secondary phenomenon (see discussion of scar cancers, chapter 7). In the scarred region, the cells may grow in distorted airspaces as irregular nests which simulate stromal invasion. Usually, the surrounding fibrous tissue is acellular and elastotic rather than the reactive cellular fibroblastic stroma typical of invasive carcinoma, and the cells are better differentiated than in ordinary adenocarcinomas.

A typical feature of nonmucinous BAC is that cells become less columnar toward the periphery of a tumor nodule and cytologic atypia fades away (fig. 13-5); at the edge of a nodule it may be impossible to separate the tumor cells from reactive type 2 cells. In such cases, the demarcation seen at scanning power and the most cytologically atypical foci at higher power are keys to

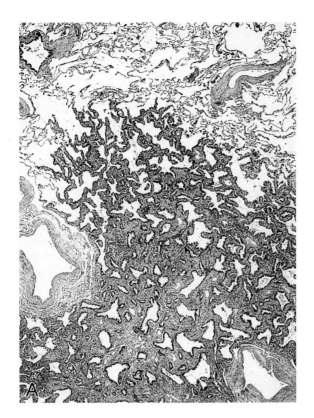

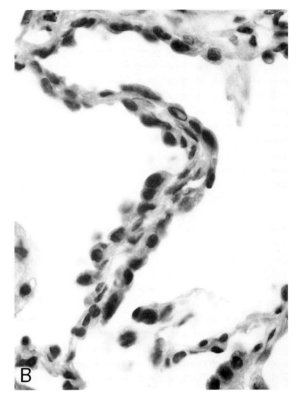

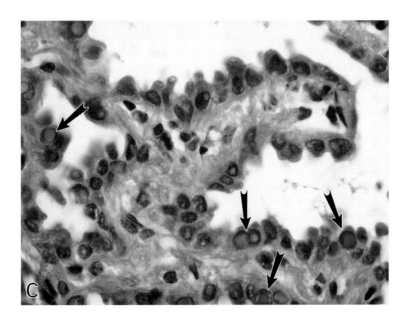

Figure 13-5
SCLEROSING NONMUCINOUS BRONCHIOLOALVEOLAR CARCINOMA
This nonmucinous BAC shows increased septal thickening toward the center of the tumor (A, bottom), with peripheral spread along intact alveolar walls and a tendency for the cells to become smaller and less cuboidal toward the periphery (B). Some nuclear inclusions are apparent (C) in the more atypical cells nearer to the center of the lesion (arrows).

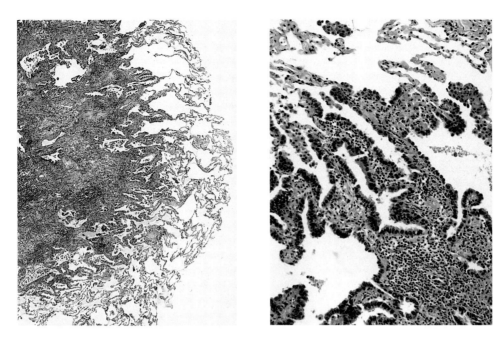

Figure 13-6
SCLEROSING NONMUCINOUS BRONCHIOLOALVEOLAR CARCINOMA
Left: This sclerosing nonmucinous BAC has prominent central scarring, although necrosis and stromal infiltration by tumor cells are not apparent.
Right: The cellular proliferation at the periphery shows growth along intact alveolar walls with accompanying alveolar septal thickening and inflammation.

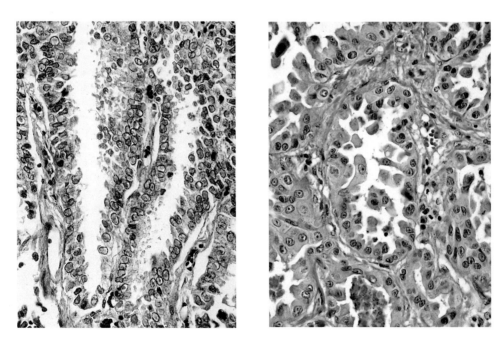

Figure 13-7
NONMUCINOUS BRONCHIOLOALVEOLAR CARCINOMA
These cases illustrate some of the variations in cytologic appearance of BAC. On the left there are numerous intranuclear inclusions that might be misinterpreted as viral inclusions (contrast with figure 13-25). On the right there is prominent cytologic atypia and considerable variation in the amount of cytoplasm present.

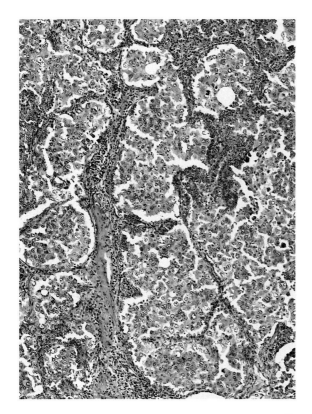 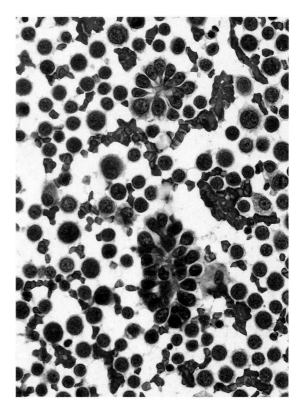

Figure 13-8
NONMUCINOUS BRONCHIOLOALVEOLAR CARCINOMA
Left: There is flooding of alveolar spaces by individual cells reminiscent of desquamative interstitial pneumonia. Elsewhere in the same case there was typical nonmucinous BAC.
Right: A fine needle aspiration of a similar case with occasional papillary clusters and numerous single cells.

making the diagnosis. Likewise, nonmucinous BACs may have satellite lesions lined by considerably less atypical cells than those in the main lesion. These satellites are often considered carcinomatous simply because of their proximity to the main lesion, although when evaluated independently, such small lesions are diagnostic dilemmas. Satellite foci of nonmucinous BAC may be impossible to separate from bronchioloalveolar cell adenomas and atypical adenomatous hyperplasia (chapter 7).

Clara cell differentiation may be suggested by the presence of apical periodic acid–Schiff (PAS)-positive granules and type 2 cell differentiation by the presence of PAS-positive intranuclear inclusions (6,7); PAS-positive intracytoplasmic vacuoles (lumina) and glycogen may also be found in either cell type (fig. 13-11). Clara cell differentiation is the most common cell type in nonmucinous BAC, seen in 90 percent of cases

(fig. 13-12) (6,7); a small percentage of BACs are composed primarily of cells with type 2 cell differentiation (fig. 13-13); and some cases show a mixture of the two cell types. Light microscopically, it may be difficult to distinguish between Clara cell and type 2 cell differentiation in individual cases.

Most nonmucinous BACs have mild interstitial thickening and fibrosis and a modest interstitial infiltrate of lymphocytes and plasma cells (figs. 13-5, 13-6). The lymphocytes are primarily T cells (1). Electron microscopy and immunohistochemistry have also identified Langerhans cells in the interstitial infiltrate (20). Occasional cases show a non-necrotizing granulomatous reaction in the lung tissue around a nonmucinous BAC. Infections and sarcoidosis should be included in the differential diagnosis when these changes are seen, although in most cases the granulomas are a nonspecific incidental finding.

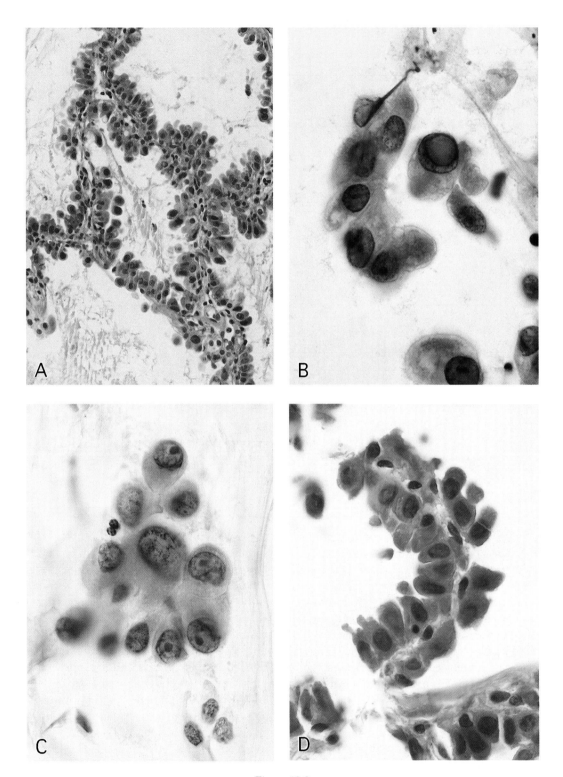

Figure 13-9
NONMUCINOUS BRONCHIOLOALVEOLAR CARCINOMA

A histologic section shows a proliferation of atypical cells along the alveolar walls (A). Cytologically (B), cells from the prior fine needle aspirate show only mild nuclear atypia. The cells have a columnar shape with basal nuclei and prominent cyanophilic cytoplasm. An intranuclear inclusion is present. Bronchial brush cytology (C) from another case shows cells with nuclear hyperchromasia and prominent eosinophilic nucleoli. The transbronchial biopsy (D) shows a typical nonmucinous BAC.

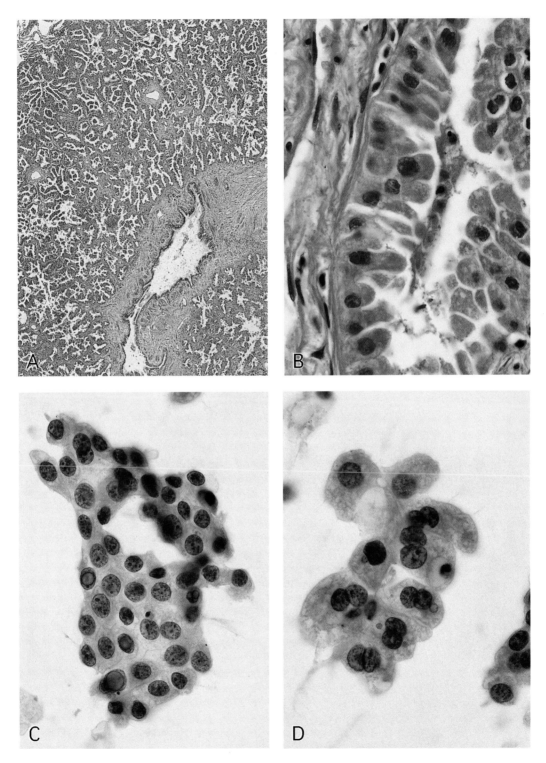

Figure 13-10
NONMUCINOUS BRONCHIOLOALVEOLAR CARCINOMA

Resection specimen (A,B) and previous fine needle aspiration (C,D) from a Clara cell BAC. There is a proliferation of eosinophilic cells with cytoplasmic protrusions lining alveolar walls (A,B). The fine needle aspiration shows monolayer sheets (C) and cells with mild nuclear atypia, cuboidal shape, and somewhat vacuolated cyanophilic cytoplasm, which has a tendency to protrude apically, even in the cytologic preparation (D).

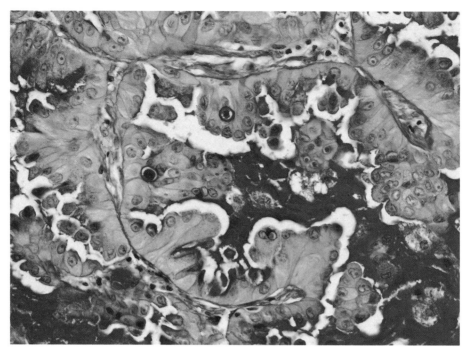

Figure 13-11
MUCIN STAINING IN BRONCHIOLOALVEOLAR CARCINOMA
Despite the fact that this BAC does not have obvious goblet cell features and the cells are eosinophilic, there is abundant luminal mucus secretion, in addition to occasional cells with intracytoplasmic mucin production as seen with a digested PAS stain.

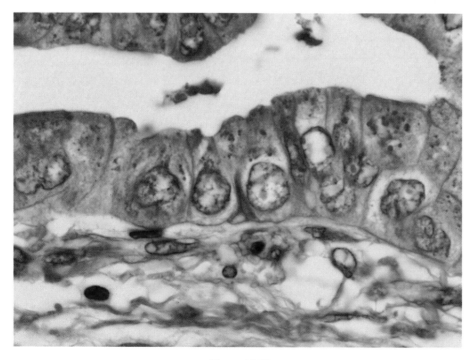

Figure 13-12
CLARA CELL BRONCHIOLOALVEOLAR CARCINOMA
Digested PAS stain shows apical PAS-positive granules.

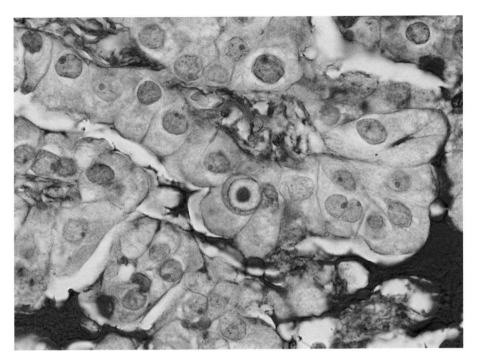

Figure 13-13
INTRANUCLEAR INCLUSION IN BRONCHIOLOALVEOLAR CARCINOMA
Digested PAS stain in this nonmucinous BAC shows an occasional cell with a PAS-positive intranuclear inclusion, probably indicative of type 2 cell differentiation.

Sclerosing nonmucinous BACs have prominent interstitial fibrosis. The lung architecture is distorted but not destroyed and stromal invasion by single cells or irregular nests of carcinoma is not present. A significant proportion of scar carcinomas are sclerosing BACs (see chapter 7). When the stroma of a sclerosing BAC is heavily infiltrated by inflammatory cells, the distinction from post-inflammatory honeycombing may be difficult.

Mucinous Bronchioloalveolar Carcinoma. The mucinous variant of BAC is composed of tall, uniform, columnar mucinous cells that are well differentiated and lack cilia (figs. 13-14–13-19). The nuclei are uniform and lack significant hyperchromasia, although clefting may be seen. Less well-differentiated examples show a greater degree of nuclear atypia, larger nucleoli, and more nuclear hyperchromasia. The cytoplasm is clear, grayish, or foamy in appearance and stains positively with mucin stains. Copious mucus is typically produced which floods the alveoli both within and at a considerable distance from the tumor cell nests. Muciphages and a few neutrophils are common in the mucus.

The pulmonary interstitium is usually normal without any inflammatory infiltrate. Axiotis and Jennings (1) have shown that these tumors may be associated with a B-cell lymphocytic response in the form of lymphoid hyperplasia along bronchovascular bundles.

A helpful diagnostic feature in small biopsies from mucinous BACs is the sharp demarcation of the tumor cells: tumor growth along alveolar septa stops abruptly, and this feature, along with the uniformity of the cells and their lack of cilia, allows for a diagnosis of malignancy, even in the absence of appreciable cytologic atypia.

Mucinous Cystic Tumors. Mucinous cystic tumors, including *mucinous cystadenoma* (chapter 5), *mucinous tumors of borderline malignancy,* and *mucinous adenocarcinomas,* have massive pooling of mucus and a relative paucity of mucinous epithelium (figs. 13-20–13-22). One may have to search several sections to find a few neoplastic mucinous cells. These foci are often indistinguishable from typical mucinous BACs. In mucinous tumors of borderline malignancy and mucinous cystadenomas, there is a partial

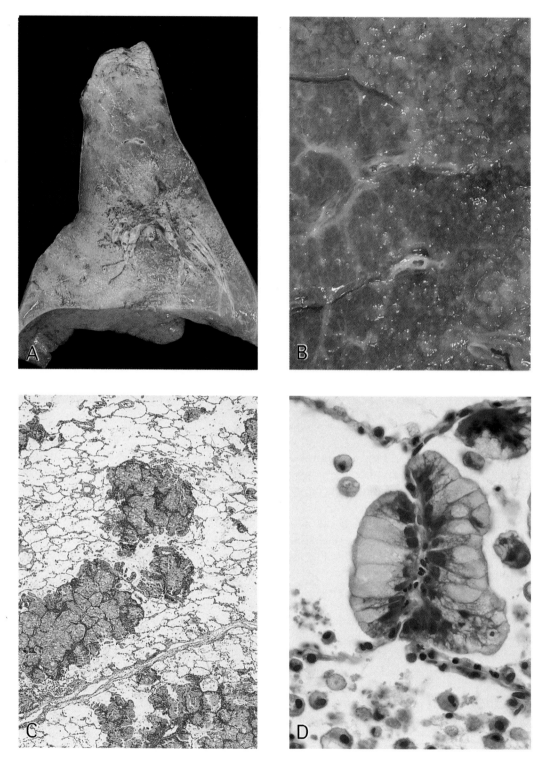

Figure 13-14
MUCINOUS BRONCHIOLOALVEOLAR CARCINOMA

This mucinous BAC shows consolidation of the entire left lower lobe (A), and careful gross examination reveals multiple tiny mucinous nodules (B) which are seen histologically in multiple discrete micronodules. Histology from a similar case shows neoplastic involvement of the alveolar walls by extremely well-differentiated mucinous epithelium (C,D). The previous fine needle aspiration specimens (E,F) show monolayer sheets of cells with mild nuclear atypia and abundant finely vacuolated cytoplasm.

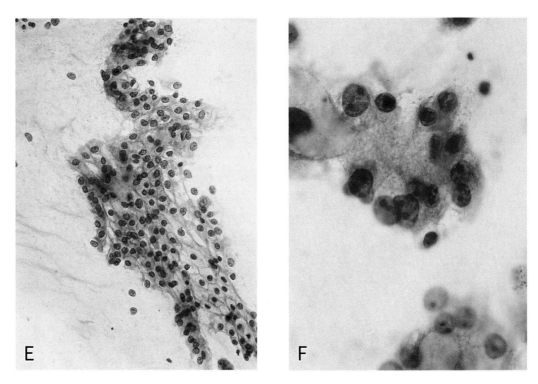

Figure 13-14 (continued)

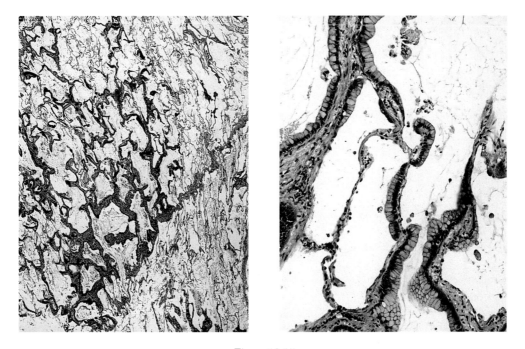

Figure 13-15
MUCINOUS BRONCHIOLOALVEOLAR CARCINOMA
There is mild septal sclerosis and inflammation, unusual features in mucinous BAC.

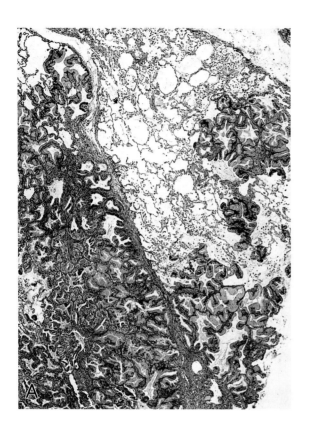

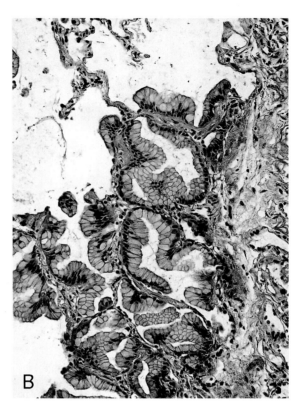

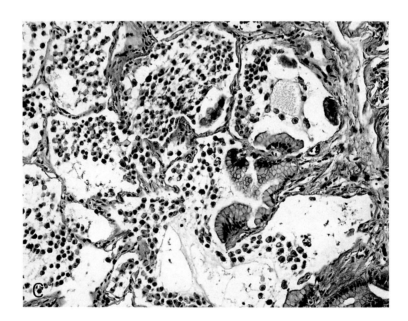

Figure 13-16
MUCINOUS BRONCHIOLOALVEOLAR CARCINOMA

The tumor cells line intact alveolar septa (A,B,C) with preservation of lung architecture, as noted by the growth along, but without destroying, a septum (A). In some foci (C) there are abundant accumulations of mucin and alveolar macrophages within alveolar spaces.

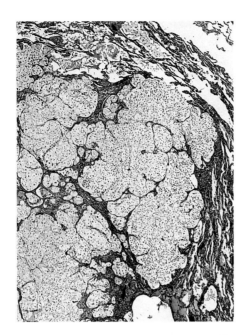

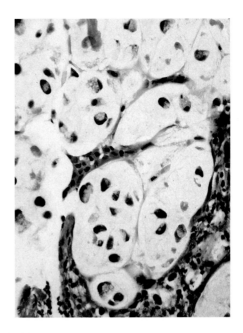

Figure 13-17
MUCINOUS BRONCHIOLOALVEOLAR CARCINOMA VARIANT

This mucinous carcinoma manifested as mucin pooling within intact alveolar spaces (left) with signet ring carcinoma cells floating in the mucus (right). Such a case could arbitrarily be called a mucinous BAC, although tumor cells are not actually seen lining alveolar spaces, or a variant of mucinous (colloid) carcinoma.

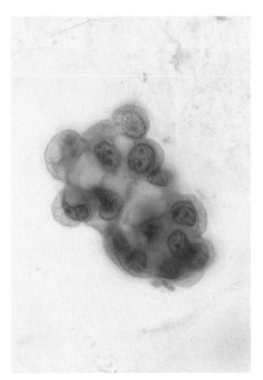

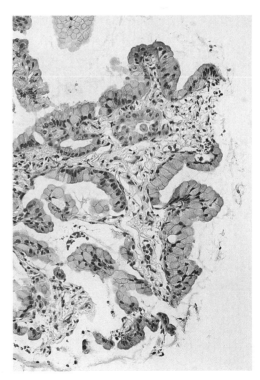

Figure 13-18
MUCINOUS BRONCHIOLOALVEOLAR CARCINOMA

Left: Sputum specimen shows a cohesive cluster of vacuolated cells with relatively uniform nuclear cytology.
Right: Corresponding transbronchial biopsy shows a uniform proliferation of mucinous cells lining alveolar walls.

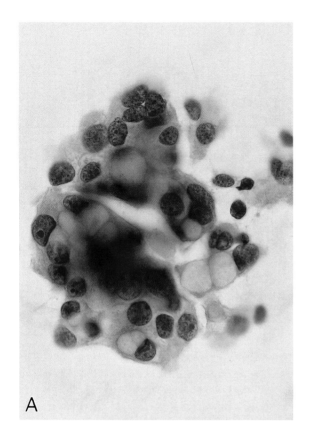

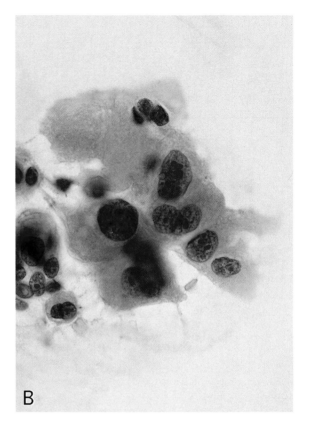

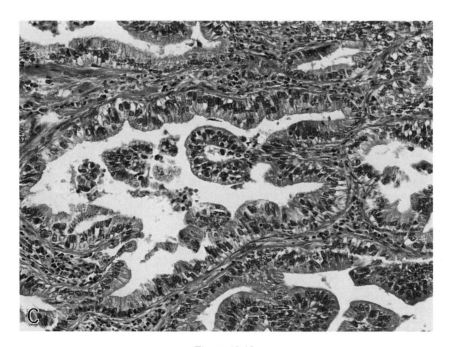

Figure 13-19
MUCINOUS BRONCHIOLOALVEOLAR CARCINOMA

Bronchial wash cytology shows some cells containing prominent vacuoles (A) whereas other cells lack such vacuolization (B). Nuclear atypia is prominent in some cells (B). The corresponding resection specimen (C) shows a mucinous BAC that is somewhat less well differentiated than is typical.

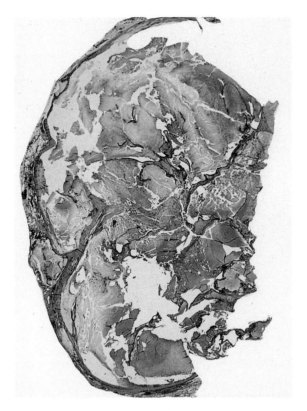 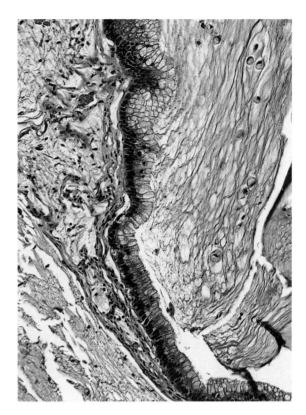

Figure 13-20
MUCINOUS CYSTADENOMA
Left: This solitary pulmonary nodule is composed of pools of mucus surrounded by fibrous tissue.
Right: The only epithelium identified was well-differentiated mucinous epithelium partially lining some of the fibrous walls.
This case could be considered a mucinous cystadenoma or a very well-differentiated mucinous adenocarcinoma.

or complete fibrous wall surrounding the mucus. The wall is lined by well-differentiated mucinous cells resembling those seen in BAC. Of the 11 borderline mucinous tumors described by Graeme-Cook (18), mucus dissected into the adjacent alveolar parenchyma in 7, resembling typical mucinous BAC. In practice, most lung lesions composed of large pools of mucus with even a few well-differentiated mucinous cells should be regarded as mucinous carcinomas, even when extremely well-differentiated, and closely aligned to mucinous BAC.

There is an uncommon subset of BAC in which many of the airspaces are filled by single neoplastic cells reminiscent of desquamative interstitial pneumonia (fig. 13-8) (16). In such cases, foci of typical BAC may present only focally.

Psammoma bodies are found in slightly over 10 percent of BACs, usually of the nonmucinous type (3). Blood vessel and lymphatic invasion may also be seen (3).

Not uncommonly, BACs have a mixed cellular composition or are difficult to classify as either mucinous or nonmucinous. Many of these mixed BACs are less differentiated than the classic mucinous or nonmucinous forms (figs. 13-7 right, 13-19C).

Papillae protruding into airspaces may be seen in both mucinous and nonmucinous types of BAC. The papillae may be a focal finding or a very prominent feature (figs. 13-23–13-25). Distinguishing BAC with papillae from papillary adenocarcinoma (chapter 12) may be difficult. Silver and Askin (33) suggest that when more than 75 percent of the tumor contains complex papillae with fibrovascular cores that markedly distort or replace airspaces (fig. 13-26), the designation of papillary adenocarcinoma is appropriate and that this lesion has a worse prognosis than BAC.

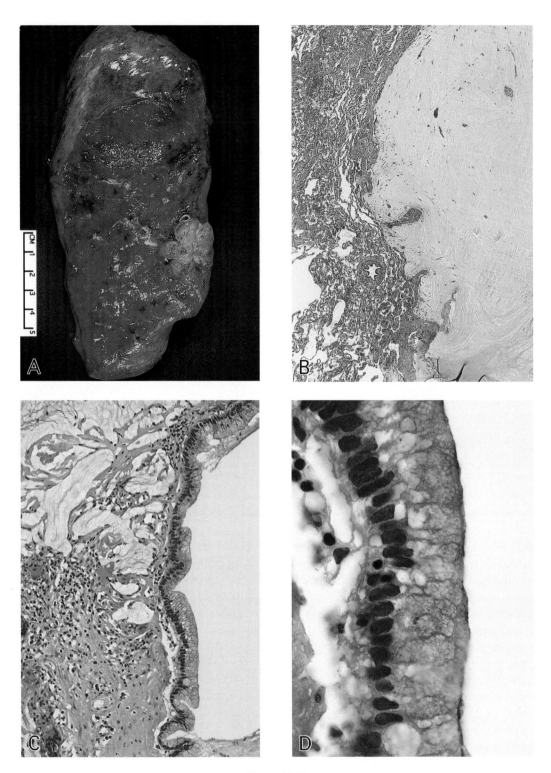

Figure 13-21
MUCINOUS CYSTADENOCARCINOMA

A resection specimen of a mucinous cystadenocarcinoma shows a well-circumscribed lobulated mucinous nodule (A, upper right) composed of relatively acellular mucin dissecting into lung parenchyma (B). Focal well-differentiated mucinous epithelium can be identified (C,D). The previous fine needle aspiration specimen showed monolayer sheets of well-differentiated glandular cells with columnar shape (E) and mild nuclear atypia including some grooving (F).

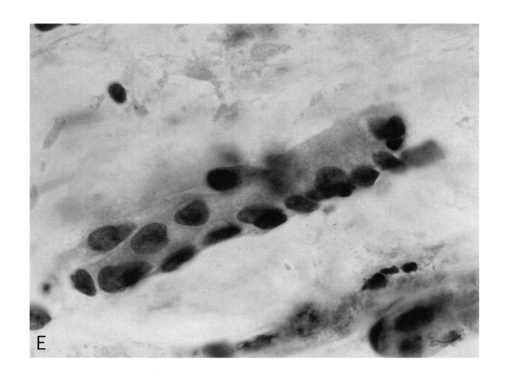

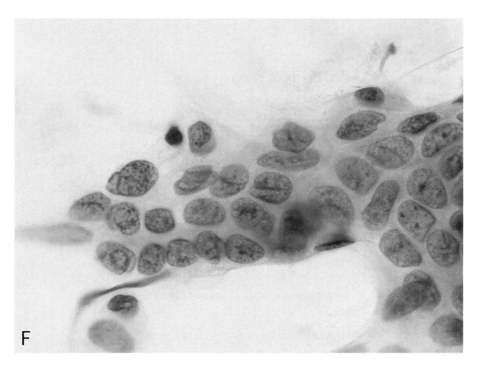

Figure 13-21 (Continued)

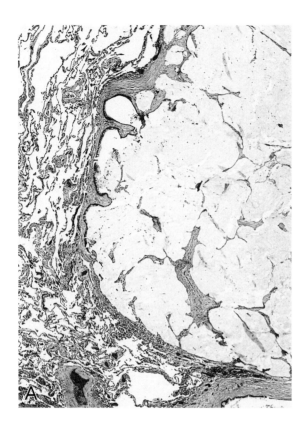

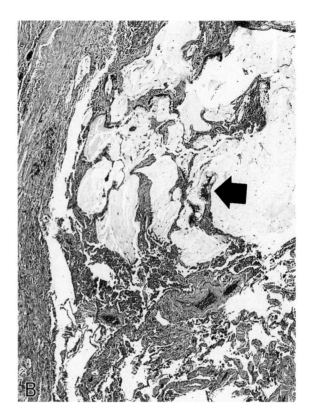

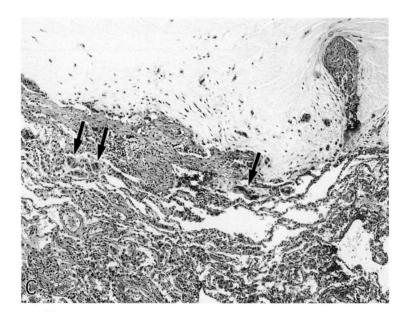

Figure 13-22
MUCINOUS CYSTADENOCARCINOMA

This solitary nodule is composed of pools of mucin with some fibrous walls (A) lined by well-differentiated mucinous epithelium. Elsewhere (B) the mucin dissects into intact lung parenchyma with occasional islands of epithelium lining alveolar septa (arrow). In other foci (C), neoplastic epithelium could be seen floating freely in alveolar spaces adjacent to the mucin pools (arrows).

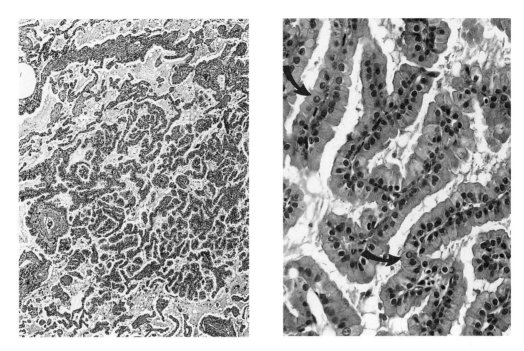

Figure 13-23
BRONCHIOLOALVEOLAR CARCINOMA WITH PAPILLARY FEATURES
In addition to growth along intact alveolar walls, there is a definite tendency to form papillae (left) which are lined by uniform eosinophilic cells (right) manifesting only mild nuclear atypia and occasional intranuclear inclusions (arrows).

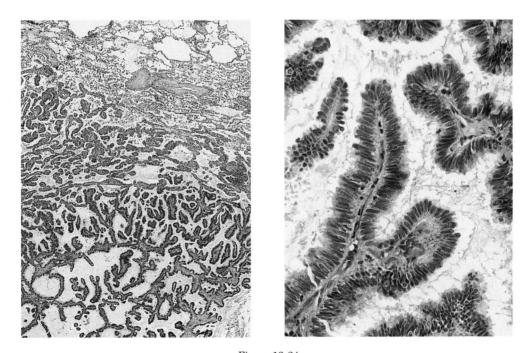

Figure 13-24
BRONCHIOLOALVEOLAR CARCINOMA WITH PAPILLARY FEATURES
Left: In this papillary BAC, growth along intact alveolar walls is apparent in some foci (top) whereas elsewhere (bottom) there are papillary structures. Mild architectural distortion is apparent.
Right: The papillae are lined by columnar cells with elongated nuclei reminiscent of papillary carcinoma of the breast.

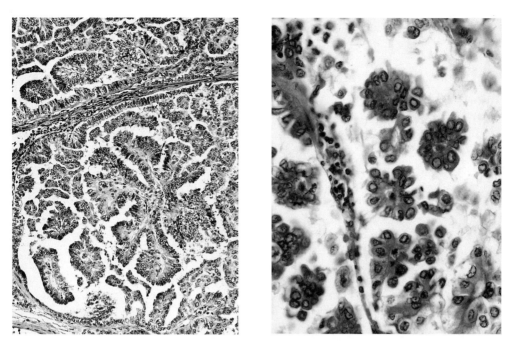

Figure 13-25
BRONCHIOLOALVEOLAR CARCINOMA WITH FOCAL PAPILLARY FEATURES
These two cases illustrate prominent papillary growth patterns. The cells on the left are cuboidal with vesicular nuclei and prominent nucleoli. The cytologic features of the cells on the right include nuclear clearing (contrast with figure 13-7) and are reminiscent of those seen in papillary carcinoma of the thyroid.

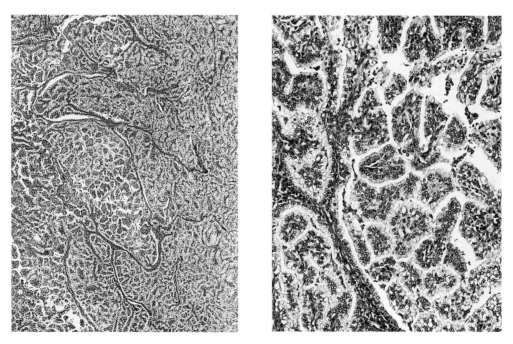

Figure 13-26
PAPILLARY ADENOCARCINOMA
This carcinoma shows complex papillae with sufficient architectural distortion to designate this case as a papillary adenocarcinoma rather than BAC with papillae (see text). Necrosis, hemorrhage, architectural destruction, and stromal invasion are not present, and the papillae are lined by relatively uniform cells with some cytoplasmic clearing and mildly atypical vesicular nuclei.

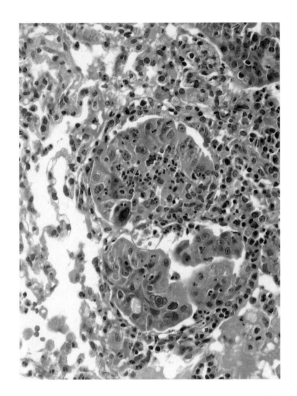 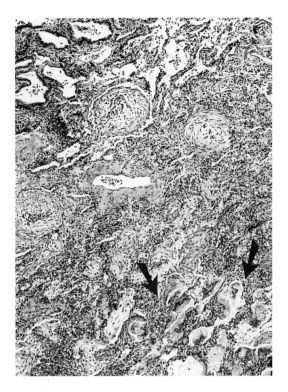

Figure 13-27
INFLAMMATORY CHANGES IN BRONCHIOLOALVEOLAR CARCINOMA
Left: There is marked acute inflammation of the intra-alveolar tumor cell clusters.
Right: The lesion was obscured by extensive airspace organization (organizing pneumonia). The foci of organization (top) obscured the tumor cells which can be seen as a uniform proliferation of mucinous cells in adjacent alveolar spaces (arrows).

Inflammatory and fibrotic changes involving the lung parenchyma sometimes obscure an associated BAC (fig. 13-27). Pulmonary fibrosis with honeycombing, foci of organizing pneumonia, interstitial inflammatory infiltrates, obstructive pneumonia, and inflammation in the pools of mucus all may obscure an associated BAC. Nevertheless, the key finding remains a monotonous proliferation of nonciliated cuboidal to columnar cells lining the airspaces.

Cytologically, BACs are well-differentiated adenocarcinomas (figs. 13-9, 13-10, 13-14, 13-18, 13-19, 13-21), and as such, cytologic diagnosis may be difficult (13,22,25,35). In exfoliated specimens, three-dimensional groups and papillae with few single cells are characteristic. There is cytologic uniformity, and the nuclei are generally round, have fine chromatin, occasionally prominent nucleoli, and minimal nuclear atypia. Nuclear folds are a common finding. The cytoplasm is voluminous and foamy, clear, or vacuolated in

mucinous BACs. The cells nearly always lack cilia. Psammoma bodies may be present. The usual differential diagnostic consideration is reactive bronchial and alveolar lining cells, and sometimes macrophages. According to Elson (13), the presence of numerous nonpigmented cells that look like pulmonary alveolar macrophages should make one suspect BAC.

Fine needle aspiration (FNA) specimens from nonmucinous BACs show monolayer sheets and three-dimensional papillary groups with a common cell border at the periphery (25,35). Few single cells are present. The chromatin is fine and uniform, and the cells have a high nuclear-cytoplasmic ratio. The cells look deceptively bland, although their number and uniformity suggest a neoplasm. Specific clues are many monolayer sheets and occasional papillae composed of cells lacking cilia. While mesothelial cells may form sheets, they are generally larger than the cells of nonmucinous BAC.

FNA specimens from mucinous BACs show large numbers of nonciliated cells in cohesive clusters and three-dimensional groups of large uniform cells with central nuclei, fine chromatin, small nucleoli, and abundant foamy to clear cytoplasm. Signet ring cells are uncommon, and their absence helps distinguish mucinous BAC cells from goblet cells. In less differentiated tumors, the cells are similar to those in ordinary adenocarcinoma of the lung.

Immunohistochemical Findings. Immunohistochemistry is not necessary for a diagnosis of BAC; occasionally it helps exclude certain metastatic carcinomas. While carcinomas of the breast, ovary, colon, and other areas may have distinctive immunohistochemical profiles that may help in their recognition as metastases in the lung, the findings should not replace knowledge of the clinical history, clinicopathologic correlation, and comparison of the lung tumor with prior tumors.

The immunohistochemical features of BACs are similar to those of other adenocarcinomas of the lung (see chapter 12). BACs with type 2 cell differentiation often stain with anti-surfactant antibodies, and those with Clara cell differentiation stain for Clara cell antigens.

Ohori et al. (32) compared the extracellular matrix in BAC with that of ordinary adenocarcinoma using immunohistochemical techniques. An intact basement membrane was found in BAC and at the periphery of conventional adenocarcinoma. In sclerosing BAC there was disruption or even absence of basement membrane components, similar to conventional adenocarcinoma. Type IV collagenase was also noted near the center of such tumors. These findings were thought to explain, in part, the more aggressive behavior seen with sclerosing BAC. Although mucinous BAC showed no basement membrane disruption, there were increased levels of type IV collagenase and low levels of alpha II integrin receptor expression; these findings may explain the ability of cells from mucinous BAC to detach from the basement membrane and spread aerogenously.

Ultrastructural Findings. Electron microscopy is also not necessary for a diagnosis of BAC. In general, the ultrastructural features of BAC (figs. 13-28–13-31) are indistinguishable from those of other adenocarcinomas of the lung (2,4-7,14). Tumors showing Clara cell differentiation

(approximately 90 percent of nonmucinous BACs) have apical, electron-dense, 600- to 1500-nm granules and a few microvilli at the cell apex (fig. 13-28). BAC cells with type 2 cell differentiation have cytoplasmic lamellar granules resembling surfactant (fig. 13-29). Nuclear inclusions composed of 40-nm branching microtubules are also characteristic of type 2 cell differentiation (fig. 13-30). About one third of nonmucinous BACs show some degree of type 2 cell differentiation, even though only 10 percent or less of nonmucinous BACs are composed predominantly of type 2 cells. In cases showing only occasional type 2 cells, distinguishing reactive from neoplastic type 2 cells is impossible. Mucinous BACs are composed of cells with central and apical vacuoles containing pale, flocculent, or electron-dense mucin (fig. 13-31). Apical microvilli with rootlets and glycocalyceal bodies, identical to those seen in colonic or ovarian carcinoma, are also common.

Rare BACs have ciliated cells (26). Squamous differentiation in the form of desmosomes or tonofilaments may also be seen ultrastructurally when not recognized light microscopically. Dekmezian et al. (9) described the presence of myoepithelial cells in a BAC. In a study of 37 BACs, Hammar (20) found 7 with prominent Langerhans cells in the interstitium.

Differential Diagnosis. The differential diagnosis of BAC includes reactive and metaplastic epithelial proliferations (honeycombing); nodules resembling BAC in young patients following chemotherapy; bronchioloalveolar cell adenomas; ordinary lung adenocarcinomas with an extensive BAC growth pattern and papillary adenocarcinoma; metastatic adenocarcinomas to the lung; and miscellaneous lesions with prominent type 2 cells including alveolar adenoma, papillary adenoma with type 2 cells, atypical adenomatous hyperplasia, and sclerosing hemangioma.

Foci of honeycombing may be confused with sclerosing BAC, and the two may occur together. The cells comprising a honeycomb pattern are generally mixed in composition and many have cilia. Squamous metaplasia, inflammation in the surrounding parenchyma, and neutrophils in the mucus pools within the honeycombing are also frequent. Cytologic atypia is not prominent and when present, is usually associated with squamous metaplasia.

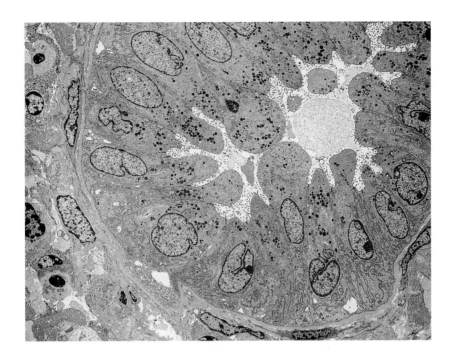

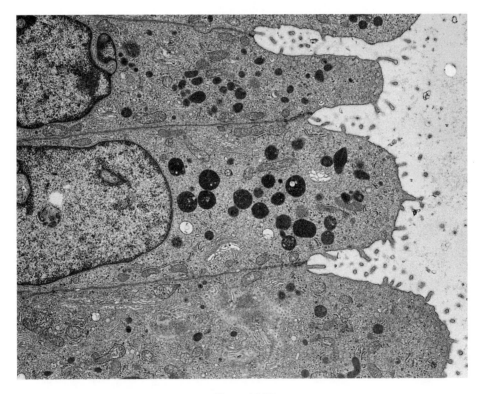

Figure 13-28
NONMUCINOUS BRONCHIOLOALVEOLAR CARCINOMA

This nonmucinous BAC showed Clara cell differentiation ultrastructurally.

Top: There is a proliferation of columnar cells forming an acinar structure within an alveolar space. (X1200)

Bottom: The cells are columnar with prominent apical protrusion and electron-dense granules oriented toward the apex of the cells. The cells have a few apical microvilli, intercellular attachments, and a moderate number of intracellular organelles. (X5000) (Courtesy of Dr. B. Mackay, Houston, TX.)

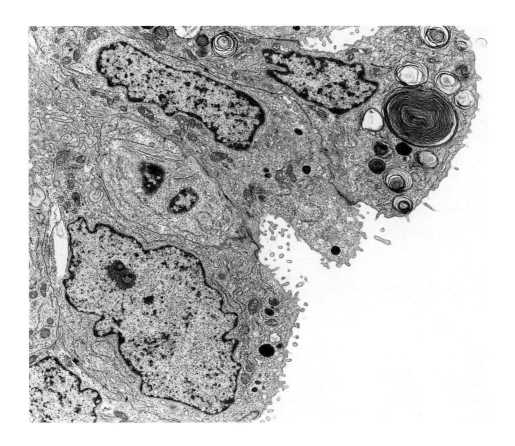

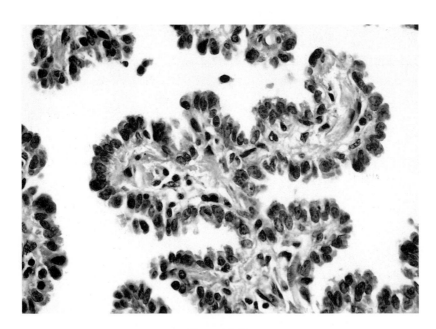

Figure 13-29
NONMUCINOUS BRONCHIOLOALVEOLAR CARCINOMA

Electron microscopic features (top) of the case illustrated at the bottom show alveolar septa lined by low cuboidal cells with a few surface microvilli, occasional apical electron-dense granules, apical junctions, and occasional cells (upper right) with features of type 2 cell differentiation.

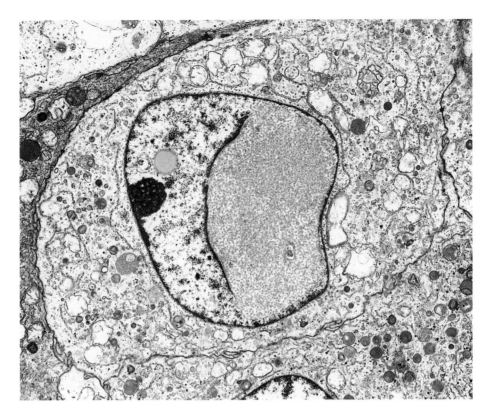

Figure 13-30
NONMUCINOUS BRONCHIOLOALVEOLAR CARCINOMA
Ultrastructurally, some intranuclear inclusions seen in nonmucinous BACs (see figure 13-7) comprise abundant microtubular arrays. (X5000) (Courtesy of Dr. B. Mackay, Houston, TX.)

Healed bronchiolar inflammatory lesions with peribronchiolar scarring and bronchiolization (metaplastic bronchiolar epithelium extending onto adjacent alveolar walls) may closely simulate BAC, however, cytologic atypia is not marked and cilia are usually readily identified. The fact that the lesion is anatomically limited to bronchioles and peribronchiolar regions is helpful.

Organizing diffuse alveolar damage is associated with peribronchiolar squamous metaplasia, which sometimes suggests BAC but more commonly is confused with squamous cell carcinoma. Organizing diffuse alveolar damage (particularly that due to chemotherapy or radiation therapy) may also be associated with many atypical type 2 cells. The cells are usually not as numerous and closely packed as in BAC, they have more variation in the amount of cytoplasm and degree of nuclear atypia, and they do not show the relatively abrupt transition to uninvolved alveolar walls so characteristic of BAC.

Miller (30) described bronchioloalveolar cell adenomas in resected lungs of patients with lung cancer (figs. 13-32, 13-33). The lesions were multiple, 1 to 7 mm in diameter, and were found in 9.3 percent of consecutive resections for lung carcinoma. The nodules were composed of type 2 cells with a minor degree of nuclear atypia lining an intact, slightly thickened alveolar wall. The authors noted that the cytologic features in some of the cases were identical to those seen at the periphery of nonmucinous BACs. They concluded that bronchioloalveolar cell adenomas were a premalignant phase of pulmonary glandular neoplasia (chapter 7).

Travis et al. (36) described nodules resembling BAC occurring in two patients following chemotherapy for childhood cancers (fig. 13-34). The lesions could not be distinguished from BAC by morphology, immunohistochemistry, or DNA content, and the possibility was raised that these might represent second malignancies in pediatric

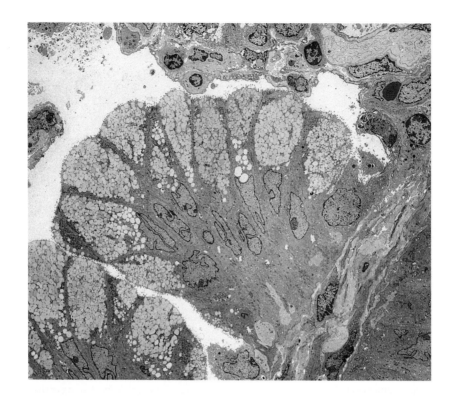

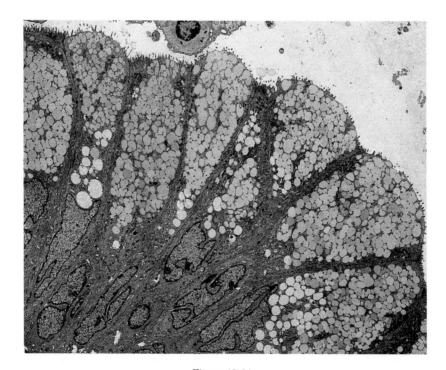

Figure 13-31
MUCINOUS BRONCHIOLOALVEOLAR CARCINOMA

Top: Ultrastructurally, this mucinous BAC shows a tuft of tall columnar mucinous cells growing along an alveolar septum. (X1000)

Bottom: The cells have apical, pale, flocculent, mucinous vacuoles and numerous short microvilli. (X2000) (Courtesy of Dr. B. Mackay, Houston, TX.)

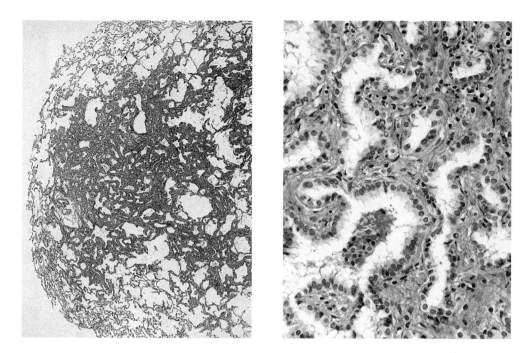

Figure 13-32
BRONCHIOLOALVEOLAR CELL ADENOMA

This incidental 3-mm nodule (left) in a resection specimen for carcinoma shows mild thickening of the alveolar septa which are lined by a uniform population of cuboidal cells (right) lacking nuclear atypia and demonstrating occasional cells with intranuclear vacuoles.

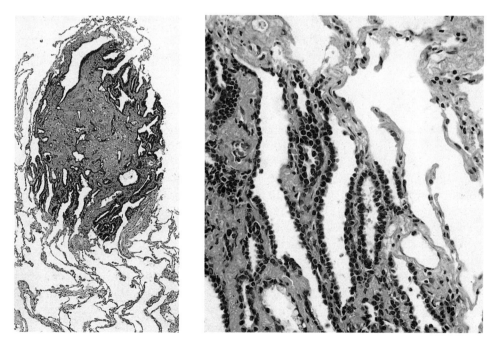

Figure 13-33
BRONCHIOLOALVEOLAR CELL ADENOMA

Left: This 2-mm nodule was an incidental finding in a specimen resected for rounded atelectasis. The lesion shows relatively prominent central scarring, and one could argue it is simply an old scar with surrounding metaplasia.

Right: The surrounding alveolar septa are lined by uniform local cuboidal cells typical of type 2 cells.

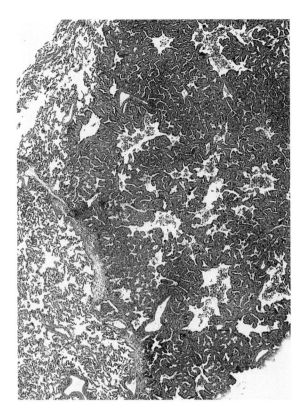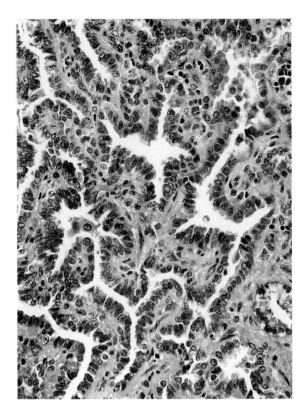

Figure 13-34
NODULE RESEMBLING BRONCHIOLOALVEOLAR CARCINOMA
Left: This nodular proliferation shows preservation of lung architecture although the alveolar septa are thickened.
Right: Cytologically, there is a proliferation of cuboidal to low columnar cells with mild nuclear atypia. Such a field would be indistinguishable from nonmucinous BAC. This case was reported by Travis et al. (36) as a pulmonary nodule resembling BAC in an adolescent cancer patient.

cancer patients. Clearly, BAC-like lesions occurring in pediatric cancer patients and bronchioloalveolar cell adenomas represent lesions that, in individual cases, may be impossible to distinguish from BAC.

Ordinary adenocarcinomas of the lung commonly have foci resembling BAC, and their distinction from BAC is simply a matter of adequate tumor sampling. The distinction between papillary adenocarcinoma and BAC with papillae is arbitrary, but the criteria of Silver and Askin (33) are reasonable (see above).

Just as conventional adenocarcinomas may show foci of BAC, so (rarely) may metastatic carcinomas. Separating BAC from metastatic carcinoma requires some knowledge of the clinical history and, where appropriate, comparison of the tumor in the lung with the prior tumor.

Metastatic mucin-producing carcinomas of the ovary and gastrointestinal tract (including the pancreas and biliary tract) may closely mimic mucinous BAC. Nonmucinous BACs, particularly those showing Clara cell and type 2 cell differentiation, are sufficiently distinctive in their histology and immunohistochemistry (positivity with antibodies to surfactant apoprotein or Clara cell antigen) that they are usually not a problem in the differential diagnosis.

A number of other miscellaneous lesions may resemble BAC. Alveolar adenomas are described in chapter 5. Papillary adenomas of type 2 cells are circumscribed and papillary in appearance, and are also discussed in chapter 5. Atypical adenomatous hyperplasia often accompanies BAC and some believe it is a precursor of BAC (chapter 7). Sclerosing hemangiomas commonly have papillary foci lined by cuboidal type 2 cells, and these foci may be reminiscent of BAC or papillary adenocarcinoma (chapter 23).

Spread and Metastases. A distinctive feature of BACs and one of the major reasons for segregating them from ordinary adenocarcinomas is their pattern of spread. While hematogenous, lymphatic, and pleural invasion may all be seen in BAC, spread of the tumor cells within airspaces is characteristic. Aerogenous dissemination has lead to descriptions such as "lepidic spread," calling forth the image of a butterfly (genus: lepidoptera) alighting on intact alveolar walls. It is extremely common in BACs to see tumor cells lying free within airspaces or floating in mucus, and these cells are thought to be the source of the aerogenous spread. The result of aerogenous spread in some cases is extensive bilateral consolidative disease that ultimately leads to respiratory failure in the absence of extrapulmonary tumor spread.

Staging, Treatment, and Prognosis. The treatment for BAC is resection, and curative surgery can be performed in half to two thirds of cases (11,12). Overall, the 5-year relative survival for bronchioloalveolar carcinoma is 42.1 percent (see fig. 8-16). Most patients with solitary peripheral nodules are candidates for resection, and an excellent prognosis may be expected. Daly et al. (8) found an over 90 percent 5-year survival for T1N0M0 tumors compared to a 55 percent 5-year survival for individuals with T2N0M0 tumors. In Daly's series, the 5-year survival for stage I disease was close to 80 percent.

Higher stage disease has a worse prognosis and approaches that of other forms of lung cancer. A recent report by Feldman et al. (15) states that patients with BAC who developed evidence of metastatic disease had a course and prognosis similar to a corresponding group of patients with ordinary adenocarcinoma.

Patients with a solitary BAC have a better prognosis than those with the pneumonic form or multicentric disease. Patients with mucinous BAC have a worse prognosis than those with nonmucinous BAC, since the former tends to be larger and more widespread at the time of diagnosis. Clayton (6,7) has suggested that it is aerogenous spread rather than histologic subtype that appears to be the major factor leading to multifocal and widespread disease; he showed that nonmucinous BACs with evidence of aerogenous spread had a prognosis similar to mucinous BACs.

REFERENCES

1. Axiotis CA, Jennings TA. Observations on bronchioloalveolar carcinomas with special emphasis on localized lesions. A clinicopathological, ultrastructural and immunohistochemical study of 11 cases. Am J Surg Pathol 1988;12:918–31.
2. Bedrossian CW, Weilbaecher DG, Bentinck DC, Greenberg SD. Ultrastructure of human bronchiolo-alveolar cell carcinoma. Cancer 1975;36:1399–413.
3. Bennett DE, Sasser WF. Bronchiolar carcinoma: a valid clinicopathologic entity? A study of 30 cases. Cancer 1969;24:876–87.
4. Bolen JW, Thorning D. Histogenetic classification of pulmonary carcinomas. Pathol Annu 1982;17(Pt 1):77–100.
5. Bonikos DS, Hendrickson M, Bensch KG. Pulmonary alveolar cell carcinoma. Fine structural and in vitro study of a case and critical review of this entity. Am J Surg Pathol 1977;1:93–108.
6. Clayton F. Bronchioloalveolar carcinomas. Cell types, patterns of growth, and prognostic correlates. Cancer 1986;57:1555–64.
7. _____. The spectrum and significance of bronchioloalveolar carcinomas. Pathol Annu 1988;23(Pt 2):361–94.
8. Daly RC, Trastek VF, Pairolero PC. Bronchoalveolar carcinoma: factors affecting survival. Ann Thorac Surg 1991;51:368–77.
9. Dekmezian R, Ordóñez NG, Mackay B. Bronchioloalveolar adenocarcinoma with myoepithelial cells. Cancer 1991;67:2356–60.
10. Dixon AY, Moran JF, Wesselius LJ, McGregor DH. Pulmonary mucinous cystic tumor. Case report with review of the literature. Am J Surg Pathol 1993;17:722–8.
11. Edgerton F, Rao U, Takita H, Vincent RG. Bronchio-alveolar carcinoma. A clinical overview and bibliography. Oncology 1981;38:269–73.
12. Edwards CW. Alveolar carcinoma: a review. Thorax 1984;39:166–74.
13. Elson CE, Moore SP, Johnston WW. Morphologic and immunocytochemical studies of bronchioloalveolar carcinoma at Duke University Medical Center, 1968-1986. Anal Quant Cytol Histol 1989;11:261–74.

14. Espinoza CG, Balis JU, Saba SR, Paciga JE, Shelley SA. Ultrastructural and immunohistochemical studies of bronchiolo-alveolar carcinoma. Cancer 1984;54:2182–9.

15. Feldman ER, Eagan RT, Schaid DJ. Metastatic bronchioloalveolar carcinoma and metastatic adenocarcinoma of the lung: comparison of clinical manifestations, chemotherapeutic responses, and prognosis. Mayo Clin Proc 1992;67:27–32.

16. Feldman PS, Innes DJ Jr. Pulmonary alveolar cell carcinoma: a new variant [Abstract]. Lab Invest 1980;42:116.

17. Gazdar AF, Linnoila RI. The pathology of lung cancer—changing concepts and newer diagnostic techniques. Semin Oncol 1988;15:215–25.

18. Graeme-Cook F, Mark EJ. Pulmonary mucinous cystic tumors of borderline malignancy. Hum Pathol 1991;22:185–90.

19. Greco RJ, Steiner RM, Goldman S, Cotler H, Patchefsky A, Cohn HE. Bronchoalveolar cell carcinoma of the lung. Ann Thorac Surg 1986;41:652–6.

20. Hammar SP, Bockus D, Remington F, et al. Langerhans cells and serum precipitating antibodies against fungal antigens in bronchioloalveolar cell carcinoma: possible association with pulmonary eosinophilic granuloma. Ultrastruct Pathol 1980;1:19–37.

21. Higashiyama M, Doi O, Kodama K, Yokouchi H, Tateishi R. Cystic mucinous adenocarcinoma of the lung. Two cases of cystic variant of mucus-producing lung adenocarcinoma. Chest 1992;101:763–6.

22. Johnston WW, Frable WJ. The cytopathology of the respiratory tract. A review. Am J Pathol 1976;84:372–424.

23. Kragel PJ, Devaney KO, Meth BM, Linnoila I, Frierson HF Jr, Travis WD. Mucinous cystadenoma of the lung. A report of two cases with immunohistochemical and ultrastructural analysis. Arch Pathol Lab Med 1990;114:1053–6.

24. Liebow AA. Bronchiolo-alveolar carcinoma. Adv Int Med 1960;10:329–58.

25. Lozowski W, Hajdu SI. Cytology and immunocytochemistry of bronchioloalveolar carcinoma. Acta Cytol 1987;31:717–25.

26. Mackay B, Lukeman JM, Ordonez NG. Tumors of the lung. In: Major problems in pathology, Vol 24. Philadelphia: WB Saunders, 1991:100–64.

27. Manning JT Jr, Spjut HJ, Tschen JA. Bronchioloalveolar carcinoma: the significance of two histopathologic types. Cancer 1984;54:525–34.

28. Marzano MJ, Deschler T, Mintzer RA. Alveolar cell carcinoma. Chest 1984;86:123–8.

29. Matthews MJ, Mackay B, Lukeman J. The pathology of non-small cell carcinoma of the lung. Semin Oncol 1983;10:34–55.

30. Miller RR. Bronchioloalveolar cell adenomas. Am J Surg Pathol 1990;14:904–12.

31. Moran CA, Hochholzer L, Fishback N, Travis WD, Koss MN. Mucinous (so-called colloid) carcinomas of lung. Mod Pathol 1992;5:634–8.

32. Ohori NP, Yousem SA, Griffin J, et al. Comparison of extracellular matrix antigens in subtypes of bronchioloalveolar carcinoma and conventional pulmonary adenocarcinoma. An immunohistochemical study. Am J Surg Pathol 1992;16:675–86.

33. Silver SA, Askin FB. True papillary carcinoma of the lung—a distinct clinicopathologic entity [Abstract]. Mod Pathol 1994;7:154A.

34. Sobin L, Yesner R. Histological typing of lung tumors. International Histological Classification of Tumors, Vol 1. 2nd ed. Geneva: World Health Organization, 1981.

35. Tao LC, Weisbrod GL, Pearson FG, Sanders DE, Donat EE, Filipetto L. Cytologic diagnosis of bronchioloalveolar carcinoma by fine-needle aspiration biopsy. Cancer 1986;57:1565–70.

36. Travis WD, Linnoila RI, Horowitz M, et al. Pulmonary nodules resembling bronchioloalveolar carcinoma in adolescent cancer patients. Mod Pathol 1988;1:372–7.

❖❖❖

14

SMALL CELL CARCINOMA AND
LARGE CELL NEUROENDOCRINE CARCINOMA

Small cell carcinoma (SCC) is discussed in this chapter as one of the four major subtypes of lung carcinoma, but it also is regarded as part of the spectrum of neuroendocrine lung tumors. An overall discussion of neuroendocrine neoplasms is found in chapter 17. While large cell neuroendocrine carcinoma (LCNEC) is much less common than SCC, these tumors are grouped together in this chapter because based on their morphologic and clinical features, they appear more closely related to each other than to typical and atypical carcinoids.

SMALL CELL CARCINOMA

Definition. SCC of the lung is a high-grade malignant epithelial tumor with characteristic cytologic features of scant cytoplasm, finely granular chromatin, absent or inconspicuous nucleoli, and frequent mitoses (16). The clinical course is very aggressive with frequent widespread metastases. SCC is considered a distinct clinicopathologic entity due to its many characteristic clinical manifestations, unique pathologic features, and sensitivity to chemotherapy, which is a major difference from nonsmall cell carcinomas (NSCCs). SCC is regarded as a systemic disease since almost all patients have metastases to regional lymph nodes and extrathoracic sites at the time of initial presentation (27). Although special techniques such as immunohistochemistry and electron microscopy can be very useful in the evaluation of SCC, the final diagnosis should rest on the routine morphologic features since the World Health Organization (WHO) and the International Association for the Study of Lung Cancer (IASLC) define SCC purely by light microscopic criteria (16,54).

Clinical Features. SCC accounts for 20 to 25 percent of all lung cancers and approximately 34,000 new cases occur in the United States each year. It is separated from NSCC by its clinical behavior and responsiveness to chemotherapy (27). The median age for patients with SCC is 60 years (range, 32 to 79 years). Males predominate but the percentage of affected women is increasing: the male to female ratio used to be 10 to 1, but more recently it has been reported to be 2 to 1. There is a strong association with smoking (27).

Due to the rapid growth and widespread metastases of SCC, most patients are symptomatic and the duration of symptoms is less than 3 months. Since most tumors are proximal, the most common pulmonary symptoms are cough, dyspnea, wheezing, hemoptysis, chest pain, or postobstructive pneumonitis (27). Mediastinal involvement is very common, as are its manifestations: superior vena cava (SVC) syndrome, recurrent laryngeal nerve paralysis, and dysphagia. SVC syndrome occurs in up to 10 percent of patients at presentation (27). A variety of clinical manifestations are distinctive for SCC including the syndrome of inappropriate secretion of antidiuretic hormone, ectopic Cushing syndrome, and the Eaton-Lambert or myasthenic-like syndrome (27). Symptoms may also be due to metastatic tumor involving sites such as the central nervous system, bone, and liver.

The system for limited and extensive staging of SCC is discussed in chapter 8. At presentation, approximately 30 percent of patients have limited stage and 70 percent extensive stage disease (27). In less than 5 percent of cases, SCC presents as a solitary pulmonary nodule or as limited stage I disease as staged by the TNM method (18).

Up to 5 percent of SCC patients have no apparent pulmonary or mediastinal lesions on chest X ray. These patients either have an extrapulmonary primary tumor in organs such as the larynx, esophagus, colon, bladder, and cervix, or they have disseminated metastases but no detectable primary tumor (27).

Gross Findings. Most of the gross pathology of SCC is encountered at autopsy (fig. 14-1) rather than in surgical specimens (fig. 14-2), since these patients are typically treated with chemotherapy rather than surgery. Approximately 70 percent of cases present as a perihilar mass. Extensive lymph node metastases are common. The tumor is white-tan, soft, friable

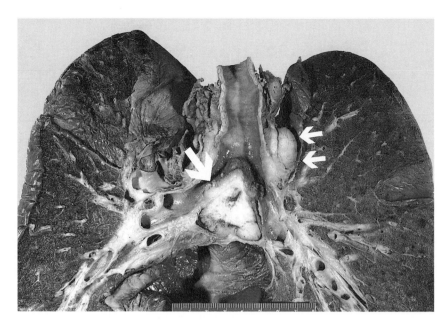

Figure 14-1
SMALL CELL CARCINOMA

A posterior view of this autopsy lung specimen shows the cut surface of a 4-cm white mass infiltrating the bronchial submucosa and compressing the left mainstem bronchus (arrow). The bulk of the mass extends to involve the adjacent hilar lymph nodes. A right paratracheal lymph node is enlarged due to metastatic tumor (double arrow).

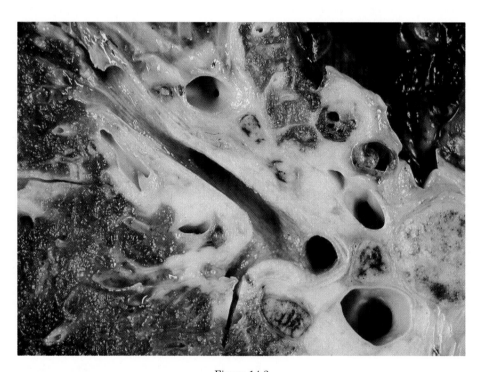

Figure 14-2
SMALL CELL CARCINOMA

Cross section of this surgically resected tumor shows peribronchial and perivascular infiltration by a white soft tumor which also involves a hilar lymph node.

Table 14-1

CLASSIFICATION OF SMALL CELL CARCINOMA*

Kreyberg (1962)	WHO (1967)	WHO (1981)	IASLC (1988)**
Oat cell	Lymphocyte-like	Oat cell	Small cell carcinoma
Polygonal	Polygonal	Intermediate	Small cell carcinoma
	Fusiform		Mixed small cell/large cell carcinoma
	Other	Combined oat cell carcinoma	Combined small cell carcinoma

*Modified from reference 16.
**IASLC = International Association for the Study of Lung Cancer.

and frequently shows extensive necrosis. SCC is typically situated in a peribronchial location. Submucosal and circumferential infiltration may occur along bronchi. Early SCC may appear as a submucosal infiltrate with normal overlying mucosa or plaque-like lesions. With advanced disease, the bronchial lumen may be obstructed by extrinsic compression. Endobronchial lesions are unusual, but have been reported. In up to 5 percent of cases, SCC presents as a peripheral coin lesion, which may be resected (18).

Histopathologic Findings. The histologic classification of SCC has evolved substantially over the past several decades (Table 14-1) (23). In 1967, the WHO defined four types of SCC: 1) lymphocyte-like or oat cell type; 2) a fusiform type, with elongated nuclei, often growing in bundles; 3) a polygonal cell type with larger nuclei; and 4) other types, containing additional squamous and glandular foci (16). In 1981, the WHO modified this classification to three types of SCC: 1) oat cell, 2) intermediate, and 3) combined types (16,54). However, this classification was difficult to reproduce by different pathologists, and various studies could not demonstrate a consistent relationship between survival and histologic subtype (16). In fact, the oat cell subtype is considered by some to be an artifact due to necrosis or processing for histology. More recently, the IASLC proposed that SCC be divided into three categories: 1) SCC, 2) mixed small cell/large cell carcinoma, and 3) combined SCC, which also has components of squamous cell and/or adenocarcinoma (Table 14-1) (16).

At low-power light microscopy, SCC often shows extensive necrosis. Within necrotic areas, hematoxyphilic encrustation of vessel walls by DNA from necrotic tumor cells (Azzopardi effect) is often seen (fig. 14-3, left) (1). Occasionally, the necrosis may be inconspicuous, consisting of single necrotic cells. Some SCCs have a prominent desmoplastic stroma (fig. 14-3, right). SCCs frequently do not grow with a specific pattern, but they can form nests (fig. 14-4, left), streams, ribbons, and rarely, tubules or ductules (1). Palisading may be seen at the periphery of nests of cells (fig. 14-4, right). Occasionally, rosettes are formed (fig. 14-5).

SCC is composed of small tumor cells with a round to fusiform shape, scant cytoplasm, finely granular nuclear chromatin, and absent or inconspicuous nucleoli (figs. 14-5, right, 14-6) (1,16). The tumor has a very hyperchromatic appearance since the cells have little cytoplasm and are situated very close to each other (figs. 14-3, right, 14-4). Nuclear molding may be conspicuous, but is more difficult to visualize in histologic sections than in cytologic preparations (fig. 14-5, right, 14-6, left). Mitotic rates are characteristically high, sometimes exceeding 10 per single high-power field.

SCC does not involve the bronchial mucosa with a pattern of carcinoma in situ. However, pagetoid infiltration of the bronchial mucosa may occur, or in cases of combined SCC-squamous cell carcinoma, squamous cell carcinoma in situ may be seen.

Crush artifact is a frequent finding in small transbronchial or mediastinal biopsy specimens

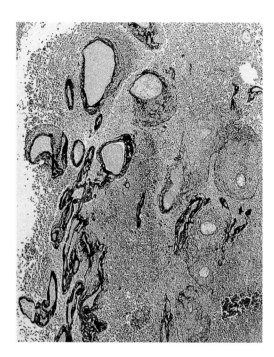
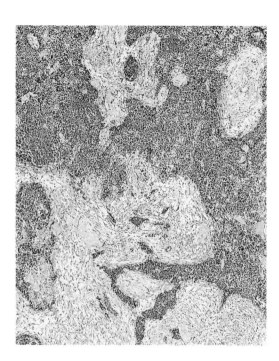

Figure 14-3
SMALL CELL CARCINOMA

Left: This extensively necrotic tumor shows prominent hematoxylin staining due to DNA encrustation of vascular walls (Azzopardi effect). (Courtesy of Dr. Donald Guinee, Sacramento, CA.)

Right: Prominent desmoplastic stroma is present, but necrosis is minimal. The tumor appears very hyperchromatic at low power due to its cellularity in addition to the compact arrangement and scant cytoplasm of the tumor cells.

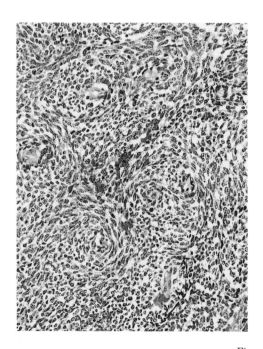
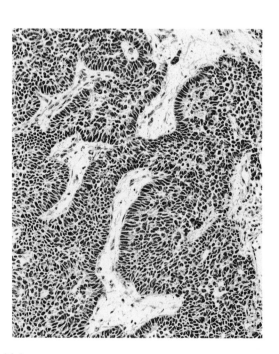

Figure 14-4
SMALL CELL CARCINOMA

Left: These round to oval and spindle-shaped tumor cells are arranged in nests and whorls.
Right: Prominent palisading is present in this case.

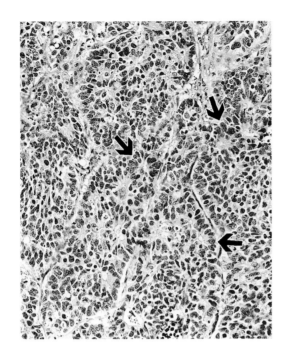
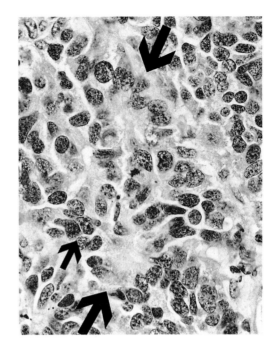

Figure 14-5
SMALL CELL CARCINOMA
Left: Multiple rosettes are present in this tumor (arrows).
Right: At higher power two rosettes are seen (large arrows). Nuclear molding is present (small arrow).

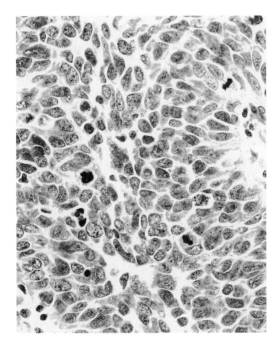
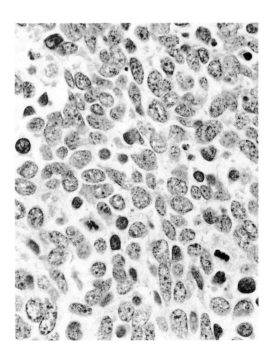

Figure 14-6
SMALL CELL CARCINOMA
Left: These tumor cells have scant cytoplasm, finely granular nuclear chromatin, and absent or inconspicuous nucleoli. Mitoses are frequent.
Right: These tumor cells are slightly larger but still have the cytologic features of small cell carcinoma.

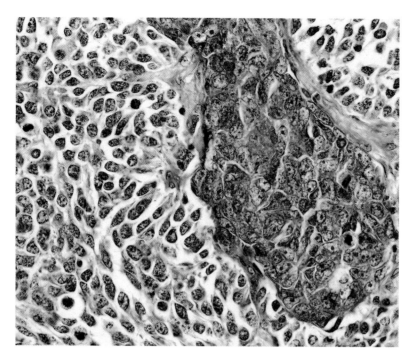

Figure 14-7
MIXED SMALL CELL/LARGE CELL CARCINOMA
This tumor consists of a mixture of small cell carcinoma (left) and large cell carcinoma (right). The cells of the large cell carcinoma component are larger with more prominent cytoplasm and prominent nucleoli.

and can make pathologic interpretation very difficult. The tumor cells of SCC have a tendency to show a streaming artifact, but this can also occur with NSCC, lymphoma, and chronic inflammation (see fig. 9-2).

Rarely, ductular structures in SCC may contain eosinophilic granular material that stains with diastase digested periodic acid–Schiff (DPAS) and mucicarmine (1); however, the cells making up these ductules have the morphology of SCC rather than adenocarcinoma. Intracellular mucin is not seen in pure SCC, and its presence indicates a combined SCC-adenocarcinoma.

The spectrum of cell morphology in SCC includes larger cells that approach the size of large cell carcinoma (fig. 14-6, right). SCC with these larger cells used to be referred to as the intermediate subtype under the 1981 WHO classification (16). Morphometric data have demonstrated a continuous spectrum of cell size from the smallest SCC to large cell carcinoma (49). Thus, cases that fall into the middle of the spectrum may not be distinguishable based on cell size alone. Since it is not reasonable for morphometry to be required

for the routine diagnosis of SCC, a practical rule is that the tumor cells of SCC should measure approximately the diameter of two to three small resting lymphocytes. Tumor cells of SCC have been reported to range up to 35 to 45 μm (49).

The size of the biopsy specimen can also affect the tumor cell size. Morphometric data indicate that the cells of SCC appear larger in larger specimens, especially open lung biopsies (49). This should be kept in mind when reviewing well-fixed open biopsies, since the most familiar morphologic image of SCC is in transbronchial biopsy specimens where the cells are smaller and often not well preserved.

Mixed Small Cell/Large Cell Carcinoma. According to the IASLC, mixed small cell/large cell (SC/LC) carcinoma is defined histologically as a tumor with a mixture of small and large cells (fig. 14-7) (16). It may consist of interspersed populations of small and large cells or sharply demarcated clusters of large cells within a SCC (fig. 14-7). This subtype has not been uniformly accepted by all lung cancer experts (20) and there is poor interobserver agreement on this subtype

Table 14-2

COMPARISON OF CLASSIC AND VARIANT SMALL CELL CARCINOMA CELL LINES*

	Classic	Variant
Cell morphology	Floating, tightly packed, spherical or amorphous, irregular aggregates	Floating, loosely adherent aggregates in small clumps and cords, or attached to substrate
L-DOPA**	Increased	Undetectable in most cell lines
Neuron-specific enolase	Increased	Increased but less concentrated
Creatine kinase-BB	Increased	Increased
Gastrin-releasing peptide	Increased	Undetectable in most cell lines
Neurosecretory type granule	Present	None in most lines
Population doubling time: mean/range (hours)	79/45-149	32/26-36
Colony forming efficiency: mean/range (percent)	2.0/0.1-5.2	14.0/0.1-30.5
Radiosensitivity	Sensitive	Resistant
C-*myc* amplification no.: amplified/no. tested (fold)	1/23 (6)	7/9 (5-76)

*From references 6,10.
**L-DOPA = L-amino acid decarboxylase.

(9). It has been suggested that at least 1 percent of the total cell population should consist of large cells to classify as mixed SC/LC carcinoma (9). Although initial reports found a frequency of 12 to 14 percent, more recent studies have suggested that this subtype comprises only about 4 to 5 percent of SCCs (9).

Justification for considering SC/LC a distinct subtype was originally based on evidence of a significantly worse prognosis than for pure SCC and data from cell lines of SCC (Table 14-2) (6,10). Significantly different biochemical and molecular features were identified in cell lines derived from SC/LC carcinomas than those derived from pure SCC; these cell lines were called variant and classic, respectively. The properties of variant SCC cell lines indicated a more malignant phenotype than the classic SCC, a finding that supported the clinical impression that SC/LC carcinoma had a worse prognosis. Recent studies, however, show a better prognosis for SC/LC carcinoma or no significant difference in survival (9).

Combined Small Cell Carcinoma. Combined SCC, as defined by the IASLC, consists of SCC with a component of squamous cell carcinoma or adenocarcinoma (16). The extent of the squamous (fig. 14-8, left) or adenocarcinoma (fig. 14-8, right) component can vary, but often is 5 percent or less (9). It is the least common of the subtypes, reported to occur in 1 to 3 percent of

SCCs (9,16,22). This frequency varies depending on the tumor sample size, number of histologic sections studied, type of specimen (autopsy versus surgical), and variation in interpretation (9,39). In addition to squamous cell or adenocarcinoma, combinations can occur with spindle cell carcinoma (fig. 14-9) (47) and giant cell carcinoma (fig. 14-10).

The clinical characteristics of combined SCC are similar to pure SCC: there are no differences in patient median age, sex, performance status, and stage of disease (22). Patients with combined SCC may have a higher incidence of peripheral lung tumors that are resected and therefore more extensively examined, and a lower median lactate dehydrogenase level (22). The response to chemotherapy and median survival period is similar to other SCC patients; however, surgical treatment may be important since, in one study, a prolonged survival of 5 years or more was observed in 22 percent of patients who underwent resection (22).

Therapeutic Effect on SCC. Following therapy, biopsy specimens from 13 to 45 percent of patients with pure SCC demonstrate a different morphology, of either SC/LC carcinoma, or SCC combined with squamous cell carcinoma, adenocarcinoma (fig. 14-11), or giant cell carcinoma (2,3,39). It is not known why these histologic changes are observed, but possible explanations

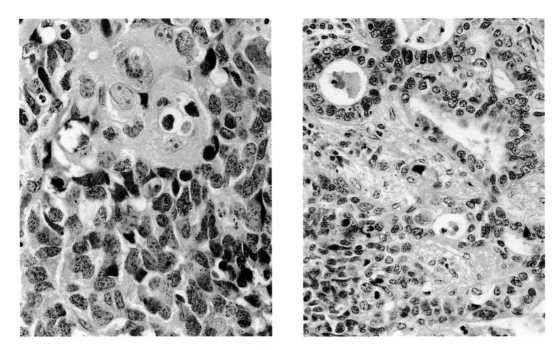

Figure 14-8
COMBINED SMALL CELL CARCINOMA
Left: This tumor consists of a combination of squamous cell carcinoma (top) and small cell carcinoma (bottom).
Right: This tumor consists of a combination of adenocarcinoma (top) and small cell carcinoma (bottom).

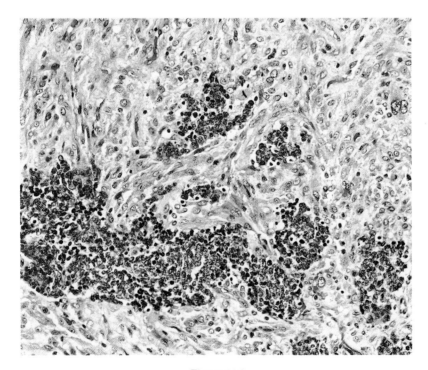

Figure 14-9
COMBINED SMALL CELL CARCINOMA
This tumor consists of a combination of spindle cell carcinoma (top) and small cell carcinoma (bottom). (Courtesy of Dr. Yukari Tsubota, Wakayama, Japan.)

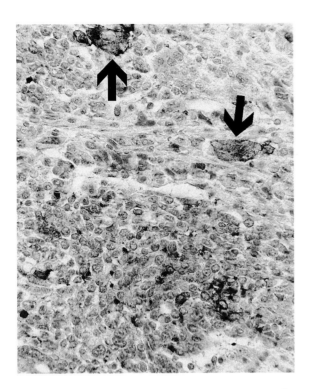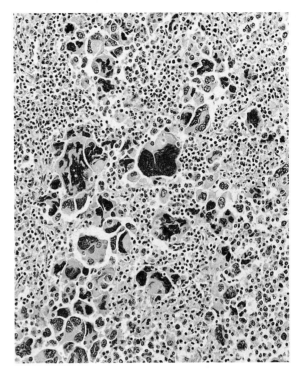

Figure 14-10
COMBINED SMALL CELL CARCINOMA

Left: This tumor consists of a combination of small cell carcinoma and giant cell carcinoma. Chromogranin focally decorates both the small cells and giant cells (arrows).

Right: Other areas of this tumor show very prominent giant cells.

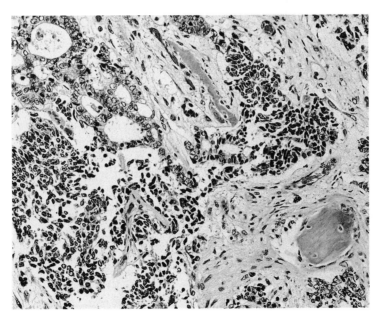

Figure 14-11
SMALL CELL CARCINOMA: POST-THERAPY

This vertebral bone marrow metastasis shows a combination of adenocarcinoma (top left) and small cell carcinoma. This was found in an autopsy of a patient who had previously received chemotherapy for small cell carcinoma.

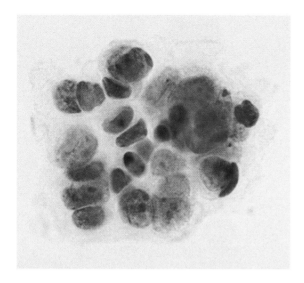

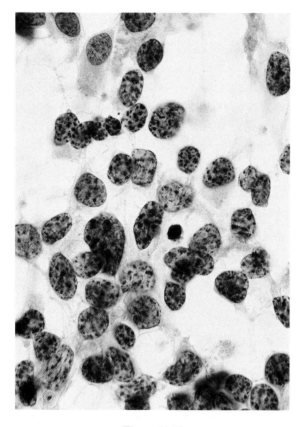

Figure 14-12
SMALL CELL CARCINOMA: CYTOLOGIC FEATURES

Top: The tumor cells from this pleural fluid show bare nuclei with finely granular chromatin, nuclear molding, and no nucleoli.

Bottom: The tumor cells from this touch preparation vary in size and shape but demonstrate scant cytoplasm, finely granular chromatin, and absent nucleoli.

include: sampling differences in a mixed or combined SCC, development of a second tumor, or a shift in the histologic type induced by therapy (2).

Interobserver Agreement. Recent evaluation of the 1988 IASLC classification scheme for the subtyping of SCC has shown that pathologists are more likely to agree on a diagnosis of pure SCC than the combined or mixed subtypes (9). Interobserver agreement between two pathologists was only 45 percent for the mixed subtype and only three of five pathologists agreed with the diagnosis in each of five cases.

Cytology. Cytology is a very reliable method for diagnosing SCC and often is a valuable supplement to transbronchial biopsies, particularly when there is significant crush artifact. In fact, since the cytology of the tumor cells is a crucial aspect of the diagnosis of SCC, cytologic preparations often allow greater diagnostic certainty than tissue sections. The features of scant cytoplasm, finely granular nuclear chromatin, faint nucleoli, and nuclear molding are evident in good cytologic preparations (fig. 14-12). The tumor cells tend to form small clusters, but may be loosely cohesive (fig. 14-12). Background necrosis and nuclear karyorrhectic debris are often prominent.

Ultrastructural Findings. By electron microscopy, most SCCs have scant cytoplasm with few organelles (fig. 14-13). The nuclei have moderately and uniformly dense chromatin. Nucleoli are small or absent, although they are more apparent than by light microscopy (21). Cytoplasmic dense core granules are usually few and small (100 to 130 nm) and occasionally situated in small dendritic cytoplasmic processes (fig. 14-13) (21). They are absent in 10 to 35 percent of cases (14,21,31). Some investigators prefer not to subdivide SCC by ultrastructural characteristics (21), while others have described ultrastructural subtypes of SCC (13,31). Minute glandular or acinar structures are seen in 15 to 33 percent of SCCs (31). Tripartite differentiation has been observed with ultrastructural evidence of squamous cell carcinoma, adenocarcinoma, and SCC within a single cell (24).

Immunohistochemical Findings. Many antibodies can be used to immunohistochemically stain SCC and other neuroendocrine lung tumors. These include an extensive list of neuroendocrine, hormonal, and other markers (Table 14-3). The most useful neuroendocrine markers

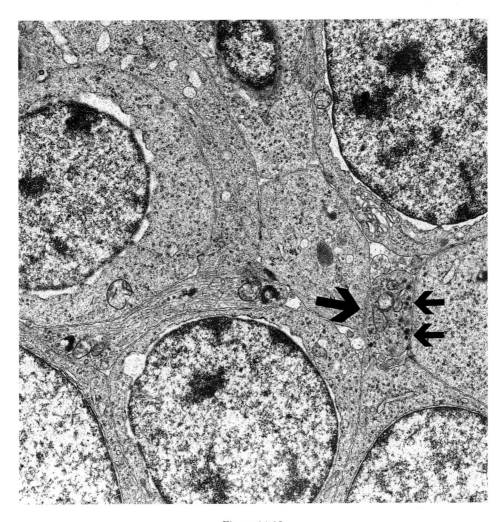

Figure 14-13
SMALL CELL CARCINOMA: ULTRASTRUCTURE
The tumor cells demonstrate finely granular nuclear chromatin, well-formed cell processes (large arrow), microtubules, and dense core granules (small arrows). (Courtesy of Dr. Samuel Hammar, Bremerton, WA.)

in formalin-fixed, paraffin-embedded tissue sections are chromogranin A (fig. 14-10, left), synaptophysin, and Leu-7 (12,46). In open lung and transbronchial biopsy specimens, chromogranin was observed in 60 and 47 percent, respectively; neuron-specific enolase (NSE) in 60 and 33 percent; Leu-7 in 40 and 24 percent; and synaptophysin in 5 and 19 percent of cases (12). NSE is not specific for neuroendocrine differentiation since it stains up to 60 percent of NSCCs (46). Gastrin-related peptide (GRP), also known as bombesin, is an autocrine growth factor for SCC, and can be demonstrated immunohistochemically in a high percentage of cases (12,46).

Keratin staining can be very useful, especially when the differential diagnosis includes malignant lymphoma, which can be difficult to differentiate from SCC on small transbronchial biopsy specimens. The results of keratin staining vary with the antibody or methods used, the type of specimen (transbronchial versus open biopsy), and the preservation of the material. For these reasons, the reported frequency of keratin staining varies from 25 to 100 percent (43,46). A recent study by Guinee et al. (12) found that both keratin (cocktail of AE1/AE3 and CAM 5.2) and epithelial membrane antigen (EMA) stained 100 percent of open lung biopsy and 95 percent of

Table 14-3

IMMUNOHISTOCHEMICAL MARKERS OF NEUROENDOCRINE PULMONARY TUMORS*

GENERAL NEUROENDOCRINE MARKERS
  Neuron-specific enolase
  Chromogranin
  Leu-7
  Synaptophysin
  Phosphorylated neurofilament subunits
  Tachykinins
    Substance P; Neurokinin A
  Opioid peptides
    Pan-opioid, α-endorphin, [met]enkephalin;
      Leu-enkephalin
  S-100 protein
  MOC1
  Cluster antigens; neural cell adhesion molecule
    (NCAM)
HORMONAL MARKERS
  Corticotropin
  Alpha-melanocyte–stimulating hormone
  Bombesin/gastrin-releasing peptide
  Calcitonin
  Corticotropin-releasing hormone
  Gastrin
  Glucagon
  Growth hormone–releasing factor
  Human chorionic gonadotropin-α
  Insulin
  Pancreatic polypeptide
  Serotonin
  Somatostatin
  Substance P
  Vasoactive intestinal peptide
OTHER TUMOR MARKERS
  Carcinoembryonic antigen
  Cytokeratin
    pK, CK 18 (RGE 53)
    SK56-23 and SK60-61
    KG8.13, PKK1, CK (Guinea pig serum), CK-4
  Prealbumin

*Primarily small cell carcinoma. Modified from reference 45.

transbronchial biopsy specimens. A "dot-like" staining pattern for keratin has been noted in some SCCs, but occurs in the minority of cases.

The majority of SCCs stain with carcinoembryonic antigen (CEA) (12,46). As with keratin, there are a variety of antibodies to CEA, including both monoclonal and polyclonal antibodies. Studies comparing CEA immunoreactivity in SCC with clinical outcome have reported both favorable and unfavorable correlations (46).

Many monoclonal antibodies against a group of neuroendocrine antigens, called cluster anti-

gens, have been developed in an attempt to identify a marker that will reliably distinguish SCC from NSCC (30,41). So far, none have proven reliable in formalin-fixed, paraffin-embedded tissue sections (44).

Molecular Biology. Much is known about the molecular biology of SCC. This is addressed in chapter 3.

Differential Diagnosis. The differential diagnosis of SCC includes NSCC, malignant lymphoma, chronic inflammation, other neuroendocrine lung tumors including carcinoids and large cell neuroendocrine carcinoma, metastatic carcinoma of the breast or prostate, and metastatic neuroendocrine carcinomas from other sites.

Since there are major differences in the therapeutic approach to patients with SCC versus NSCC, the major question asked of pathologists interpreting lung biopsy specimens is whether the tumor is a SCC or a NSCC. The major criteria for separating SCC from large cell carcinoma, including large cell neuroendocrine carcinoma (LCNEC), are listed in Table 14-4. Distinguishing these tumors from SCC should not rest on a single feature such as cell size or nucleoli, but on incorporation of multiple features including nuclear-cytoplasmic ratio, nuclear chromatin, nucleoli, nuclear molding, cell shape (fusiform versus polygonal), and hematoxylin vascular staining (46).

Morphologic separation of SCC from NSCC can be difficult. Lung cancer pathologists disagree over the distinction in 5 to 7 percent of cases (50). Several factors contribute to interobserver variability including small crushed biopsy specimens, ischemic changes, poor fixation, and poor histologic sections. The morphometric data discussed above is also important to keep in mind, since there probably is a continuum of cell size that does not allow a sharp separation of SCC from NSCC in all cases. Several practical considerations, however, may be helpful: 1) never diagnose SCC on a crushed specimen unless well-preserved tumor cells are also present since NSCC, carcinoids, and lymphocytic infiltrates can show the same crush artifact; 2) look for in situ involvement of the bronchial mucosa since its presence indicates NSCC, probably squamous cell carcinoma; 3) correlate with any available cytology specimens that may show better morphology than the biopsy material; 4) papillary growth favors the diagnosis of NSCC; and

Table 14-4

LIGHT MICROSCOPIC CRITERIA FOR DISTINGUISHING SMALL CELL CARCINOMA AND LARGE CELL CARCINOMA*

Histologic Features	Small Cell Carcinoma	Large Cell Carcinoma**
Cell size	Smaller (less than diameter of 3 lymphocytes)	Larger
Nuclear-cytoplasmic ratio	Higher	Lower
Nuclear chromatin	Finely granular, uniform	Coarsely granular or vesicular, less uniform
Nucleoli	Absent or faint	Often (not always) present, may be prominent or faint
Nuclear molding	Characteristic	Uncharacteristic
Fusiform shape	Common	Uncommon
Polygonal shape with ample pink cytoplasm	Uncharacteristic	Characteristic
Nuclear smear	Frequent	Uncommon
Basophilic staining of vessels and stroma	Occasional	Rare

*Modified from reference 49.
**Includes large cell neuroendocrine carcinoma.

5) if a biopsy specimen is insufficient to make a definitive diagnosis or if the biologic behavior of a tumor raises doubts about the diagnosis, additional studies such as radionuclide scans or bone marrow and other biopsies may be necessary.

Lymphoid infiltrates, whether due to small lymphocytic lymphoma or chronic inflammation, can be distinguished by their dyscohesive pattern of growth contrasting with the epithelial clustering and nuclear molding of SCC. In addition, immunohistochemistry for keratin and lymphoid markers such as common leukocyte antigen are useful.

Both typical and atypical carcinoid tumors are histologically of much lower grade than SCC. In SCC, mitotic rates are high and necrosis tends to be extensive while in carcinoid tumors the rates are low, with only up to 10 mitoses per 10 high-power fields, and necrosis tends to be focal. In a small crushed specimen, it may be difficult to identity mitoses. SCC cells have less cytoplasm than carcinoid cells thus the tumor appears more hyperchromatic.

SCC and LCNEC are best separated by consideration of the same morphologic features that are used to distinguish large cell carcinoma (Table 14-4).

Treatment and Prognosis. The median survival period for untreated patients with limited stage SCC is 3 months and 1.5 months for extensive stage disease. With combination chemotherapy and chest radiotherapy, the median survival is improved to 10 to 16 months for patients with limited stage disease and 6 to 11 months for patients with extensive stage disease. Since combination chemotherapy is capable of inducing a complete remission of SCC (32), oncologists rely heavily on pathologists to distinguish SCC from NSCC. Some studies show improved complete response and survival rates with the addition of radiotherapy to the chemotherapy regimen.

It is controversial whether surgical resection should be performed in patients with limited stage disease in addition to chemotherapy or radiation therapy (8,26,40). Patients with surgically resected, pathologically confirmed stage I SCC have been reported to have a 30 to 60 percent survival rate (35).

Six to 13 percent of SCC patients survive 2 or more years and up to 5 percent survive 10 years (42). Long-term survival is correlated with limited stage, female sex, and the occurrence of herpes zoster. If followed for 5 to 10 years, over one third of these long-term survivors will die of recurrent SCC, another type of lung cancer, or other malignancies. SCC has recurred as late as 8 years after presentation (17,27).

LARGE CELL NEUROENDOCRINE CARCINOMA

Definition. Large cell neuroendocrine carcinoma (LCNEC) is a poorly differentiated, high-grade lung carcinoma that has a neuroendocrine appearance by light microscopy, with organoid, palisading, trabecular, and rosette-like arrangements. The light microscopic impression of neuroendocrine differentiation should be confirmed by immunohistochemistry or electron microscopy.

LCNEC corresponds most closely with those tumors classified as intermediate-cell differentiated neuroendocrine carcinoma by Gould and colleagues (11,51,52) or the reclassified tumors with neuroendocrine features reported by Mooi (28). They have also been classified as atypical carcinoid, the intermediate subtype of SCC, large cell carcinoma, and large cell neuroendocrine tumor.

Clinical Features. The median age for patients with LCNEC is 64 years (range, 35 to 75 years). Most are cigarette smokers with a 50 pack/year smoking history (46). Ectopic hormone production has not been observed in any reported cases (46).

Gross Findings. LCNECs may be central, peripheral, or extensively replace the lung (fig. 14-14). They average 3 cm in size, ranging from 1.3 to 10 cm. Although they are usually circumscribed, unencapsulated nodular masses, occasionally they may be multinodular. The cut surface is yellow, white, or tan (fig. 14-14, top). Necrosis is frequently extensive and areas of hemorrhage may be present (fig. 14-14, bottom). Lymph node metastases are frequent.

Histopathologic Findings. LCNECs are characterized by the following histopathologic criteria: 1) light microscopic features commonly associated with neuroendocrine tumors such as organoid, palisading, trabecular, or rosette-like growth patterns (figs. 14-15, 14-16); 2) tumor cells of large size, polygonal shape, low nuclear-cytoplasmic ratio, coarse or vesicular nuclear chromatin, and frequent nucleoli (figs. 14-15–14-17); 3) high mitotic rate (greater than 10 per 10 high-power fields) and frequent necrosis (figs. 14-15A, C, 14-16B); and 4) neuroendocrine features by immunohistochemistry (fig. 14-16C) or electron microscopy (fig. 14-18) (46). Rounded nests of tumor cells with central necrosis are common. The description "large cell carcinoma, probably LCNEC" can be used for tumors resembling LCNEC by light microscopy, if tissue samples are not available for special studies to confirm the diagnosis. As one might expect, LCNEC may be encountered with mixtures of other histologic types of lung carcinoma such as adenocarcinoma or squamous cell carcinoma.

LCNEC has taken longer to be recognized as a distinct entity than the other neuroendocrine tumors such as typical carcinoid, atypical carcinoid, and SCC for several reasons: 1) diagnosis requires confirmation with special studies such as immunohistochemistry or electron microscopy; 2) only in the past decade have reliable neuroendocrine markers such as chromogranin, synaptophysin, and Leu-7 become widely available for routine use on paraffin-embedded tissue. Such immunohistochemical stains can be obtained in many hospital laboratories, increasing the likelihood of a correct diagnosis; 3) LCNEC is uncommon; 4) LCNEC is harder to diagnose than other neuroendocrine lung tumors based on small transbronchial biopsy and cytology specimens because the essential light microscopic neuroendocrine pattern can be difficult to discern and immunohistochemistry can be difficult to interpret; and 5) due to lack of precise criteria in the past, many of these cases were diagnosed as atypical carcinoid, large cell carcinoma, and SCC, especially the intermediate variant.

Ultrastructural Findings. By electron microscopy, LCNEC differs from atypical carcinoid in that dense core granules are fewer and often focal or patchy in distribution (fig. 14-18). Unlike SCC, dense core granules are not observed within cytoplasmic processes (21,46) and well-developed cytoplasmic lumina suggestive of glandular differentiation (fig. 14-18, top) and marked desmosomal intercellular attachments reminiscent of squamous differentiation may be found (46).

Immunohistochemical Findings. LCNECs stain immunohistochemically with NSE (100 percent), chromogranin (80 percent), Leu-7 (40 percent), synaptophysin (40 percent), bombesin (40 percent), CEA (100 percent), and keratin (100 percent) (46). The staining is often focal (fig. 14-16C). NSE is not regarded as a reliable marker for neuroendocrine differentiation since it stains up to 60 percent of NSCCs (38). Hormonal markers such as corticotropin (ACTH) and calcitonin are positive in only a few cases. In

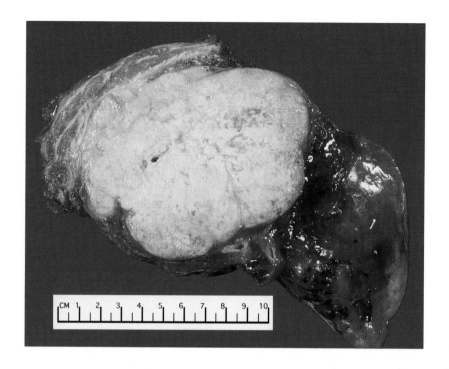

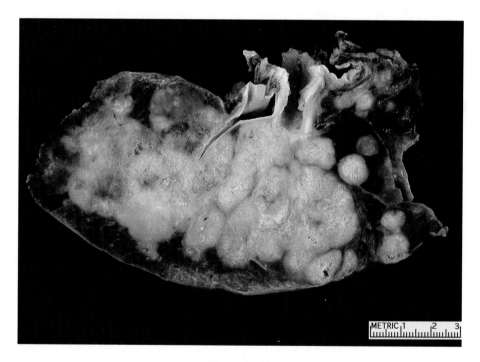

Figure 14-14
LARGE CELL NEUROENDOCRINE CARCINOMA

Top: This 10-cm tumor invades through the pleura into the adjacent chest wall. The cut surface shows a yellow-white mass with extensive necrosis and focal areas of hemorrhage.

Bottom: This lung is extensively replaced by multiple white nodules of tumor. Areas of grey discoloration are also focally present.

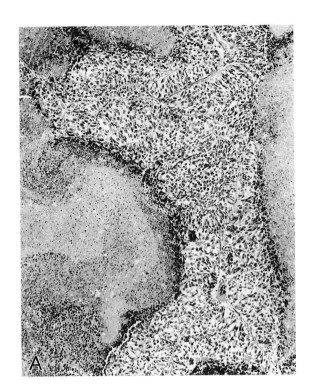

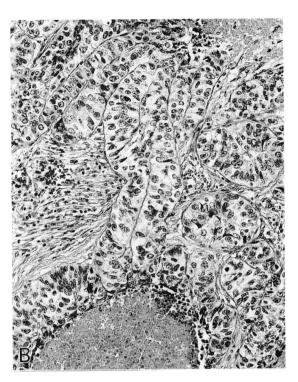

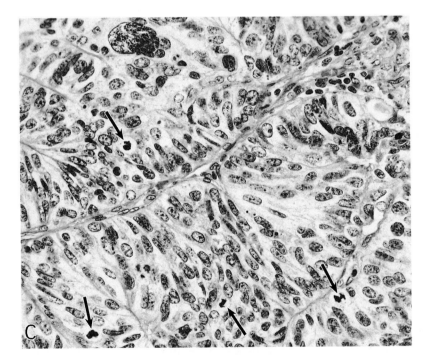

Figure 14-15
LARGE CELL NEUROENDOCRINE CARCINOMA

A: This tumor is extensively necrotic.

B: The tumor cells are arranged in organoid nests (right) and trabeculae (upper left).

C: The tumor cells are oval to spindle shaped with a single large pleomorphic cell (top left). Mitoses are frequent (arrows). The abundant cytoplasm, vesicular chromatin, and occasional nucleoli favor a nonsmall cell carcinoma.

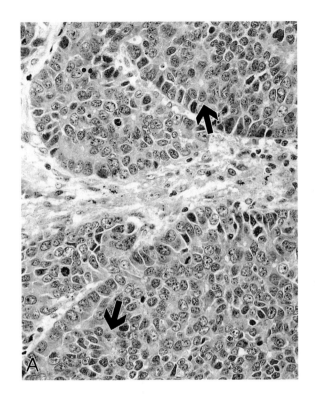

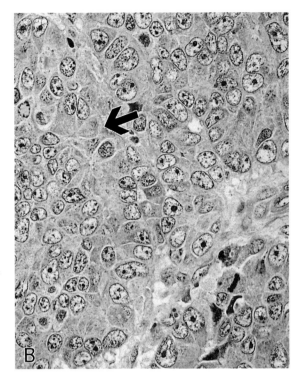

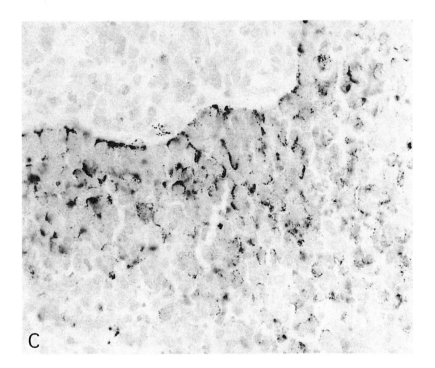

Figure 14-16
LARGE CELL NEUROENDOCRINE CARCINOMA

A: Prominent organoid nests of tumor cells with peripheral palisading and rosette-like structures (arrows) are present in this tumor. Mitoses are frequent.

B: Higher magnification reveals that these tumor cells have prominent nucleoli and focally form rosette-like structures (arrow).

C: The tumor cells stain focally, but intensely, for chromogranin.

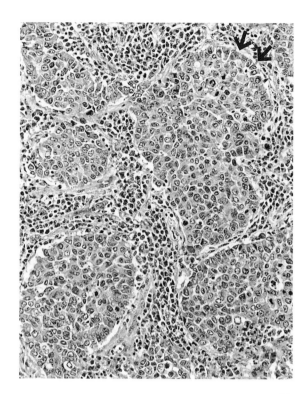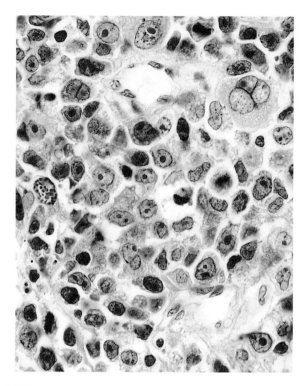

Figure 14-17
LARGE CELL NEUROENDOCRINE CARCINOMA

Left: This case shows a less striking neuroendocrine pattern, but the tumor cells show a nesting pattern surrounded by a chronically inflamed stroma and there is a hint of palisading at the edge of the tumor cell nests (arrows). Although this case was referred as an atypical carcinoid tumor, and thus regarded morphologically as a neuroendocrine tumor by the contributor, it actually represents one end of the morphologic spectrum of large cell neuroendocrine carcinomas that approaches ordinary large cell carcinoma. This tumor stained intensely with chromogranin.

Right: At high power the tumor cells show abundant cytoplasm, prominent nucleoli, and focal multinucleation.

general, the distribution and intensity of immunohistochemical staining for neuroendocrine markers is greater for typical and atypical carcinoid tumors than it is for LCNEC. However, a higher percentage of LCNECs stain for keratin and CEA (46). CEA immunoreactivity was predictive of treatment failure in one study of atypical carcinoid (37); perhaps LCNECs were included in this study, accounting for this observation.

Flow Cytometry. Aneuploidy is present in 75 percent of cases (46). This is comparable to SCC and much higher than for atypical carcinoid (46).

Molecular Biology. Recent data for the P53 phosphoprotein product showed diffuse and intense staining in the majority of LCNECs and SCCs (34). In contrast, all typical carcinoid tumors were negative for P53 and only a few atypical carcinoids had weak and focal staining. Similar data was reported for a spectrum of neuroendo-

crine lung tumors classified according to a different scheme (36). P53 mutations were found in several LCNECs and SCCs but not in typical and atypical carcinoid tumors (34). This data is consistent with the concept that LCNECs are more closely related to SCCs than to carcinoid tumors. Future studies of the molecular characteristics of neuroendocrine lung tumors may better define the relationship between these tumors.

Differential Diagnosis. LCNEC must be distinguished from SCC, atypical carcinoid, large cell carcinoma (LCC), and large cell carcinoma with neuroendocrine differentiation (LCC-NE). Separation of LCNEC from SCC requires consideration of multiple histologic features rather than a single criterion (Table 14-4). Artifacts introduced by frozen sections can distort cellular morphology, resulting in confusion with SCC (fig. 14-19).

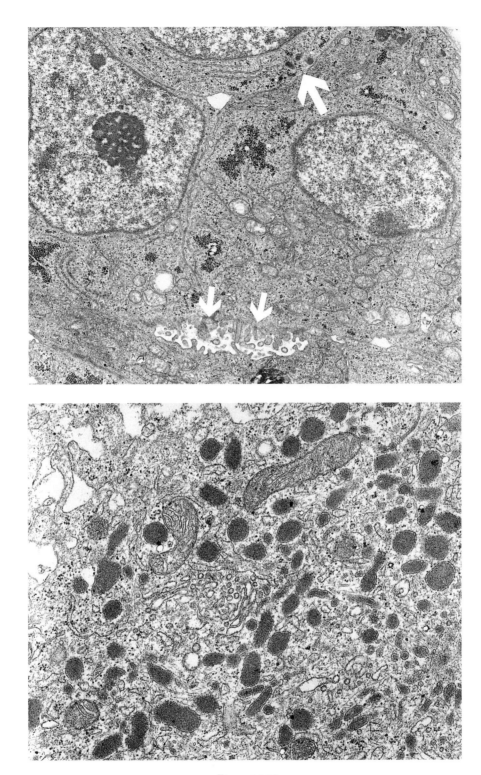

Figure 14-18
LARGE CELL NEUROENDOCRINE CARCINOMA: ELECTRON MICROSCOPY

Top: This tumor shows focal dense core granules (large arrow) and a cytoplasmic lumen surrounded by microvilli (small arrows).
Bottom: Focally, this tumor showed numerous cytoplasmic neuroendocrine granules which vary in size and shape. (Fig. 6 from Travis WD, Linnoila RI, Tsokos MG, et al. Neuroendocrine tumors of the lung with proposed criteria for large-cell neuroendocrine carcinoma. An ultrastructural, immunohistochemical, and flow cytometric study of 35 cases. Am J Surg Pathol 1991;15:529–53.)

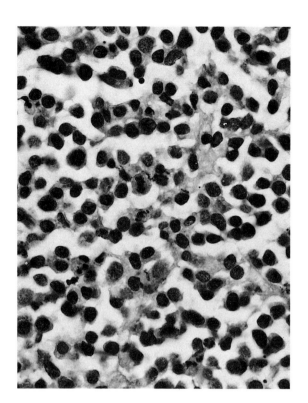
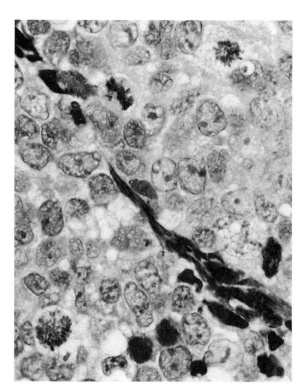

Figure 14-19
LARGE CELL NEUROENDOCRINE CARCINOMA: FROZEN SECTION ARTIFACT

Left: The frozen control section of this mediastinal lymph node metastasis was misinterpreted as small cell carcinoma due to the poor preservation of the tumor cells.

Right: The permanent section from this lymph node metastasis shows that many of the tumor cells have prominent nucleoli, excluding the diagnosis of small cell carcinoma. Many mitoses are also present. This patient had a peripheral large cell neuroendocrine carcinoma associated with a scar.

Mitotic counts are one of the most important criteria for distinguishing atypical carcinoid from LCNEC (45,46). In atypical carcinoids the mitotic rate is less than 10 per 10 high-power fields while in LCNEC it ranges between 30 to 100 mitoses per 10 high-power fields. Mitoses may be difficult to identify in small, crushed specimens. Necrosis tends to be focal in atypical carcinoids and extensive in LCNEC.

If a large cell carcinoma has no neuroendocrine pattern by light microscopy, but immunohistochemistry or electron microscopy demonstrates neuroendocrine features, the tumor is classified as LCC-NE. These cases are similar to the 10 to 15 percent of NSCCs in which neuroendocrine differentiation (NSCC-NE) can be found by electron microscopy or immunohistochemistry despite the absence of neuroendocrine features by light microscopy (4,5,7,15, 19,25,28,29,33,48,53).

Separation of LCNEC from LCC is based on whether or not a light microscopic neuroendocrine pattern is present. In most cases, distinction is not difficult because the neuroendocrine morphologic features are so distinctive (figs. 14-15, 14-16). However, in some tumors these neuroendocrine features are more subtle and separation from LCC or LCC-NE may be more difficult (fig. 14-17). Thus large cell carcinomas can be separated into those that have neuroendocrine features by light microscopy as well as immunohistochemistry or electron microscopy (LCNEC), large cell carcinomas with neuroendocrine features by special studies (LCC-NE), and large cell carcinomas with no neuroendocrine pattern by light microscopy or special studies (LCC) (46).

Treatment and Prognosis. LCNEC is an aggressive malignancy with a prognosis approaching the dismal outlook for SCC. The 5- and 10-year

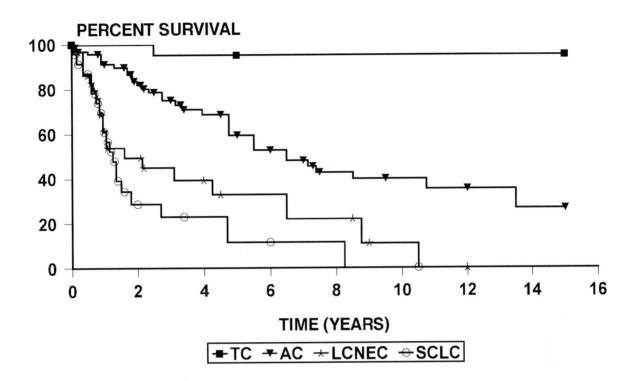

Figure 14-20
SURVIVAL OF NEUROENDOCRINE LUNG TUMORS
Kaplan-Meier survival curves for 158 neuroendocrine lung tumors from the AFIP (p<0.001): typical carcinoid (TC, n=37), atypical carcinoid (AC, n=69), large cell neuroendocrine carcinoma (LCNEC, n=29), small cell lung carcinoma (SCLC, n=23).

survival for LCNEC was found to be 33 percent and 11 percent, respectively (fig. 14-20). This is significantly worse than the survival for atypical carcinoid (AC) (p<0.001), but not significantly different from the survival for SC/LC carcinoma (p=.28). The optimal therapy remains to be defined since these are rare tumors and few institutions have accumulated enough data to make definite therapeutic recommendations. Until more is known about the clinical behavior and response to chemotherapy of LCNEC, resectable tumors should probably be removed surgically. Some patients with advanced stage disease have responded to chemotherapy; adjunctive chemotherapy may be of benefit following surgery.

REFERENCES

1. Azzopardi JG. Oat-cell carcinoma of the bronchus. J Pathol Bacteriol 1959;78:513–9.

2. Bégin P, Sahai S, Wang NS. Giant cell formation in small cell carcinoma of the lung. Cancer 1983;52:1875–9.

3. Bepler G, Neumann K, Holle R, Havemann K, Kalbfleisch H. Clinical relevance of histologic subtyping in small cell lung cancer. Cancer 1989;64:74–9.

4. Berendsen HH, de Leij L, Poppema S, et al. Clinical characterization of non-small-cell lung cancer tumors showing neuroendocrine differentiation features. J Clin Oncol 1989;7:1614–20.

5. Brambilla E, Veale D, Moro D, Morel F, Dubois F, Brambilla C. Neuroendocrine phenotype in lung cancers. Comparison of immunohistochemistry with biochemical determination of enolase isoenzymes. Am J Clin Pathol 1992;98:88–97.

6. Carney DN, Gazdar AF, Bepler G, et al. Establishment and identification of small cell lung cancer cell lines having classic and variant features. Cancer Res 1985;45:2913–23.

7. Dhillon AP, Rode J, Dhillon DP, et al. Neural markers in carcinoma of the lung. Br J Cancer 1985;51:645–52.

8. Elias AD, Ayash L, Frei E III, et al. Intensive combined modality therapy for limited-stage small-cell lung cancer. JNCI 1993;85:559–66.

9. Fraire AE, Johnson EH, Yesner R, Zhang XB, Spjut HJ, Greenberg SD. Prognostic significance of histopathologic subtype and stage in small cell lung cancer. Hum Pathol 1992;23:520–8.

10. Gazdar AF, Carney DN, Nau MM, Minna JD. Characterization of variant subclasses of cell lines derived from small cell lung cancer having distinctive biochemical, morphological, and growth properties. Cancer Res 1985;45:2924–30.

11. Gould VE, Linnoila RI, Memoli VA, Warren WH. Neuroendocrine cells and neuroendocrine neoplasms of the lung. Pathol Annu 1983;18(Pt 1):287–330.

12. Guinee D, Fishback NF, Koss MN, Abbondanzo S, Travis WD. Diagnostic utility of immunohistochemistry in small cell lung carcinoma in transbronchial and open lung biopsies. Am J Clin Pathol 1994;102:406–14.

13. Hage E, Hansen M, Hirsch FR. Electron microscopic sub-classification of small cell carcinoma of the lung. Acta Pathol Jpn 1983;33:671–81.

14. Hammar SP, Bockus D, Remington F, Friedman S. Small cell undifferentiated carcinomas of the lung with nonneuroendocrine features. Ultrastruct Pathol 1985;9:319–30.

15. Hammond ME, Sause WT. Large cell neuroendocrine tumors of the lung. Clinical significance and histopathologic definition.. Cancer 1985;56:1624–9.

16. Hirsch FR, Matthews MJ, Aisner S, et al. Histopathologic classification of small cell lung cancer. Changing concepts and terminology. Cancer 1988;62:973–7.

17. Johnson BE. Management of small-cell lung cancer. Clin Chest Med 1993;14:173–87.

18. Kreisman H, Wolkove N, Quoix E. Small cell lung cancer presenting as a solitary pulmonary nodule. Chest 1992;101:225–31.

19. Linnoila RI, Mulshine JL, Steinberg SM, et al. Neuroendocrine differentiation in endocrine and nonendocrine lung carcinomas. Am J Clin Pathol 1988;90:641–52.

20. Mackay B, Lukeman JM, Ordóñez NG. Tumors of the lung. Philadelphia: WB Saunders, 1991.

21. _____, Ordóñez NG, Bennington JL, Dugan CC. Ultrastructural and morphometric features of poorly differentiated and undifferentiated lung tumors. Ultrastruct Pathol 1989;13:561–71.

22. Mangum MD, Greco FA, Hainsworth JD, Hande KR, Johnson DH. Combined small-cell and non-small-cell lung cancer. J Clin Oncol 1989;7:607–12.

23. McCue PA, Finkel GC. Small-cell lung carcinoma: an evolving histopathological spectrum. Semin Oncol 1993;20:153–62.

24. McDowell EM, Trump BF. Pulmonary small cell carcinoma showing tripartite differentiation in individual cells. Hum Pathol 1981;12:286–94.

25. _____, Wilson TS, Trump BF. Atypical endocrine tumors of the lung. Arch Pathol Lab Med 1981;105:20–8.

26. Mentzer SJ, Reilly JJ, Sugarbaker DJ. Surgical resection in the management of small-cell carcinoma of the lung. Chest 1993;103:349S–51S.

27. Minna JD, Pass HI, Glatstein E, Ihde DC. Cancer of the lung. In: DeVita VT, Hellman S, Rosenberg SA, eds. Cancer. Principles and practice of oncology, Vol. 3. Philadelphia: JB Lippincott, 1989:591–705.

28. Mooi WJ, Dewar A, Springall D, Polak JM, Addis BJ. Non-small cell lung carcinomas with neuroendocrine features. A light microscopic, immunohistochemical and ultrastructural study of 11 cases. Histopathology 1988;13:329–37.

29. Neal MH, Kosinski R, Cohen P, Orenstein JM. Atypical endocrine tumors of the lung: a histologic, ultrastructural, and clinical study of 19 cases. Hum Pathol 1986;17:1264–77.

30. Noguchi M, Hirohashi S, Shimosato Y. Immunohistochemical detection of cluster 1 small cell lung cancer antigen and chromogranin A in lung carcinomas. Jpn J Clin Oncol 1992;22:6–9.

31. Nomori H, Shimosato Y, Kodama T, Morinaga S, Nakajima T, Watanabe S. Subtypes of small cell carcinoma of the lung: morphometric, ultrastructural, and immunohistochemical analyses. Hum Pathol 1986;17:604–13.

32. Perry MC, Eaton WL, Propert KJ, et al. Chemotherapy with or without radiation therapy in limited small-cell carcinoma of the lung. N Engl J Med 1987;316:912–8.

33. Piehl MR, Gould VE, Warren WH, et al. Immunohistochemical identification of exocrine and neuroendocrine subsets of large cell lung carcinomas. Pathol Res Pract 1988;183:675–82.

34. Pryzygodzki R, Finkelstein S, Zeren H, et al. p53 analysis of neuroendocrine (NE) tumors: discriminating factors in atypical carcinoid (AC) within the NE spectrum [Abstract]. Mod Pathol 1994;7:153A.

35. Quoix E, Fraser R, Wolkove N, Finkelstein H, Kreisman H. Small cell lung cancer presenting as a solitary pulmonary nodule. Cancer 1990;66:577–82.

36. Roncalli M, Doglioni C, Springall DR, et al. Abnormal p53 expression in lung neuroendocrine tumors. Diagnostic and prognostic implications. Diagn Mol Pathol 1992;1:129–35.

37. Rozenberg I, Wechsler J, Koenig F, et al. Erdheim-Chester disease presenting as malignant exophthalmos. Br J Radiol 1986;59:173–7.

38. Said JW, Vimadalal S, Nash G, et al. Immunoreactive neuron-specific enolase, bombesin, and chromogranin as markers for neuroendocrine lung tumors. Hum Pathol 1985;16:236–40.

39. Sehested M, Hirsch FR, Osterlind K, Olsen JE. Morphologic variations of small cell lung cancer. A histopathologic study of pretreatment and posttreatment specimens in 104 patients. Cancer 1986;57:804–7.

40. Shepherd FA, Ginsberg RJ, Haddad R, et al. Importance of clinical staging in limited small-cell lung cancer: a valuable system to separate prognostic subgroups. The University of Toronto Lung Oncology Group. J Clin Oncol 1993;11:1592–7.

41. Souhami RL, Beverley PC, Bobrow LG. Antigens of small-cell lung cancer. First International Workshop. Lancet 1987;2:325–6.

42. _____, Law K. Longevity in small cell lung cancer. A report to the Lung Cancer Subcommittee of the United Kingdom Coordinating Committee for Cancer Research. Br J Cancer 1990;61:584–9.

43. Tabatowski K, Vollmer RT, Tello JW, et al. The use of a panel of monoclonal antibodies in ultrastructurally characterized small cell carcinomas of the lung. Acta Cytol 1988;32:667–74.

44. Tome Y, Hirohashi S, Noguchi M, Matsuno Y, Shimosato Y. Comparison of immunoreactivity between two different monoclonal antibodies recognizing peptide and polysialic acid chain epitopes on the neural cell adhesion molecule in normal tissues and lung tumors. Acta Pathol Jpn 1993;43:168–75.

45. Travis WD. Carcinoid and other neuroendocrine tumors. In: Saldana MJ, ed. Pathology of pulmonary disease. Philadelphia: JB Lippincott, 1994:581–96.

46. _____, Linnoila RI, Tsokos MG, et al. Neuroendocrine tumors of the lung with proposed criteria for large-cell neuroendocrine carcinoma. An ultrastructural, immunohistochemical, and flow cytometric study of 35 cases. Am J Surg Pathol 1991;15:529–53.

47. Tsubota YT, Kawaguchi T, Hoso T, Nishino E, Travis WD. A combined small cell and spindle cell carcinoma of the lung. Report of a unique case with immunohistochemical and ultrastructural studies. Am J Surg Pathol 1992;16:1108–15.

48. Visscher DW, Zarbo RJ, Trojanowski JQ, Sakr W, Crissman JD. Neuroendocrine differentiation in poorly differentiated lung carcinomas. a light microscopic and immunohistologic study. Mod Pathol 1990;3:508–12.

49. Vollmer RT. The effect of cell size on the pathologic diagnosis of small and large cell carcinomas of the lung. Cancer 1982;50:1380–3.

50. _____, Ogden L, Crissman JD. Separation of small-cell from non-small-cell lung cancer. The Southeastern Cancer Study Group pathologists' experience. Arch Pathol Lab Med 1984;108:792–4.

51. Warren WH, Faber LP, Gould VE. Neuroendocrine neoplasms of the lung. A clinicopathologic update. J Thorac Cardiovasc Surg 1989;98:321–32.

52. _____, Memoli VA, Gould VE. Immunohistochemical and ultrastructural analysis of bronchopulmonary neuroendocrine neoplasms. II. Well-differentiated neuroendocrine carcinomas. Ultrastruct Pathol 1984;7:185–99.

53. Wick MR, Berg LC, Hertz MI. Large cell carcinoma of the lung with neuroendocrine differentiation. A comparison with large cell "undifferentiated" pulmonary tumors. Am J Clin Pathol 1992;97:796–805.

54. World Health Organization. Histological typing of lung tumors. Geneva: World Health Organization, 1981.

❖❖❖

15

LARGE CELL CARCINOMA

Definition. Large cell carcinoma, also called *large cell anaplastic carcinoma* and *large cell undifferentiated carcinoma*, is defined as a malignant epithelial tumor with large nuclei, prominent nucleoli, abundant cytoplasm, and usually well-defined cell borders without the characteristic features of squamous cell, small cell, or adenocarcinoma (40). This definition is one of exclusion and is dependent upon extensive sampling of a given tumor. Further, the definition is based purely on light microscopic features and histochemistry (absence of mucin). While small biopsies may be interpreted as large cell carcinoma, extensive sampling of the same tumor, if resected, might reveal foci of differentiation. It is well known that fields in otherwise typical squamous cell carcinoma and adenocarcinoma may lack differentiation and qualify as large cell carcinoma when assessed alone. Combined adenocarcinoma/large cell carcinoma and squamous cell/large cell carcinoma are not recognized and are simply designated as adenocarcinoma and squamous cell carcinoma, respectively. Small cell carcinomas may contain appreciable numbers of large cells (individually or in sheets), and the category of mixed small cell/large cell carcinoma is recognized (see chapter 14).

In addition to ordinary large cell carcinoma, with sheets of relatively uniform large neoplastic cells, there are a number of less common patterns. *Giant cell carcinoma* has a prominent component of huge (sometimes several hundred microns in diameter), highly pleomorphic and often multinucleated cells. *Spindle cell carcinoma* is another variant. The term *pleomorphic carcinoma* has been proposed to include cases showing components of spindle cell or giant cell carcinoma (13). Pleomorphic carcinoma is discussed below. *Clear cell carcinoma* is a large cell carcinoma composed of cells with clear or foamy cytoplasm without mucin. *Lymphoepithelioma-like carcinoma* is a subset of large cell carcinoma identical to undifferentiated nasopharyngeal carcinoma (lymphoepithelioma). *Large cell neuroendocrine carcinoma* is discussed in chapter 14 and *large cell carcinoma with neuroendocrine features* is discussed in chapter 17.

Clinical Features. The clinical features of large cell carcinoma are summarized in chapter 8. Large cell carcinomas comprise 10 to 20 percent of lung carcinomas (26,27,42). Nearly all patients are smokers and median age at presentation is approximately 60 years (8,9). Most symptoms are due to local effects of the tumor. A minority of patients present with paraneoplastic or endocrine syndromes. Radiographically, large cell carcinomas may be central or peripheral, and are rarely occult.

Gross Findings. Large cell carcinomas are typically large necrotic masses which may invade the overlying pleura and other contiguous structures (figs. 15-1, 15-2) (14,24,26,27).

Microscopic Findings. There is a wide histologic spectrum (14,24,27,40,42). Some tumors have a squamoid (figs. 15-3, 15-4) or glandular growth pattern but without definitive squamous or glandular differentiation, or histochemical evidence of mucin production. Others are composed of intermediate-sized polygonal cells (figs. 15-5, 15-6), with extensive necrosis reminiscent of small cell carcinoma, but containing cells too large, nucleoli too prominent, and too much cytoplasm for small cell carcinoma as defined in chapter 14. The separation of large cell carcinoma from large cell neuroendocrine carcinoma is discussed in chapter 14.

Most typically, large cell carcinomas grow as sheets and nests of large polygonal cells with large vesicular nuclei containing prominent nucleoli (figs. 15-3, 15-4). The cell borders are often prominent, imparting a squamoid appearance. The stroma varies from absent to extensive. Invasive and destructive growth is often associated with a desmoplastic stroma. Hemorrhage and necrosis may be prominent. Some cases show marked acute or chronic inflammatory cell infiltrates. A giant cell or granulomatous reaction may be present. Kodama (22) described a case that was associated with peripheral eosinophilia and eosinophil tumor infiltrates. Occasionally there is marked cellular dyscohesion,

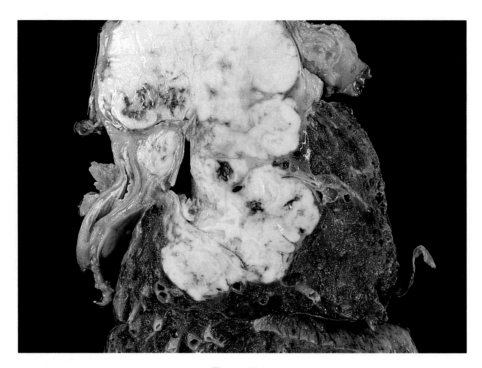

Figure 15-1
LARGE CELL CARCINOMA

This large cell carcinoma at autopsy shows a large multilobulated tumor adjacent to the hilum. A metastatically involved lymph node is present next to the bronchus.

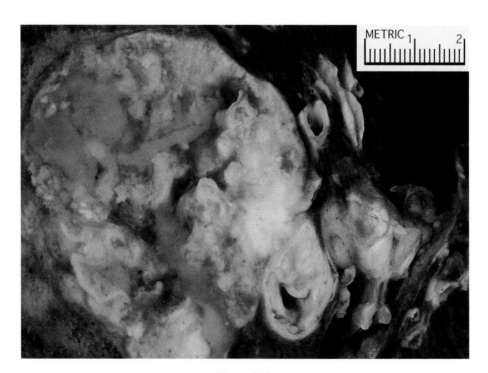

Figure 15-2
LARGE CELL CARCINOMA

This tumor is an extensively necrotic, well-circumscribed mass adjacent to a large bronchus. Foci of giant cell carcinoma were present in this case.

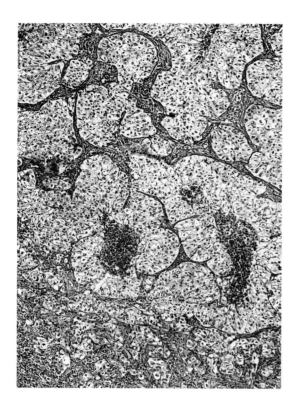
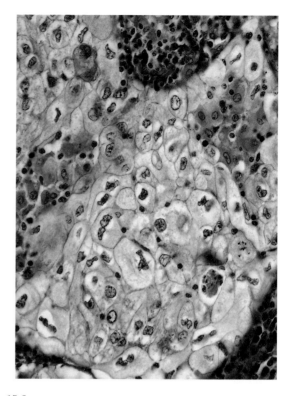

Figure 15-3
LARGE CELL CARCINOMA
Left: Nests of cells showing clear cell change and central necrosis are present.
Right: Detail shows abundant cytoplasm with some clearing. Sharp cell borders impart a squamoid appearance.

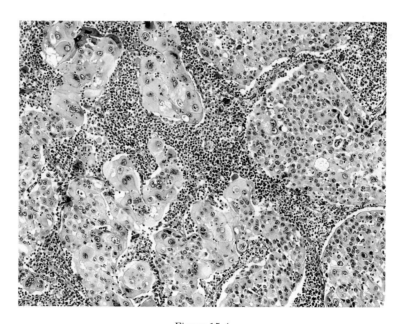

Figure 15-4
LARGE CELL CARCINOMA
This case shows focal giant cell change (left) with cells that are three to four times as large as the conventional large cell carcinoma cells at the right.

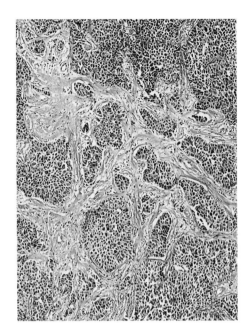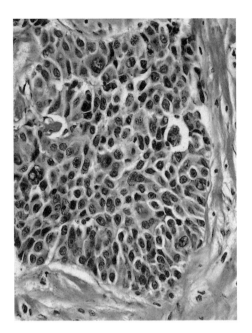

Figure 15-5
LARGE CELL CARCINOMA

Left: A dense fibrous stroma surrounds nests of cells that have a suggestion of peripheral pallisading imparting a basaloid or neuroendocrine appearance.

Right: Cytologically, the cells have a moderate amount of cytoplasm and nuclei which vary from small and hyperchromatic to large and vesicular with prominent nucleoli.

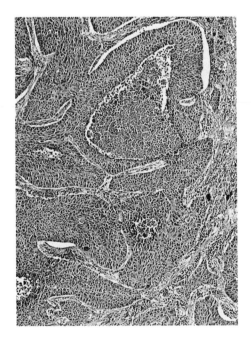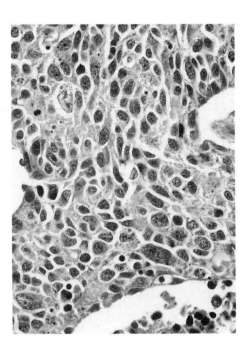

Figure 15-6
LARGE CELL CARCINOMA

Left: Sheets of tumor cells show central necrosis. Some pallisading at the periphery of the cell nests is present.

Right: Cytologically, the tumor cells have a moderate amount of cytoplasm and considerable nuclear variation with some small hyperchromatic forms resembling small cell carcinoma and others that are larger and vesicular containing prominent nucleoli. The features suggest the possibility of neuroendocrine differentiation, but it was not proven in this case.

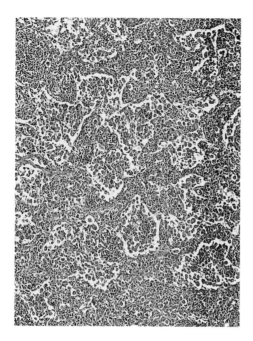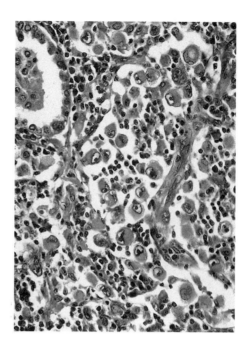

Figure 15-7
LARGE CELL CARCINOMA
Left: There is a prominent interstitial inflammatory infiltrate and the carcinoma cells flood the alveoli as individual cells reminiscent of desquamative interstitial pneumonia.
Right: Cytologically, the cells have abundant eosinophilic cytoplasm and large vesicular nuclei with very prominent nucleoli. A portion of an alveolus lined by metaplastic type 2 cells is present (upper left). Other fields in this case showed characteristic cohesive nests of large cell carcinoma.

with the neoplastic cells floating in pools of inflammatory cells, often neutrophils; emperipolesis of inflammatory cells (lymphocytes, plasma cells, or neutrophils) into the neoplastic cells is common in such cases. Some cases flood alveolar spaces (fig. 15-7) or grow along interstitial planes (fig. 15-8). Cellular dyscohesion noted by light microscopy correlates with a paucity of cell attachments ultrastructurally (1).

The cytoplasm of large cell carcinomas may be eosinophilic, clear, or foamy and is usually abundant. The nuclei may be single or multiple, with a variable degree of hyperchromatism. Nucleoli may be single or multiple and are often very prominent and eosinophilic.

When mucin-positive cells are present (usually they are relatively numerous), the designation *solid adenocarcinoma with mucin production* is appropriate. At present this pattern is not clinically significant.

Several other patterns of large cell carcinoma are discussed below. One extremely rare pattern is *pseudoangiosarcomatous carcinoma*: the cells

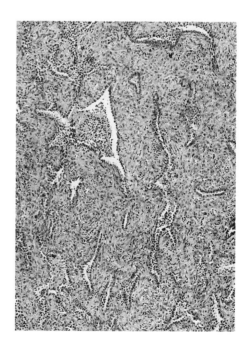

Figure 15-8
LARGE CELL CARCINOMA
Interstitial growth by large cell carcinoma imparts a pseudobiphasic appearance with preserved alveoli lined by reactive type 2 cells.

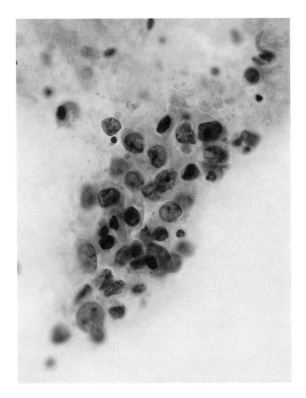 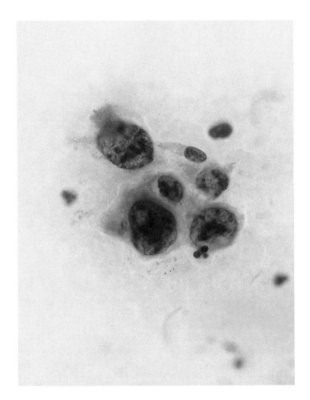

Figure 15-9
LARGE CELL CARCINOMA
Bronchial wash cytology specimen (left and right) shows clusters of neoplastic cells with large nuclei, prominent nucleoli, and abundant cytoplasm.

are positive for keratin and negative for endothelial markers (2).

The cytologic findings parallel the histologic findings (figs. 15-9, 15-10) (18,26,27). The cells generally are large with obvious malignant nuclear features: hypochromasia, irregular nuclear contours, and prominent nucleoli. Cells occur singly or in groups, and marked dyscohesion (single cells) characterizes some cases. The cytoplasm may be abundant and finely vacuolated.

While the diagnosis of malignancy may be readily apparent cytologically, it is more difficult to definitively exclude poorly differentiated squamous cell carcinoma, poorly differentiated adenocarcinoma, and other tumors, such as lymphomas, especially in small specimens. Distinguishing large cell carcinoma, small cell carcinoma, and combined small cell/large cell carcinoma also can be difficult (see chapter 14).

Immunohistochemical Findings. There have been several immunohistochemical studies of large cell carcinoma, and a number of markers

have been assessed (7,17,21,25,29,33,38). The results can be summarized as follows: cytokeratins and CAM 5.2, positive in half to three fourths of cases; epithelial membrane antigen (EMA), positive in over half the cases; carcinoembryonic antigen (CEA), positive in half to two thirds of cases; vimentin, positive in slightly less than half of cases; neuron-specific enolase (NSE), positive in less than half of cases; B72.3, positive in less than one fourth of cases; secretory component, positive in about one third of cases; and surfactant apoprotein, negative. Markers that are rarely positive include bombesin, serotonin, substance P, corticotropin (ACTH), leu-enkephalin, calcitonin, melanocyte stimulating hormone (MSH), chromogranin, vasopressin, neurotensin, neurofilament, Leu-M1, and lactoferrin (25,33,37). The presence of neuroendocrine markers suggests either large cell carcinoma with neuroendocrine features (LCC-NE) or large cell neuroendocrine carcinoma (LCNEC) (see chapter 14).

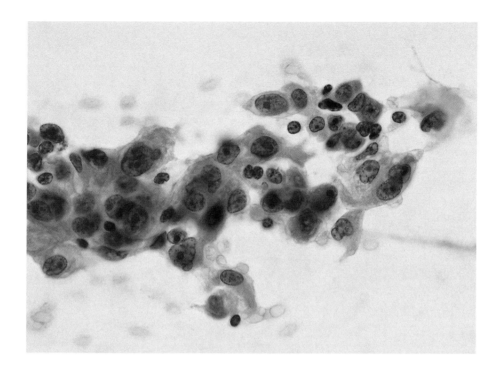

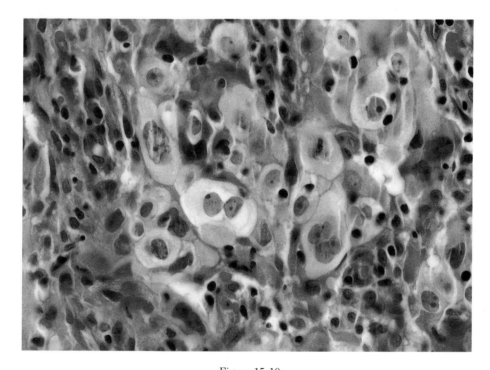

Figure 15-10
LARGE CELL CARCINOMA
Top: Fine needle aspiration shows a group of partially cohesive neoplastic cells with large nuclei, relatively prominent nucleoli, and abundant cytoplasm.
Bottom: The corresponding surgical resection shows neoplastic cells with abundant pale eosinophilic cytoplasm and a surrounding infiltrate of inflammatory cells which can also be seen among the tumor cells in the fine needle aspirate specimen.

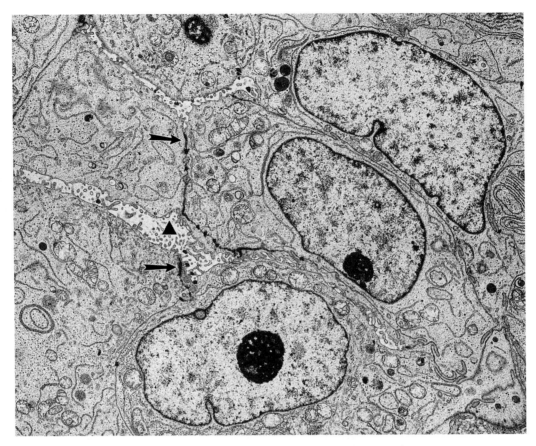

Figure 15-11
LARGE CELL CARCINOMA
This tumor was undifferentiated light microscopically. Electron microscopic examination shows lumen formation (black triangle) with microvilli extending into the luminal space and prominent cell junctions (arrows) between the cells. The ultrastructural features suggest adenocarcinomatous differentiation. (X5750) (Courtesy of Dr. Bruce MacKay, Houston, TX.)

In general, immunohistochemical positivity for epithelial markers parallels ultrastructural evidence of differentiation (7). Cases showing cellular dyscohesion (the "loose" type of Ishida et al. (17)) are less likely to stain for epithelial markers. In up to one third of cases studied, staining for all markers was negative (7,17,21).

Delmonte et al. (7) found that the immunohistochemical staining pattern correlated with the ultrastructural findings: cases showing neurosecretory granules stained positively with NSE; cases showing glandular or squamous differentiation stained positively with CEA and keratin.

Ultrastructural Findings. The heterogeneity of large cell carcinoma has been confirmed ultrastructurally in several studies; large cell carcinomas diagnosed light microscopically frequently show evidence of differentiation at the ultrastructural level (fig. 15-11) (6,7,10,21,23, 36). In these studies, the presence of desmosomes and tonofilaments is indicative of squamous differentiation; lumina, microvilli, tight junctions, and secretory granules are evidence of adenocarcinomatous differentiation; the presence of both is evidence of adenosquamous carcinoma; and neurosecretory-type granules are indicative of neuroendocrine differentiation. The results of a number of these studies are shown in Table 15-1.

It is apparent from Table 15-1 that the majority of large cell carcinomas show ultrastructural evidence of differentiation along one or more lines, but just as with immunohistochemistry, there remain a small number of cases that are truly undifferentiated, even at the ultrastructural level (fig. 15-12).

Table 15-1

ULTRASTRUCTURAL ASSESSMENT OF LARGE CELL CARCINOMA

Author	No. Cases	Squamous Differen- tiation	Adenocar- cinomatous Differen- tiation	Adeno- squamous Differen- tiation	Neuro- endocrine Differen- tiation (+/- adeno- or squamous features)	Undiffer- entiated	Other*
Churg (6)	7	3	4	—	—	—	—
Leong (23)	16	6	4	1	3	1	1
Saba (36)	5	0	1	1	2	1	—
Kodama (21)	18	1	8	4	1	4	—
Delmonte (7)	41	5	8	12	8	8	—
Dunnill (10)	9	2	7	—	—	—	—
Totals	96	17 (18%)	32 (34%)	18 (19%)	14 (14%)	14 (14%)	1 (1%)

*Other tumors (e.g., lymphoma).

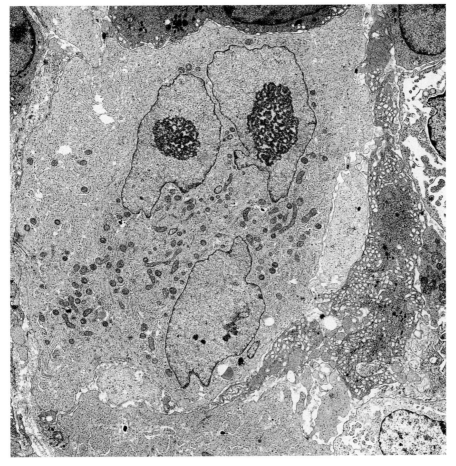

Figure 15-12
LARGE CELL CARCINOMA
Ultrastructural examina-
tion of this tumor showed no
evidence of differentiation. Anaplastic tumor cells with lobulated nuclei and markedly enlarged nucleoli are present.
Squamous and glandular differentiation were lacking. (X
4650) (Courtesy of Dr. Bruce
MacKay, Houston, TX.)

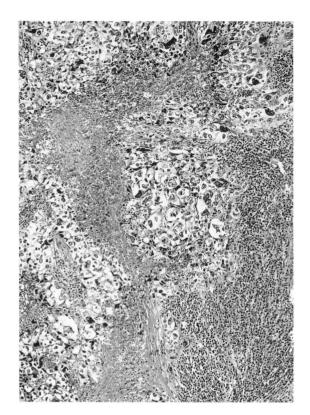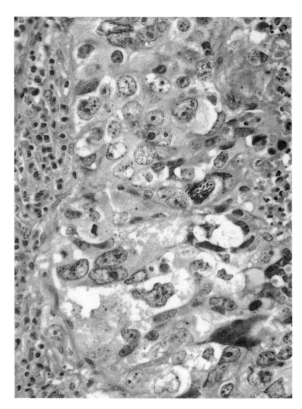

Figure 15-13
GIANT CELL CARCINOMA
Left: Sheets of tumor cells associated with necrosis are surrounded by a stroma rich in inflammatory cells.
Right: The giant size of the tumor cells can be appreciated by comparing them to the inflammatory cells.

Histologic Variants of Large Cell Carcinoma. *Giant cell carcinoma* is a distinctive morphologic variant of large cell carcinoma with huge, bizarre, pleomorphic and multinucleated tumor giant cells of up to 700 or 800 μm in diameter (figs. 15-13–15-17). Focal giant cell change is not uncommon in many lung carcinomas and radiated tumors may have giant cell features (fig. 15-18). According to the World Health Organization (WHO) criteria (40), there must be a "prominent component" of giant cell carcinoma in order to designate a case as such; however, no consistent percentage has been used as a criterion in the literature. A minimum component of 10 percent for a diagnosis of giant cell carcinoma is reasonable (13). There is a quantitative requirement for the cell size: the cells should be at least two to three times the size of cells of ordinary nonsmall cell carcinomas; there is size gradation in many cases (fig. 15-5).

Marked cellular dyscohesion is often prominent and is usually associated with an inflammatory infiltrate of neutrophils, both within and surrounding the neoplastic cells.

Giant cell carcinomas of the lung were initially reported in 1958 by Nash and Stout (31). They are considered a rare and highly malignant form of lung cancer. Addis et al. (1) found only one pure giant cell carcinoma among the 10 cases they described, and Fishback et al. (13) found only 2 among 78 cases of pleomorphic carcinoma. According to WHO criteria, giant cell carcinomas are classified as a subset of large cell carcinoma (40). Nevertheless, foci of giant cell carcinoma may be seen in carcinomas with identifiable squamous or glandular differentiation (see below).

The incidence of giant cell carcinoma in different studies has varied: 0.8 percent in the series of Ginsberg et al. (15), 2 percent in the series of Flanagan and Roeckel (12), and 4 percent in the

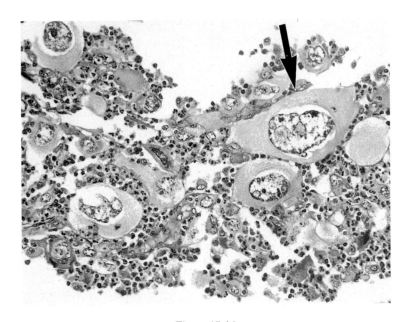

Figure 15-14
GIANT CELL CARCINOMA
Gigantic carcinoma cells, nearly 750 μm in size (arrow), are set in an inflammatory background.

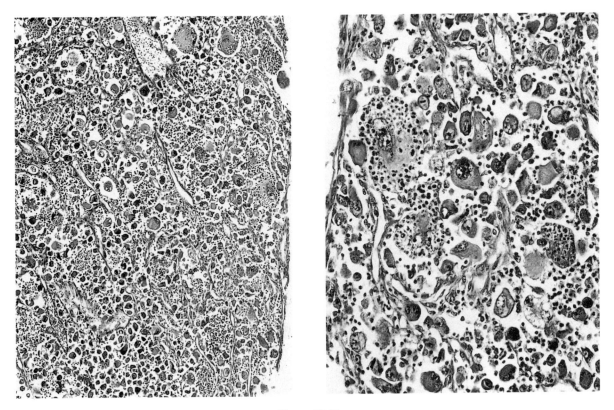

Figure 15-15
GIANT CELL CARCINOMA
These two figures illustrate marked cellular dyscohesion with neutrophils surrounding the tumor giant cells. The higher power (right) shows prominent emperipolesis of neutrophils into the tumor cells.

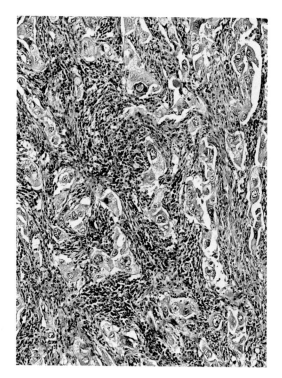

Figure 15-16
GIANT CELL CARCINOMA
This endobronchial tumor was composed of a stroma rich in inflammatory cells surrounded by cords and nests of giant cell carcinoma. The size of the tumor cells can be appreciated by comparing them to the inflammatory cells in the stroma.

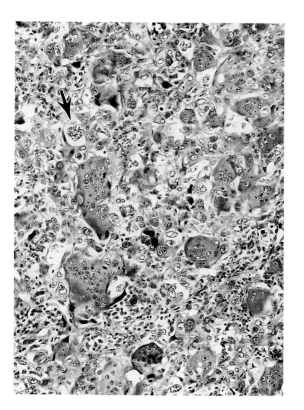

Figure 15-17
GIANT CELL CARCINOMA
This giant cell carcinoma contains scattered tumor giant cells (arrow) as well as osteoclastic giant cells.

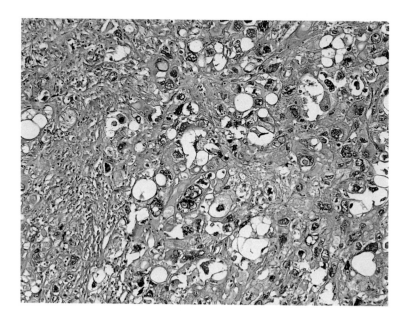

Figure 15-18
RADIATED CARCINOMA
Following radiation therapy, this large cell carcinoma showed giant cell change in the neoplastic cells. Such a field is indistinguishable from giant cell carcinoma.

series of Kallenberg and Jaqué (19). A figure of 1 percent or less is probably reasonable (15) although Fishback et al. give a figure of 0.3 percent for pleomorphic carcinoma overall (see below).

Giant cell carcinomas are similar to large cell carcinomas in terms of age, sex ratio, duration of symptoms, and smoking history. They are only rarely discovered as an incidental radiographic finding.

Grossly, giant cell carcinomas are similar to large cell carcinomas. They may be central but frequently present as a peripheral mass lesion. Giant cell carcinomas are recognized microscopically by the presence of pleomorphic and often multinucleated tumor giant cells (which may be seen either as cohesive nests or as dyscohesive cells infiltrated by inflammatory cells) comprising more than 10 percent of a given tumor. The tumor cells may have single or multiple large nuclei with one or several nucleoli. Nuclear inclusions are occasionally seen. Signet cell forms may be present. Some cases of giant cell carcinoma resemble choriocarcinoma and may even produce human chorionic gonadotropin (hCG) (see fig. 23-37). An accompanying spindle cell carcinoma component is present in 30 to 40 percent of cases (13).

Immunohistochemically, giant cell carcinomas are similar to large cell carcinomas. In the series of Addis et al. (1) and Chejfec et al. (5), the following staining patterns were seen: cytokeratin and CAM 5.2, usually positive; vimentin, usually positive; and EMA, occasionally positive. Staining was focal or widespread, and sometimes most marked at the periphery of the giant cells. Chejfec et al. (5) noted positive staining with a monoclonal antibody for mucinous glycoprotein in all 10 cases studied.

Ultrastructurally, giant cell carcinomas are characterized by abundant mitochondria, whorls of tonofilament-like fibrils, multiple pairs of centrioles, and emperipolesis of inflammatory cells (1,41). In individual cases features of squamous differentiation (desmosomes and tonofilaments) or adenocarcinomatous differentiation (secretory granules, microvilli, lumen formation) can be identified. Addis (1) noted the accumulation of dense filament bundles in a perinuclear distribution and thought these corresponded to vimentin intermediate filaments. He also noted that a paucity of desmosomes

correlated with the cellular dyscohesion seen by light microscopy. Kodama et al. (21) studied 9 cases of giant cell carcinoma ultrastructurally and found adenocarcinomatous differentiation in 6, squamous carcinomatous differentiation in 2, and no differentiation in 1.

While a number of series have suggested that giant cell carcinoma is one of the most highly malignant forms of lung cancer (12,35,39), with a short median survival and a greater number of metastatic sites, some recent studies report a prognosis similar to (15), or better than (17), other nonsmall cell lung carcinomas. Ginsberg et al. (15) noted a propensity for giant cell carcinoma to metastasize to the gastrointestinal tract.

Spindle cell carcinomas lacking squamous or glandular differentiation can also be included as a subset of large cell carcinoma (although in the WHO classification spindle cell carcinomas are included only with squamous carcinomas (40)). Carcinomatous differentiation must be present either histologically, immunohistochemically, or ultrastructurally; this definition, therefore, departs to some extent from a pure light microscopic classification. Spindle cell foci may be the sole component or they may be associated with giant cell carcinoma or ordinary large cell carcinoma (figs. 15-19–15-21). The spindle cells may suggest a sarcoma, but the cell fascicles tend to be plumper and the nuclei more vesicular than in sarcomas, and the foci often coexist with or merge with more recognizable cohesive carcinomatous cell nests. Nevertheless, spindle cell foci may resemble fibrosarcoma, leiomyosarcoma, and malignant fibrous histiocytoma. Immunohistochemistry and electron microscopy are necessary to recognize carcinomatous features in some cases. Vascular invasion is particularly prominent in spindle cell carcinomas. Spindle cell carcinoma and carcinosarcoma are discussed further in chapter 21.

Pleomorphic (spindle/giant cell) carcinoma accounts for only 0.3 percent of all lung malignancies. This subset consists of lung carcinomas that exhibit a spindle cell component, a giant cell component, or both, of 10 percent or more. Recently, the Armed Forces Institute of Pathology (AFIP) reviewed 78 cases of pleomorphic carcinoma of the lung (13). Epithelial differentiation was confirmed in all spindle cell carcinomas by positive immunohistochemical staining for epithelial markers

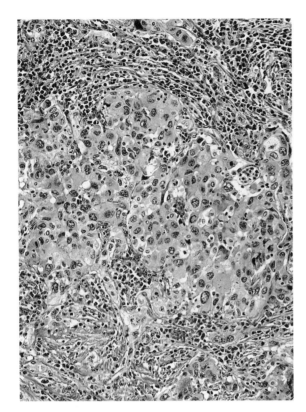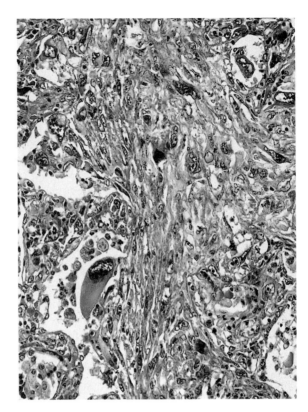

Figure 15-19
LARGE CELL CARCINOMA WITH SPINDLE CELL FOCI
Left: Some regions of this tumor showed ordinary large cell carcinoma.
Right: Other regions, comprising approximately 80 percent of the lesion, showed bizarre neoplastic spindle cells mimicking a sarcoma.

such as keratin or EMA. The reasons for proposing this category include the frequent coexistence of spindle and giant cell components (in 40 percent of cases), the frequent association with other histologic types of lung carcinoma (over 90 percent for spindle cell carcinoma and over 97 percent for giant cell carcinoma), and the poor survival (about 10 percent) regardless of the associated histologic type. These tumors usually presented in older male smokers with large peripheral lung tumors, chest wall invasion, and metastases. The most common associated histologic type was adenocarcinoma (45 percent), followed by ordinary large cell carcinoma (25 percent), squamous cell carcinoma (8 percent), and small cell carcinoma (1 percent). Ten percent (eight cases) had giant cell and spindle cell carcinomas as the only components. Only 9 percent were pure spindle cell carcinoma (7 cases) and only 3 percent were pure giant cell carcinoma (2

cases). The spindle cell component resembled fibrosarcoma, leiomyosarcoma, malignant fibrous histiocytoma, or undifferentiated sarcoma. The peripheral location of pleomorphic carcinoma and its poor survival (about 10 percent; see fig. 8-16) closely mimic the clinical presentation and biologic behavior of large cell carcinoma.

The current WHO guidelines classify such tumors according to the best differentiated component (40), for example, poorly differentiated adenocarcinoma if adenocarcinoma is present. According to the concept proposed by Fishback et al. (13), such a tumor would be called pleomorphic adenocarcinoma with spindle and/or giant cell features, mentioning each histologic type present. If the spindle or giant cell components coexist with large cell carcinoma, they suggest the term pleomorphic (spindle and/or giant cell) carcinoma. There is precedent for such an approach in the WHO classification of thyroid tumors where

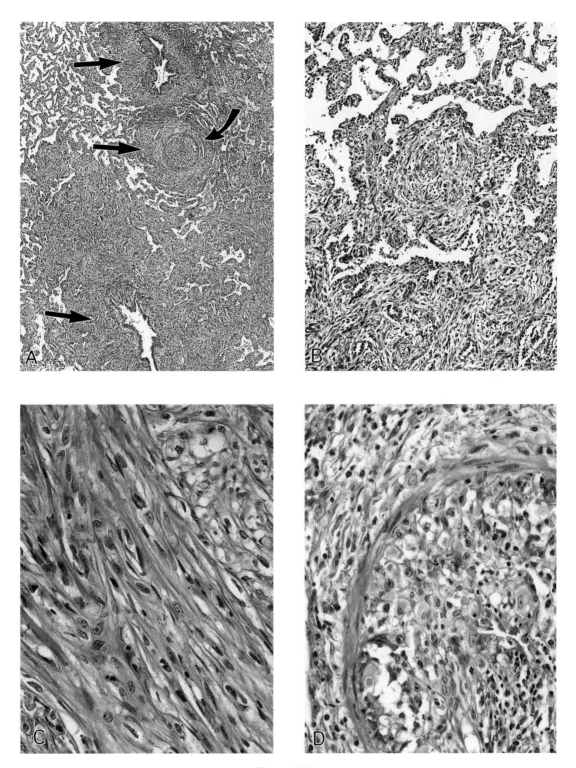

Figure 15-20
SPINDLE CELL CARCINOMA
This spindle cell carcinoma shows extensive peribronchiolar and perivascular infiltration (A, arrows) as well as invasion of the pulmonary artery branches (curved arrow). The infiltrate extends along alveolar septa (B). The tumor is composed almost entirely of spindle cells (C). Focally, in one of the invaded vessels, the epithelial nature of the tumor cells is apparent in the polygonal shaped cells with prominent cytoplasmic borders (D, center). In this case the spindle cells were uniformly keratin positive.

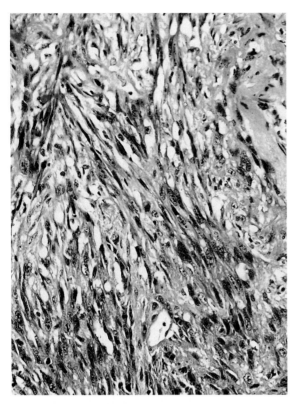

Figure 15-21
SPINDLE CELL CARCINOMA
This solitary tumor was composed entirely of spindle cells and was thought on the basis of light microscopy to be a high-grade sarcoma. Electron microscopy showed cell junctions characteristic of epithelial cells.

highly malignant tumors composed in part or wholly of undifferentiated cells with spindle or giant cell features are considered "undifferentiated (anaplastic) carcinoma" (16). While in the thyroid many of these tumors are considered to represent dedifferentiation of follicular or papillary carcinomas, they are classified according to the undifferentiated component since this appears to dictate the poor prognosis in these patients. In the lung, the term "undifferentiated" has long been applied to both small cell carcinomas and large cell carcinomas, and therefore the term "pleomorphic" seems more reasonable.

Until the WHO decides how to modify the classification of these tumors in the lung, it is appropriate to identify each histologic subtype present and primarily classify the tumor according to the best differentiated component. When heterologous mesenchymal elements are identi-

fied, the possibility of carcinosarcoma has to be considered (chapter 21). In the case of a pure spindle cell malignancy in which an epithelial component cannot be identified by morphology, immunohistochemistry, or ultrastructure, a sarcoma has to be considered.

Clear cell change is common in carcinomas of the lung (20). Rare tumors are composed entirely of clear cells and lack squamous or glandular differentiation; these represent a subset of large cell carcinoma (fig. 15-22). Mucin is lacking, although glycogen is often present.

Katzenstein et al. (20) studied 348 consecutive resections for lung carcinoma and found clear cell change in 105 (30 percent): 33 percent of squamous carcinomas, 27 percent of adenocarcinomas, 33 percent of adenosquamous carcinomas, and 71 percent of large cell carcinomas. Of the 105 carcinomas with clear cell change, 15 had clear cell foci comprising more than 50 percent of the tumor and were designated as clear cell carcinomas. Of these 15, 10 showed squamous foci and were classified as squamous carcinoma with clear cells and 4 showed adenocarcinomatous foci and were classified as adenocarcinoma with clear cells. Only 1 case (0.3 percent of the total) was a pure clear cell carcinoma qualifying also as a large cell carcinoma.

Edwards and Carlile (11) studied 6 cases diagnosed as clear cell carcinoma by light microscopy. Further sampling of the tumors and electron microscopy led to a diagnosis of adenocarcinoma in 3, squamous carcinoma in 2, and large cell carcinoma in 1.

It is clear from these two studies that pure clear cell carcinomas are extremely rare but that they do exist. The cells are large with abundant clear cytoplasm and prominent cell borders, and have large nuclei with prominent nucleoli. Abundant cytoplasmic glycogen is usually present.

Lymphoepithelioma-like carcinomas of the lung are identical to their nasopharyngeal counterparts and are a subset of large cell carcinoma (figs. 15-23, 15-24) (3,4,32,34). Nests of undifferentiated neoplastic cells are surrounded and infiltrated by a dense lymphoplasmacytic cell population. The tumor cells have moderate amounts of cytoplasm and prominent vesicular nuclei with modest nucleoli. The cells lack squamous or glandular differentiation. Foci showing dense lymphoid infiltrates may merge with foci of infiltrating cell

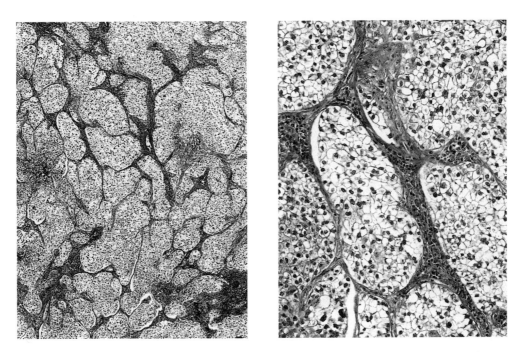

Figure 15-22
CLEAR CELL CARCINOMA
This large cell carcinoma is composed entirely of clear cells. There was no evidence of squamous or glandular differentiation and a primary renal cell carcinoma was excluded clinically.

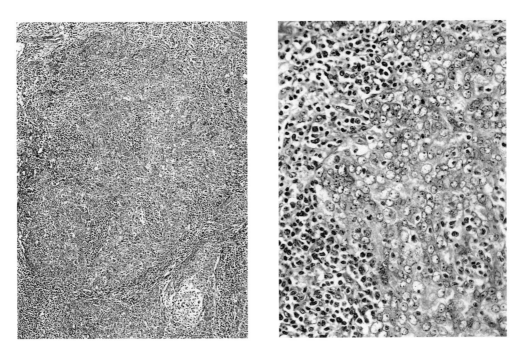

Figure 15-23
LYMPHOEPITHELIOMA-LIKE CARCINOMA
Left: This is an example of a large cell carcinoma showing features identical to a nasopharyngeal lymphoepithelioma. The cell nests are difficult to discern and are heavily infiltrated by lymphoid cells.
Right: Detail shows the characteristic vesicular nuclei with small nucleoli in the carcinomatous nests adjacent to the lymphoid stroma.

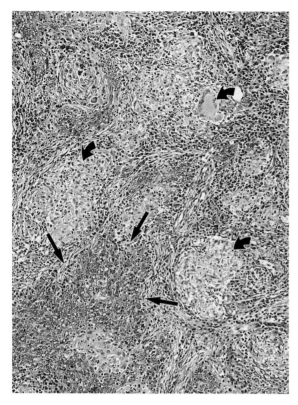

Figure 15-24
LYMPHOEPITHELIOMA-LIKE CARCINOMA
The tumor cell nests, which are relatively inconspicuous cells (arrows), are composed of cells with vesicular nuclei. The surrounding stroma shows several epithelioid cell granulomas and an occasional giant cell (curved arrows). Similar granulomatous features are occasionally seen in nasopharyngeal lymphoepitheliomas.

nests in a fibrous stroma with relatively little lymphoid infiltrate. Most reported cases occur within the lung parenchyma (3,4,34); Onizuka (32) reported a case presenting as an intratracheal mass. Butler et al. (4) found the Epstein-Barr virus (EBV) genome by in situ hybridization in one of four cases. Bégin et al. (3) also noted an association with EBV. This pattern of carcinoma of the lung is relatively more common in the Far East: the study by Pittaluga et al. (34) from Hong Kong showed that 5 of 137 resections for lung carcinoma were lymphoepithelioma-like carcinomas. Since EBV was seen in all 5 tumors by in situ hybridization, the authors postulated an association between EBV infection and this tumor.

Differential Diagnosis. The differential diagnosis of large cell carcinoma primarily centers on other malignancies: other lung carcinomas, including squamous carcinoma, adenocarcinoma, small cell carcinoma; primary nonepithelial malignancies of the lung: sarcomas, lymphomas, melanoma; metastatic neoplasms: carcinomas, sarcomas, melanoma, lymphomas; and miscellaneous lesions.

The distinction of large cell carcinoma from squamous carcinoma and adenocarcinoma is mainly a function of sampling. In general, the more extensively a tumor is sampled, the more likely foci of squamous or adenocarcinomatous differentiation will be found. As noted above, such differentiation is frequent at the ultrastructural level, but classification of a tumor as large cell carcinoma is based on light microscopic features. The distinction of large cell carcinoma from small cell carcinoma and large cell neuroendocrine carcinoma is discussed in chapter 14.

Since large cell carcinomas may show spindled foci and cellular dyscohesion, the differential diagnosis includes sarcomas and lymphomas. In fact, in some studies (38), lymphoma was mistaken for large cell carcinoma on initial evaluation. The lymphoma cells tend to be smaller, and the nuclei show a greater degree of hyperchromasia and membrane irregularity than those in large cell carcinoma. Nodular sclerosing Hodgkin disease, with sheets of lacunar cells infiltrated by leukocytes and malignant fibrous histiocytomas may mimic giant cell carcinoma. Anaplastic large cell (CD30 positive) lymphomas may closely mimic large cell or giant cell carcinoma. Some large cell carcinomas may have fields indistinguishable from malignant melanoma; if there is a question, immunohistochemical staining for epithelial and melanoma markers is appropriate. Primary sarcomas of the lung tend to have cells that are not quite as large and plump as spindle cell carcinomas, and smaller and more elongated nuclei. In difficult cases, immunohistochemical staining may be useful. Distinguishing metastatic carcinoma from large cell carcinoma primarily depends on knowledge of the prior tumor(s) and comparison of the tumor in the lung with the other known primaries. In selected cases, immunohistochemical studies may be helpful, however, some cases will remain insoluble. In the case of clear cell carcinoma, the possibility of metastatic renal cell carcinoma should always be considered and a radiographic evaluation of the kidneys suggested. Metastatic nasopharyngeal lymphoepithelioma may produce a solitary nodule indistinguishable from primary lymphoepithelioma-like carcinoma of the lung.

Large cell carcinomas are occasionally mistaken for a number of other lesions. Clear cell carcinoma may be mistaken for a clear cell tumor (see chapter 23) unless careful attention is paid to the features of malignancy in the former. Spindle carcinomas with central necrosis and abundant fibroblastic reaction may be mistaken for an abscess, focal organizing pneumonia, or inflammatory pseudotumor. Attention to cytologic detail and immunohistochemical staining of the atypical cells for epithelial markers are both useful in such cases. Giant cell carcinoma may resemble choriocarcinoma and may be associated in hCG production.

Spread and Staging. See chapter 8.

Treatment and Prognosis. Large cell carcinomas are generally grouped with squamous cell carcinoma and adenocarcinoma as nonsmall cell lung cancers, and therapy and prognosis are generally similar (see chapter 8). In one study, large cell carcinoma was found to have a dismal prognosis with frequent presentation at high stage: of 96 consecutive cases studied by RS Downey et al. (9), only 10 tumors were resectable, and only 1 patient was alive at 5 years (5-year survival of slightly over 1 percent). In the Surveillance Epidemiology End Result (SEER) data (see fig. 8-16), there was an overall 5-year relative survival of 11.4 percent for large cell carcinoma, worse than for squamous cell carcinoma and adenocarcinoma (see fig. 8-16). However, other studies have shown a prognosis similar to other nonsmall cell carcinomas (8,17). Of 61 cases (preselected as surgical candidates) reported by RJ Downey et al. (8), 52 were resectable, and there was a 38 percent 5-year survival. Ishida et al. (17) reported a similar survival (approximately 37 percent) and a better prognosis for cases showing a compact or cohesive growth pattern in comparison to those showing a loose or dyscohesive pattern. They suggested that the better prognosis correlated with more intercellular attachments. McDonagh et al. (28) noted similar findings.

REFERENCES

1. Addis BJ, Dewar A, Thurlow NP. Giant cell carcinoma of the lung—immunohistochemical and ultrastructural evidence of dedifferentiation. J Pathol 1988;155:231–40.
2. Banerjee SS, Eyden BP, Wells S, McWilliam LJ, Harris M. Pseudoangiosarcomatous carcinoma: a clinicopathological study of seven cases. Histopathology 1992;21:13–23.
3. Bégin LR, Eskandari J, Joncas J, Panasci L. Epstein-Barr virus related lymphoepithelioma-like carcinoma of lung. J Surg Oncol 1987;36:280–3.
4. Butler AE, Colby TV, Weiss L, Lombard C. Lymphoepithelioma-like carcinoma of the lung. Am J Surg Pathol 1989;13:632–9.
5. Chejfec G, Candel A, Jansson DS, et al. Immunohistochemical features of giant cell carcinoma of the lung: patterns of expression of cytokeratins, vimentin, and the mucinous glycoprotein recognized by monoclonal antibody A-80. Ultrastruct Pathol 1991;15:131–8.
6. Churg A. The fine structure of large cell undifferentiated carcinoma of the lung. Evidence for its relation to squamous cell carcinomas and adenocarcinomas. Hum Pathol 1978;9:143–56.
7. Delmonte VC, Alberti O, Saldiva PH. Large cell carcinoma of the lung. Ultrastructural and immunohistochemical features. Chest 1986;90:524–7.
8. Downey RJ, Deschamps C, Asakura S, et al. Large cell carcinoma of the lung: results of surgical treatment. Lung Cancer 1994;11(Suppl):153.
9. Downey RS, Sewell CW, Mansour KA. Large cell carcinoma of the lung: a highly aggressive tumor with dismal prognosis. Ann Thorac Surg 1989;47:806–8.
10. Dunnill MS, Gatter KC. Cellular heterogeneity in lung cancer. Histopathology 1986;10:461–75.
11. Edwards C, Carlile A. Clear cell carcinoma of the lung. J Clin Pathol 1985;38:880–5.
12. Flanagan P, Roeckel IE. Giant cell carcinoma of the lung. Am J Med 1964;36:214–21.
13. Fishback N, Travis W, Moran C, Guinee DG, McCarthy W, Koss MN. Pleomorphic (spindle/giant cell) carcinoma of the lung: a clinicopathologic study of 78 cases. Cancer 1994;73:2936–45.
14. Gazdar AF, Linnoila RI. The pathology of lung cancer—changing concepts and newer diagnostic techniques. Semin Oncol 1988;15:215–25.
15. Ginsberg SS, Buzaid AC, Stern H, Carter D. Giant cell carcinoma of the lung. Cancer 1992;70:606–10.
16. Hedinger C, Williams ED, Sobin LH. Undifferentiated (anaplastic) carcinoma. In: Anonymous, ed. World Health Organization. Histological Typing of Thyroid Tumors. Berlin: Springer-Verlag, 1988:13–4.

17. Ishida T, Kaneko S, Tateishi M, et al. Large cell carcinoma of the lung. Prognostic implications of histopathologic and immunohistochemical subtyping. Am J Clin Pathol 1990;93:176–82.

18. Johnston WW, Frable WJ. The cytopathology of the respiratory tract. A review. Am J Pathol 1976;84:372–424.

19. Kallenberg F, Jaqué J. Giant-cell carcinoma of the lung. Clinical and pathological assessment. Comparison with other large-cell anaplastic bronchogenic carcinomas. Scand J Thor Cardiovasc Surg 1979;13:343–6.

20. Katzenstein AL, Prioleau PG, Askin FB. The histologic spectrum and significance of clear-cell change in lung carcinoma. Cancer 1980;45:943–7.

21. Kodama T, Shimosato Y, Koide T, Watanabe S, Teshima S. Large cell carcinoma of the lung—ultrastructural and immuno-histochemical studies. Jpn J Clin Oncol 1985;15:431–41.

22. _____, Takada K, Kameya T, Shimosato Y, Tsuchiya R, Okabe T. Large cell carcinoma of the lung associated with marked eosinophilia. A case report. Cancer 1984;54:2313–7.

23. Leong AS. The relevance of ultrastructural examination in the classification of primary lung tumours. Pathology 1982;14:37–46.

24. Linnoila I. Pathology of non-small cell lung cancer. New diagnostic approaches. Hematol Oncol Clin North Am 1990;4:1027–51.

25. Linnoila RI, Mulshine JL, Steinberg SM, et al. Neuroendocrine differentiation in endocrine and nonendocrine lung carcinomas. Am J Clin Pathol 1988;90:641–52.

26. Matthews MJ. Morphology of lung cancer. Semin Oncol 1974;1:175–82.

27. _____, Mackay B, Lukeman J. The pathology of non-small cell carcinoma of the lung. Semin Oncol 1983;10:34–55.

28. McDonagh D, Vollmer RT, Shelburne JD. Intercellular junctions and tumor behavior in lung cancer. Mod Pathol 1991;4:436–40.

29. Mizutani Y, Nakajima T, Morinaga S, et al. Immunohistochemical localization of pulmonary surfactant apoproteins in various lung tumors. Special reference to nonmucus producing lung adenocarcinomas. Cancer 1988;61:532–7.

30. Mooi WJ, Dingemans KP, Wagenaar SS, Hart AA, Wagenvoort CA. Ultrastructural heterogeneity of lung carcinomas. Representativity of samples for electron microscopy in tumor classification. Hum Pathol 1990;21:1227–34.

31. Nash AD, Stout AP. Giant cell carcinoma of the lung: report of 5 cases. Cancer 1958;11:359–68.

32. Onizuka M, Doi M, Mitsui K, Ogata T, Hori M. Undifferentiated carcinoma with prominent lymphocytic infiltration (so-called lymphoepithelioma) in the trachea. Chest 1990;98:236–7.

33. Piehl MR, Gould VE, Warren WH, et al. Immunohistochemical identification of exocrine and neuroendocrine subsets of large cell lung carcinomas. Pathol Res Pract 1988;183:675–82.

34. Pittaluga S, Wong MP, Chung LP, Loke SL. Clonal Epstein-Barr virus in lymphoepithelioma-like carcinoma of the lung. Am J Surg Pathol 1993;17:678–82.

35. Razzuk MA, Urschel HC Jr, Albers JE, Martin JA, Paulson DL. Pulmonary giant cell carcinoma. Ann Thorac Surg 1976;21:540–5.

36. Saba SR, Espinoza CG, Richman AV, Azar HA. Carcinomas of the lung: an ultrastructural and immunocytochemical study. Am J Clin Pathol 1983;80:6–13.

37. Said JW. Immunohistochemistry of lung tumors. Lung Biol Health Dis 1990;44:635–51.

38. Schulte MA, Ramzy I, Greenberg SD. Immunocytochemical characterization of large cell carcinomas of the lung. Role, limitations and technical considerations. Acta Cytol 1991;35:175–9.

39. Shin MS, Jackson LK, Shelton RW Jr, Greene RE. Giant cell carcinoma of the lung. Chest 1986;89:366–9.

40. Sobin L, Yesner R. Histological typing of lung tumors. International Histological Classification of Tumors, Vol. 1. 2nd ed. Geneva: World Health Organization, 1981.

41. Wang NS, Seemayer TA, Ahmed MN, Knaack J. Giant cell carcinoma of the lung. A light and electron microscopic study. Hum Pathol 1976;7:3–16.

42. Yesner R. Large cell carcinoma of the lung. Semin Diagn Pathol 1985;2:255–69.

✧✧✧

16

ADENOSQUAMOUS CARCINOMA, CARCINOMAS ASSOCIATED WITH CYSTS, AND PAGET DISEASE OF THE BRONCHUS

ADENOSQUAMOUS CARCINOMA

Definition. According to World Health Organization (WHO) criteria, adenosquamous carcinomas contain both squamous carcinomatous and adenocarcinomatous components (3). While the proportions of each subtype required for a diagnosis are not defined, a minimum amount of 5 percent for one component, as suggested by Takamori et al. (5), is reasonable. For most investigators, the presence of acini, tubules, or papillary structures is indicative of glandular differentiation; the sole finding of mucin production with mucin stains is insufficient. The diagnosis of adenosquamous carcinoma should be restricted to carcinomas that show unequivocal squamous differentiation in the form of keratin or intercellular bridges, and unequivocal glandular differentiation in the form of acini, tubules, or papillary structures (1,3). Squamous cell carcinomas with mucin-positive cells can be labeled squamous carcinomas with mucin production. For cases with less than 5 percent of one component, the diagnosis should reflect the major component with a comment about focal glandular or squamous differentiation as appropriate. The definition of adenosquamous carcinoma is sampling-dependent, since the larger the sample, the greater the likelihood of finding both components in a given tumor. For this reason, studies of adenosquamous carcinomas are probably biased in favor of surgically resected tumors.

Small cell carcinoma with a squamous cell carcinoma component, an adenocarcinoma component, or both are recognized and discussed in chapter 14.

Clinical Features. The incidence of adenosquamous carcinoma has varied from .04 to 4.0 percent of lung carcinomas in different series; a figure of 2.0 percent is reasonable (1,2,4). In one review the incidence appeared to be on the rise (4).

In two recent large series of adenosquamous carcinoma (127 and 56 cases), the clinical and radiographic features were found to be similar to those of other nonsmall cell carcinomas (4,5). The majority of patients are smokers.

Pathologic Findings. Grossly, adenosquamous carcinomas are similar to other nonsmall cell carcinomas. They are more frequently peripheral (2), and they may contain a central scar.

Well-defined squamous cell carcinoma and adenocarcinoma are identified histologically (fig. 16-1) with each component comprising at least 5 percent of the tumor (1–5). Squamous carcinoma is as described in chapter 11, and adenocarcinoma is identified on the basis of acinar, papillary, and tubular structures as described in chapters 12 and 13. The two components may be separate and discrete or they may merge and mingle. The squamous or the glandular component may be dominant or they may be equal in proportion. The degree of differentiation of the two components is not interdependent, and all combinations of well-, moderate, and poorly differentiated squamous cell carcinoma have been associated with well-, moderate, and poorly differentiated adenocarcinoma. A component of large cell carcinoma may be present in addition to the other two components. Mucin may be demonstrable with mucin stains. Other histologic features, including stromal inflammation and secondary changes in the lung parenchyma, occur as described for squamous cell carcinoma and adenocarcinoma individually.

Yousem (6) described two cases of adenosquamous carcinoma with amyloid-like stroma (fig. 16-2). In addition to adenocarcinomatous and squamous carcinomatous differentiation, there was deposition of extracellular eosinophilic material that resembled amyloid. The cells in both components were positive with stains for keratin, epithelial membrane antigen (EMA), carcinoembryonic antigen (CEA), vimentin, and S-100 protein. Electron microscopy showed that the eosinophilic material was not amyloid and had features of basement membrane–like material and collagen. Yousem thought that these tumors were more closely aligned histogenetically to salivary gland type neoplasms.

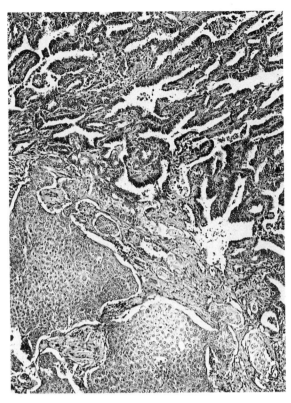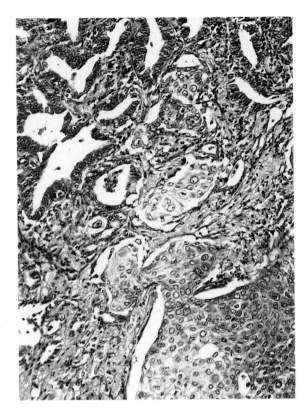

Figure 16-1
ADENOSQUAMOUS CARCINOMA
This tumor is composed of two well-defined components comprising well-differentiated adenocarcinoma growing in a bronchioloalveolar fashion and large nests of well-differentiated squamous carcinoma with squamous pearls.

Adenosquamous carcinomas may be graded. Each component should be graded separately, and the dominant component identified.

Immunohistochemical Findings. Results of immunohistochemical studies of adenosquamous carcinomas are similar to those described for each component separately. Generally, adenosquamous carcinomas are keratin, CEA, and EMA positive. Ishida et al. (2) noted that the glandular component may stain for secretory component or lactoferrin.

Ultrastructural Findings. The ultrastructural features are the same as for squamous carcinoma and adenocarcinoma individually. Adenosquamous carcinomas are defined on the basis of light microscopy, and finding adenosquamous features in a tumor ultrastructurally (a not uncommon finding in a variety of lung carcinomas) does not confirm a diagnosis of adenosquamous carcinoma.

Differential Diagnosis. The differential diagnosis of adenosquamous carcinoma includes squamous cell carcinoma or adenocarcinoma with metaplastic epithelial changes and high-grade mucoepidermoid carcinoma.

Any carcinoma of the lung may infiltrate interstitially or subepithelially in airspaces and surround small acinar structures lined by reactive type 2 cells. These acinar structures may be misinterpreted as adenocarcinomatous differentiation and lead to an overdiagnosis of adenosquamous carcinoma. Examples of such cases are illustrated in figures 8-3, 11-3, and 15-11. Similarly, adenocarcinoma may be associated with squamous metaplasia in areas of necrosis, inflammation, or scarring.

High-grade mucoepidermoid carcinomas (see chapter 6) may be difficult to distinguish from adenosquamous carcinomas with poorly differentiated components, but generally the two are

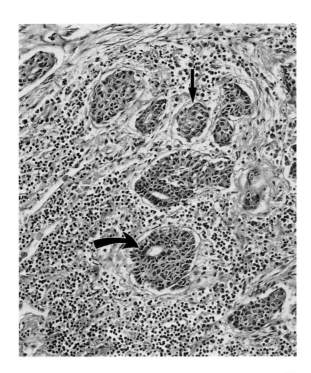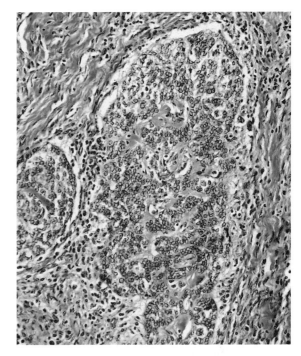

Figure 16-2
ADENOSQUAMOUS CARCINOMA WITH AMYLOID-LIKE STROMA
Left: Cell nests showing squamous (arrow) and glandular features (curved arrow) are apparent.
Right: Some fields showed amyloid-like stroma associated with the tumor cells. (Courtesy of Dr. S. A. Yousem, Pittsburgh, PA.)

separable. According to the criteria outlined by Yousem and Hochholzer (7), a high-grade mucoepidermoid carcinoma is an exophytic tumor in the proximal bronchial tree that lacks carcinoma in situ in the surface epithelium; is composed of a random mixture of sheet-like and glandular cells lacking individual cell keratinization and squamous pearl formation; and shows areas of low-grade mucoepidermoid carcinoma. Most adenosquamous carcinomas are peripheral, and all produce keratin or have intercellular bridges. In mucoepidermoid carcinomas, glandular differentiation usually manifests as scattered goblet cells rather than as tubular, acinar, or papillary growth patterns.

Spread. The spread of adenosquamous carcinoma of the lung is similar to other nonsmall cell carcinomas (see chapter 8).

Staging and Prognosis. The staging of adenosquamous carcinoma is similar to that for other nonsmall cell carcinomas and is described in chapter 8. Adenosquamous carcinomas are sufficiently rare that the number studied is limited, and the data is probably biased toward resected tumors (i.e., more likely to be low stage than lung carcinoma in general). Nevertheless, Sridhar et al. (4) noted a particularly poor prognosis in cases with regional or distant metastases; however, they found a 5-year survival rate after resection of 62.5 percent for those with localized disease. Ishida et al. (2) reported a 35 percent 5-year survival rate, similar to other resected nonsmall cell carcinomas. In a study of 56 cases, Takamori et al. (5) found that the prognosis was poorer than for adenocarcinoma or squamous carcinoma in stages I and II and thought that the histologic subtype was an independent unfavorable prognostic determinant. According to the Surveillance Epidemiology End Results (SEER) data for 1978-1986, the 5-year relative survival rate for adenosquamous carcinoma was 21.6 percent (see fig. 8-16).

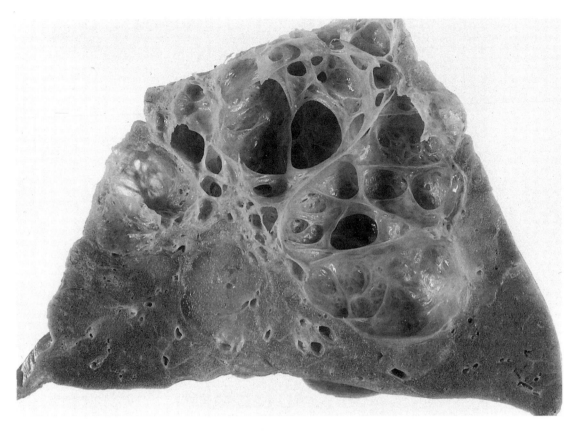

Figure 16-3
BRONCHIOLOALVEOLAR CARCINOMA COMPLICATING A LUNG CYST
This gross photograph shows a multiloculated cyst (upper portion), which had been present for at least 12 years, involving much of the lobectomy specimen. There is a consolidated focus with a mucoid appearance representing the bronchioloalveolar carcinoma. (Courtesy of Dr. G. S. Sterrett, Nedlands, Western Australia.)

CARCINOMAS ASSOCIATED WITH LUNG CYSTS

There have been a number of reports over the years describing carcinomas complicating cystic disease of the lungs. In older reports it was not always clear what the underlying cystic disease was; the term "congenital cystic emphysema" was often used (12). Some of these were probably cystic adenomatoid malformations (see chapter 2) complicated by carcinoma. Recent reports (9, 11,14–16) confirm the older literature (8,10, 12,13) and show a definite association of lung cysts and congenital cystic adenomatoid malformations with the development of carcinoma.

Most carcinomas complicating cystic disease of the lung are mucinous bronchioloalveolar carcinomas (figs. 16-3–16-5); however, all subtypes of lung carcinoma have been reported (14,16). The tumors are generally recognized when an individ-

ual known to have a lung cyst or cystic disease develops new symptoms or there is a radiographic change in the lesion. Many of the cases are seen in relatively young individuals compared to other patients with lung carcinoma; nonsmokers, as well as smokers, may be affected.

Prichard et al. (14) described two women with longstanding cysts (9 and 12 years) who developed mucinous bronchioloalveolar carcinomas. One had a solitary cyst, the other had multiple cysts in one lobe. Hurley et al. (11) described a similar case.

Sheffield et al. (15) reported an 18-year-old man with mucinous bronchioloalveolar carcinoma adjacent to a congenital cystic adenomatoid malformation (CCAM). They compared the case with two CCAMs with mucinous cells in infants and found the mucinous cells to be similar, and concluded that the mucinous epithelium may be premalignant.

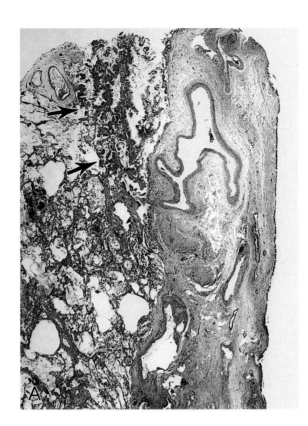

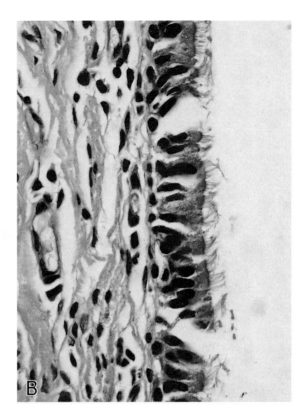

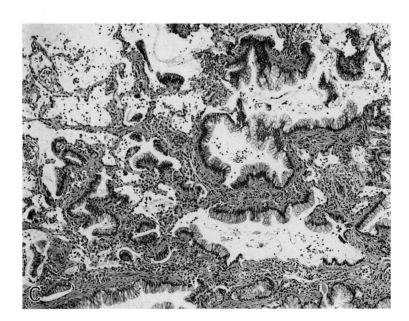

Figure 16-4

BRONCHIOLOALVEOLAR CARCINOMA COMPLICATING A LONGSTANDING LUNG CYST

The specimen shows the fibrovascular cyst wall (A) lined in part by ciliated pseudostratified columnar epithelium (B). Lung tissue adjacent to the cyst (A, arrows and C) shows a well-differentiated mucinous bronchioloalveolar carcinoma growing along intact alveolar walls.

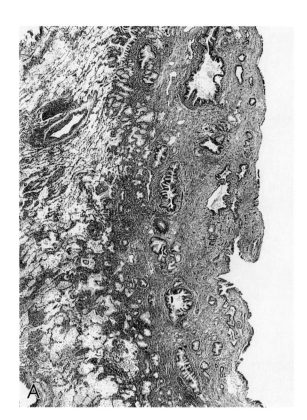

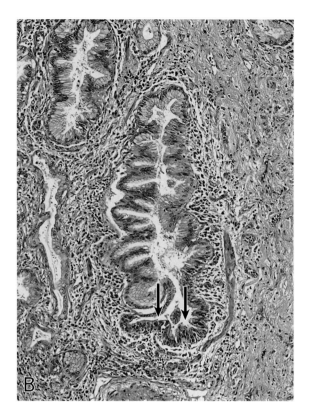

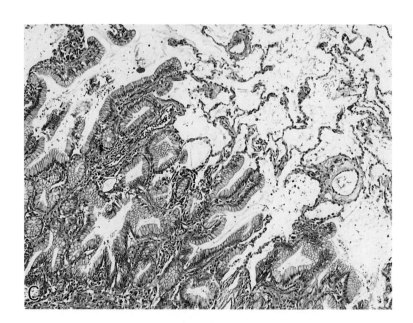

Figure 16-5
BRONCHIOLOALVEOLAR CARCINOMA COMPLICATING A LONGSTANDING LUNG CYST

In comparison with the case illustrated in figure 16-4, this lesion shows a much greater degree of proliferation of mucinous epithelium within the cyst wall (A) and the cyst lining was entirely replaced by mucinous epithelium. Many glandular structures are present in the cyst wall; some are preexisting bronchioles embedded in the cyst wall (B) which show partial replacement of the mucosa by mucinous epithelium with only focal residual ciliated epithelium (arrows). The lung tissue away from the cyst wall shows typical well-differentiated mucinous bronchioloalveolar carcinoma growing along intact alveolar walls (C).

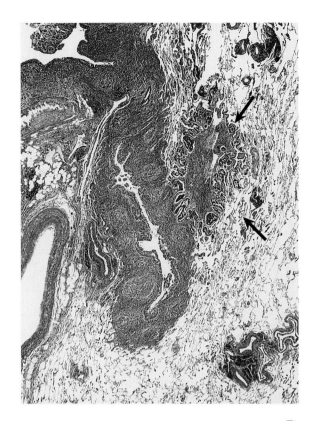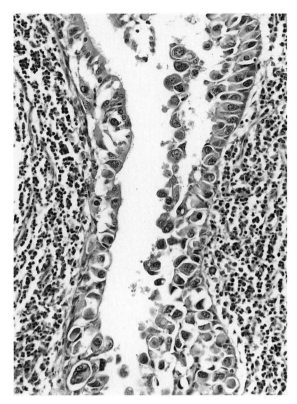

Figure 16-6
PAGETOID INFILTRATION OF ADENOCARCINOMA IN THE BRONCHIAL EPITHELIUM
Left: There is a small focus of moderately differentiated adenocarcinoma involving alveolar structures (arrows). An adjacent airway shows marked inflammation in the wall with germinal centers, and extensive pagetoid spread of carcinoma cells.
Right: Detail of bronchial epithelium. Focally, the residual ciliated pseudostratified epithelium can be identified (upper left). (Courtesy of Dr. M. Higashiyama, Osaka, Japan.)

Benjamin and Cahill (9) described a 19-year-old man who developed a mucinous bronchioloalveolar carcinoma in the left lower lobe after having had a CCAM resected from the left upper lobe in infancy.

Usui (16) described a minute squamous carcinoma in the wall of a congenital lung cyst. These authors and others (11) have stressed aggressive evaluation of patients with congenital cysts who have new symptoms or changes in the radiographic characteristics of the cyst(s).

PAGETOID SPREAD OF ADENO-CARCINOMA IN THE BRONCHUS

Pagetoid spread of carcinoma cells in the small and large airways is an occasional incidental histologic finding in biopsies and resection specimens of lung carcinoma. It is rarely more than an incidental finding.

Higashiyama et al. (17) described a case of adenocarcinoma of the lung with prominent pagetoid spread of the tumor cells in airway epithelium as "extramammary Paget disease of the bronchial epithelium" (fig. 16-6). The cells infiltrating the bronchial epithelium showed a staining pattern similar to Paget disease at other sites: periodic acid–Schiff (PAS) positive, Alcian blue (pH 2.5) positive, CEA positive, neuron-specific enolase (NSE) negative, and S-100 protein negative. The case described was associated with an adenocarcinoma in the adjacent lung tissue, and the authors concluded that pagetoid change was a histologic pattern that could be seen with adenocarcinoma of the lung.

REFERENCES

Adenosquamous Carcinoma

1. Fitzgibbons PL, Kern WH. Adenosquamous carcinoma of the lung: a clinical and pathologic study of seven cases. Hum Pathol 1985;16:463–6.
2. Ishida T, Kaneko S, Yokoyama H, Inoue T, Sugio K, Sugimachi K. Adenosquamous carcinoma of the lung. Clinicopathologic and immunohistochemical features. Am J Clin Pathol 1992;97:678–85.
3. Sobin L, Yesner R. Histological typing of lung tumors. International Histological Classification of Tumors, Vol 1. 2nd ed. Geneva: World Health Organization, 1981.
4. Sridhar KS, Bounassi MJ, Raub W Jr, Richman SP. Clinical features of adenosquamous lung carcinoma in 127 patients. Am Rev Respir Dis 1990;142:19–23.
5. Takamori S, Noguchi M, Morinaga S. Clinicopathologic characteristics of adenosquamous carcinoma of the lung. Cancer 1991;6:649–54.
6. Yousem SA. Pulmonary adenosquamous carcinomas with amyloid-like stroma. Mod Pathol 1989;2:420–6.
7. _____, Hochholzer L. Mucoepidermoid tumors of the lung. Cancer 1987;60:1346–52.

Carcinoma Associated with Lung Cysts

8. Bauer S. Carcinoma arising in a congenital lung cyst. Chest 1961;40:552–5.
9. Benjamin DR, Cahill JL. Bronchioloalveolar carcinoma of the lung and congenital cystic adenomatoid malformation. Am J Clin Pathol 1991;95:889–92.
10. Huntington HW, Poppe JK, Goodman MJ. Carcinoma arising in a congenital cyst of the lung. Chest 1963;44:329–32.
11. Hurley P, Corbishley C, Pepper J. Bronchioloalveolar carcinoma arising in longstanding lung cysts [Letter]. Thorax 1985;40:960.
12. Korol E. The correlation of carcinoma and congenital cystic emphysema of the lungs. Chest 1953;23:403–11.
13. Larkin JC, Phillips S. Carcinoma complicating cyst of lung. Chest 1955;27:453–7.
14. Prichard MG, Brown PJ, Sterrett GF. Bronchioloalveolar carcinoma arising in longstanding lung cysts. Thorax 1984;39:545–9.
15. Sheffield EA, Addis BJ, Corrin B, McCabe MM. Epithelial hyperplasia and malignant change in congenital lung cysts. J Clin Pathol 1987;40:612–4.
16. Usui Y, Takabe K, Takayama S, Miura H, Kimula Y. Minute squamous cell carcinoma arising in the wall of a congenital lung cyst. Chest 1991;99:235–6.

Paget Disease

17. Higashiyama M, Doi O, Kodama K, Tateishi R, Kurokawa E. Extramammary Paget's disease of the bronchial epithelium. Arch Pathol Lab Med 1991;115:185–8.

17
CARCINOID AND OTHER NEUROENDOCRINE TUMORS

UNIFYING CONCEPT OF PULMONARY NEUROENDOCRINE TUMORS

Neuroendocrine Cells

Neuroendocrine cells, also known as *Kulchitsky cells*, named after the Russian histologist, Nicholas Kulchitsky (1856-1925), are normally present within the bronchial and bronchiolar respiratory epithelium. In the human fetus and neonate they are numerous (43), but are rare in adults (72). In rabbits they have been observed in the epithelium of respiratory bronchioles, alveolar ducts, and alveoli (6,72). Neuroendocrine cells are nonciliated, cylindrical cells situated in the basal aspect of the mucosa; rarely, cytoplasmic processes reach the airway lumen (72). These cells have a clear cytoplasm with an eosinophilic hue; ovoid nuclei with finely granular, homogeneous chromatin; and a small nucleolus (63).

Ultrastructurally, neuroendocrine cells contain electron-dense neurosecretory granules with a dense core surrounded by a light halo and averaging 1400 to 1500 Å in diameter (6,72). The cytoplasm may also contain lipofuscin granules, bundles of thick filaments (about 100 Å in diameter), and microtubules (6,72). Prominent pseudopod-like cytoplasmic processes often contain neurosecretory granules and pinocytotic vesicles (6). These processes may be knob shaped and resemble synapses or endorgans of nonmyelinated nerves (6). Although light microscopic studies by Frölich (30) and Lauweryns (64) suggested attachments between nerves and neuroendocrine cells, this was not confirmed ultrastructurally by Bensch (6). Not only do neuroendocrine cells have neuroendocrine features when examined ultrastructurally, but they also react with argyrophilic stains (97) and neuroendocrine immunohistochemical markers. In bronchial epithelium showing dysplastic changes, neuroendocrine cells have fewer secretory granules and smaller Golgi vesicles than in normal mucosa (41). Increased numbers of neuroendocrine cells in the epithelium of the bronchial or bronchiolar mucosa can result in either linear hyperplasia, in which solitary neuroendocrine cells form continuous rows, or neuroendocrine bodies, which consist of clusters of neuroendocrine cells (40).

Many consider the Kulchitsky cell to be the cell of origin for most neuroendocrine tumors of the lung (5,40,72). Neuroendocrine granules and neuroendocrine immunohistochemical markers can be demonstrated ultrastructurally in neuroendocrine cells in the bronchial mucosa as well as in virtually all of the neuroendocrine tumors listed in Table 17-1 (5,35,72). This concept impacts not only on histogenesis, but also on classification. Pulmonary neuroendocrine tumors are a group of distinct lesions with a spectrum of differentiation and clinical behavior ranging from benign to high-grade malignant.

The amine precursor uptake and decarboxylation (APUD) concept, which proposed that all neuroendocrine cells were derived embryologically from the neural crest, was once popular. Currently, the dispersed neuroendocrine system (DNS) theory is accepted. According to this concept, neuroendocrine cells in different sites of the body are linked by a common neuroendocrine phenotype, originating from pluripotent cells that differentiate locally under the control of factors unique to a specific site or organ (81).

Although some considered Kulchitsky cells to be the cell of origin for both carcinoid tumorlets and small cell carcinoma (11), there is no established clinical association between these tumors or with other bronchogenic carcinomas. Although early studies speculated that carcinoid tumorlets might represent early or in situ small cell carcinoma (84), the simultaneous occurrence of these two lesions is rare.

Classification

The classification of pulmonary neuroendocrine tumors of the lung is complex and potentially confusing. For many years, carcinoid tumor and small cell lung carcinoma were the only two recognized types. In 1972, Arrigoni et al. (2) proposed that bronchial carcinoids be separated into typical and atypical variants, with the latter having more malignant histologic characteristics and clinical behavior. Since that

Table 17-1

**TERMINOLOGY FOR PULMONARY TUMORS
WITH NEUROENDOCRINE DIFFERENTIATION***

Spectrum of Pulmonary Neuroendocrine Lesions	Other Published Terminology
I. Common neoplasms with a neuroendocrine light microscopic appearance	I. Common primary neuroendocrine neoplasms
A. Typical carcinoid	A. Mature carcinoid, Kulchitsky cell carcinoma-I
B. Atypical carcinoid	B. Malignant carcinoid, well-differentiated neuroendocrine carcinoma, Kulchitsky cell carcinoma-II, peripheral small cell carcinoma resembling carcinoid tumor
C. Large cell neuroendocrine carcinoma (LCNEC) 1. LCNEC (if confirmed by immunohistochemistry or electron microscopy) 2. Poorly differentiated carcinoma, probably LCNEC (if special studies not available)	C. Neuroendocrine carcinoma of intermediate cell type, nonsmall cell carcinoma with neuroendocrine features
D. Small cell lung carcinoma 1. Pure small cell carcinoma 2. Mixed small cell/large cell carcinoma 3. Combined small cell carcinoma	D. Small cell undifferentiated carcinoma, small cell neuroendocrine carcinoma, Kulchitsky cell carcinoma-III, oat cell carcinoma, neuroendocrine carcinoma of small cell type
II. Nonsmall cell lung carcinoma with neuroendocrine features (NSCLC-NE) (adenocarcinoma, squamous cell carcinoma or large cell carcinoma with neuroendocrine features not seen by light microscopy but detected by immunohistochemistry or ultrastructurally)	II. Atypical endocrine tumor Large cell neuroendocrine tumor, neuroendocrine differentiation in poorly differentiated carcinomas
III. Uncommon primary neuroendocrine neoplasms	
A. Amphicrine neoplasms	
B. Blastomas with focal neuroendocrine differentiation	
C. Primitive neuroepithelial tumors	
D. Neuroendocrine carcinoma with anemone features	
E. Primary pulmonary paraganglioma	

*Modified from reference 100.

time, a number of studies have confirmed the importance of recognizing atypical carcinoid as a distinct entity (100). Although Arrigoni et al. did not specifically propose a three-category classification system, many pathologists who adhere to his concept consider neuroendocrine lung tumors to encompass three categories: typical carcinoid, atypical carcinoid, and small cell carcinoma.

Over the past two decades, a broader spectrum of pulmonary neuroendocrine neoplasia has been recognized since occasional neuroendocrine lung tumors do not fit into one of these three categories. A variety of additional categories have been proposed, including large cell neuroendocrine tumor, large cell neuroendocrine carcinoma, neuroendocrine carcinoma of intermediate differentiation, peripheral small cell carcinoma of the lung resembling carcinoid

tumor, and nonsmall cell carcinoma with neuroendocrine features (Table 17-1). The diversity of terminology and inconsistent histopathologic criteria are confusing for pathologists trying to understand how to classify neuroendocrine lung tumors, especially the more malignant types.

A recent review of a series of pulmonary neuroendocrine tumors at the National Cancer Institute (100) revealed a spectrum of neuroendocrine tumors with high and low histologic grades that fall between the traditional criteria for typical carcinoid and small cell carcinoma. Since most pathologists using Arrigoni's criteria use a three-category scheme, the term atypical carcinoid has come to include a heterogeneous group of tumors. A review of the literature on atypical carcinoid tumors reveals the diversity of tumors often grouped into this category.

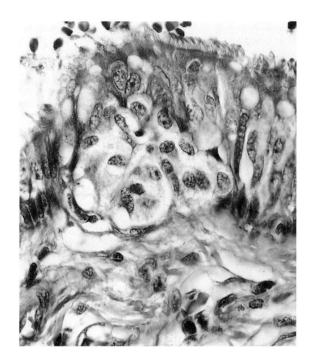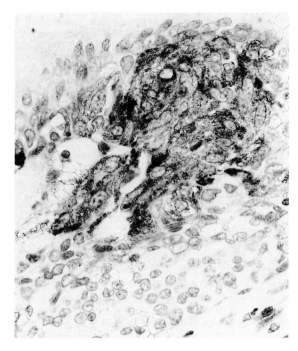

Figure 17-1
NEUROENDOCRINE BODY
Left: This cluster of neuroendocrine cells is situated mostly at the base of the bronchiolar mucosa. The cells of this neuroendocrine body do not reach the surface of the epithelium. The cells closely resemble those seen in carcinoid tumors, having a moderate amount of eosinophilic cytoplasm and finely granular nuclear chromatin.
Right: This neuroendocrine body stains strongly for chromogranin.

The traditional three-category histologic classification system can be expanded to include a fourth category: large cell neuroendocrine carcinoma (Table 17-1). As discussed, neuroendocrine lung tumors that morphologically fall between criteria for typical carcinoid and small cell carcinoma are called atypical carcinoid in the three-category scheme. However, these tumors seem to be too heterogeneous to be grouped into one category. As a result, pathologists are sometimes faced with classifying malignant neuroendocrine tumors as either atypical carcinoid or small cell carcinoma when criteria are not met for either. Although a four-category classification scheme has been proposed, its use has been limited. Large cell neuroendocrine carcinoma represents a high histologic grade neuroendocrine carcinoma, while Arrigoni's criteria for atypical carcinoid preserves the low histologic grade that he originally defined. As discussed in chapter 14, large cell neuroendocrine carcinoma should be distinguished from large cell carcinoma with neuroendocrine features.

Neuroendocrine differentiation can be seen by electron microscopy or immunohistochemistry in 10 to 20 percent of nonsmall cell carcinomas that do not show morphologic neuroendocrine features (NSCC-NE) (45,69,109). Evidence is accumulating suggesting that NSCC-NE may be responsive to small cell carcinoma chemotherapy regimens (42,68), and that expression of neuroendocrine markers may be an unfavorable prognostic factor (7,55).

Neuroendocrine Body

Neuroendocrine bodies were illustrated by Frölich in 1949 (30) in his description of neuroendocrine cells ("helle zelle" or clear cells) in the bronchiolar mucosa. Feyrter (28) showed that these cells were argyrophilic. However, not until 1972 did Lauweryns (64) describe the neuroendocrine body in human infants. Neuroendocrine bodies consist of a cluster of 4 to 10 neuroendocrine cells (fig. 17-1, left). On well-oriented sections, they can extend from the subepithelial basement membrane to the airway lumens (63). They are found not only in the epithelium of bronchi and bronchioles, but also in alveoli (63). Neuroendocrine bodies stain with neuroendocrine immunohistochemical markers (fig. 17-1, right) (66,101). They are increased in the lungs of patients with hypertensive pulmonary vascular disease (39,49) and infants with bronchopulmonary dysplasia (53); and reduced in infants with hyaline membrane disease (53).

The function of neuroendocrine bodies is not known. A chemoreceptor or tactile receptor function has been proposed (6,62,64). Since the neuroendocrine body contacts the airway lumens and capillaries, it has been suggested that they may play a role in vasoconstriction during hypoxia. They have also been shown to proliferate following exposure of animal lungs to nitroso compounds, particularly dinitrosoamine (56).

CARCINOID TUMORLET

Definition. Carcinoid tumorlets consist of small proliferations of neuroendocrine cells and are typically incidental pathologic findings of no clinical significance. As radiologic imaging techniques have become more sophisticated and smaller pulmonary nodules detected, an increasing number of carcinoid tumorlets are found as incidental radiographic findings. Carcinoid tumorlets have also been called *peripheral adenomas, atypical hyperplasia of bronchiolar epithelium, minute peripheral pulmonary tumors, multicentric carcinomas, microscopic oat cell carcinomas, early bronchogenic carcinomas, bronchiolargenic carcinomas, multiple microscopic bronchiolar carcinomas, basal cell carcinomas, carcinoid atypical proliferations,* and *pulmonary tumorlets* (11,17,86).

Incidence and Histogenesis. The incidence of carcinoid tumorlets is difficult to determine. They were observed in 20 percent of bronchiectatic surgical lung specimens in one study in which serial sections were performed with a deliberate search for tumorlets (19). Carcinoid tumorlets were found in 17 of 7800 or 0.22 percent of autopsies at one institution (17), and in 2 of 1400 or 0.1 percent of autopsies in another study (108). Often they are found in lung specimens showing bronchiectasis (19,84,108), interstitial fibrosis (89), chronic abscesses (108), or

tuberculosis (70): in surgically resected lung specimens, tumorlets were found in 2.1 percent of cases of bronchiectasis, 0.17 percent of cases of tuberculosis, and 5 percent of abscessed lungs (108). In one study (19), carcinoid tumorlets were found in 32.1 percent of bronchiectatic specimens removed from patients over 20 years of age and 6 percent of similar specimens from patients under 20 years of age. They have also been reported in a case of diffuse panbronchiolitis (105). Restrictive and obstructive lung disease has been reported in a patient with multiple peripheral carcinoids and tumorlets (73). It has been suggested that proliferation of bronchiolar neuroendocrine cells and tumorlets may cause airway injury and destructive disease (1).

On the basis of light and electron microscopic observations, carcinoid tumorlets have been shown to originate from the same bronchial Kulchitsky cells that are found in carcinoid tumors (11,17,86,99). The neuroendocrine nature of these cells can also be demonstrated by positive reactivity with argyrophil stains (35) and immunohistochemical stains such as chromogranin and synaptophysin (38).

Clinical Features. Carcinoid tumorlets are typically incidental microscopic findings in surgical or autopsy specimens and do not cause symptoms. One patient with multiple, bilateral tumorlets presented with Cushing syndrome due to the ectopic atypical corticotropin (ACTH) syndrome (89). They are found most often in adults, rarely in children, and more commonly in women (19). With improved radiographic imaging techniques, they present on rare occasion as a coin lesion (85).

Lymph node metastases have been reported in several cases (20,21,89,94), sometimes in the setting of multiple tumorlets (21). Other putative cases of carcinoid tumorlets with lymph node metastases are actually carcinoid tumors (48).

Gross Findings. Traditionally, carcinoid tumorlets have been incidental microscopic findings and there is little information available about the gross pathology of these lesions. However, careful examination of the gross specimen may reveal millimeter-sized grey-tan nodules. The size of carcinoid tumorlets has been defined as "not more than 3 or 4 mm" (14). However, some reported "tumorlets" have included proliferations of neuroendocrine cells measuring up to about 1.5 cm (48).

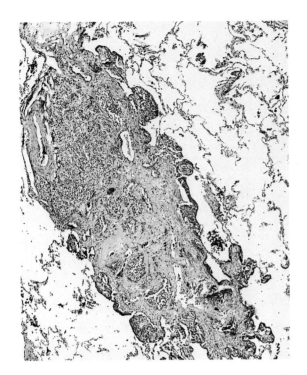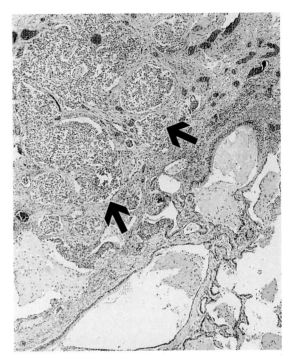

Figure 17-2
CARCINOID TUMORLET
Left: There is a small nodular proliferation of neuroendocrine cells with a dense fibrous stroma.
Right: This tumorlet (arrows) is associated with endstage fibrosis characterized by cystic remodelling of the lung architecture.

We regard a neuroendocrine lesion larger than 0.5 cm to be a carcinoid tumor. This size distinction is somewhat arbitrary, since these small nodules probably represent a continuum of neuroendocrine cell proliferation.

According to Churg and Warnock (17), approximately one third of carcinoid tumorlets occur in association with fibrotic lung disease; in the other cases, the lungs show little or no scarring. Thus, carcinoid tumorlets may be difficult to discern by gross examination due to the associated fibrotic and inflammatory changes associated with bronchiectasis, interstitial fibrosis, or abscesses.

Histologic Findings. Carcinoid tumorlets are usually peripherally situated in the lung, beneath or within the pleura or adjacent to bronchioles (84). They may be found in relatively normal lung parenchyma (fig. 17-2, left) or in the setting of interstitial fibrosis (fig. 17-2, right) or bronchiectasis. Rarely, they form a polypoid plug within the lumen of bronchioles (fig. 17-3) (84). The cells are often embedded in a fibrotic stroma which may resemble a scar (fig. 17-2, left). Although often circumscribed, the edge of the

tumorlets may be ill-defined, resulting in an infiltrative appearance. The neuroendocrine cells may spill over into alveolar spaces (figs. 17-4, 17-5). Carcinoid tumorlets may be multifocal and resemble metastatic malignancy, especially in a patient with a known primary cancer.

The proliferating cells in carcinoid tumorlets are uniform in appearance, with a moderate amount of eosinophilic cytoplasm (fig. 17-6); occasionally the cytoplasm is clear (fig. 17-4). The nuclei have finely granular chromatin. The cells are often round or oval, but they may also be spindle shaped.

Differential Diagnosis. Carcinoid tumorlets must be distinguished from neuroendocrine cell hyperplasia (multiple neuroendocrine bodies), typical carcinoid, bronchiolar epithelial hyperplasia or metaplasia associated with interstitial fibrosis, minute pulmonary meningothelial-like nodules (so-called chemodectomas), lymphangitic carcinoma, and small cell carcinoma.

Neuroendocrine cell hyperplasia consists of multiple neuroendocrine cells and/or bodies which proliferate within the bronchial or bronchiolar

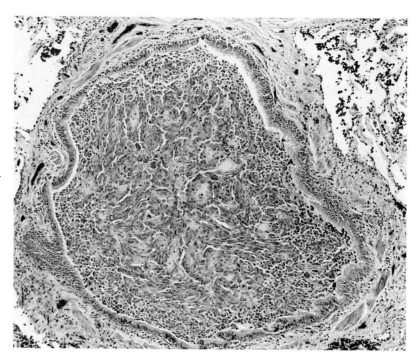

Figure 17-3
CARCINOID TUMORLET
The tumorlet shows intrabronchiolar growth.

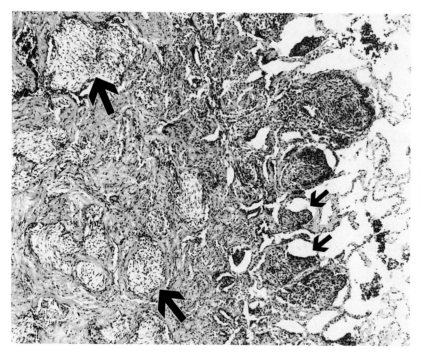

Figure 17-4
CARCINOID TUMORLET
Many of the neuroendocrine cells in the center of this tumorlet (large arrows) have clear cytoplasm. At the periphery, the tumor cells protrude into the alveolar spaces in a polypoid fashion (small arrows).

epithelium. The hyperplasia may accompany carcinoid tumorlets, especially when they are multiple. Carcinoid tumorlets, however, form discrete nodular proliferations.

Distinguishing a carcinoid tumorlet from typical carcinoid tumor may be difficult. It has been proposed that tumorlets never exceed 3 to 4 mm in greatest dimension (14), however, others accept as tumorlets lesions up to about 1.0 cm in size. With careful examination of gross specimens and improved radiographic techniques, some of these lesions may be discovered prior to

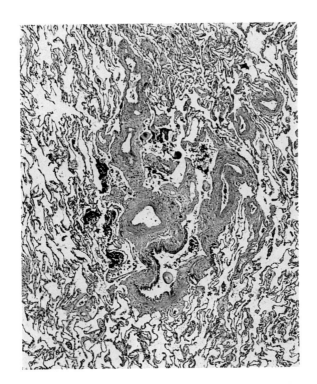
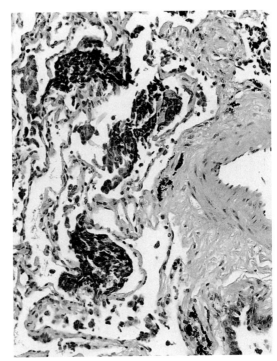

Figure 17-5
CARCINOID TUMORLET

Left: The tumorlet consists of clusters of cells scattered in the peribronchiolar and perivascular alveolar spaces and interstitium.

Right: At higher power the cells are crushed. This led to concern for possible small cell carcinoma or metastatic carcinoma. The cells stained strongly with chromogranin.

Figure 17-6
CARCINOID TUMORLET

These neuroendocrine cells are arranged in organoid nests separated by a fibrous stroma. The cells have a moderate amount of eosinophilic cytoplasm and uniform nuclei.

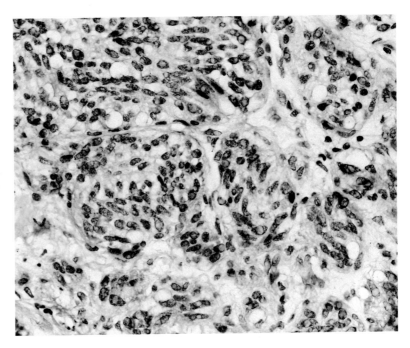

microscopic examination. Recognizing that any size cut-off is arbitrary, we suggest using 0.5 cm to distinguish between a tumorlet and a carcinoid tumor.

Bronchiolar epithelial hyperplasia/metaplasia associated with scarring can be mistaken for a carcinoid tumor. Although carcinoid tumorlets can be seen in this setting, the proliferating epithelium in these cases represents pseudostratified bronchiolar epithelium, sometimes with squamous metaplasia, rather than neuroendocrine cells.

Minute pulmonary chemodectomas have a distinct "zellenballen" pattern and are interstitial lesions that differ from carcinoid tumorlets, which do not have as striking a swirling nesting pattern and may contact air spaces directly. Chemodectomas characteristically are situated around veins while tumorlets are frequently around bronchioles. Immunohistochemically and ultrastructurally, chemodectomas lack neuroendocrine features and show characteristics of meningothelial cells (see chapter 23).

Tumorlets should also be distinguished from metastatic carcinoma or lymphangitic carcinomatosis, especially if they are found in tumor resection specimens.

TYPICAL AND ATYPICAL CARCINOID TUMORS

Definition. Carcinoid tumors are low-grade malignant neoplasms of neuroendocrine cells and comprise 1 to 2 percent of all lung tumors (14). They are divided into typical and atypical subtypes, with the latter possessing more malignant histologic and clinical features (2).

Clinical Features. Carcinoid tumors are indolent: 51 percent of patients are asymptomatic at presentation and 9 percent of cases are incidental findings at surgery or autopsy (71). The most common pulmonary manifestations include hemoptysis in 18 percent, postobstructive pneumonitis in 17 percent, and dyspnea in 2 percent of patients (71). The symptoms vary depending on whether the tumor is situated in the center, middle, or periphery of the lung. Central carcinoids tend to cause obstructive pneumonitis and hemoptysis while peripheral carcinoids are discovered incidentally on a routine chest X ray in an asymptomatic patient (12).

Bronchial carcinoids occur with equal frequency in men and women (24,65,71,95). The mean age of patients is 55 years, with a range up to 82 years (71). Bronchial carcinoids occur in childhood and adolescence and are the most common lung tumor of childhood (59).

A variety of paraneoplastic syndromes occur with carcinoid tumors, including carcinoid syndrome (71), Cushing syndrome (80), and acromegaly. Bronchial carcinoids occasionally occur in patients with multiple neuroendocrine neoplasia (MEN), type I (26). Carcinoid syndrome has been reported in 2 to 7 percent of bronchial carcinoids and most (86 percent) are associated with liver metastases (71). Cushing syndrome is usually due to ectopic production of ACTH, but it can also occur with ectopic corticotropin-releasing hormone (CRH) production (112). Rarely, a paraneoplastic syndrome consisting of central nervous system symptoms (51), paraneoplastic encephalomyelitis (102), and subacute dysautonomia (102) is seen in pulmonary carcinoid patients.

Atypical carcinoid represented 11 to 24 percent of pulmonary carcinoid tumors in several large single institutional series (2,71). Other terms applied to atypical carcinoid are listed in Table 17-2.

Gross Findings. Carcinoid tumors are frequently subdivided into central and peripheral tumors. Sixteen to 40 percent are peripheral (71, 77,95); the remainder are central. A review of computerized tomography (CT) studies shows, however, that about one third of carcinoid tumors are located centrally, one third peripherally, and one third in the mid-portion of the lung (100). Thus the location of carcinoids may be more evenly distributed in the lung than the broad categories of central and peripheral imply. Although there does not appear to be any significant predilection for the right or left lung, for unknown reasons, a disproportionate number of carcinoid tumors occur in the periphery of the right middle lobe (71,87).

Central carcinoids frequently have a large endobronchial component with a fleshy, smooth, polypoid mass protruding into the bronchial lumen (fig. 17-7A,B). Endobronchial growth is more common in typical than atypical carcinoid (74). A variable amount of tumor may infiltrate beyond the cartilage plates into the surrounding lung parenchyma. The cut surface may appear tan-yellow or red depending on the extent of

Table 17-2
TYPICAL AND ATYPICAL CARCINOID: DISTINGUISHING FEATURES

Histologic or Clinical Features	Typical Carcinoid	Atypical Carcinoid
Histologic patterns: organoid, trabecular, palisading, and spindle cell	Characteristic	Characteristic
Mitoses	Absent or rare	Increased, up to 10 per 10 high-power fields
Necrosis	Uncharacteristic	Characteristic, usually focal or punctate
Nuclear pleomorphism, hyperchromatism	Usually absent, not sufficient by itself for diagnosis of atypical carcinoid	Often present
Regional lymph node metastases at presentation	5-15%	40-48%
Distant metastases at presentation	Rare	20%
Disease-free survival at 5 years	100%	69%
Disease-free survival at 10 years	87%	52%

vascularity. Necrosis or extensive hemorrhage are characteristic of atypical carcinoid. A specimen X ray may highlight bone in an extensively ossified lesion (fig. 17-7C). The lung parenchyma distal to endobronchial carcinoids may show changes due to postobstructive pneumonia (fig. 17-7A).

Peripheral carcinoids are situated in the subpleural parenchyma and are often not anatomically related to a bronchus (fig. 17-7D). They are circumscribed, but not encapsulated, nodules which may infiltrate into the surrounding parenchyma. Peripheral carcinoids may be multiple and associated with multiple tumorlets (35,87).

Central carcinoids tend to be larger than peripheral tumors, with a mean diameter of 3.1 cm (range, 0.5 to 10 cm) versus 2.4 cm (range, 0.5 to 6 cm) and atypical carcinoids are larger than typical ones, with a mean diameter of 3.6 cm compared to 2.3 cm (71).

Histologic Findings. Both typical and atypical carcinoids are characterized histologically by an organoid growth pattern and uniform cytologic features consisting of moderate eosinophilic, finely granular cytoplasm and nuclei possessing a finely granular chromatin pattern (fig. 17-8). Nucleoli are inconspicuous in most typical carcinoids, but may be more prominent in atypical carcinoids (fig. 17-9). The chromatin may be somewhat coarse in atypical carcinoids.

A variety of histologic patterns occur in both atypical and typical carcinoids including spindle cell (fig. 17-9), trabecular (fig. 17-10A), palisading (fig. 17-10B), glandular (fig. 17-10B), follicular (fig. 17-10C), rosette-like, papillary (fig. 17-11), and sclerosing papillary patterns (12,87, 100). These histologic patterns are frequently focal and most tumors exhibit more than one pattern. The majority of tumors with spindle cell histology are peripheral carcinoids (87). Eosinophilic hyaline globules have been described in an atypical carcinoid associated with marked alpha-fetoprotein production (76).

A diffusely infiltrating pattern has been described (92). In such cases, metastases from another site such as the thyroid should be excluded since metastatic medullary carcinoma can present as multifocal bronchial carcinoid (18). A case reported as medullary carcinoma of the lung with amyloid stroma probably represents a form of pulmonary carcinoid tumor (37).

The cells of pulmonary carcinoid tumors may have oncocytic (fig. 17-12, left), acinic cell-like, signet-ring, mucin-producing, or melanocytic features (fig. 17-13) (32,100). They may appear ciliated ultrastructurally, or have type 2 pneumocyte features (100). There may be a stromal deposition of amyloid, or ossification (figs. 17-7C, 17-12, right) or calcification (100).

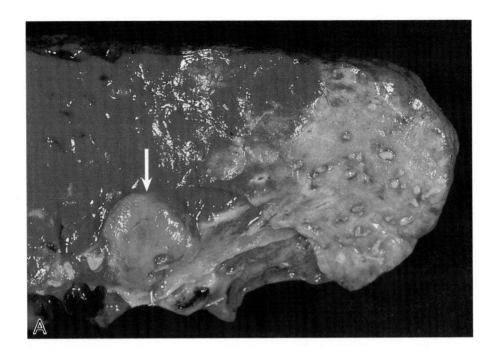

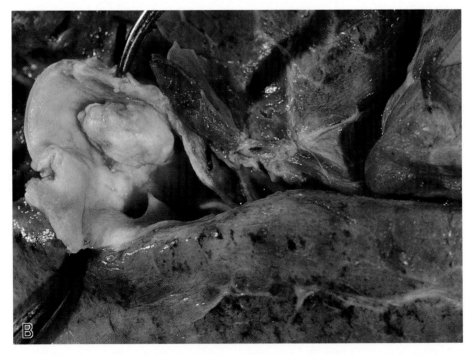

Figure 17-7
CARCINOID TUMOR: GROSS PATHOLOGY

A: This 2.0-cm, circumscribed, central carcinoid tumor impinges on the proximal bronchus to the left upper lobe. The cut surface of the tumor shows a smooth, tan-yellow mass. The lung parenchyma distal to the tumor shows postobstructive pneumonia.

B: This tumor has a prominent endobronchial component.

C: The nodular opacity seen on this specimen X ray reflects the extensive ossified stroma of this tumor.

D: This peripheral carcinoid consists of a 1.0-cm circumscribed nodular mass with a solid tan cut surface. This tumor was found on a chest CT scan after an extensive search for an occult source of ectopic ACTH production in a patient who presented with Cushing syndrome.

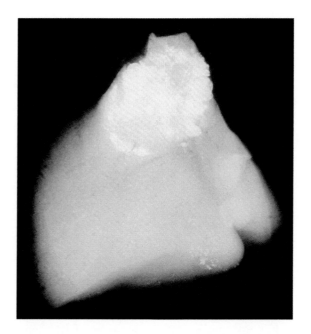

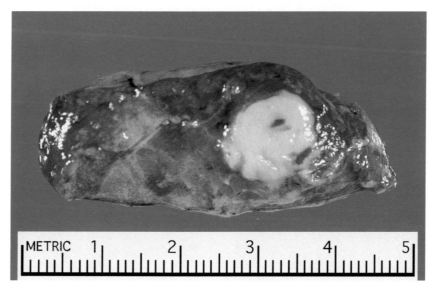

Figure 17-7 (Continued)

Atypical carcinoid, as defined by Arrigoni et al. (2), is distinguished from typical carcinoid by the following criteria: 1) increased mitotic activity, with 1 mitotic figure per 1 to 2 high-power fields (or 5 to 10 mitoses per 10 high-power fields) (fig. 17-14); 2) nuclear pleomorphism, hyperchromatism, and an abnormal nuclear-cytoplasmic ratio (fig. 17-14, left); 3) areas of increased cellularity with disorganization of the architec-

ture; and 4) tumor necrosis (fig. 17-15). Both atypical (fig. 17-15, left) and typical carcinoids (fig. 17-16) may have lymphatic invasion. Uncommonly, there may be prominent cytologic pleomorphism in the absence of necrosis and mitoses in typical carcinoids (fig. 17-17). The necrosis usually consists of small foci centrally located within organoid nests of tumor cells (fig. 17-15); uncommonly, the necrosis forms larger

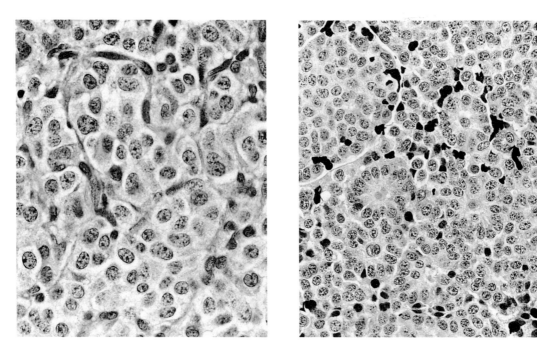

Figure 17-8
TYPICAL CARCINOID TUMOR

Left: Prominent organoid nesting pattern. The tumor cells have a moderate amount of cytoplasm and nuclei with finely granular chromatin. Faint nucleoli are also present.

Right: Prominent rosettes.

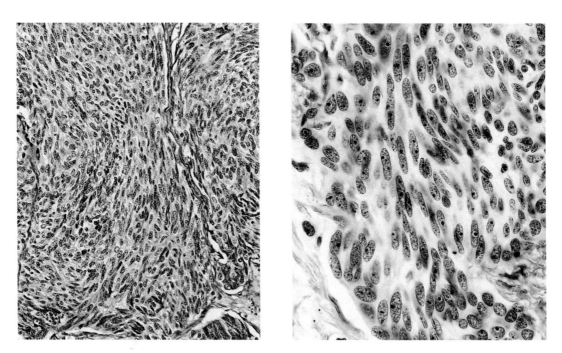

Figure 17-9
SPINDLE CELL CARCINOID TUMOR

Left: Spindle cell pattern.

Right: Higher power of spindle-shaped tumor cells. Small nucleoli are also present. This tumor was an atypical carcinoid, but spindle cell patterns can also be seen in typical carcinoids.

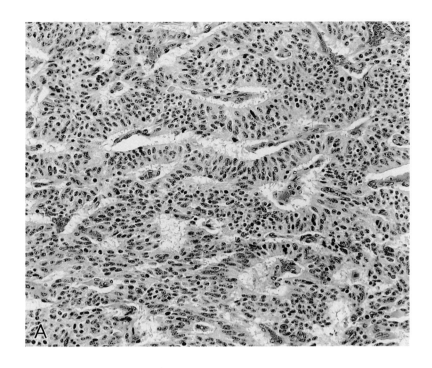

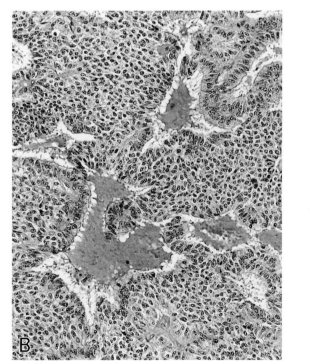
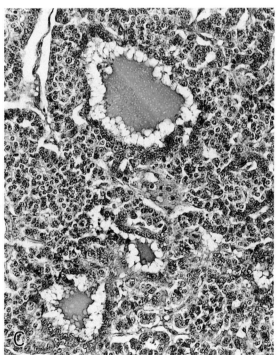

Figure 17-10
TYPICAL CARCINOID TUMOR

A: Trabecular pattern.

B: Pseudoglandular pattern. Prominent peripheral palisading of tumor cells at the edge of the spaces gives a gland-like appearance.

C: Follicular pattern with colloid-like eosinophilic material within glandular spaces. The eosinophilic material is scalloped around the edges, similar to thyroid follicles.

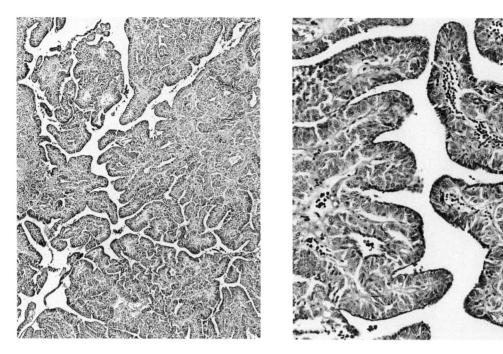

Figure 17-11
TYPICAL CARCINOID TUMOR

Left: Papillary pattern.
Right: The cells within the papillae have a carcinoid appearance. This tumor stained intensely with chromogranin.

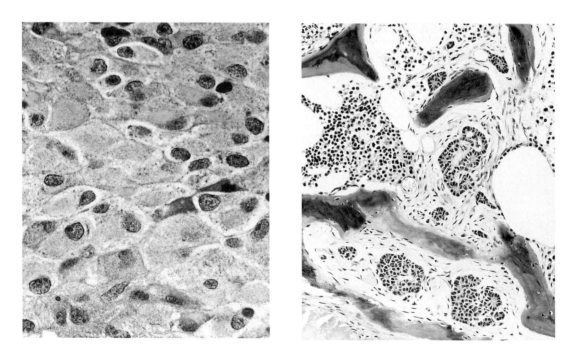

Figure 17-12
TYPICAL CARCINOID TUMOR

Left: Oncocytic carcinoid with abundant oxyphilic tumor cell cytoplasm.
Right: Prominent stromal ossification.

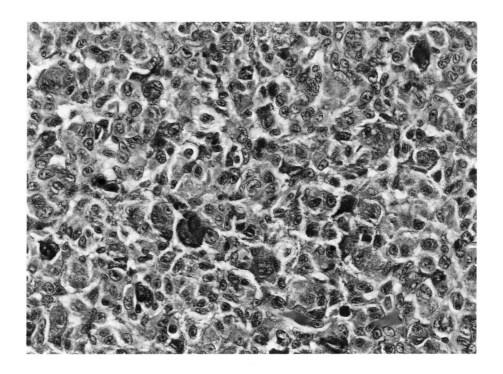

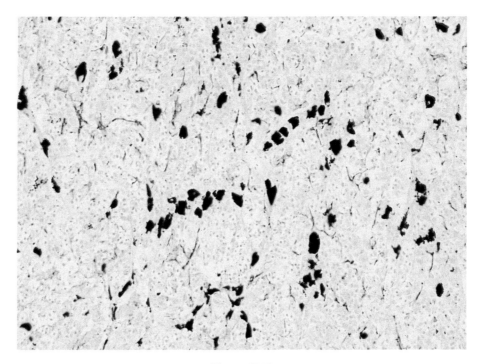

Figure 17-13
MELANOCYTIC CARCINOID
Top: This atypical carcinoid shows a prominent organoid nesting pattern of tumor cells with oxyphilic cytoplasm containing brown pigment.
Bottom: The pigment deposits stain positively with the Fontana-Masson stain. (Courtesy of Dr. Anthony A. Gal, Atlanta, GA.)

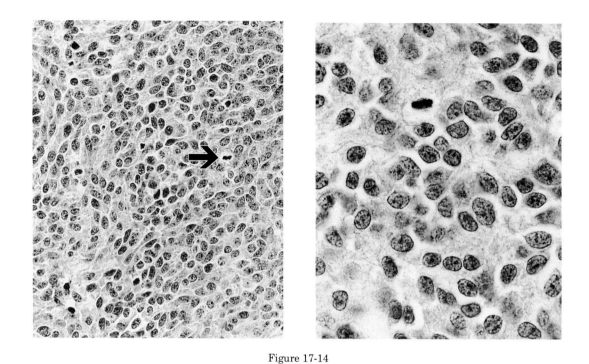

Figure 17-14
ATYPICAL CARCINOID TUMOR
Left: Tumor cells have slight pleomorphism. A single mitotic figure is present (arrow).
Right: The cells have a neuroendocrine appearance with finely granular nuclear chromatin. A single mitotic figure is present.

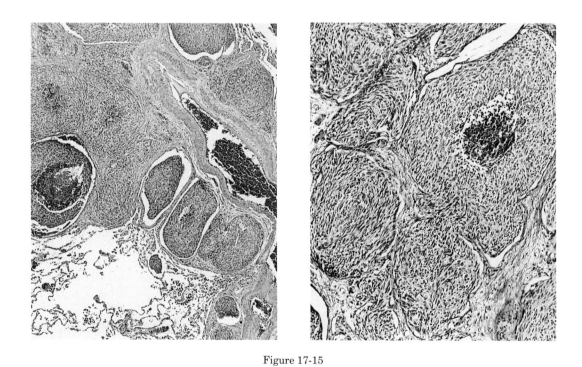

Figure 17-15
ATYPICAL CARCINOID TUMOR
Left: Lymphatic invasion is prominent. Necrosis is present in the center of tumor cell nests.
Right: This type of focal necrosis in the center of a nest of tumor cells is characteristic of atypical carcinoid.

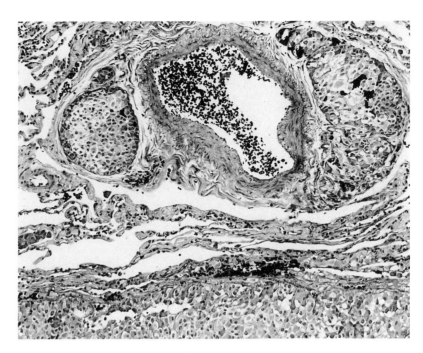

Figure 17-16
TYPICAL CARCINOID TUMOR
Lymphatic invasion can also occur in typical carcinoids.

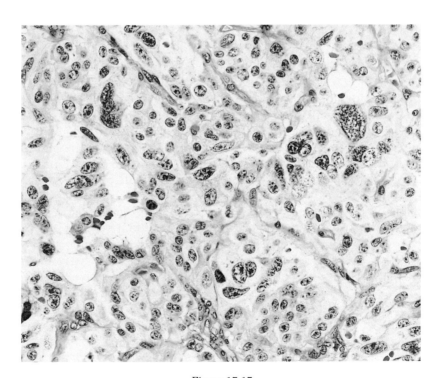

Figure 17-17
CARCINOID TUMOR WITH CYTOLOGIC ATYPIA
Marked cytologic atypia was seen in this carcinoid, however, no necrosis or mitoses were found and the patient survived 10 years without recurrence. Further cases are needed to establish whether such a tumor should be regarded as a typical or atypical carcinoid.

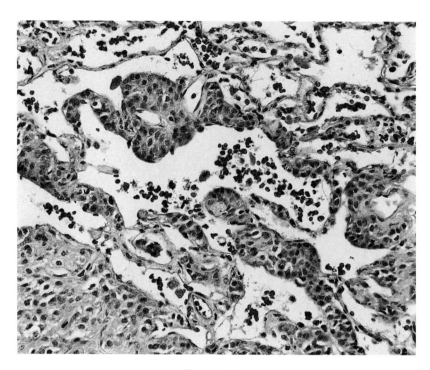

Figure 17-18
ATYPICAL CARCINOID TUMOR
These tumor cells infiltrate the interstitium of the alveolar septa.

confluent zones. Infiltration of the alveolar septal interstitium can also occur (fig. 17-18). Criteria for separation of typical from atypical carcinoid are summarized in Table 17-2.

The criteria outlined above for atypical carcinoid are more restrictive than those used in many articles subsequent to Arrigoni's original paper. Arrigoni defined a histologically low-grade tumor and other authors have included tumors of higher histologic grade in the category of atypical carcinoid (100). According to the criteria proposed by Gould and colleagues (104), well-differentiated neuroendocrine carcinoma includes atypical carcinoid at one end of the spectrum as well as histologically high-grade tumors which could be classified as large cell neuroendocrine carcinoma.

Cytology. Sputum cytology is rarely helpful in evaluation of typical and atypical carcinoids since few tumor cells are shed into the bronchi. Fine needle aspiration cytology of carcinoid tumors is distinctive (29,96). The tumor cells have small, round, oval or spindle-shaped nuclei (fig. 17-19). The cells may be single or in loose or tight syncytial aggregates. There is typically a moder-

ate amount of finely granular eosinophilic cytoplasm, but cytoplasm may be absent in single cells and "stripped" nuclei are common in fine needle aspiration biopsy material. Acinar arrangements of cells may be seen. Typical carcinoids have finely granular chromatin, small nucleoli, a clean background without necrotic debris, and no mitoses. Nuclear molding may be seen in spindle cell carcinoids.

Atypical carcinoid cells have greater pleomorphism, with more uneven, coarsely granular chromatin and small to prominent nucleoli. A background of necrotic debris or single cell necrosis may be seen. Nuclear molding is common and a few mitoses are characteristic (96).

Ultrastructural Findings. Typical carcinoids have numerous dense core granules which vary considerably in shape and size (fig. 17-20A). Oncocytic carcinoids have numerous cytoplasmic mitochondria as well as dense core granules (33,93); these differ from pulmonary oncocytomas which do not have neuroendocrine granules (fig. 17-20C) (93). There are fewer dense core granules in atypical than typical carcinoids and the granules are slightly smaller and less varied in

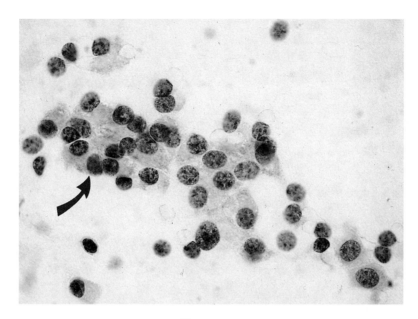

Figure 17-19
CARCINOID TUMOR: FINE NEEDLE ASPIRATION CYTOLOGY
These clusters of tumor cells show the characteristic cytologic features of carcinoid tumor cells: uniform size and shape, moderate amount of eosinophilic cytoplasm, and finely granular nuclear chromatin. The tumor cells focally form a rosette-like arrangement (arrow).

size (fig. 17-20B). The granules in atypical carcinoid tumors are usually diffusely distributed in the cytoplasm.

Immunohistochemical Findings. Of the various types of pulmonary neuroendocrine tumors, typical carcinoids have the highest percentage, distribution, and intensity of immunohistochemical staining for neuroendocrine and hormonal markers. These are slightly less for atypical carcinoids (fig. 17-21A,B). Chromogranin is the most useful immunohistochemical marker of neuroendocrine differentiation, followed by synaptophysin and Leu-7.

Hormonal markers have been used to confirm ectopic hormone production in neuroendocrine tumors that cause Cushing syndrome (fig. 17-21C) and acromegaly. Positive staining for ACTH may also occur in pulmonary carcinoids in the absence of clinical evidence of Cushing syndrome; similarly, growth-hormone releasing hormone (GHRH) may be detected by immunohistochemistry in the absence of elevated serum GHRH or acromegaly.

Flow Cytometry. A variety of forms of DNA analysis have been used in bronchial carcinoid tumors including flow cytometry (24,52,54,98, 100,111), cell image analysis of cytomorpho-

nuclear parameters (integrated optical density [IOD] and nuclear optical density variance [VOD]) (60), nuclear morphometry (mean nuclear area) (98), cytogenetic studies (25), and fluorescent cytophotometric DNA measurements (10). Aneuploidy has been found in 5 to 32 percent of typical carcinoids and 16 to 79 percent of atypical carcinoids (24,52,54,98,100,111), and correlates with poor prognosis (54). However, all aneuploid carcinoid tumors do not behave aggressively: in one study, 58 percent of patients with aneuploid carcinoid tumors survived 5 years (54). Aneuploidy is more common in carcinoid tumors larger than 3 cm (24), with undifferentiated growth patterns (54), atypical versus typical histology (24), pleomorphic nuclei (54), lymph node metastases (24,54), vascular invasion (24,111), and necrosis (54).

The cell proliferation index (the sum of the percentage of cells in the S and G2/M of the cell cycle) may provide a useful supplement to aneuploidy data (100).

Differential Diagnosis. It can be difficult to distinguish typical carcinoid from atypical carcinoid (and occasionally, small cell carcinoma) in small, crushed biopsy specimens; therefore, one

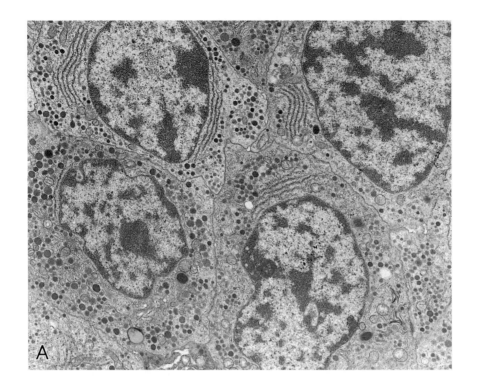

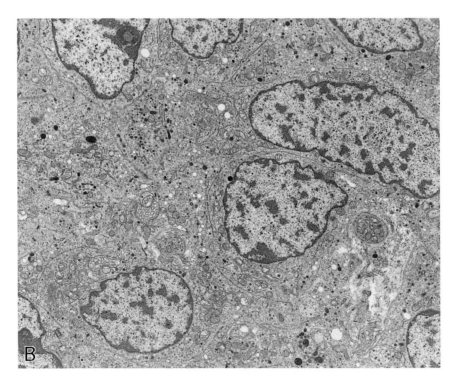

Figure 17-20
CARCINOID TUMOR: ELECTRON MICROSCOPY
A: Typical carcinoid has numerous neuroendocrine granules. Stacks of rough endoplasmic reticulum are also present.
B: Atypical carcinoid with fewer and smaller dense core granules.
C: Oncocytic carcinoid has numerous mitochondria as well as neuroendocrine granules in the cytoplasm. (Courtesy of Dr. Maria Tsokos, Bethesda, MD.)

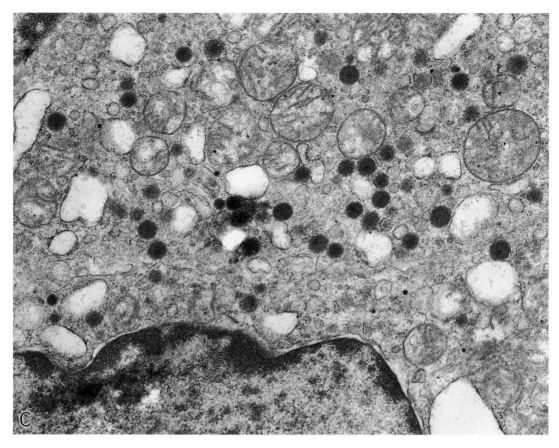

Figure 17-20 (Continued)

should be careful when interpreting transbronchial biopsies if the tumor cells are not well preserved. The criteria for distinguishing typical from atypical carcinoid are reviewed in Table 17-2.

Depending on the histologic pattern or cytology, the differential diagnosis may vary. The spindle cell pattern frequently causes difficulty. Although a spindle cell pattern is more common in atypical carcinoid and small cell carcinoma, it should not be used as a criterion for malignancy since it also occurs in typical carcinoid. Spindle cell carcinoids differ from other non-neuroendocrine tumors composed of spindle-shaped cells such as smooth muscle tumors (leiomyoma, hemangiopericytoma, leiomyosarcoma), chemodectoma, schwannoma, fibrous mesothelioma, spindle cell carcinoma, metastatic sarcoma, or metastatic melanoma. The oncocytic features raise the question of oncocytoma. A papillary pattern may be confused with sclerosing hemangioma. A glandular pattern may lead to confusion with adenoid cystic carcinoma or adenocarcinoma. A melanocytic carcinoid may be confused with a melanoma. Carcinoid is distinguished by an organoid pattern, finely granular nuclear chromatin, and positive immunohistochemical staining for neuroendocrine markers or dense core granules by electron microscopy.

Carcinoid tumors can also be difficult to separate cytologically from metastatic carcinoma, especially from the breast and prostate. Breast or prostate carcinomas also occasionally stain for neuroendocrine immunohistochemical markers. In this situation, the presence of multiple pulmonary nodules favors metastases. If a patient has had previous biopsies of prostate or breast tumors, they should be reviewed for comparison. Immunohistochemistry for prostate-specific antigen may be helpful if the question of prostate carcinoma arises, although immunoreactivity for prostatic acid phosphatase can be found in bronchial carcinoids.

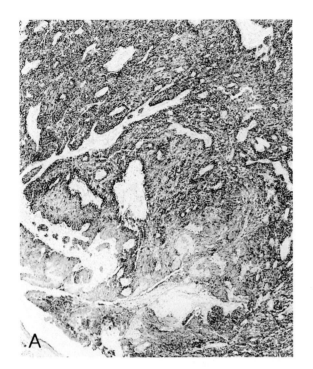

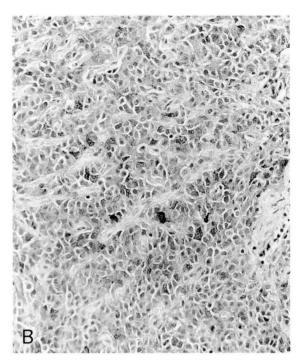

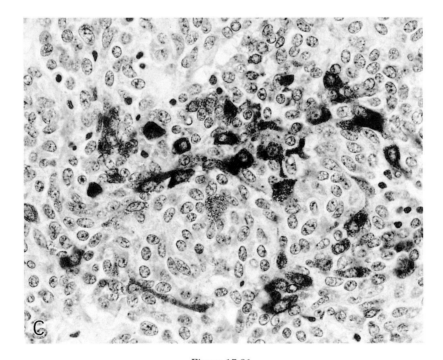

Figure 17-21
CARCINOID TUMOR: IMMUNOHISTOCHEMISTRY

A: Typical carcinoid stains diffusely and intensely with chromogranin.

B: Atypical carcinoid stains focally and less intensely with chromogranin.

C: Focal immunohistochemical staining for ACTH in typical carcinoid. Patient had Cushing syndrome due to ectopic production of ACTH by this bronchial carcinoid. Patient was cured following surgical removal.

Treatment and Prognosis. Surgery is the primary management of bronchial carcinoids (71,95). Lobectomy is the treatment of choice in most cases, particularly for central tumors. Segmentectomy or wedge excision may be adequate for small peripheral tumors. Bronchial sleeve resection may be possible in some cases; but some proximal tumors may require pneumonectomy (95). Regardless of the type of procedure, lymph node sampling is important even for small peripheral tumors, since all carcinoid tumors have the potential to metastasize to regional lymph nodes. These tumors are relatively resistant to chemotherapy and radiation therapy; therefore, when possible, metastatic disease is best managed surgically. Radiation may relieve pain in some cases of bone metastases.

Patients with typical carcinoids have an excellent prognosis and rarely die of tumor (71,103). Metastases should not be used as a criteria for distinguishing typical from atypical carcinoids since 5 to 20 percent of typical carcinoids have regional lymph node involvement. Rarely, distant metastases of typical carcinoids occur, sometimes many years after initial diagnosis. Even patients with distant metastases survive long term. Although it has been suggested that the spindle cell variant of carcinoid tumor is more aggressive, this does not appear to be the case (87). Most peripheral carcinoids are typical carcinoids (87).

Compared to typical carcinoids, atypical carcinoids are larger, with a higher rate of metastasis and a significantly reduced survival. The mortality reported in most series is approximately 30 percent, ranging from 27 to 47 percent (2,71). Mean survival is slightly over 2 years, with a range up to 10 years. According to one study, the 5- and 10-year disease-free survival for typical carcinoids is 100 percent and 87 percent, and for atypical carcinoids is 69 percent and 52 percent, respectively (p<0.001) (71).

Poor prognosis is correlated with a variety of clinical and pathologic features including lack of surgical therapy, advanced stage, large tumor size (equal to or greater than 3 cm), lymph node metastasis, vascular invasion, atypical versus typical histology, intraluminal versus extrabronchial spread, aneuploidy, elevated S-phase, and increased nuclear DNA content measured by integrated optical density (24,71,79).

Unusual sites of metastasis include the skin (78), ovaries (13), the choroid of both eyes (31), and breast (47).

UNUSUAL LUNG TUMORS WITH NEUROENDOCRINE DIFFERENTIATION

Paraganglioma

The existence of paragangliomas as primary tumors of the lung is somewhat controversial. Although carcinoid tumors are common and paragangliomas rare, there is considerable overlap in the histologic features of these two tumors and no specific discriminating features by electron microscopy or immunohistochemistry. Other reported terms for paraganglioma (8,23,46,75, 91), include *carotid body-like tumor* (50), *glomus tumor* (8), and *chemodectoma* (27,36,61,67). We are not convinced that all of the reported cases are paragangliomas of the lung: the authors of this Fascicle have never seen a bone fide case, nor have Lack et al. (58). However, the work of Blessing and Hora (9) indicates the potential existence of paragangliomas since paraganglia-like structures exist in the periarterial interstitium of the lungs in the newborn.

Histologically, paragangliomas have a characteristic zellenballen pattern of organoid nesting. However, carcinoid tumors may have this same pattern. Paraganglioma cells show nuclear pleomorphism with vesicular or hyperchromatic, ovoid or round nuclei. The cytoplasm is pale, homogeneous or vacuolated. Tumor cells may appear syncytial since their cytoplasmic borders are poorly defined. There may be interdigitation of adjoining cells or cell processes, giving the appearance of cells embracing one another (34).

Based on a light microscopic comparison of over 100 head and neck paragangliomas and 30 carcinoid tumors the following criteria are suggested for paraganglioma: 1) a diffuse zellenballen pattern throughout the tumor; 2) absence of the histologic features distinctive of carcinoid tumors (trabecular pattern, pseudoglandular acini, ossification, perivascular pseudorosettes, oncocytic change, spindle cells); 3) presence of features distinctive of paragangliomas (cytoplasmic vacuoles, cell-in-cell embracing phenomenon); and 4) absence of immunohistochemical staining for keratin. The presence of the carcinoid syndrome (1 to 2 percent of bronchial carcinoids) favors a carcinoid tumor. Since

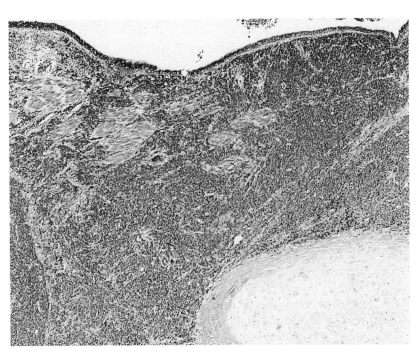

Figure 17-22
PRIMITIVE
NEUROECTODERMAL
TUMOR
This small round cell tumor extensively infiltrates the bronchial submucosa.

there is no one discriminating feature, multiple parameters must be used for distinction (58). Up to 80 percent of carcinoids stain with keratin, while paragangliomas are virtually always keratin negative. S-100 protein–positive cells can be found in carcinoids as well as paragangliomas (3,4).

Finally, the diagnosis of primary pulmonary paraganglioma requires exclusion of an extrapulmonary paraganglioma or pheochromocytoma. Multifocal malignant pheochromocytoma can present as a lung tumor (90), and cervical paraganglioma can present with extensive pulmonary metastases (83). The case reported as multiple pulmonary paragangliomas in a patient with neurofibromatosis may actually be metastases from either a left adrenal pheochromocytoma or a left jugular foramen paraganglioma (22). Since both carcinoid tumors and paragangliomas are low-grade malignant tumors with a similar prognosis, there is probably little clinical significance to making the pathologic distinction.

Primitive Neuroectodermal Tumor (Malignant Small Round Cell Tumor of the Thoracopulmonary Region)

Primitive neuroectodermal tumor (PNET) is closely related to, if not the same as, malignant small round cell tumor of the thoracopulmonary

region. These tumors primarily involve the chest wall, but occasionally present as a primary pulmonary neoplasm (44,110). They usually occur in young adults. They grow rapidly and can cause pulmonary or chest wall symptoms such as cough, dyspnea, and chest pain. PNETs tend to be large and have a soft, fleshy, gross appearance with frequent hemorrhage and necrosis.

Histologically, the tumors are composed of small cells growing in sheets or lobules (figs. 17-22, 17-23). The cells are dyscohesive, with virtually no reticulin between the tumor cells. In better differentiated tumors, rosette formation may be seen. The Homer Wright rosette is the most common, with cells surrounding a central core of fibrillary material; less often they may be of the Flexner-Wintersteiner type with a central lumen or vesicle. The tumor cells are small and may be round to oval or spindle shaped. They are hyperchromatic with indistinct cytoplasm and most cells do not have prominent nucleoli. PNETs often stain for neuron-specific enolase (NSE), but can be distinguished from other neuroendocrine lung tumors since they are usually negative for chromogranin, synaptophysin, Leu-7, S-100 protein, and keratin. PNETs also stain positively with antibodies to the MIC II gene product (12E7 or HBA 71). In rare cases, occasional keratin-positive tumor cells may be present. PNETs are

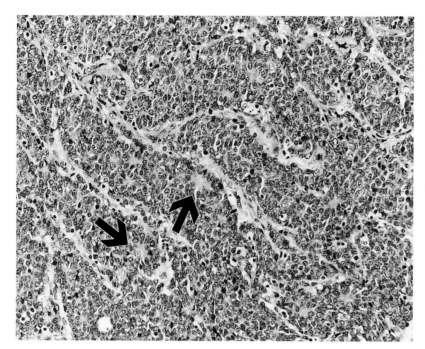

Figure 17-23
PRIMITIVE
NEUROECTODERMAL TUMOR
The tumor cells grow in diffuse
sheets with focal rosettes (arrows).

distinguished from lymphomas by cells that tend grow in a pattern and do not stain for common leukocyte antigen. A reciprocal translocation may be present between chromosomes 11 and 22. The diagnosis should be strongly considered if a small round cell tumor in a young adult fails to stain with most immunohistochemical markers and shows evidence of chest wall or rib involvement.

Neuroendocrine Carcinoma with Rhabdoid Phenotype

Rarely, neuroendocrine carcinomas of the lung may exhibit a rhabdoid phenotype that is characterized by cytoplasmic inclusions corresponding immunohistochemically and ultrastructurally to whorls of intermediate filaments. To our knowledge, only one such tumor has occurred, in a 24-year-old female who had a right upper lobe lung mass. Grossly, the tumor formed a dominant mass but diffusely infiltrated the lung. Histologically, the tumor was composed of diffuse sheets and nests of cells with a focal organoid pattern. Many of the tumor cells had a round to oval eosinophilic cytoplasmic inclusion (fig. 17-24). Immunohistochemistry showed positive staining for keratin, vimentin, chromogranin (fig. 17-25), NSE, desmin, and actin. Electron microscopy demonstrated numerous intermediate filaments in a whorl-like pattern characteristic of rhabdoid tumors (fig. 17-26). In addition, neuroendocrine granules and desmosomes were found focally.

The rhabdoid tumor was first described as a childhood renal tumor; subsequently, however, extrarenal rhabdoid tumors have been reported in a wide variety of sites (107). It has never been described as a pulmonary tumor. It is also known that rhabdoid features may be encountered in a wide variety of tumors including soft tissue sarcomas, adenomas, carcinomas, mesotheliomas, and melanomas; thus, the term rhabdoid phenotype is often applied for such tumors (106).

Amphicrine Neoplasms

Amphicrine cells exhibit both exocrine and endocrine differentiation (15,44). These neoplasms typically appear as adenocarcinomas by routine light microscopy and histochemical stains show mucin either within well-defined lumens or in intracytoplasmic droplets (88). However by electron microscopy, neuroendocrine granules are often seen concentrated in the basal pole or in cytoplasmic processes (fig. 17-27). Immunohistochemistry may demonstrate chromogranin, bombesin, or other neuroendocrine markers (44).

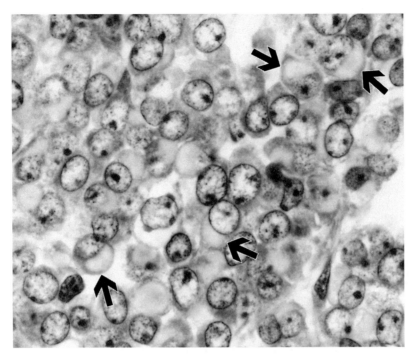

Figure 17-24
NEUROENDOCRINE CARCINOMA WITH RHABDOID PHENOTYPE
These tumor cells have prominent eosinophilic cytoplasmic globules (arrows).

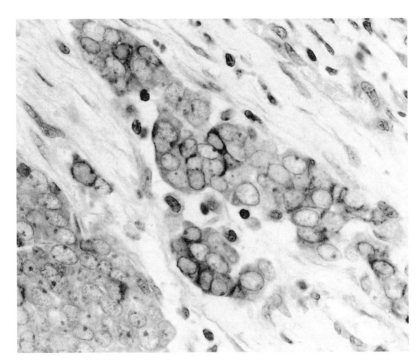

Figure 17-25
NEUROENDOCRINE CARCINOMA WITH RHABDOID PHENOTYPE
Focal positive staining of tumor cells with chromogranin.

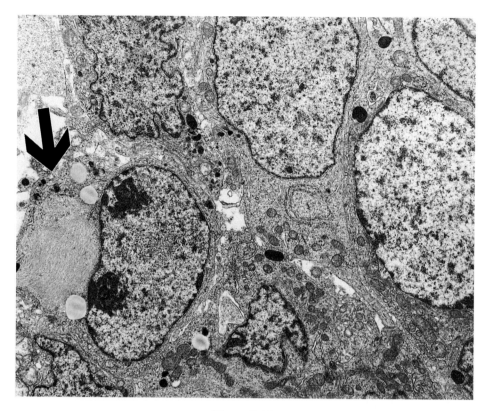

Figure 17-26
NEUROENDOCRINE CARCINOMA WITH RHABDOID PHENOTYPE
Electron microscopy shows a nodular paranuclear bundle of cytoplasmic intermediate filaments (arrow). (Courtesy of Dr. Maria Tsokos, Bethesda, MD.)

Neuroendocrine Carcinoma with Anemone Features

Anemone or *porcupine cell tumors* are rare neoplasms which by ultrastructure have prominent circumferential microvilli (44,82). Both epithelial and hematopoietic malignant neoplasms can exhibit this unusual feature (82). One neuroendocrine lung carcinoma has been reported to have the morphology of anemone cells (44).

Pulmonary Blastoma with Neuroendocrine Differentiation

Neuroendocrine differentiation can occur in pulmonary blastomas, particularly in cell morules that resemble neuroepithelial bodies (16,57). These morular cells stain for chromogranin, NSE, synaptophysin, gastrin, calcitonin, bombesin, somatostatin, and serotonin (16). Pulmonary blastoma is discussed in more detail in chapter 21.

REFERENCES

1. Aguayo SM, Miller YE, Waldron JA Jr, et al. Brief report: idiopathic diffuse hyperplasia of pulmonary neuroendocrine cells and airways disease. N Engl J Med 1992;327:1285–8.
2. Arrigoni MG, Woolner LB, Bernatz PE. Atypical carcinoid tumors of the lung. J Thorac Cardiovasc Surg 1972;64:413–21.
3. Barbareschi M, Ferrero S, Frigo B, Mariscotti C, Mosca L. Bronchial carcinoid with S-100 positive sustentacular cells. Tumori 1988;74:705–11.
4. _____, Mauri MF, Muscara M, Mauri FA, Lo Re V. S-100 protein in human lung neuroendocrine neoplasms. Immunohistochemical study of 14 cases and review of the literature. Histol Histopathol 1987;2:185–92.

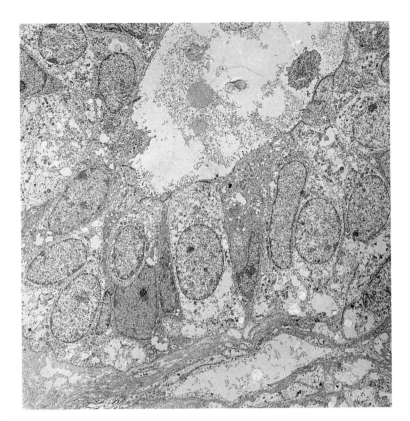

Figure 17-27
AMPHICRINE CARCINOMA: UL-
TRASTRUCTURE

A: This tumor shows glandular formation with tumor cells oriented around a
central lumen and secretory-like structures at the apical aspect of the cells.

B: The tumor cells have distinct
dense core granules in the base of the
cells (arrow). (Courtesy of Dr. Samuel
Hammar, Bremerton, WA.)

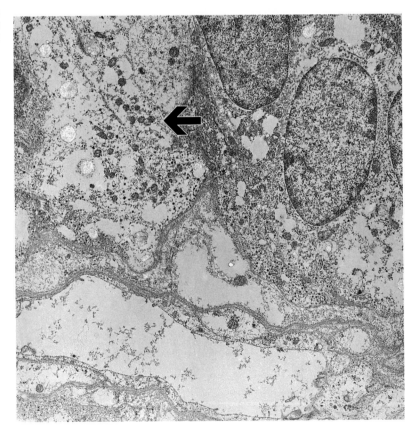

5. Bensch KG, Corrin B, Pariente R, et al. Oat-cell carcinoma of the lung: its origin and relationship to bronchial carcinoid. Cancer 1968;22:1163–72.

6. _____, Gordon GB, Miller LR. Studies on the bronchial counterpart of the Kultchitzky (argentaffin) cell and innervation of bronchial glands. J Ultrast Res 1965;12:668–86.

7. Berendsen HH, de Leij L, Poppema S, et al. Clinical characterization of non-small-cell lung cancer tumors showing neuroendocrine differentiation features. J Clin Oncol 1989;7:1614–20.

8. Blessing MH, Borchard F, Lenz W. Glomus tumour (so-called chemodectoma) of the lung. Pathological and biochemical findings. Virchows Arch [A] 1973;359:315–29.

9. _____, Hora BI. Glomera in the human lung. Z Zellforsch Mikrosk Anat 1968;87:562–70.

10. Blöndal T, Arnorsson T, Bengtsson A, Wilander E. Nuclear DNA in carcinoid tumours of the lung. Eur J Respir Dis 1983;64:298–305.

11. Bonikos DS, Archibald R, Bensch KG. On the origin of the so-called tumorlets of the lung. Hum Pathol 1976;7:461–9.

12. _____, Bensch KG, Jamplis RW. Peripheral pulmonary carcinoid tumors. Cancer 1976;37:1977–98.

13. Brown BL, Scharifker DA, Gordon R, Deppe GG, Cohen CJ. Bronchial carcinoid tumor with ovarian metastasis: a light microscopic and ultrastructural study. Cancer 1980;46:543–6.

14. Carter D, Eggleston JC. Tumors of the lower respiratory tract. Atlas of Tumor Pathology, Second Series, Fascicle 17. Washington, D.C.: Armed Forces Institute of Pathology, 1980.

15. Chejfec G, Capella C, Solcia E, Jao W, Gould VE. Amphicrine cells, dysplasias, and neoplasias. Cancer 1985;56:2683–90.

16. _____, Cosnow I, Gould NS, Husain AN, Gould VE. Pulmonary blastoma with neuroendocrine differentiation in cell morules resembling neuroepithelial bodies. Histopathology 1990;17:353–8.

17. Churg A, Warnock ML. Pulmonary tumorlet. A form of peripheral carcinoid. Cancer 1976;37:1469–77.

18. Clague JE, Pearson MG, Sharma A, Taylor W. Medullary carcinoma of the thyroid presenting as multifocal bronchial carcinoid tumour. Thorax 1991;46:67–8.

19. Cunningham GJ, Nassau E, Walter JB. The frequency of tumor-like formations in bronchiectatic lungs. Thorax 1958;13:64–8.

20. Cureton RJR, Hill IM. Malignant change in bronchiectasis. Thorax 1955;10:131–6.

21. D'Agati VD, Perzin KH. Carcinoid tumorlets of the lung with metastasis to a peribronchial lymph node. Report of a case and review of the literature. Cancer 1985;55:2472–6.

22. DeAngelis LM, Kelleher MB, Post KD, Fetell MR. Multiple paragangliomas in neurofibromatosis: a new neuroendocrine neoplasia. Neurology 1987;37:129–33.

23. Düsseldorf M, Straaten HG. Primary pulmonary paraganglioma. Zentralbl Chir 1990;115:1575–8.

24. el-Naggar AK, Ballance W, Karim FW, et al. Typical and atypical bronchopulmonary carcinoids. A clinicopathologic and flow cytometric study. Am J Clin Pathol 1991;95:828–34.

25. Falor WH. Chromosomes in bronchial adenomas and in bronchogenic carcinomas. Am Rev Respir Dis 1971;104:198–205.

26. Farhangi M, Taylor J, Havey A, O'Dorisio TM. Neuroendocrine (carcinoid) tumor of the lung and type I multiple endocrine neoplasia. South Med J 1987;80:1459–62.

27. Fawcett FJ, Husband EM. Chemodectoma of lung. J Clin Pathol 1967;20:260–2.

28. Feyrter F. Über die Argyrophilie des Helle-Zelle-Systems im Bronchialbaum des Menschen. Z Mikrosk Anat Forsch 1954;61:73–81.

29. Frierson HF Jr, Covell JL, Mills SE. Fine needle aspiration cytology of atypical carcinoid of the lung. Acta Cytol 1987;31:471–5.

30. Frölich F. Die "Helle Zelle" der Bronchialschleimhaut und ihre Beziehungen zum Problem der Chemoreceptoren. Frankfurter Z Pathol 1949;60:517–59.

31. Fu YS, McWilliams NB, Stratford TP, Kay S. Bronchial carcinoid with choroidal metastasis in an adolescent. Case report and ultrastructural study. Cancer 1974;33:707–15.

32. Gal AA, Koss MN, Hochholzer L, DeRose PB, Cohen C. Pigmented pulmonary carcinoid tumor. An immunohistochemical and ultrastructural study. Arch Pathol Lab Med 1993;117:832–6.

33. Ghadially FN, Block HJ. Oncocytic carcinoid of the lung. J Submicrosc Cytol 1985;17:435–42.

34. Glenner GG, Grimley PM. Tumors of the extra-adrenal paraganglion system (including chemoreceptors). Atlas of Tumor Pathology, 2nd Series, Fascicle 9. Washington, D.C.: Armed Forces Institute of Pathology, 1974.

35. Gmelich JT, Bensch KG, Liebow AA. Cells of Kultschitzky type in bronchioles and their relation to the origin of peripheral carcinoid tumor. Lab Invest 1967;17:88–98.

36. Goodman ML, Laforet EG. Solitary primary chemodectomas of the lung. Chest 1972;61:48–50.

37. Gordon HW, Miller R Jr, Mittman C. Medullary carcinoma of the lung with amyloid stroma: a counterpart of medullary carcinoma of the thyroid. Hum Pathol 1973;4:431–6.

38. Gosney J, Green AR, Taylor W. Appropriate and inappropriate neuroendocrine products in pulmonary tumourlets. Thorax 1990;45:679–83.

39. Gosney J, Heath D, Smith P, Harris P, Yacoub M. Pulmonary endocrine cells in pulmonary arterial disease. Arch Pathol Lab Med 1989;113:337–41.

40. Gould VE, Linnoila RI. Pulmonary neuroepithelial bodies, neuroendocrine cells, and pulmonary tumors. Hum Pathol 1982;13:1064–6.

41. _____, Yannopoulos AD, Sommers SC, Terzakis JA. Neuroendocrine cells in dysplastic bronchi: ultrastructural observations and quantitative analysis of secretory granules and the golgi complex. Am J Pathol 1978;90:49–56.

42. Graziano SL, Mazid R, Newman N, et al. The use of neuroendocrine immunoperoxidase markers to predict chemotherapy response in patients with non-small-cell lung cancer. J Clin Oncol 1989;7:1398–406.

43. Hage E. Electron microscopic identification of several types of endocrine cells in the bronchial epithelium of human foetuses. Z Zellforsch Mikrosk Anat 1973;141:401–12.

44. Hammar S, Bockus D, Remington F, Cooper L. The unusual spectrum of neuroendocrine lung neoplasms. Ultrastruct Pathol 1989;13:515–60.

45. Hammond ME, Sause WT. Large cell neuroendocrine tumors of the lung. Clinical significance and histopathologic definition. Cancer 1985;56:1624–9.

46. Hangartner JR, Loosemore TM, Burke M, Pepper JR. Malignant primary pulmonary paraganglioma. Thorax 1989;44:154–6.

47. Harrist TJ, Kalisher L. Breast metastasis: an unusual manifestation of a malignant carcinoid tumor. Cancer 1977;40:3102–6.

48. Hausman DH, Weimann RB. Pulmonary tumorlet with hilar lymph node metastasis. Report of a case. Cancer 1967;20:1515–9.

49. Heath D, Yacoub M, Gosney JR, Madden B, Caslin AW, Smith P. Pulmonary endocrine cells in hypertensive pulmonary vascular disease. Histopathology 1990;16:21–8.

50. Heppleston A. A carotid-body-like tumour in the lung. J Pathol Bacteriol 1958;75:461–4.

51. Hussein AM, Feun LG, Savaraj N, East D, Hussein DT. Carcinoid tumor presenting as central nervous system symptoms. Case report and review of the literature. Am J Clin Oncol 1990;13:251–5.

52. Jackson-York GL, Davis BH, Warren WH, Gould VE, Memoli VA. Flow cytometric DNA content analysis in neuroendocrine carcinoma of the lung. Correlation with survival and histologic subtype. Cancer 1991;68:374–9.

53. Johnson DE, Kulik TJ, Lock JE, Elde RP, Thompson TR. Bombesin-, calcitonin-, and serotonin-immunoreactive pulmonary neuroendocrine cells in acute and chronic neonatal lung disease. Pediatr Pulmonol 1985;1(3 Suppl):S13–S20.

54. Jones DJ, Hasleton PS, Moore M. DNA ploidy in bronchopulmonary carcinoid tumours. Thorax 1988;43:195–9.

55. Kibbelaar RE, Moolenaar KE, Michalides RJ, et al. Neural cell adhesion molecule expression, neuroendocrine differentiation and prognosis in lung carcinoma. Eur J Cancer 1991;27:431–5.

56. Kleinerman J, Marchevsky A. Quantitative studies of argyrophilic APUD cells in airways: II. The effects of transplacental diethylnitrosamine. Am Rev Respir Dis 1982;126:152–5.

57. Koss MN, Hochholzer L, O'Leary T. Pulmonary blastomas. Cancer 1991;67:2368–81.

58. Lack EE. Pathology of adrenal and extra-adrenal paraganglia. Philadelphia: WB Saunders, 1994.

59. _____, Harris GB, Eraklis AJ, Vawter GF. Primary bronchial tumors in childhood. A clinicopathologic study of six cases. Cancer 1983;51:492–7.

60. Larsimont D, Kiss R, de Launoit Y, Melamed MR. Characterization of the morphonuclear features and DNA ploidy of typical and atypical carcinoids and small cell carcinomas of the lung. Am J Clin Pathol 1990;94:378–83.

61. Laustela E, Mattila S, Franssila K. Chemodectoma of the lung. Scand J Thorac Cardiovasc Surg 1969;3:59–62.

62. Lauweryns JM, Cokelaere M. Hypoxia-sensitive neuroepithelial bodies. Intrapulmonary secretory neuroreceptors, modulated by the CNS. Z Zellforsch Mikrosk Anat 1973;145:521–40.

63. _____, Goddeeris P. Neuroepithelial bodies in the human child and adult lung. Am Rev Respir Dis 1975;111:469–76.

64. _____, Peuskens JC. Neuro-epithelial bodies (neuroreceptor or secretory organs?) in human infant bronchial and bronchiolar epithelium. Anat Rec 1972;172:471–81.

65. Lawson RM, Ramanathan L, Hurley G, Hinson KW, Lennox SC. Bronchial adenoma: review of 18-year experience at the Brompton Hospital. Thorax 1976;31:245–53.

66. Lee I, Gould VE, Moll R, Wiedenmann B, Franke WW. Synaptophysin expressed in the bronchopulmonary tract: neuroendocrine cells, neuroepithelial bodies, and neuroendocrine neoplasms. Differentiation 1987;34:115–25.

67. Lee YT, Hori JM. Chemodectoma of the lung. J Surg Oncol 1972;4:33–7.

68. Linnoila RI, Jensen SM, Steinberg SM, Minna JD, Gazdar AF, Mulshine JL. Neuroendocrine (NE) differentiation in non-small cell lung cancer (NSCLC) correlates with favorable response to chemotherapy (CT) [Abstract]. Proc Am Soc Clin Oncol 1989;8:248

69. _____, Mulshine JL, Steinberg SM, et al. Neuroendocrine differentiation in endocrine and nonendocrine lung carcinomas. Am J Clin Pathol 1988;90:641–52.

70. Marchevsky A, Nieburgs HE, Olenko E, Kirschner P, Teirstein A, Kleinerman J. Pulmonary tumorlets in cases of tuberculoma of the lung with malignant cells in brush biopsy. Acta Cytol 1982;26:491–4.

71. McCaughan BC, Martini N, Bains MS. Bronchial carcinoids. Review of 124 cases. J Thorac Cardiovasc Surg 1985;89:8–17.

72. McDowell EM, Barrett LA, Trump BF. Observations on small granule cells in adult human bronchial epithelium and in carcinoid and oat cell tumors. Lab Invest 1976;34:202–6.

73. Miller MA, Mark GJ, Kanarek D. Multiple peripheral pulmonary carcinoids and tumorlets of carcinoid type, with restrictive and obstructive lung disease. Am J Med 1978;65:373–8.

74. Mills SE, Cooper PH, Walker AN, Kron IL. Atypical carcinoid tumor of the lung. A clinicopathologic study of 17 cases. Am J Surg Pathol 1982;6:643–54.

75. Mostecky H, Lichtenberg J, Kalus M. A non-chromaffin paraganglioma of the lung. Thorax 1966;21:205–8.

76. Ohtsuki H, Midorikawa O, Okada H, Morikawa S, Sakaguchi H. Pulmonary atypical carcinoid tumor with marked alphafetoprotein production and features of an adenocarcinoma differentiation. Pathol Res Pract 1988;184:86–97.

77. Okike N, Bernatz PE, Woolner LB. Carcinoid tumors of the lung. Ann Thorac Surg 1976;22:270–7.

78. Oleksowicz L, Morris JC, Phelps RG, Bruckner HW. Pulmonary carcinoid presenting as multiple subcutaneous nodules. Tumori 1990;76:44–7.

79. Paladugu RR, Benfield JR, Pak HY, Ross RK, Teplitz RL. Bronchopulmonary Kulchitzky cell carcinomas. A new classification scheme for typical and atypical carcinoids. Cancer 1985;55:1303–11.

80. Pass HI, Doppman JL, Nieman L, et al. Management of the ectopic ACTH syndrome due to thoracic carcinoids. Ann Thorac Surg 1990;50:52–7.

81. Pearse AG, Takor T. Embryology of the diffuse neuroendocrine system and its relationship to the common peptides. Fed Proc 1979;38:2288–94.

82. Phillips JI, Murray J, Verhaart S. Squamous cell carcinoma with anemone cell features. Ultrastruct Pathol 1987;11:47–52.

83. Pinsker KL, Messinger N, Hurwitz P, Becker NH. Cervical chemodectoma with extensive pulmonary metastases. Chest 1973;64:116–8.

84. Prior JT. Minute peripheral pulmonary tumors. Observations on their histogenesis. Am J Pathol 1953;29:703–12.

85. Prior JT, Bonk JP. Pulmonary tumorlet with coin lesion symptom. N Y State J Med 1978;78:2086–8.

86. Ranchod M. The histogenesis and development of pulmonary tumorlets. Cancer 1977;39:1135–45.

87. _____, Levine GD. Spindle-cell carcinoid tumors of the lung: a clinicopathologic study of 35 cases. Am J Surg Pathol 1980;4:315–31.

88. Reddy V, Gattuso P, Reyes CV, Chinoy M. Amphicrine carcinoma of the lung. Diagnosis by fine needle aspiration cytology. Cytopathology 1990;1:45–8.

89. Rodgers-Sullivan RF, Weiland LH, Palumbo PJ, Hepper NG. Pulmonary tumorlets associated with Cushing's syndrome. Am Rev Respir Dis 1978;117:799–806.

90. Shamsuddin AM, Edelman B, Nguyen TH, Toker C. Multifocal malignant pheochromocytoma presenting as a lung tumor. Hum Pathol 1981;12:475–8.

91. Singh G, Lee RE, Brooks DH. Primary pulmonary paraganglioma: report of a case and review of the literature. Cancer 1977;40:2286–9.

92. Skinner C, Ewen SW. Carcinoid lung: diffuse pulmonary infiltration by a multifocal bronchial carcinoid. Thorax 1976;31:212–9.

93. Sklar JL, Churg A, Bensch KG. Oncocytic carcinoid tumor of the lung. Am J Surg Pathol 1980;4:287–92.

94. Spain DM, Parsonnet V. Multiple origin of minute bronchiolargenic carcinomas. Cancer 1951;4:277–85.

95. Stamatis G, Freitag L, Greschuchna D. Limited and radical resection for tracheal and bronchopulmonary carcinoid tumour. Report on 227 cases. Eur J Cardiothorac Surg 1990;4:527–32.

96. Szyfelbein WM, Ross JS. Carcinoids, atypical carcinoids, and small-cell carcinomas of the lung: differential diagnosis of fine-needle aspiration biopsy specimens. Diagn Cytopathol 1988;4:1–8.

97. Tateishi R. Distribution of argyrophil cells in adult human lungs. Arch Pathol 1973;96:198–202.

98. Thunnissen FB, Van Eijk J, Baak JP, et al. Bronchopulmonary carcinoids and regional lymph node metastases. A quantitative pathologic investigation. Am J Pathol 1988;132:119–22.

99. Torikata C. Tumorlets of the lung—an ultrastructural study. Ultrastruct Pathol 1991;15:189–95.

100. Travis WD, Linnoila RI, Tsokos MG, et al. Neuroendocrine tumors of the lung with proposed criteria for large-cell neuroendocrine carcinoma. An ultrastructural, immunohistochemical, and flow cytometric study of 35 cases. Am J Surg Pathol 1991;15:529–53.

101. Tsutsumi Y, Osamura RY, Watanabe K, Yanaihara N. Immunohistochemical studies on gastrin-releasing peptide- and adrenocorticotropic hormone-containing cells in the human lung. Lab Invest 1983;48:623–32.

102. Veilleux M, Bernier JP, Lamarche JB. Paraneoplastic encephalomyelitis and subacute dysautonomia due to an occult atypical carcinoid tumour of the lung. Can J Neurol Sci 1990;17:324–8.

103. Warren WH, Gould VE. Long-term follow-up of classical bronchial carcinoid tumors. Clinicopathologic observations. Scand J Thorac Cardiovasc Surg 1990;24:125–30.

104. Warren WH, Memoli VA, Gould VE. Well differentiated and small cell neuroendocrine carcinomas of the lung. Two related but distinct clinicopathologic entities. Virchows Arch [Cell Pathol] 1988;55:299–310.

105. Watanabe H, Kobayashi H, Honma K, Ohnishi Y, Iwafuchi M. Diffuse panbronchiolitis with multiple tumorlets. A quantitative study of the Kultschitzky cells and the clusters. Acta Pathol Jpn 1985;35:1221–31.

106. Weeks DA, Beckwith JB, Mierau GW. Rhabdoid tumor. An entity or a phenotype?. Arch Pathol Lab Med 1989;113:113–4.

107. _____, Beckwith JB, Mierau GW, Zuppan CW. Renal neoplasms mimicking rhabdoid tumor of kidney. A report from the National Wilms' Tumor Study Pathology Center. Am J Surg Pathol 1991;15:1042–54.

108. Whitwell F. Tumourlets of the lung. J Pathol Bacteriol 1955;70:529–41.

109. Wick MR, Berg LC, Hertz MI. Large cell carcinoma of the lung with neuroendocrine differentiation. A comparison with large cell "undifferentiated": pulmonary tumors. Am J Clin Pathol 1992;97:796–805.

110. Yellin A, Benfield JR. Pneumothorax associated with lymphoma. Am Rev Respir Dis 1986;134:590–2.

111. Yousem SA, Taylor SR. Typical and atypical carcinoid tumors of lung: a clinicopathologic and DNA analysis of 20 tumors. Mod Pathol 1990;3:502–7.

112. Zárate A, Kovacs K, Flores M, Morán C, Félix I. ACTH and CRF-producing bronchial carcinoid associated with Cushing's syndrome. Clin Endocrinol (Oxf) 1986;24:523–9.

18

HAMARTOMA

Definition. Hamartoma is defined as an abnormal mixture of tissue elements, or an abnormal proportion of a single element, normally present in an organ (14). *Pulmonary hamartoma* refers to a mass consisting of varying combinations of cartilage, connective tissue, fat, smooth muscle, and respiratory epithelium derived from entrapped lung epithelium. Despite the name, hamartoma of lung is now considered to be a benign neoplasm derived from peribronchial mesenchyme, so that an alternative name, *mesenchymoma*, has been proposed (17). We will continue to use the term hamartoma in this Fascicle because of its familiarity to both clinicians and pathologists. Pulmonary hamartoma has also been called *hamartochondroma, chondromatous hamartoma, adenochondroma,* and *fibroadenoma of lung* (1,16,17).

Clinical Features. The population incidence of pulmonary hamartoma is 0.25 percent (8). Pulmonary hamartomas are reported in males two to four times as often as in females. Despite the name, they are rare in children, typically occurring in adult life (peak age in the sixth decade) and progressively increasing in size after discovery (2,6,8,17). They can be divided into parenchymal and central en-

dobronchial types (2). *Parenchymal hamartoma* is more frequent, usually measures less than 4 cm in diameter, and typically presents as an asymptomatic round nodule in the lung periphery on routine chest X ray films or at autopsy. By contrast, central or *endobronchial hamartoma* produces symptoms due to airway obstruction, such as cough, hemoptysis, dyspnea, or obstructive pneumonia (1,2,11). Most hamartomas are solitary, but multiple lesions can occur (7,9).

Hamartomas account for 7 to 14 percent of pulmonary coin lesions (17). A characteristic popcorn pattern of calcification on X ray films is seen in up to 30 percent of cases.

Gross Findings. Pulmonary parenchymal hamartomas typically present as a solitary (or occasionally multiple), well-circumscribed, bulging, white or grey nodule with a cartilaginous consistency (fig. 18-1). They measure from 1 to 7 cm (average, 2 cm) in diameter (17). The nodule or mass often contains gritty flecks of calcium and bone. Most parenchymal hamartomas do not have an obvious connection to a bronchus and typically shell out easily from the surrounding lung.

Endobronchial hamartomas represent only 10 to 20 percent of all hamartomas (17). They are

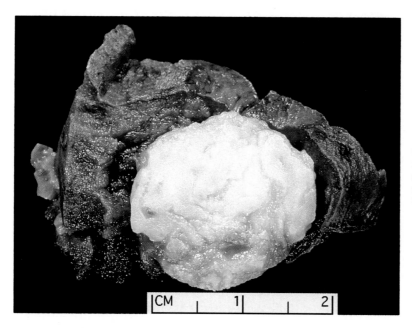

Figure 18-1
GROSS APPEARANCE OF
PARENCHYMAL HAMARTOMA
The surrounding lung falls away from the well-circumscribed mass, a typical feature of these lesions. The hamartoma shows a variegated yellow and white appearance, which corresponds respectively to fat and cartilage.

319

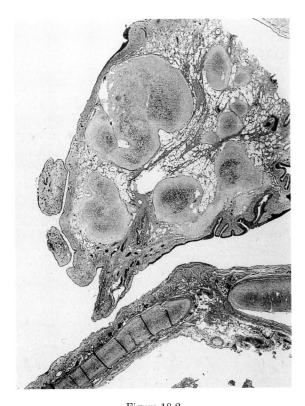

Figure 18-2
ENDOBRONCHIAL HAMARTOMA
The lesion protrudes into the bronchial lumen as a polypoid nodule composed of islands of cartilage and fat.

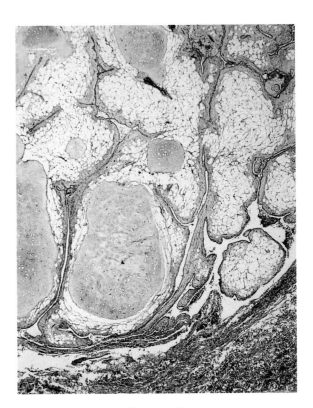

Figure 18-3
PULMONARY PARENCHYMAL HAMARTOMA
This hamartoma is well circumscribed with islands of cartilage readily visible. At its periphery, respiratory epithelial-lined clefts can be seen. However, a bronchus is typically not found in these parenchymal lesions.

usually broad-based, lobulated nodules within the lumen of a large bronchus (fig. 18-2). Distal obstructive or golden pneumonia, or atelectasis can also be present.

Microscopic Findings. Pulmonary parenchymal hamartomas are generally well circumscribed and composed predominantly of cartilage (fig. 18-3). Other components include fibromyxoid connective tissue, fat, bone, and smooth muscle, in descending order of abundance (1,2,17). The cartilage is usually centrally located and consists of irregular, broad masses (figs. 18-3, 18-4). It is surrounded by the other mesenchymal elements, such as islands of fat, strands of smooth muscle, and a rim of fibromyxoid connective tissue. At the periphery of the lesion, there are usually in-branching, cleft-like spaces of variable length lined by ciliated, nonciliated, and mucus-producing epithelium (fig. 18-5). In parenchymal hamartomas, this epithelial component, which apparently de-

rives from entrapped respiratory epithelium, may be prominent, but evidence of an originating bronchus is usually absent. Occasionally, cartilage is completely absent, and the dominant element is fat, a primitive fibromyxoid stroma, or smooth muscle (figs. 18-6–18-8). Still, a mixture of two or more of the these mesenchymal elements is present to support the diagnosis of hamartoma. The surrounding lung may show obstructive pneumonia.

In central or endobronchial lesions, a similar mixture of mesenchymal tissues can be seen, but fat may be more abundant and there is constant association with the bronchial wall (fig. 18-9). Seromucous glands may be present superficial to the hamartomatous mass, while epithelial inclusions similar to those seen in parenchymal hamartomas may also be found. Sometimes, the cartilage shows cytologic atypia in the form of increased cellularity and nuclear hyperchromasia.

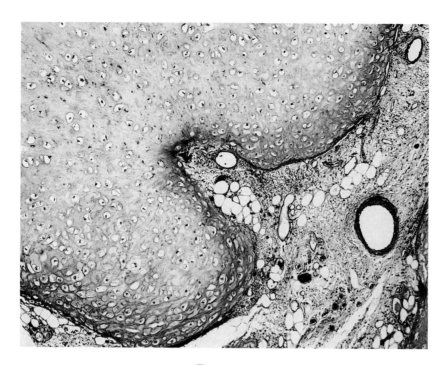

Figure 18-4
PULMONARY PARENCHYMAL HAMARTOMA
An irregular, broad island of central cartilage shows an outer rim of fat and primitive mesenchyme.

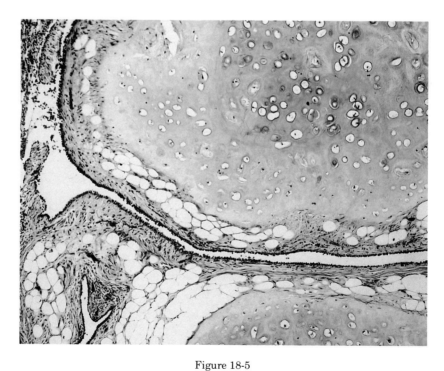

Figure 18-5
PULMONARY PARENCHYMAL HAMARTOMA
The periphery of the lesion shows a deeply invaginated, cleft-like space lined by cuboidal (predominantly respiratory) epithelium.

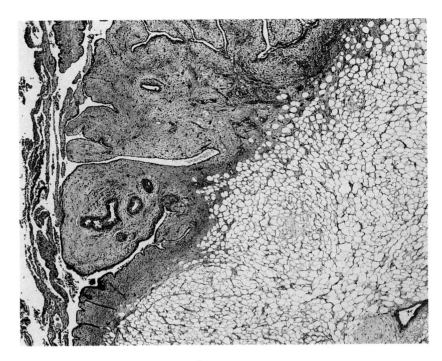

Figure 18-6
PULMONARY PARENCHYMAL HAMARTOMA COMPOSED LARGELY OF FAT
This unusual variant of hamartoma consists of a mixture of fibromyxoid stroma and fat, without evidence of cartilage.

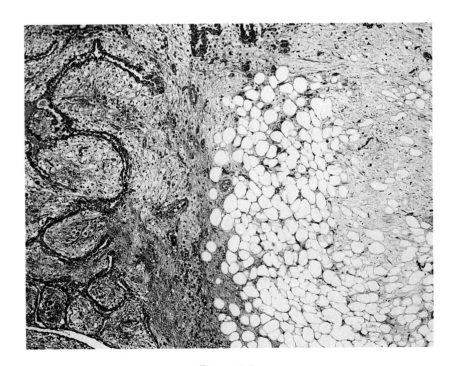

Figure 18-7
PULMONARY PARENCHYMAL HAMARTOMA COMPOSED LARGELY OF FAT
Higher magnification of case shown in figure 18-6. A fibromyxoid stroma surrounds an island of fat and extends into the border of the hamartoma. Note the typical branching epithelial-lined clefts.

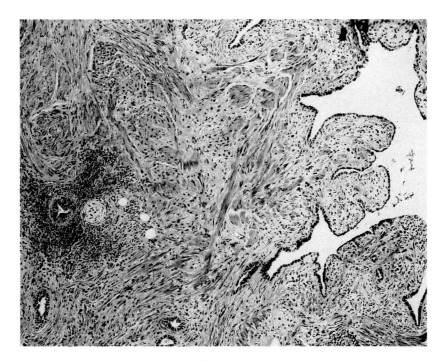

Figure 18-8
PULMONARY PARENCHYMAL HAMARTOMA SHOWING EXTENSIVE SMOOTH MUSCLE COMPONENT
The lesion demonstrates peripheral entrapment of glandular elements, numerous bundles of smooth muscle, and a small amount of admixed fat.

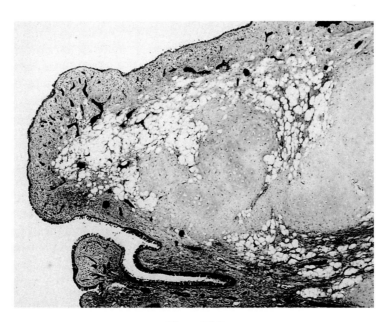

Figure 18-9
BRONCHIAL HAMARTOMA
The lesion protrudes as a broad-based polyp into the bronchial lumen. There is relatively abundant fat but also large islands of cartilage.

Ultrastructural Findings. The cells within the cartilage show the typical ultrastructural features of cartilage, while the stromal spindle cells are primitive mesenchymal cells (15). The epithelium is composed of a mixture of airway cell types including ciliated respiratory cells, mucin-secreting cells, and Clara cells; even occasional type 2 pneumocytes are reported.

Cytologic Findings. Needle aspiration biopsy can be used to establish the diagnosis of hamartoma in 86 percent of cases (6). Sputum cytology is usually of little diagnostic use (8).

Differential Diagnosis. Bronchial chondromas occur in young patients, primarily women, in the setting of Carney triad (chapter 20) (3). The triad consists of pulmonary chondromas, gastric epithelioid tumors, and extra-adrenal paragangliomas (particularly of head and neck) (3,10,13). On occasion, only two elements of the triad, such as gastric and pulmonary tumors, are present. Chondromas can also occur in lung as an isolated finding in patients without Carney triad. Chondromas, by definition, arise from and lie in continuity with bronchial cartilage, a feature not typical of hamartomas, and they lack the mixture of mesenchymal elements (fat, smooth muscle, or immature fibromyxoid tissue) found in hamartomas.

Glandular inclusions that simulate those of hamartomas are found in both benign and low-grade malignant mesenchymal tumors of the lung such as leiomyomatous or fibroleiomyomatous proliferations. These are termed *leiomyomatous hamartoma* or *benign metastasizing leiomyoma*, depending on whether one considers them to be hormonally-induced hyperplasias (5) or slow-growing sarcomas metastatic to lung (18) (see chapter 20). The term leiomyomatous hamartoma seems a poor choice here, not only because of the disputed histogenesis of these smooth muscle proliferations but also because it increases the possibility for confusion with pulmonary hamartoma. Microscopically, these lesions consist of multiple, or occasionally, solitary circumscribed nodules of smooth muscle that often contain spaces lined by respiratory epithelium similar to that found in hamartomas (18). Still, they lack other mesenchymal elements, such as cartilage, fat, or fibromyxoid connective tissue, that are typical of pulmonary hamartomas.

When a hamartoma consists largely of fat, lipoma should be considered. This is discussed further in chapter 20, but once again, it is the admixture of different mesenchymal elements that suggests hamartoma.

As noted above, central bronchial hamartomas sometimes show the cellularity and cytologic atypia of chondrosarcoma (chapter 20). Not only are chondrosarcomas of lung exceedingly rare, but the presence of other differentiated mesenchymal elements of mature histologic appearance supports a diagnosis of hamartoma.

Chondromatous hamartomas are readily distinguished from so-called mesenchymal cystic hamartomas or cystic blastomas. A cambium layer of embryonic mesenchyme underlying epithelial-lined cysts is typical of these lesions and is not seen in hamartomas. Further, when cartilage, fat, or muscle is present in cystic blastomas, it is immature or frankly malignant.

There are a few reported cases of placental transmogrification of lung, a papillary and cystic lesion that bears both gross and microscopic resemblance to placental villi (4). The papillae contain blood vessels, lymphoid nodules, smooth muscle, and fat, but the papillary and cystic appearances differ from hamartomas. The lesion may be a peculiar complication of emphysema and bullae.

Treatment and Prognosis. Pulmonary hamartomas grow slowly, ranging from 1 to 10 mm per year according to serial chest X rays (7,8). Adenocarcinomas arising in or adjacent to hamartomas are exceptional (12). The typical treatment is conservative surgery: wedge resection or enucleation of peripheral lesions and sleeve excision of endobronchial lesions. Lobectomy may be necessary because of the size and location of a hamartoma and the presence of recurrent obstructive pneumonia.

REFERENCES

1. Bateson EM. Relationship between intrapulmonary and endobronchial cartilage-containing tumours (so-called hamartomata). Thorax 1965;20:447–61.

2. Butler C, Kleinerman J. Pulmonary hamartoma. Arch Pathol 1969;88:584–92.

3. Carney JA. The triad of gastric epithelioid leiomyosarcoma, pulmonary chondroma, and functioning extra-adrenal paraganglioma: a five year review. Medicine (Baltimore) 1983;62:159–69.

4. Fidler MY, Koomen M, Sebek B, Greco MA, Rizk CC, Askin FB. Placental transmogrification of the lung: a clinicopathologic study of three further cases [Abstract]. Mod Pathol 1993;6:130A

5. Gal AA, Brooks JS, Pietra GG. Leiomyomatous neoplasms of the lung: a clinical, histologic, and immunohistochemical study. Mod Pathol 1989;2:209–16.

6. Hamper UM, Khouri NF, Stitik FP, Siegelman SS. Pulmonary hamartoma: diagnosis by transthoracic needle-aspiration biopsy. Radiology 1985;155:15–8.

7. King TE, Christopher KL, Schwarz MI. Multiple pulmonary chondromatous hamartomas. Hum Pathol 1982;13:496–7.

8. Koutras P, Urschel HJ Jr, Paulson DL. Hamartoma of the lung. J Thor Cardiovasc Surg 1971;61:768–76.

9. Minasian H. Uncommon pulmonary hamartomas. Thorax 1977;32:360–4.

10. Perez-Atayde AR, Shamberger RC, Kozakewich HW. Neuroectodermal differentiation of the gastrointestinal tumors in the Carney triad. Am J Surg Pathol 1993;17:706–14.

11. Poirier TJ, Van Ordstrand HS. Pulmonary chondromatous hamartomas: report of seventeen cases and review of the literature. Chest 1971;59:50–5.

12. Poulsen JT, Jacobsen M, Francis D. Probable malignant transformation of a pulmonary hamartoma. Thorax 1979;34:557–8.

13. Raafat F, Salman WD, Roberts K, Ingram L, Rees R, Mann JR. Carney's triad: gastric leiomyosarcoma, pulmonary chondroma and extra-adrenal paraganglioma in young females. Histopathology 1986;10:1325–33.

14. Stedman's Medical Dictionary, 24th ed., s. v. "hamartoma."

15. Stone FJ, Churg AM. The ultrastructure of pulmonary hamartoma. Cancer 1977;39:1064–70.

16. Tomashefski JF Jr. Benign endobronchial mesenchymal tumors: their relationship to parenchymal pulmonary hamartomas. Am J Surg Pathol 1982;6:531–40.

17. van den Bosch JM, Wagenaar SS, Corrin B, Westermann CJ. Mesenchymoma of the lung (so-called hamartoma): a review of 154 parenchymal and endobronchial cases. Thorax 1987;42:790–3.

18. Wolff M, Kaye G, Silva F. Pulmonary metastases (with admixed epithelial elements) from smooth muscle neoplasms. Report of nine cases, including three males. Am J Surg Pathol 1979;3:325–42.

19

FIBROUS AND FIBROHISTIOCYTIC TUMORS
AND TUMOR-LIKE CONDITIONS

INFLAMMATORY PSEUDOTUMOR (PLASMA CELL GRANULOMA-HISTIOCYTOMA COMPLEX)

Definition. Inflammatory pseudotumor is a circumscribed, usually single, tumefactive lesion that destroys the underlying lung architecture and is composed of a variable mixture of collagen, inflammatory cells, and benign mesenchymal cells, including spindled myofibroblasts, fibroblasts, plasma cells, lymphocytes, foam cells, giant cells, and macrophages. The histologic spectrum that results can be divided into two major categories: fibrohistiocytic and plasma cell granuloma subtypes. Although most lesions can be placed in one of these categories, individual cases may have microscopic features that overlap more than one group; this, as well as similarities in the clinical presentation and behavior between the groups, suggests that they be treated as one clinicopathologic entity (26). Spencer (29), in appreciation of this, used the term *plasma cell granuloma-histiocytoma complex* as a synonym for inflammatory pseudotumor to suggest the histologic spectrum of disease.

As might be expected, the polymorphous microscopic appearance of inflammatory pseudotumors has also led to a variety of other diagnostic terms: *fibroxanthoma, histiocytoma, xanthofibroma, xanthoma, xanthogranuloma, sclerosing hemangioma* (a misnomer), and *mast cell granuloma*. We view these as outdated terms. Recent synonyms for plasma cell granuloma include *inflammatory myofibroblastic tumor* (26) and *inflammatory pseudotumor, lymphoplasmacytic type* (21). For this Fascicle, we will use the term plasma cell granuloma, since it is deeply embedded in the literature.

Inflammatory pseudotumors occur principally in lung but lesions with the same name have been reported in almost every organ system in the body as well as in the mediastinum and retroperitoneum (12).

Clinical Features. Patients range in age from 1 to 77 years, but approximately 60 percent are under the age of 40 years (3,21,26). Inflammatory pseudotumors account for the majority (56 percent) of benign lung "tumors" in children (10). There is no sex predilection (21).

Most patients (44 to 74 percent) present with an asymptomatic mass found in a routine chest X ray. Symptoms, when present, include cough, fever, chest pain, hemoptysis, and shortness of breath. A history of an antecedent respiratory infection is obtained in 5 to 50 percent of adults and up to 20 percent of children. This is significant in view of the suggestion that these lesions arise from preexisting pulmonary infections.

The chest X ray shows a solitary, well-defined mass in nearly 70 percent of cases. Other roentgenologic findings include a solitary, poorly circumscribed mass with spiculation, pneumonic consolidation and atelectasis, multiple (up to three) separate lesions (26), and involvement of both lung and mediastinum (3). Infrequently, focal calcification or cavitation may be found. Follow-up chest films usually show the mass to be constant in size or to grow smaller, but slow enlargement occurs in less than 10 percent of cases. The most frequent clinical diagnosis in adults is carcinoma.

Routine cultures of sputum and tissue for organisms are negative. There are reports of an endobronchial location with subsequent obstructive pneumonia (2,34). In about 30 percent of cases, the diagnosis can be made by bronchoscopic biopsy (23).

Gross Findings. The lesions are typically solitary, round, well-circumscribed but unencapsulated intrapulmonary masses (fig. 19-1). Rarely, they show poor circumscription. They vary in diameter from 0.8 to 36 cm (3); most are 1 to 6 cm (26). In about 12 percent of cases, they occur as polypoid endobronchial masses (fig. 19-2)(21). Inflammatory pseudotumors (usually the plasma cell granuloma subtype) grossly penetrate the pleura and extend into adjacent mediastinal structures in about 6 percent of cases.

Tumor color varies depending on the major histologic component. Lesions rich in xanthoma cells and lipid are yellow; those with large numbers of

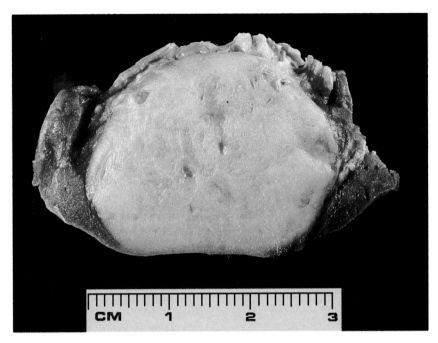

Figure 19-1
GROSS APPEARANCE OF INFLAMMATORY PSEUDOTUMOR
This lesion is a fibroxanthoma rich in lipid, imparting a distinct yellow color. Note the sharp demarcation from surrounding lung.

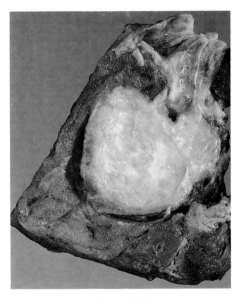

Figure 19-2
INFLAMMATORY PSEUDOTUMOR IMPINGING ON
A BRONCHUS

The lesion presented as a broad-based mass protruding into the bronchial lumen, but the cut section shows an "iceberg" configuration with much of the mass actually within lung parenchyma. Note the sharp demarcation between it and lung, from which the lesion was easily shelled out.

plasma cells and lymphocytes are tan; and those with abundant fibrous connective tissue are white (fig. 19-1). Foci of red or brown, denoting areas of recent or old hemorrhage, are common (29). Calcification and small foci of necrosis can be seen in up to 10 percent of cases.

Microscopic Findings. At low magnification, peripheral lesions are usually circumscribed, with a pushing border but no capsule (fig. 19-3) (36). Small numbers of residual airways or vessels may be present, particularly at the periphery of the lesion, but the alveolar parenchyma underlying the lesion is largely destroyed. Masson bodies, typical of organized or organizing pneumonia, can be present at the margin of the lesion (21). Endobronchial pseudotumors often have a polypoid or sessile appearance.

In general, inflammatory pseudotumors consist of a mixture of chronic inflammatory cells, particularly plasma cells; lymphocytes; macrophages; a few eosinophils; fibroblasts; and fibrous connective tissue. The mix of these components vary, and has allowed separation of the lesions into two broad categories, but there can also be considerable overlap in a given case (21,29).

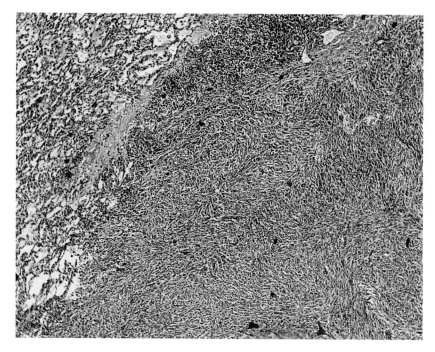

Figure 19-3
INFLAMMATORY PSEUDOTUMOR, FIBROHISTIOCYTIC TYPE
The alveolar architecture within the lesion is obliterated, a characteristic finding in inflammatory pseudotumors. Note the sharp demarcation from surrounding lung. A thin pseudocapsule is present focally at the margin of the lesion.

The *fibrohistiocytic* subtype of inflammatory pseudotumor consists of spindle cells (myofibroblasts and fibroblasts), collagen, macrophages, foamy macrophages (xanthoma cells), and Touton giant cells (fig. 19-4). The spindle cells are arrayed in a characteristic pinwheel or storiform pattern (figs. 19-4, 19-5) (21,25). They are typically admixed with a variable number of lymphocytes and plasma cells (fig. 19-5) (32). There may be prominent foci of xanthoma cells (fig. 19-6). Touton giant cells may be abundant (fig. 19-7). Rarely, histiocytes predominate without spindle cells (*benign histiocytic tumor of lung*) (14). Foci of osseous metaplasia and calcification can also be present. Mitoses are infrequent and extensive necrosis and cellular anaplasia are unusual; when present they point to diagnoses other than inflammatory pseudotumor (see Differential Diagnosis). The lipid found in the xanthomatous lesions consists of ethanolamine and N-acetyl neuraminic acid. It is believed to be endogenous in origin (16,37).

The *plasma cell granuloma* subtype shows a mixture of spindled fibroblasts, myofibroblasts, collagen, and inflammatory cells, principally lymphocytes and abundant plasma cells (fig. 19-8). The term granuloma in this context is misleading, since epithelioid cells, multinucleated giant cells of Langhans or foreign body types, or granulomas are not seen. The spindled cells may be arrayed in long columns or in short interlacing fascicles (fig 19-9). They usually have oval, plump nuclei with small nucleoli and eosinophilic cytoplasm. Mild nuclear atypia is occasionally present. Clusters of plasma cells, some with Mott or Russell bodies, are admixed with lymphocytes (fig. 19-9). Lymphoid follicles are sometimes seen at the margin of the lesion. Other inflammatory cells, including foamy macrophages, neutrophils, eosinophils, and surprisingly large numbers of mast cells, can also be found.

While fibrous connective tissue is a component of most inflammatory pseudotumors, largely sclerotic or fibrosed inflammatory pseudotumors may occur (fig. 19-10). In addition, some idiopathic focal organizing pneumonias may take on the appearance of pseudotumors when they show central loss of alveolar

329

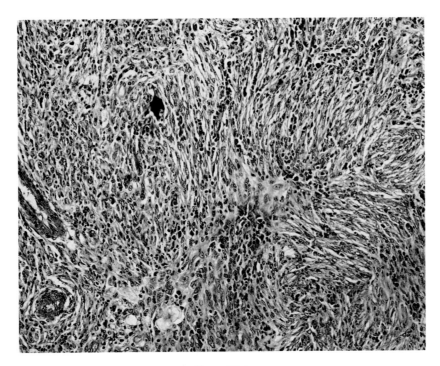

Figure 19-4
INFLAMMATORY PSEUDOTUMOR, FIBROHISTIOCYTIC TYPE

A spindle cell population with a distinct storiform (pinwheel) appearance is typical of this form of pseudotumor. A scattering of small, dark, chronic inflammatory cells and a few foamy cells can also be appreciated.

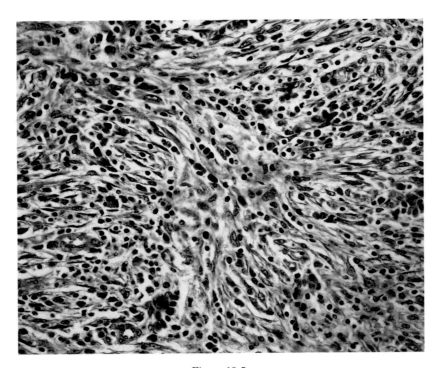

Figure 19-5
INFLAMMATORY PSEUDOTUMOR, FIBROHISTIOCYTIC TYPE

Higher magnification of lesion in figure19-4. Note again the distinct pinwheel pattern of the spindled fibroblastic cells and the diffuse admixture of chronic inflammatory cells that are hallmarks of this particular lesion.

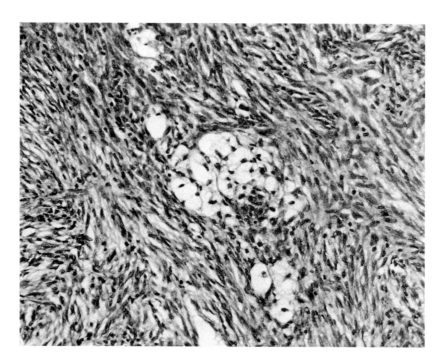

Figure 19-6
INFLAMMATORY PSEUDOTUMOR, FIBROHISTIOCYTIC TYPE
Well-delimited foci of xanthoma cells are present.

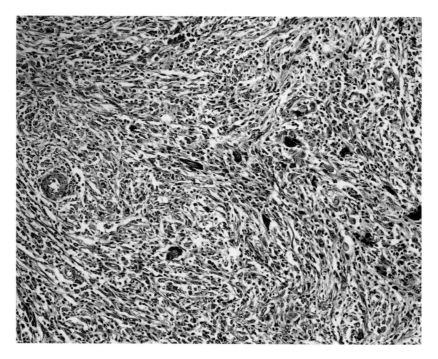

Figure 19-7
INFLAMMATORY PSEUDOTUMOR, FIBROHISTIOCYTIC TYPE
Numerous Touton giant cells are scattered haphazardly among the spindle cells.

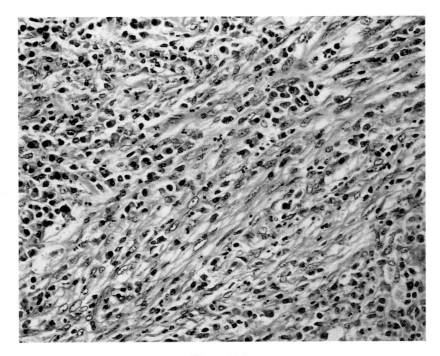

Figure 19-8
INFLAMMATORY PSEUDOTUMOR, PLASMA CELL GRANULOMA TYPE
Numerous plasma cells are interspersed among spindled fibroblastic cells arranged in fascicles.

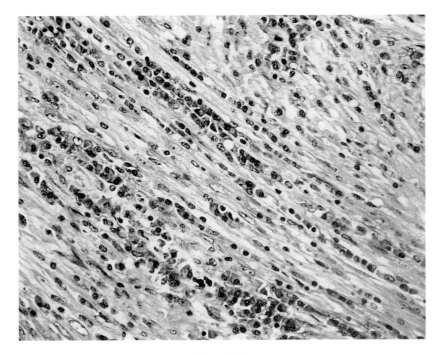

Figure 19-9
INFLAMMATORY PSEUDOTUMOR, PLASMA CELL GRANULOMA TYPE
Fascicles of spindled fibroblasts/myofibroblasts course through the field. Plasma cells are arrayed linearly and in clusters along the course of the spindled cells.

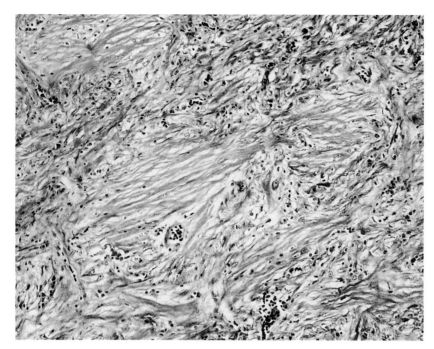

Figure 19-10
INFLAMMATORY
PSEUDOTUMOR WITH
EXTENSIVE FIBROSIS
In this example, the pseudotumor
might have shown fibrohistiocytic or
plasma cell granuloma features earlier
in the clinical course.

architecture (figs. 19-11–19-13) (see Focal Organizing Pneumonia, chapter 24) (6,21). Matsubara and associates (21) have used the term *inflammatory pseudotumor, organizing pneumonia type* for some of these cases. The authors prefer to restrict the term inflammatory pseudotumor to those cases in which the inflammatory process extensively obliterates lung parenchyma.

Abscesses are unusual in inflammatory pseudotumors and should suggest alternative diagnoses, such as infection. Small zones of infarct-like necrosis can occur in up to 15 percent of pseudotumors (21). Eosinophils may be present in the tissue adjacent to such areas.

Infiltration of small peripheral vessels, particularly veins, by lymphocytes and plasma cells is common, and thrombosis and recanalization of vessels may occur. Warter and associates (36) also reported luminal invasion of pulmonary vessels at a distance from the main mass. One of their patients died following extension of plasma cell granuloma into pulmonary veins and pericardium. Microscopic invasion of pleura and involvement of mediastinum can also occur. In these cases, the lesions are appropriately considered to be plasma cell granulomas when they are cytologically bland, but if they show cellularity or cytologic atypia, the possibility of inflammatory fibrosarcoma must be considered (see Differential Diagnosis).

Ultrastructural and Immunohistochemical Findings. Ultrastructurally, inflammatory pseudotumors consist of numerous myofibroblasts and fibroblasts with an admixture of lymphocytes, plasma cells, macrophages, and entrapped pneumocytes (4,15,26–28). Endothelial cells of small vessels and pericytes have also been reported (4).

Immunohistochemical studies demonstrate vimentin, muscle-specific actin, and focally, desmin within the cytoplasm of the spindle cells, findings in keeping with myofibroblastic differentiation. Staining for cytokeratin may be present, but it is probably due to staining of entrapped bronchoalveolar cells. Staining for lysozyme and alpha-1-antichymotrypsin may be prominent when xanthoma cells are abundant. The plasma cells are typically polyclonal (23,26,33,36).

Cytology. The cytologic appearance of inflammatory pseudotumor is rarely described. Bronchoscopic brushings in one case yielded short, spindled cells with basophilic cytoplasm and enlarged, mildly atypical, oval nuclei (35). The cells are usually arrayed in a storiform pattern. Fine needle aspiration biopsies have also been performed in a small number of cases (17). They show a mixture of histiocytes, fibroblasts, lymphocytes, and

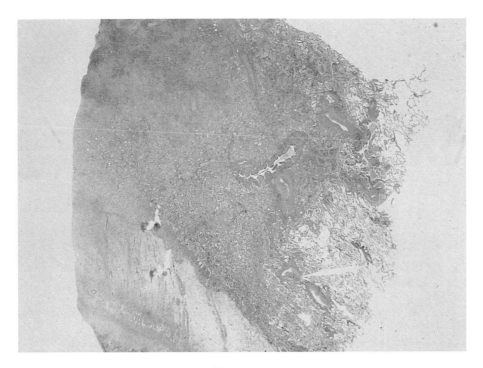

Figure 19-11
FOCAL ORGANIZING PNEUMONIA
A localized unencapsulated area of consolidation is present. (Figures 9-11–9-13 are from the same case.)

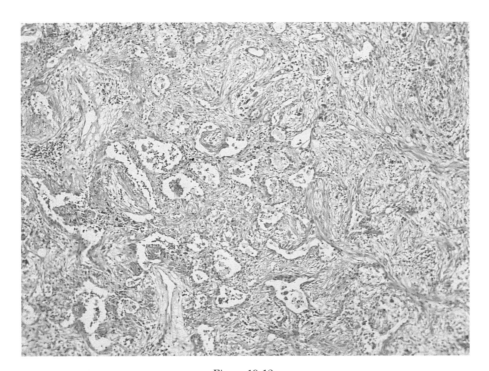

Figure 19-12
FOCAL ORGANIZING PNEUMONIA
Much of the lesion shows typical features of an interstitial and organized pneumonia, with polypoid tufts of fibrous tissue in the alveoli.

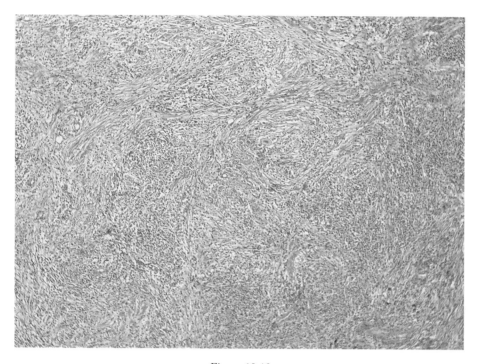

Figure 19-13
FOCAL ORGANIZING PNEUMONIA
The center of the lesion shows a focus of obliteration of the underlying alveolar structure with replacement by an inflammatory fibrous mass, reminiscent of the features seen in pseudotumor.

plasma cells. There may also be isolated atypical cells with characteristics of both histiocytes and fibroblasts. These findings should be viewed as nonspecific, since inflammatory lesions of diverse origin may produce the same appearance. Surgical biopsy remains the most accurate method of making a diagnosis of inflammatory pseudotumor.

Differential Diagnosis. Each of the categories of pseudotumor presents its own differential diagnostic problems.

Fibrohistiocytic Variant. The histologic resemblance of the fibrohistiocytic variant to fibrous histiocytoma of the soft tissues, the enlargement of the lesions in a minority of cases, and rare reports of recurrence and invasion raise the possibility that some "pseudotumors" are actually neoplasms, in particular fibrous histiocytomas that are benign or malignant. For example, Spencer (29) reported two cases of "inflammatory pseudotumor" that had foci suggestive of malignant fibrous histiocytoma. From our own experience and that of others (7,27), there appears to be a small group of

lesions that are true fibrous histiocytomas of lung. These low-grade tumors show the storiform pattern of spindled and Touton-type giant cells of inflammatory pseudotumors, but they further show increased cellularity, loss of the admixed lymphoid component, poor histologic circumscription, focal necrosis, increased mitoses (up to 2 per 50 high-power fields), or invasion of blood vessels (fig. 19-14) (7,9,27). The small number of cases reported to date have had a benign course, but additional experience is necessary to determine their ultimate prognosis and relationship to the invasive "inflammatory pseudotumors" reported in published cases.

If a fibrohistiocytic lesion has a storiform pattern of growth and also demonstrates cellular anaplasia in the form of nuclear hyperchromatism and pleomorphism, bizarre multinucleated cells, necrosis of greater than 15 percent of the tumor, and frequent mitoses (more than 3 per 50 high-power fields) it is best diagnosed as malignant fibrous histiocytoma (discussed later in this chapter) (38). Malignant fibrous histiocytoma more frequently metastasizes to lung from sites in

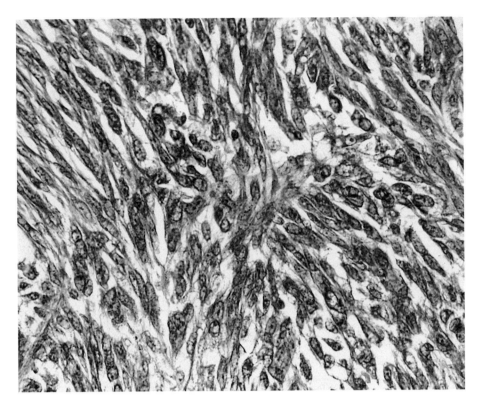

Figure 19-14
DIFFERENTIAL DIAGNOSIS OF INFLAMMATORY PSEUDOTUMOR:
"ATYPICAL FIBROHISTIOCYTIC LESION" OR FIBROUS HISTIOCYTOMA
The lesion shows greater cellularity and less inflammatory infiltrate in comparison to inflammatory pseudotumor, fibrohistiocytic type.

the soft tissues, but it may arise in the lung (30, 38). It typically presents as a solitary large mass.

As for other malignancies, pleomorphic (spindle cell) carcinomas are far more common in lung than malignant fibrous histiocytoma. They may have a prominent storiform pattern with interspersed chronic inflammation (chapter 15). The presence of cellular anaplasia, frequent mitoses, extensive necrosis, extensive angioinvasion, or distant metastasis should alert one to this possibility. A careful search for foci of epithelial differentiation and application of immunohistochemical stains for epithelial markers (e.g., keratin, carcinoembryonic antigen, etc.) support the diagnosis.

Pulmonary hyalinizing granuloma is in the differential diagnosis of sclerosed pseudotumors, but hyalinizing granulomas are usually multiple rather than solitary (chapter 24). In addition, as the name indicates, they have distinctive hyalinization due to lamellar collagen, which is the key to diagnosis. Still, there may be marked chronic inflammation at the periphery of hyalinizing granulomas and areas suggestive of focal organized pneumonia, indicating a possible link between this entity and pseudotumor.

Plasma Cell Granuloma Variant. The plasma cell granuloma subtype must be distinguished from inflammatory fibrosarcoma, a tumor recently described by Meis and Enzinger (22) that may occasionally involve the thorax (fig. 19-15). We have seen several possible examples of this tumor in lung. The tumor is composed of fascicles or whorls of fibroblastic and myofibroblastic cells with admixed plasma cells and variable amounts of collagen. Mitoses are rare, but the tumor is more cellular and the spindle cells show significant nuclear atypia, which are the main differentiating features. Since in a given lesion these features may be focal, we recommend extensive sampling of "plasma cell granulomas," particularly those that are invasive into large vessels, pleura, etc.

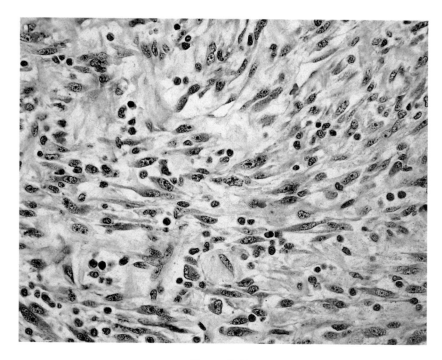

Figure 19-15
DIFFERENTIAL DIAGNOSIS OF PLASMA CELL GRANULOMA: INFLAMMATORY FIBROSARCOMA
These spindled fibroblastic cells show far greater nuclear atypia than is seen in plasma cell granuloma.

Tan-Liu and associates (31) described a rare spindle cell fibroblastic tumor of the major bronchi and trachea under the term *invasive fibrous tumor of the tracheobronchial tree*. Histologically, the tumor invaded the airway wall and consisted of fibroblast-like cells growing in fascicles with a focal storiform pattern, slight to moderate nuclear atypia and enlarged nucleoli, occasional multinucleated cells, and mitotic counts of less than 2 mitoses per 10 high-power fields. The authors noted that the key difference from inflammatory pseudotumor was the absence of an inflammatory component in the form of either xanthoma cells or an intimately admixed lymphoplasmacytic infiltrate. More experience with this lesion is necessary to assure that it is a separate entity.

Extramedullary plasmacytomas are neoplastic proliferations of plasma cells occurring outside of bone (chapter 22). They are exceedingly rare in lung, more commonly occurring in the head and neck (1,13). They may be difficult to distinguish from plasma cell granulomas, particularly in small biopsies or in fine needle aspirates (5,13). Microscopically, they are composed largely of plasma cells, but their nuclear pleomorphism, abundant mitoses, scant fibrous stroma, and monoclonal pattern of staining for immunoglobulin light chains help to distinguish them from plasma cell granuloma.

The term sclerosing hemangioma was at one time a synonym for inflammatory pseudotumor, but it is now recognized as a completely separate entity whose areas of fibrosis, foci of hemorrhage, and aggregates of foamy macrophages only superficially microscopically resemble inflammatory pseudotumor. Sclerosing hemangiomas are either benign neoplasms or hamartomas, possibly arising from epithelial cells (presumably pneumocytes) (see chapter 23). At least in some areas, they show typical interstitial collections of uniform, round or polygonal cells. Ultrastructurally, these cells have a simplified cytoplasm without the features of either myofibroblasts or fibroblasts. Further, they are stained by antibodies for epithelial membrane antigen but not for desmin and muscle-specific actin, as seen in inflammatory pseudotumors.

Treatment and Prognosis. Inflammatory pseudotumor is best treated by surgery. The consensus appears to favor conservative removal of peripheral lesions by segmental resection and of endobronchial nodules by bronchotomy and excision or sleeve resection, with a reasonable margin of uninvolved tissue, but there are dissenting voices (see below). There are even reports of partial excision or biopsy followed by spontaneous disappearance of the lesion on long-term follow-up (20,21). Corticosteroids may also be effective in cases in which, because of location, residual lesion is left after biopsy (8).

Most pseudotumors remain constant in size or shrink, but up to 10 percent grow slowly over years (2,3) or even enlarge rapidly (36). In fact, inflammatory pseudotumors (usually reported as plasma cell granulomas) can invade pulmonary veins (36), pleura (19), chest wall (24), hilum, spine (11), or mediastinum. Warter and associates (36), noting this aggressive behavior, suggested "radical and precocious," rather than conservative, surgical intervention. We suspect that some of these invasive plasma cell granulomas are low-grade inflammatory fibrosarcomas.

The prognosis of completely resected lesions is excellent: between 78 and 100 percent of patients are alive and well after average follow-up periods of 3.3 years (2,3,21). Intrathoracic recurrence is rare (5 percent of cases) (2,3). It usually occurs when a wide margin of excision is not obtained, as when a mass is shelled out or when an endobronchial lesion is treated by sleeve resection with a minimal margin of normal tissue. More aggressive lesions that extend into the mediastinum or chest wall, invade pulmonary veins, or involve airways extensively may become unresectable or, when resectable, may recur and lead to death (18,24,29,36).

INTRAPULMONARY LOCALIZED FIBROUS TUMOR

Definition. Intrapulmonary fibrous tumors are subpleural neoplasms contiguous to visceral pleura, grossly localized, and histologically identical to localized fibrous tumors of the pleura (localized fibrous mesothelioma). In appreciation of this microscopic resemblance, the tumors have been termed *intraparenchymal localized fibrous mesothelioma, intrapulmonary fibrous mesothelioma,* or *"inverted" fibrous tumor of the pleura* (40,41, 45,47). Yousem and Flynn (47) suggested the term *fibroma of lung* for microscopically similar tumors that are close to, but distinct from, the visceral pleura. Because of the histologic similarity to localized fibrous tumors of pleura, we believe that intrapulmonary localized fibrous tumor is the best name. A microscopically cellular and presumably malignant variant exists, but it is difficult to distinguish from fibrosarcoma of lung (40,45).

Clinical Features. An intrapulmonary location for solitary fibrous "mesotheliomas" was mentioned as early as 1942 by Stout and Murray (46). Subsequently, it has become clear that microscopically similar tumors occur in a variety of extrapulmonary locations, including retroperitoneum and mediastinum, as well as the external surfaces of the stomach and small intestine. Still, lung is the most frequent extrapleural location (42). The apparent incidence of lung involvement varies from 3 to 38 percent of cases of solitary fibrous tumors of pleura (40,41,44,45), but the true frequency of entirely intrapulmonary tumors probably lies at the lower end of the scale. For example, in one series, only 7.5 percent of solitary fibrous tumors of the pleura were wholly intrapulmonary (40). From what can be gleaned from these reports, there does not appear to be any distinction between intrapulmonary fibrous tumors and fibrous tumors of the pleura as far as age, sex, and clinical symptoms are concerned. Most patients present with an incidental coin lesion on chest X ray (42,47).

Tumors are removed with a significant margin of lung tissue, typically by segmental resection or lobectomy (44,47).

Although England et al. (41) reported that three of six "inverted" localized fibrous tumors were malignant, other authors noted no recurrence of disease or tumor-induced mortality after admittedly short-term follow-up; the prognosis is not yet accurately defined (40,47).

Gross Findings. Intraparenchymal localized fibrous tumors are usually less than 8 cm in diameter, a size on average smaller than pedunculated extrapulmonary lesions (39,45,47). The tumors are typically round or oval with a smooth covering of visceral pleura. Usually, the mass is contiguous to the pleural surface. The cut surface has a firm, well-circumscribed, white or gray, whorled appearance (fig. 19-16) (39,47).

Microscopic Findings. These tumors microscopically mimic the histologic appearance of fibrous tumors of the pleura. They are subpleural

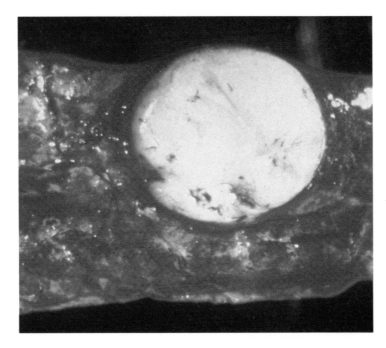

Figure 19-16
GROSS APPEARANCE OF
INTRAPULMONARY FIBROUS TUMOR
The mass is well circumscribed, abuts the
visceral pleura, and is white.

Figure 19-17
INTRAPULMONARY FIBROUS TUMOR
In this view, the tumor is close to, but
does not directly abut, the visceral pleura.

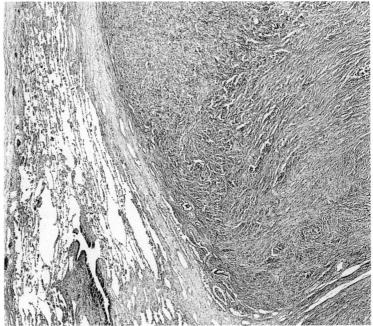

in location and are often broadly attached to the visceral pleura. Still, they may also be separated from it (fig. 19-17). At its advancing margin in lung, there are often branching clefts lined by cuboidal epithelium, presumably replicating alveolar or bronchiolar epithelium, producing a scalloped pattern (fig. 19-18) (47). This phenom- enon of epithelial-lined (mesothelial or type 2 pneumocyte) clefts has also been observed at the base of typical fibrous tumors of the visceral pleura (39–41). In general, the histologic appear- ance of these tumors is identical to fibrous tu- mors of the pleura (fig. 19-19) (42,47). They con- sist of spindle cells with oval nuclei, diffuse fine

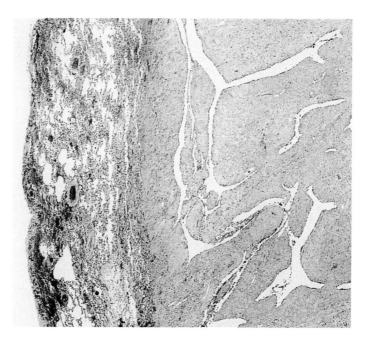

Figure 19-18
INTRAPULMONARY FIBROUS TUMOR
The advancing margin of this tumor, like many slow-growing mesenchymal tumors in lung, shows a scalloped appearance due to entrapment of bronchioloalveolar structures. Once again, the tumor is separate from the visceral pleura in this field.

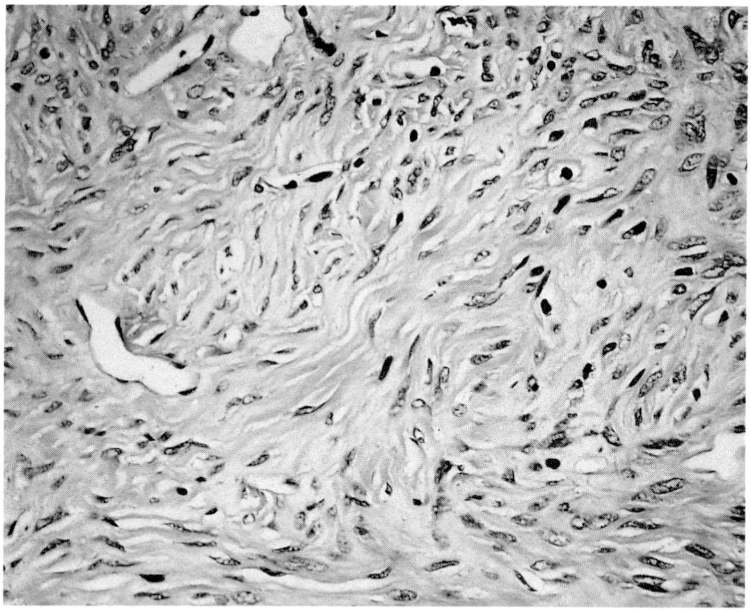

Figure 19-19
INTRAPULMONARY
FIBROUS TUMOR
High magnification view shows spindle tumor cells set among ropy bundles of collagen.

chromatin, and scant cytoplasm (fig. 19-19). The cells are most often arrayed in short fascicles or in a haphazard fashion, but they may have a focal storiform or hemangiopericytomatous pattern. As in the case of fibrous tumors of the pleura, cellularity varies and wiry lamellar collagen separates the spindle cells (fig. 19-20). Cytologic atypia and necrosis are typically absent and mitoses are usually less than 4 per 10 high-power fields.

The tumor cells may contain glycogen. They strongly express vimentin and are often positive for smooth muscle actin, but not keratin, in keeping with a myofibroblastic/fibroblastic phenotype (42,47).

Differential Diagnosis. Some intrapulmonary spindle cell tumors that have a broad visceral pleural attachment are far more cellular than those described above (the relative frequency of

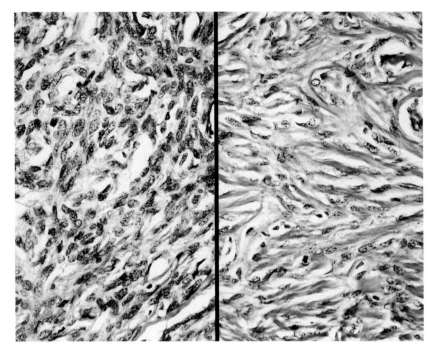

Figure 19-20
INTRAPULMONARY
FIBROUS TUMOR
The two fields show the varia-
tion in cellularity that can be seen
in the same tumor.

the two types is unclear) (40,45). These tumors consist of closely packed oval or spindled cells arranged either randomly or in fascicles; they typically lack a hemangiopericytomatous pattern (40). They may show moderate nuclear pleomorphism, prominent nucleoli, necrosis, giant tumor cells, or increased mitotic counts (4 or more figures per 10 high-power fields), as well as decreased or absent collagen (40,41,45). Whether neoplasms with this microscopic appearance are the intrapulmonary analogue of localized malignant fibrous tumors of the pleura or should be regarded as fibrosarcomas of lung secondarily impinging on visceral pleura is a matter of debate. Guccion and Rosen (43) argued that the aggressive behavior of such tumors (with a tendency towards rapid distant metastasis) significantly differs from that of localized malignant fibrous tumors of pleura and is more in keeping with intrapulmonary sarcomas, an opinion with which we agree.

Intrapulmonary fibrous tumors may be readily confused with inflammatory pseudotumors. While pseudotumors often present as solitary nodules in lung and may show abundant collagenized stroma, they also have an inflammatory component consisting of plasma cells,

macrophages, or xanthoma cells, features that are lacking in intrapulmonary fibrous tumors.

Pulmonary hyalinizing granuloma most frequently presents as multiple ill-defined nodules in lung without a predilection for the pleura, although solitary masses may occur. It has far fewer spindle cells and a more marked inflammatory infiltrate than intrapulmonary fibrous tumor, and histologically it most closely resembles sclerosing mediastinitis (48).

Intrapulmonary fibrous tumors, because they sometimes show prominent lobulation and epithelial clefts, are occasionally confused with hamartomas, but they lack the mixture of other mesenchymal components, such as cartilage, fat, and smooth muscle, that are typical of hamartomas.

Malignant fibrous histiocytomas of lung are easily distinguished from intrapulmonary fibrous tumors. The former show numerous atypical mononuclear and giant tumor cells with a prominent storiform growth pattern, numerous mitoses, and abundant necrosis.

Diffuse malignant fibrous mesotheliomas are readily distinguished by their reactivity for keratin and diffuse pattern of growth over the pleura (42).

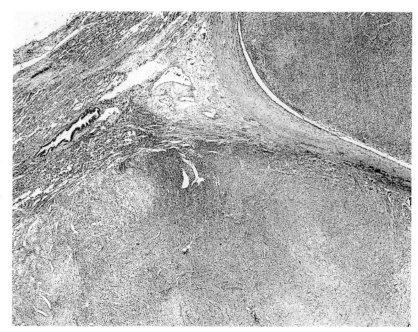

Figure 19-21
MALIGNANT FIBROUS
HISTIOCYTOMA
This lobulated tumor has a pushing border with surrounding lung. (Fig. 1 from Yousem S, Hocholzer L. Malignant fibrous histiocytoma of the lung. Cancer 1987;60:253–41.)

MALIGNANT FIBROUS HISTIOCYTOMA

Definition. Malignant fibrous histiocytoma (MFH) is a sarcoma composed of a polymorphous population of histiocyte-like cells, pleomorphic giant cells, fibroblasts, and undifferentiated mesenchymal cells and having one of several histologic patterns. It is the most common malignant soft tissue tumor of older adults, most frequently involving the extremities, retroperitoneum, and trunk, but it is rare as a primary tumor of lung. By 1988, only about 40 pulmonary cases with supporting electron microscopic or immunohistochemical studies had been reported (50–52,54a).

Clinical Findings. Patients vary from 41 to 75 years, but they are most often in the sixth and seventh decades (54a). The sex ratio is approximately one. Two thirds of patients are symptomatic, reporting cough, chest pain, shortness of breath, hemoptysis, or weight loss.

A correct diagnosis is difficult to make preoperatively. Sputum cytologies are usually negative and bronchoscopy typically shows no gross endobronchial lesions, although brushings may demonstrate malignant cells (51). There is equal difficulty in arriving at a correct frozen section diagnosis.

Chest X rays show a mass lesion. In about 5 percent of cases there is more than one tumor.

There is no predilection for either side of the lung, although the lower lobes are affected more often than the upper ones.

Gross Findings. A solitary mass (rarely, two masses) measuring 2 to 10 cm (median, 4 cm) is found. Frequently, the mass shows foci of yellow necrosis; rarely, it is cavitated. The tumor is typically intraparenchymal or subpleural in location rather than intrabronchial.

Microscopic Findings. The neoplasm may have lobulated, pushing borders as it expands into surrounding lung (fig. 19-21). MFHs in lung have microscopic features similar to those in the soft tissues. The tumor consists of a polymorphous cell population arrayed in a variety of histologic patterns: storiform, pleomorphic, or fascicular, usually in combination (54). The storiform pattern is characterized by spindle cells arranged in a pinwheel or cartwheel fashion (fig. 19-22). The pleomorphic pattern consists of sheet-like growth of spindle cells, histiocyte-like cells, and pleomorphic giant cells. The fascicular pattern consists of parallel arrays of spindle (fibroblast-like) cells; it usually occurs only focally and in association with the other patterns. There are oval and spindle-shaped cells with a fibroblastic appearance, cytologically atypical histiocyte-like cells showing moderate eosinophilic cytoplasm, single vesicular nuclei, irregular-shaped xanthoma cells, and pleomorphic

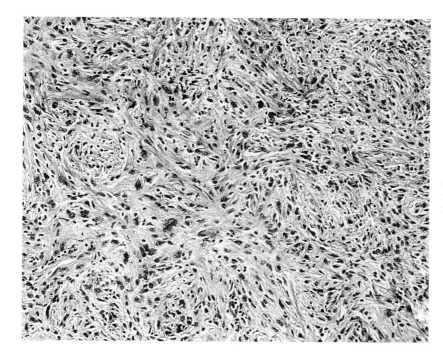

Figure 19-22
MALIGNANT FIBROUS
HISTIOCYTOMA
The tumor shows the typical storiform pattern and cytologic pleomorphism and atypia seen in these neoplasms.

Figure 19-23
MALIGNANT FIBROUS
HISTIOCYTOMA
Higher magnification of lesion shown in figure 19-22. Note the pinwheel pattern of the spindle cells, the atypical binucleated cells, and the scattering of chronic inflammatory cells. Many of the mononuclear cells also show nuclear atypia.

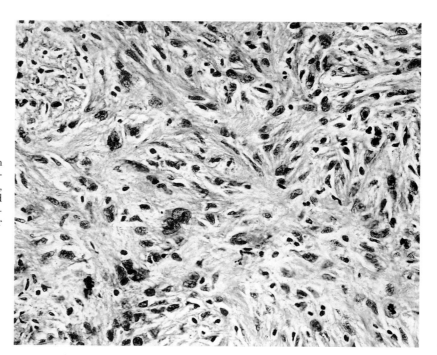

mononuclear and multinuclear giant cells (fig. 19-23). Lymphocytes and plasma cells are dispersed among the tumor cells and occasionally can be a significant proportion of the cell population, while neutrophils can be seen around areas of necrosis (fig. 19-24). A sparse collagen matrix is typical. On occasion, a prominent myxoid stroma (myxoid variant) or numerous diffusely interspersed neutrophils (inflammatory variant) are the dominant microscopic feature. Numerous mitoses (up to 48 per 10 high-power fields), including atypical mitoses, and extensive foci of necrosis are

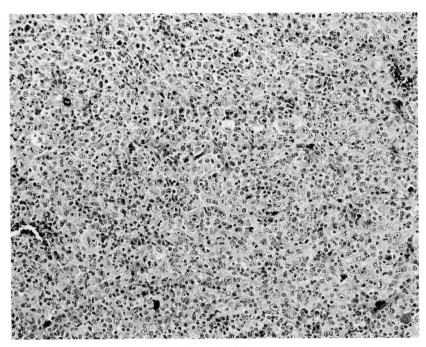

Figure 19-24
MALIGNANT FIBROUS HISTIOCYTOMA
Sheet-like array of malignant mononuclear cells with a diffusely dispersed chronic inflammatory cell infiltrate. (Fig. 5 from Yousem S, Hocholzer L. Malignant fibrous histiocytoma of the lung. Cancer 1987;60:2532–41.)

usual. Histochemical stains for mucin and glycogen are negative, except near areas of necrosis, where intracellular glycogen may be found.

Ultrastructural Findings. The ultrastructural appearance is typically polymorphous, reflecting the light microscopic diversity of this tumor (50,51). There are spindle-shaped fibroblasts with prominent, often dilated, cisternae of rough endoplasmic reticulum. Occasional simplified or intermediate-type junctions can be seen among fibroblasts. Myofibroblasts, cells combining the abundant dilated cisternae of rough endoplasmic reticulum noted in fibroblasts with cytoplasmic aggregates of thin filaments, lateral dense plaques, and pinocytotic vesicles of myocytes, are present less frequently in these pulmonary tumors than in their soft tissue counterparts (50,51). Histiocyte-like cells with numerous lysosomes, lipid droplets, occasional cisternae of rough endoplasmic reticulum, and ruffled cell surfaces (pseudopodia) are present. Finally, there can be undifferentiated mesenchymal cells and cells showing features intermediate between fibroblasts and histiocytes.

Immunohistochemical Findings. The tumor cells stain diffusely for vimentin and more focally for alpha-1-antitrypsin (49,51) and alpha-1-antichymotrypsin (51). Stains for keratin, epithelial membrane antigen (EMA), carcinoembryonic antigen (CEA), S-100 protein, desmin, and myoglobin are negative.

Differential Diagnosis. Metastatic MFH from a primary site in the soft tissues is much more common than primary MFH of lung. Still, only about 0.5 percent metastasize before the primaries are discovered (54).

Pleomorphic (spindle and giant cell) carcinoma (chapter 15) is a far more frequent primary tumor in lung than MFH. Further, it may show spindle cells arrayed in a storiform pattern, multinucleated giant cells, frequent and abnormal mitoses, and necrosis. Cohesive epithelial cell nests, squamous or glandular differentiation, or intracellular mucin support a diagnosis of carcinoma, but it is often impossible to distinguish the tumors by light microscopy alone (a fact that makes it difficult to accept some published cases as pulmonary MFH) (53). The presence of desmosomes, junctional complexes, microvilli within glands, or cytoplasmic tonofibrils by electron microscopy, or the finding of intracellular keratin or CEA by immunohistochemical methods supports carcinoma over MFH. Because of the difficulty in distinguishing spindle and giant cell carcinomas, we recommend that all cases of putative MFH be evaluated by either immunohistochemistry or electron microscopy for epithelial features.

MFH must also be distinguished from the fibrohistiocytic variant of inflammatory pseudotumor. The latter typically lacks the anaplasia, necrosis, and mitoses of MFH. As noted in the section on inflammatory pseudotumor in this chapter, cellular anaplasia in the form of nuclear hyperchromatism and pleomorphism, bizarre multinucleated cells, necrosis of greater than 15 percent of the tumor, and frequent mitoses (greater than 3 per 50 high-power fields) suggest MFH (49a).

Finally, other primary sarcomas of lung need to be considered. Light microscopic features that suggest leiomyosarcoma include elongated tumor cell nuclei with blunted or rounded ends, perinuclear vacuolization when the cells are cut in cross section, fuchsinophilic cytoplasmic fibrils in trichrome stains, and smooth muscle actin in immunohistochemical stains. A myxoid stroma and prominent nuclear palisades may suggest malignant schwannoma or malignant peripheral nerve sheath tumor; the presence of S-100 protein supports the diagnosis. Fibrosarcoma of the lung shows pointed cell bodies and nuclei arrayed in a prominent herringbone pattern. Electron microscopy may also be of aid in distinguishing these tumors.

Treatment and Prognosis. At the time of diagnosis most patients have localized disease, but between 20 and 25 percent of patients present with metastatic disease. The first line of therapy is surgical resection, most frequently lobectomy. Adjuvant chemotherapy or radiation is used in a few cases. Approximately 60 to 70 percent of patients develop recurrent or metastatic disease, most frequently in liver, mediastinum, or central nervous system; between 65 and 75 percent of them die of tumor, most often within 24 months (51,54a). The median survival is 16 months, in our experience. Only 13 percent of patients survive more than 5 years. Perhaps the most significant prognostic indicator is advanced stage of disease at diagnosis (54a).

MISCELLANEOUS FIBROUS AND FIBROHISTIOCYTIC TUMORS

Fibrosarcomas

Fibrosarcomas consist of spindle cells, often arranged in a herringbone pattern, that demonstrate a fibroblastic phenotype. Relatively few recent cases have been reported in lung, and there is controversy over the histogenesis of many of the tumors, largely because few have been examined systematically by immunohistochemistry or electron microscopy to support a fibroblastic phenotype. For example, some pediatric "fibrosarcomas" (57,64,68) have been reclassified as myofibroblastic tumors (congenital peribronchial myofibroblastic tumor) after immunohistochemical evaluation (chapter 20) (62). For that reason and because of the uniformly benign behavior of these pediatric tumors, they will not be discussed further in this section. In addition, some tumors classified as fibrosarcomas of lung are actually pulmonary artery sarcomas.

Adult patients with fibrosarcoma range from 23 to 69 years of age (median, 49 years) (56a,63). Tumors may be endobronchial or parenchymal in location and symptoms vary accordingly. Endobronchial tumors induce cough, dyspnea, and hemoptysis. Up to 55 percent of adults are asymptomatic; they most often have intrapulmonary masses.

Grossly, the tumors can be divided into two groups based on location: endobronchial and parenchymal (56a). The former consists of typically small (1 to 3 cm), tan, gray, or pink, polypoid or pedunculated lesions arising in the lobar or main stem bronchi. They may be restricted to the bronchial wall and lumen or, when larger, may invade into lung parenchyma. Parenchymal tumors measure 2 to 23 cm in diameter and are well-circumscribed, unencapsulated masses with gray-white or yellow firm cut surfaces, but areas of hemorrhage can be seen (fig. 19-25). Focal and sometimes large cysts may be found.

At low microscopic magnification, endobronchial tumors are typically polypoid growths usually confined to the bronchial wall; however, they may extend beyond the cartilage plates into contiguous lung (fig. 19-26). Intrapulmonary tumors are usually well circumscribed at scanning magnification. They surround and destroy vessels,

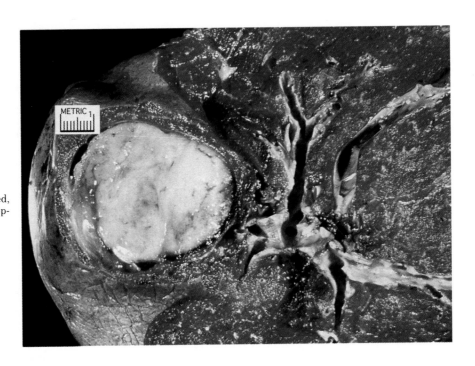

Figure 19-25
GROSS APPEARANCE
OF PERIPHERAL
FIBROSARCOMA
OF LUNG
A relatively circumscribed,
fleshy mass is present and sep-
arate from the pleura.

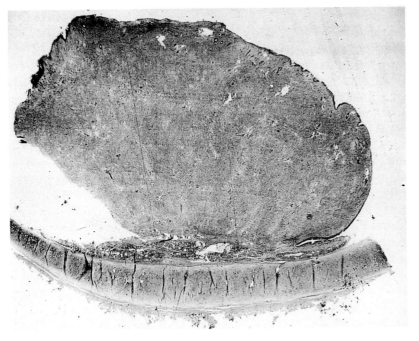

Figure 19-26
POLYPOID ENDOBRONCHIAL
FIBROSARCOMA OF LUNG
The low-power view shows the
tumor within the bronchial lumen
and confined to the bronchial wall.
(Fig. 3 from Guccion J, Rosen S.
Bronchopulmonary leiomyosarcoma
and fibrosarcoma. A study of 32 cases
and review of the literature. Cancer
1972;30:836–47.)

cartilage-bearing airways, and alveoli. Peripheral tumors may occasionally impinge on the
visceral pleura.

Fibrosarcomas are generally highly cellular.
They consist of spindle cells with pointed cell
bodies and nuclei, often growing in a herringbone
or broad fascicular pattern, with variable but
usually scant collagenized stroma (figs. 19-27,
19-28) (56a,66). Areas of necrosis can be present
and mitoses vary from 3 or less per 10 high-
power fields (particularly in endobronchial tumors) to 8 to 40 or more per 10 high-power fields.

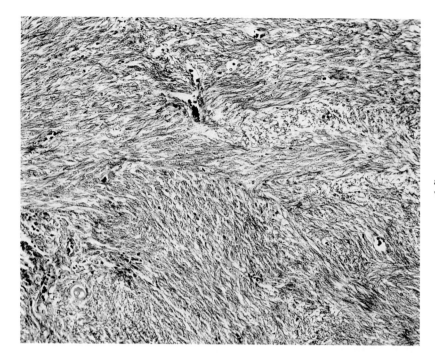

Figure 19-27
FIBROSARCOMA OF LUNG
The tumor is markedly cellular and has a broadly fascicular pattern, with scant collagenized stroma.

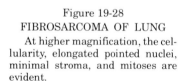

Figure 19-28
FIBROSARCOMA OF LUNG
At higher magnification, the cellularity, elongated pointed nuclei, minimal stroma, and mitoses are evident.

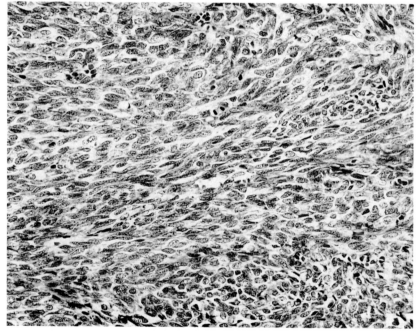

Reticulin stains show a fine network of fibers around individual cells. The malignant cells react with antibody to vimentin.

We have also encountered a few cases of inflammatory fibrosarcoma, a tumor originally described in the retroperiotoneum and omentum, in lung (62a). The tumor shows fascicles of spin-

dled fibroblastic cells admixed with plasma cells, lymphocytes, and variable amounts of collagen (fig. 19-15).

Surgical extirpation is the best opportunity for cure. Chemotherapy and radiotherapy are reserved for cases that cannot be resected. In one series of patients, only two of nine (22 percent) survived long-term and all patients with tumors larger than 5 cm died (63). Patients frequently develop distant metastases and have a high mortality rate (56a,63). The size of the tumor at clinical presentation is linked, to some extent, with its location: endobronchial tumors, because they provoke symptoms earlier in the course, tend to be smaller on discovery and have a correspondingly better prognosis. The number of mitoses (less than 8 per 10 high-power fields) may also be a prognostic factor.

Perhaps the most important point in the differential diagnosis is that metastatic sarcomas are far more frequent than primary pulmonary sarcomas. A diagnosis of sarcoma of lung should be considered only after rigorous exclusion of other primary sites. This is particularly true of metastatic monophasic synovial sarcomas, whose histologic appearance can mimic fibrosarcoma. The finding of diffuse and strong cytokeratin in a "fibrosarcoma" by immunohistochemical methods requires an exclusion of synovial sarcoma. The differential diagnosis includes other rare spindle cell sarcomas primary in lung, such as leiomyosarcoma and neurofibrosarcoma, as well as localized fibrous tumor of the pleura, intrapulmonary fibrous tumor, and inflammatory pseudotumor. A careful application of immunohistochemical stains and electron microscopic observations helps exclude the first two possibilities, while a high mitotic rate and marked cellularity excludes the latter two diagnoses.

Mesenchymal Cystic Hamartoma

Mesenchymal cystic hamartomas are cystic lesions that are lined by respiratory epithelium and surrounded by a subepithelial or cambium layer of primitive mesenchymal cells (figs. 19-29, 19-30) (61). They were initially described in adults. The combination of epithelial-lined cysts and embryonic mesenchyme suggested a hamartomatous lesion to Mark (61). However, the nosology of this lesion is undergoing revision, impelled by the finding that cystic metastatic sarcomas, such as endometrial stromal sarcomas, can closely simulate mesenchymal cystic hamartoma grossly and microscopically (55,67).

In children, cystic lesions with a light microscopic appearance similar to mesenchymal cystic hamartoma have been reported, but primitive sarcomas frequently supervene (56,58,65,69).

While some suggest that these lesions are preneoplastic with a propensity to malignant transformation (56,58), the frequency of outright sarcoma suggests to us that they should be viewed as part of the spectrum of cystic blastomas of childhood, and they are so classified in this Fascicle (see chapter 21).

Cystic Fibrohistiocytic Tumor

Cystic fibrohistiocytic tumor consists of multiple pulmonary cystic masses (60). Only two patients have been reported so far, both men (60), but there may be a third case that fits the microscopic description of the tumor (59) and we illustrate a fourth in figures 19-31 and 19-32. Still, at least two of the tumors have been subsequently identified as multifocal metastatic dermatofibrosarcoma protuberans (T. Colby, personal communication, 1993). The chest X ray shows bilateral nodules or a mixture of solid nodules and thin-walled cysts that slowly enlarge over many years without tumor-induced mortality. There may be recurrent spontaneous pneumothoraces.

Microscopically, the scanning view shows cysts of variable size lined by bronchiolar or squamous epithelium and type 2 pneumocytes (fig. 19-31). The cysts may contain old hemorrhage with hemosiderin-laden macrophages, xanthoma cells, and giant cells. The cystic lesions are associated, sometimes focally, with an interstitial spindle cell proliferation (fig. 19-32). These cells demonstrate a storiform pattern and show neither cytologic atypia nor mitoses, producing the overall impression of a fibrous histiocytoma (60).

Distinction of this lesion from cystic metastatic sarcomas may be difficult and cystic fibrohistiocytic tumor may actually be low-grade metastatic sarcoma. As noted above, thin-walled cavities have been reported in a number of metastatic low-grade sarcomas in lung, including leiomyosarcoma, synovial sarcoma, dermatofibrosarcoma protuberans, and endometrial stromal sarcoma (55,67). The amount of solid tumor present may be so scant as to produce difficulties in identifying the neoplasm at the light microscopic level. Immunohistochemical studies for smooth muscle actin, keratin, and desmin can help to identify the phenotype of some cases. Solution to the problem of whether cystic fibrohistiocytic tumor is actually a separate entity awaits additional experience with the lesion.

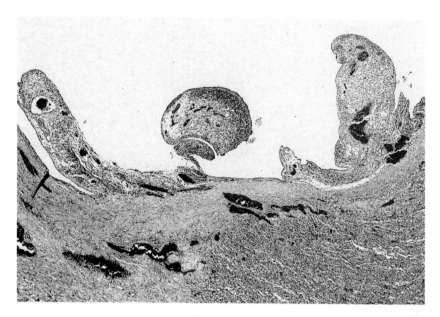

Figure 19-29
MESENCHYMAL CYSTIC HAMARTOMA
The lesion presents as a cyst containing a few polypoid projections into the lumen. A dark band of cellularity, corresponding to a cambium layer, is present beneath the cyst surface, best seen in the central polyp.

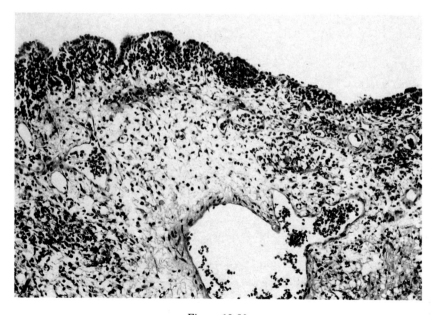

Figure 19-30
MESENCHYMAL CYSTIC HAMARTOMA
At higher magnification, the cambium layer consists of small dark cells lying in a layer just beneath the surface of the cyst.

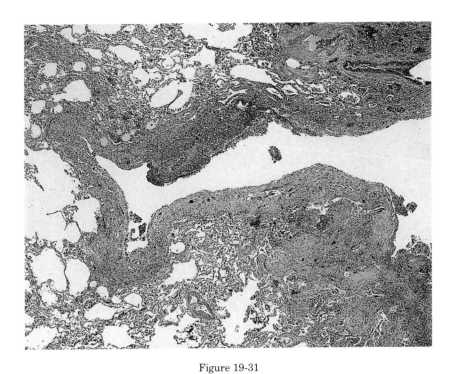

Figure 19-31
CYSTIC FIBROHISTIOCYTIC TUMOR
The tumor presents as a thin-walled cyst with only focal areas of cellularity. It lies adjacent to a small artery and bronchiole.

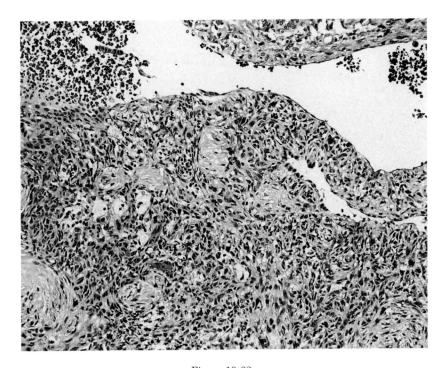

Figure 19-32
CYSTIC FIBROHISTIOCYTIC TUMOR
A cellular area within the wall of the cyst shown in figure 19-31. Note the relatively bland spindle cell proliferation. Mitoses were not seen.

REFERENCES

Inflammatory Pseudotumor (Plasma Cell Granuloma—Histiocytoma Complex)

1. Amin R. Extramedullary plasmacytoma of the lung. Cancer 1985;56:152–6.

2. Bahadori M, Liebow AA. Plasma cell granulomas of the lung. Cancer 1973;31:191–208.

3. Berardi RS, Lee SS, Chen HP, Stines GJ. Inflammatory pseudotumors of the lung. Surg Gynecol Obstet 1983;156:89–96.

4. Buell R, Wang NS, Seemayer TA, Ahmed MN. Endobronchial plasma cell granuloma (xanthomatous pseudotumor): a light and electron microscopic study. Hum Pathol 1976;7:411–26.

5. Childress W, Adie G. Plasma cell tumors of the mediastinum and lung: report of two cases. J Thorac Surg 1950;19:794–9.

6. Cordier JF, Loire R, Brune J. Idiopathic bronchiolitis obliterans organizing pneumonia. Definition of characteristic clinical profiles in a series of 16 patients. Chest 1989;96:999–1004.

7. Dail D. Uncommon tumors. In: Dail DH, Hammar SP, eds. Pulmonary pathology. 2nd ed. New York: Springer-Verlag, 1994:1384.

8. Doski JJ, Priebe CJ Jr, Driessnack M, Smith T, Kane P, Romero J. Corticosteroids in the management of unresected plasma cell granuloma (inflammatory pseudotumor) of the lung. J Pediatr Surg 1991;26:1064–6.

9. Gal AA, Koss MN, McCarthy WF, Hochholzer L. Prognostic factors in pulmonary fibrohistiocytic lesions. Cancer 1994;73:1817–24.

10. Hartman GE, Shochat SJ. Primary pulmonary neoplasms of childhood: a review. Ann Thorac Surg 1983;36:108–19.

11. Hong HY, Castelli MJ, Walloch JL. Pulmonary plasma cell granuloma (inflammatory pseudotumor) with invasion of thoracic vertebra. Mt Sinai J Med 1990;57:117–21.

12. Hurt MA, Santa Cruz DJ. Cutaneous inflammatory pseudotumor. Lesions resembling "inflammatory pseudotumors" or "plasma cell granulomas" of extracutaneous sites. Am J Surg Pathol 1990;14:764–73.

13. Joseph G, Pandit M, Korfhage L. Primary pulmonary plasmacytoma. Cancer 1992;71:721–4.

14. Katzenstein AL, Maurer JJ. Benign histiocytic tumor of lung: a light- and electron-microscopic study. Am J Surg Pathol 1979;3:61–8.

15. Kuzela D. Ultrastructural study of a postinflammatory "tumor" of the lung. Cancer 1975;19:149–56.

16. Long F, Nott D, MacArthur E. Xanthomatous tumors of the lung with identification of lipid content. Australas Ann Med 1970;19:362–5.

17. Machicao CN, Sorensen K, Abdul-Karim FW, Somrak TM. Transthoracic needle aspiration biopsy in inflammatory pseudotumors of the lung. Diagn Cytopathol 1989;5:400–3.

18. Maier HC, Sommers SC. Recurrent and metastatic pulmonary fibrous histiocytoma/plasma cell granuloma in a child. Cancer 1987;60:1073–6.

19. Makela V, Matilla S, Makinen J. Plasma cell granuloma (histiocytoma) of the lung and pleura. Acta Pathol Microbiol Immunol Scand [A] 1972;80:634–40.

20. Mandelbaum I, Brashear RE, Hull MT. Surgical treatment and course of pulmonary pseudotumor (plasma cell granuloma). J Thorac Cardiovasc Surg 1981;82:77–82.

21. Matsubara O, Tan-Liu NS, Kenney RM, Mark EJ. Inflammatory pseudotumors of the lung: progression from organizing pneumonia to fibrous histiocytoma or to plasma cell granuloma in 32 cases. Hum Pathol 1988;19:807–14.

22. Meis JM, Enzinger FM. Inflammatory fibrosarcoma of the mesentery and retroperitoneum. A tumor closely simulating inflammatory pseudotumor. Am J Surg Pathol 1991;15:1146–56.

23. Monzon CM, Gilchrist GS, Burgert EO Jr, et al. Plasma cell granuloma of the lung in children. Pediatrics 1982;70:268–74.

24. Muraoka S, Sato T, Takahashi T, Ando M, Shimoda A. Plasma cell granuloma of the lung with extrapulmonary extension. Immunohistochemical and electron microscopic studies. Acta Pathol Jpn 1985;35:933–44.

25. Nair S, Nair K, Weisbrot I. Fibrous histiocytoma of the lung (sclerosing hemangioma variant?). Chest 1974;65:465–8.

26. Pettinato G, Manivel JC, De Rosa N, Dehner LP. Inflammatory myofibroblastic tumor (plasma cell granuloma). Clinicopathologic study of 20 cases with immunohistochemical and ultrastructural observations. Am J Clin Pathol 1990;94:538–46.

27. Sajjad S, Begin L, Dail D, Lukeman J. Fibrous histiocytoma of the lung—a clinicopathologic study of two cases. Histopathology 1981;5:325–34.

28. Shirakusa T, Miyazak N, Kitagawa T, Sugiyama K. Ultrastructural study of pulmonary plasma cell granuloma—report of a case. Br J Dis Chest 1979;73:289–96.

29. Spencer H. The pulmonary plasma cell/histiocytoma complex. Histopathology 1984;8:903–16.

30. Tanino M, Odashima S, Sugiura H, Matsue T, Kajikawa M, Maeda S. Malignant fibrous histiocytoma of the lung. Acta Pathol Jpn 1985;35:945–50.

31. Tan-Liu NS, Matsubara O, Grillo HC, Mark EJ. Invasive fibrous tumor of the tracheobronchial tree: clinical and pathologic study of seven cases. Hum Pathol 1989;20:180–4.

32. Titus J, Harrison E, Clagett O, Anderson M, Knaff L. Xanthomatous and inflammatory pseudotumors of the lung. Cancer 1962;15:522–38.

33. Toccanier M, Exquis B, Groebli Y. Granuloma plasmocytaire du poumon. Neuf observations avec etude immunohistochemique. Ann Pathol 1982;2:21–8.

34. Umiker W, Iverson L. Postinflammatory "tumors" of the lung. J Thorac Surg 1954;28:55–63.

35. Usuda K, Saito Y, Imai T, et al. Inflammatory pseudotumor of the lung diagnosed as granulomatous lesion by preoperative brushing cytology. A case report. Acta Cytol 1990;34:685–9.

36. Warter A, Satge D, Roeslin N. Angioinvasive plasma cell granulomas of the lung. Cancer 1987;59:435–43.

37. Wentworth P, Lynch MJ, Fallis JC, Turner JA, Lowden JA, Conen PE. Xanthomatous pseudotumor of lung. A case report with electron microscope and lipid studies. Cancer 1968;22:345–55.

38. Yousem S, Hochholzer L. Malignant fibrous histiocytoma of the lung. Cancer 1987;60:2532–41.

Intrapulmonary Localized Fibrous Tumor

39. Briselli M, Mark EJ, Dickersin GR. Solitary fibrous tumors of the pleura: eight new cases and review of 360 cases in the literature. Cancer 1981;47:2678–89.

40. Dalton W, Zolliker A, McCaughey W, Jacques J, Kannerstein M. Localized primary tumors of the pleura. Cancer 1979;44:1465–75.

41. England D, Hochholzer L, McCarthy M. Localized benign and malignant fibrous tumors of the pleura. Am J Surg Pathol 1989;13:640–58.

42. Goodlad JR, Fletcher CD. Solitary fibrous tumour arising at unusual sites: analysis of a series. Histopathology 1991;19:515–22.

43. Guccion J, Rosen S. Bronchopulmonary leiomyosarcoma and fibrosarcoma. A study of 32 cases and review of the literature. Cancer 1972;30:836–47.

44. Okike N, Bernatz PE, Woolner LB. Localized mesothelioma of the pleura: benign and malignant variants. J Thorac Cardiovasc Surg 1978;75:363–72.

45. Stout A, Himadi G. Solitary (localized) mesothelioma of the pleura. Ann Surg 1950;133:50–64.

46. _____, Murray M. Localized pleural mesothelioma. Arch Pathol 1942;34:951–64.

47. Yousem S, Flynn S. Intrapulmonary localized fibrous tumor: intraparenchymal so-called localized fibrous mesothelioma. Am J Clin Pathol 1988;89:365–9.

48. _____, Hochholzer L. Pulmonary hyalinizing granuloma. Am J Clin Pathol 1987; 87:1–6.

Malignant Fibrous Histiocytoma

49. Chowdhury LN, Swerdlow MA, Jao W, Kathpalia S, Desser RK. Postirradiation malignant fibrous histiocytoma of the lung. Demonstration of alpha 1-antitrypsin-like material in neoplastic cells. Am J Clin Pathol 1980;74:820–6.

49a. Gal AA, Koss MN, McCarthy WF, Hochholzer L. Prognostic factors in pulmonary fibrohistiocytic lesions. Cancer 1994;73:1817–24.

50. Lee JT, Shelburne JD, Linder J. Primary malignant fibrous histiocytoma of the lung. A clinicopathologic and ultrastructural study of five cases. Cancer 1984;53:1124–30.

51. McDonnell T, Kyriakos M, Roper C, Mazoujian G. Malignant fibrous histiocytoma of the lung. Cancer 1988;61:137–45.

52. Mills SA, Breyer RH, Johnston FR, et al. Malignant fibrous histiocytoma of the mediastinum and lung: a report of three cases. J Thorac Cardiovasc Surg 1982;84:367–72.

53. Misra DP, Sunderrajan EV, Rosenholtz MJ, Hurst DJ. Malignant fibrous histiocytoma in the lung masquerading as recurrent pulmonary thromboembolism. Cancer 1983;51:538–41.

53a. Tanino M, Odashima S, Sugiura H, Matsue T, Kajikawa M, Maeda S. Malignant fibrous histiocytoma of the lung. Acta Pathol Jpn 1985;35:945–50.

54. Weiss SW, Enzinger FM. Malignant fibrous histiocytoma: an analysis of 200 cases. Cancer 1978;41:2250–66.

54a. Yousem S, Hochholzer L. Malignant fibrous histiocytoma of the lung. Cancer 1987;60:2532–41.

Miscellaneous Fibrous and Fibrohistiocytic Tumors

55. Abrams J, Talcott J, Corson JM. Pulmonary metastases in patients with low-grade endometrial stromal sarcoma. Clinicopathologic findings with immunohistochemical characterization. Am J Surg Pathol 1989;13:133–40.

56. Bove KE. Sarcoma arising in pulmonary mesenchymal cystic hamartoma. Pediatr Pathol 1989;9:785–92.

56a. Guccion J, Rosen S. Bronchopulmonary leiomyosarcoma and fibrosarcoma. A study of 32 cases and review of the literature. Cancer 1972;30:836–47.

57. Haller JO, Kauffman SL, Kassner EG. Congenital mesenchymal tumour of the lung. Br J Radiol 1977;50:217–9.

58. Hedlund GL, Bissett GS III, Bove KE. Malignant neoplasms arising in cystic hamartomas of the lung in childhood. Radiology 1989;173:77–9.

59. Holden WE, Mulkey D, Kessler S. Multiple peripheral lung cysts and hemoptysis in an otherwise asymptomatic adult. Am Rev Respir Dis 1982;126:930–2.

60. Joseph M, Colby T, Swensen S, Mikus J, Gaensler E. Multiple cystic fibrohistiocytic tumors of the lung: report of two cases. Mayo Clin Proc 1990;65:192–7.

61. Mark EJ. Mesenchymal cystic hamartoma of the lung. N Engl J Med 1986;315:1255–9.

62. McGinnis M, Jacobs G, el-Naggar A, Redline RW. Congenital peribronchial myofibroblastic tumor (so-called "congenital leiomyosarcoma"). A distinct neonatal lung lesion associated with nonimmune hydrops fetalis. Mod Pathol 1993;6:487–92.

62a. Meis JM, Enzinger FM. Inflammatory fibrosarcoma of the mesentery and retroperitoneum. A tumor closely simulating inflammatory pseudotumor. Am J Surg Pathol 1991;15:1146–56.

63. Nascimento AG, Unni K, Bernatz P. Sarcomas of the lung. Mayo Clin Proc 1982;57:355–9.

64. Pettinato G, Manivel JC, Saldana MJ, Peyser J, Dehner LP. Primary bronchopulmonary fibrosarcoma of childhood and adolescence: reassessment of a low-grade malignancy. Clinicopathologic study of five cases and review of the literature. Hum Pathol 1989;20:463–71.

65. Stephanopoulis C, Catsaras H. Myxosarcoma complicating a cystic hamartoma of the lung. Thorax 1963; 18:144–5.

66. Stout AP. Fibrosarcoma in infants and children. Cancer 1962;15:1028–40.

67. Traweek T, Rotter AJ, Swartz W, Azumi N. Cystic pulmonary metastatic sarcoma. Cancer 1990;65:1805–11.

68. Warren JS, Seo IS, Mirkin LD. Massive congenital mesenchymal malformation of the lung: a case report with ultrastructural study. Pediatr Pathol 1985;3:321–8.

69. Weinberg AG, Currarino G, Moore GC, Votteler TB. Mesenchymal neoplasia and congenital pulmonary cysts. Pediatr Radiol 1980;9:179–82.

20
MISCELLANEOUS MESENCHYMAL TUMORS

Like other organs, the lungs may be the primary site of mesenchymal (soft tissue) tumors. Some of the more distinctive tumors are discussed in chapters 18 and 19. Many of the lung tumors covered in this chapter may present as an endobronchial (or endotracheal) or parenchymal mass (Table 20-1) (2). In the former, there is often a history of recurrent pneumonia, whereas the latter may become quite large before symptoms develop. A number of studies of benign and malignant mesenchymal tumors of the lung have been published (1,3–10). These and Table 20-1 illustrate the range seen in the lung. In some, multiple mesenchymal components may be present histologically (10).

SMOOTH MUSCLE TUMORS

Smooth muscle tumors of the lung include: primary solitary leiomyoma, primary solitary leiomyosarcoma, glomus tumor, so-called benign metastasizing leiomyoma, metastatic high-grade leiomyosarcoma, and lymphangioleiomyomatosis. Lymphangioleiomyomatosis, although not a neoplasm, is included because of its importance in differential diagnosis.

Leiomyoma and Leiomyosarcoma

Primary solitary leiomyomas (2,6,9,36,42,44, 48) are either endobronchial (45 percent of cases) (fig. 20-1) or parenchymal (55 percent of cases) and comprise approximately 2 percent of benign lung tumors (44). The average age at presentation is in the fourth decade (range, 5 to 67 years), with females affected more often than males (1.5 to 1) (42). Patients with endobronchial lesions exhibit symptoms related to obstruction whereas most of the remainder (those with parenchymal masses) are asymptomatic. Two cases were recently described in HIV-infected children (18). Leiomyomas may occur in the pleura as well. The histologic, immunohistochemical, and ultrastructural features of these tumors are identical to leiomyomas at other sites. The treatment is resection, and lung-sparing surgery, such as sleeve (47) and wedge resec-

tion, is reasonable. The prognosis is excellent with complete resection. Laser therapy has been used for an endobronchial leiomyoma (12).

The differential diagnosis includes hamartomas with a prominent smooth muscle component, low-grade leiomyosarcomas (primary or metastatic), benign metastasizing leiomyoma, and other spindle cell tumors (especially spindle cell carcinoid and intrapulmonary solitary fibrous tumor).

Table 20-1

MESENCHYMAL TUMORS OF THE LUNG*

Tumor	Pulmonary Paren-chyma	Bronchi	Trachea
Leiomyoma	X	X	X
BML**	X		
Glomus tumor	X	X	X
Leiomyosarcoma	X	X	X
Rhabdomyosarcoma	X	X	X
Hemangioma	X		
Lymphangioma	X		
EH**	X		
Kaposi sarcoma	X	X	X
Angiosarcoma	X		
Hemangiopericytoma	X		
Neurilemmoma	X	X	
Neurofibroma	X	X	X
Meningioma	X		
Chondroma	X	X	
Chondrosarcoma		X	X
Osteosarcoma	X		
Lipoma	X	X	
Liposarcoma		X	X

*Modified from reference 2 with additions from the text.
**BML, benign metastasizing leiomyoma; EH, epithelioid hemangioendothelioma.

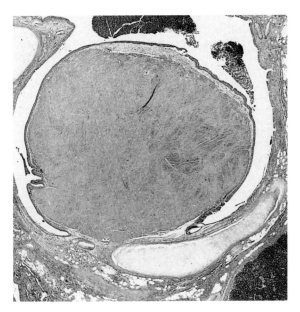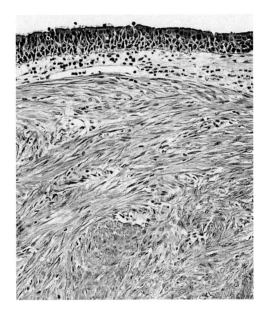

Figure 20-1
ENDOBRONCHIAL LEIOMYOMA
This leiomyoma presented as a polypoid endobronchial mass (left). It is cytologically benign (right). It was associated with recurrent pneumonias.

Primary solitary leiomyosarcomas (1–5,7,8, 24,43,48) are slightly more common than leiomyomas. Ninety-two cases were found in a 1984 review (48). The mean age at presentation is 50 (range, newborn to 83 years), and males are affected more frequently (2.5 to 1). Most are parenchymal masses, some with an endobronchial component. There is a propensity for a hilar location. Lillo-Gal (31) described a case associated with cystic change. Most patients have symptoms that include pain, cough, hemoptysis, and dyspnea. The lesions tend to be large, circumscribed masses grossly similar to their counterparts at other sites; the histologic, immunohistochemical, and ultrastructural features are similar to leiomyosarcomas at other sites as well.

The treatment is resection, and a 50 percent 5-year survival rate can be expected (43,48), but at least one fourth of patients (48) have advanced (unresectable) disease at the time of presentation.

The differential diagnosis includes primary leiomyoma, benign metastasizing leiomyoma, metastatic leiomyosarcoma, and pleuropulmonary blastoma.

There are no established criteria for the distinction between leiomyomas and leiomyosarcomas in the lung. Gal et al. (24) have proposed that an average mitotic count greater than 5 mitoses per 50 high-power fields is indicative of leiomyosarcoma; however, most cases show considerably higher counts, are large, have prominent nuclear atypia, and exhibit necrosis. Gal et al. emphasized the need for adequate sampling of such tumors. Whenever a primary leiomyosarcoma of the lung is under consideration in a woman, the possibility of a metastasis from the genital tract should be carefully excluded.

Leiomyosarcomas of the lung are occasionally seen in children (14,28). When this diagnosis is contemplated, the possibility of a pleuropulmonary blastoma (with a leiomyosarcomatous component) should be excluded. McGinnis et al. (33) have suggested that some leiomyosarcomas in children, especially so-called congenital leiomyosarcomas, may be true congenital neoplasms of peribronchial myofibroblasts that are relatively benign. They believe some of the cases reported as bronchopulmonary fibrosarcoma, congenital fibroleiomyosarcoma, hamartoma, and massive congenital mesenchymal malformation of the lung also fit in this category.

Benign metastasizing leiomyoma is a term that has been used for multiple (and rarely, single) nodules of well-differentiated smooth muscle

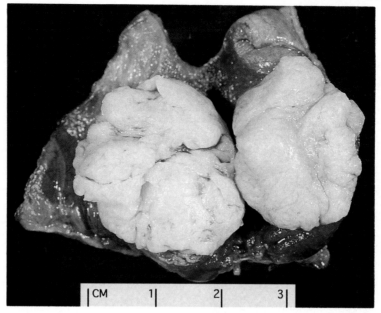

Figure 20-2
BENIGN METASTASIZING LEIOMYOMA
This gross photograph shows a gray-white 2.5 cm diameter nodule with a typical appearance of smooth muscle. The nodule is somewhat lobulated and appears to shell out from the surrounding lung parenchyma.

occurring in the lung, almost invariably in women, many of whom have a history of smooth muscle tumors in the uterus (16,21,22,24,32,45, 46). The term benign metastasizing leiomyoma is not uniformly accepted, and some argue that these tumors are actually metastatic low-grade leiomyosarcomas (46) or hormonally responsive in situ proliferations (24). While the histogenesis of this lesion remains in dispute and the name may be misleading, or in fact a misnomer, it is well recognized and conveys the essence of the condition. Multiple *fibroleiomyomatous hamartomas* of the lung are morphologically identical to, and are now recognized as the same lesion as, benign metastasizing leiomyoma (27,46).

With the exception of the three men included in Wolff's series (46), all of the patients with benign metastasizing leiomyoma have been adult women, with an average age of 47 years (range, 30 to 74 years). Blacks may be more commonly affected: 8 of 17 cases occurred in black women in a review by Gal et al. (24). The nodules vary in size from microscopic to over 10 cm (46); they are single in 10 percent of the cases, and only one lung is affected in about 30 percent of cases. About one third of patients are symptomatic, usually complaining of cough or dyspnea (27).

Grossly, the lesions have the appearance of smooth muscle (fig. 20-2); cystic change may be present both grossly (fig. 20-3) and radiographically (41). The nodules may easily enucleate from the lung tissue (21).

Histologically, the nodules have features of smooth muscle cells as seen by light microscopy, immunohistochemistry, and electron microscopy (24,46). Fibrosis may be present centrally. The nodules are well-circumscribed and do not show any discernible anatomic distribution. They start as microscopic interstitial proliferations of smooth muscle cells which expand to form circumscribed nodules with epithelial inclusions (fig. 20-4). This latter finding has led to some of the confusion with hamartomas. The epithelial inclusions are usually lined by cuboidal type 2 cells without atypia and not bronchiolar epithelium as is characteristic of hamartomas. Large cystic spaces are lined by metaplastic epithelium.

The smooth muscle cells show considerable variation histologically: some lesions are paucicellular, without atypia or mitotic figures and with abundant collagen deposition between the cells (fig. 20-4) and others are more cellular, with occasional mitotic figures (fig. 20-5). Gal et al. (24) proposed that finding more than 5 mitotic

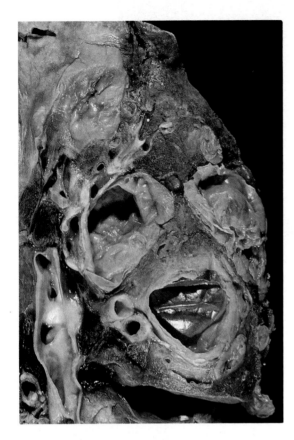

Figure 20-3
BENIGN METASTASIZING LEIOMYOMA

This case of benign metastasizing leiomyoma at autopsy is associated with marked cystic change; there had been progressive enlargement of the cysts over many years.

figures per 50 high-power fields is indicative of leiomyosarcoma. Since many cases reported as benign metastasizing leiomyoma have a greater mitotic rate than this (46), it is apparent why some favor the term metastatic low-grade leiomyosarcoma. Nevertheless, the histologic findings in benign metastasizing leiomyoma show a continuum from histologically benign to those with features of low-grade leiomyosarcoma, and any definition is arbitrary. But as a group, these lesions conform to the clinicopathologic entity of benign metastasizing leiomyoma, which is separable from metastatic high-grade leiomyosarcoma.

The differential diagnosis includes hamartoma with a prominent smooth muscle component, primary leiomyoma and leiomyosarcoma of the lung, metastatic high-grade leiomyosarcoma, lymphangioleiomyomatosis, and metaplastic smooth muscle in scars and fibrotic lung disease.

When a diagnosis of leiomyoma or leiomyosarcoma is considered, the possibility of metastasis from an extrapulmonary site should also be considered, even with solitary lesions, and in women the genital tract should be carefully evaluated. If there has been a prior hysterectomy, an effort should be made to review those slides.

The prognosis of benign metastasizing leiomyoma is variable and probably reflects a number of factors including histologic grade and degree of hormonal responsiveness in the individual patient. In some patients, the tumor is slowly progressive, with little compromise in respiratory function, whereas in others, respiratory insufficiency develops as the nodules continue to enlarge (21,27). Resected uterine smooth muscle tumors have shown features of either leiomyoma or very low-grade leiomyosarcoma (46). In the Wolff series (46), some pulmonary lesions presented prior to the presumed primary.

The treatment for benign metastasizing leiomyoma is not settled. Slowly progressive cases may simply be followed. Resection of the nodules is an option when they are few and large (22,45). Hormonal manipulation offers promise because of the apparent hormonal responsiveness of a number of tumors that have regressed during pregnancy or after castration (22).

Lymphangioleiomyomatosis

Lymphangioleiomyomatosis (LAM) is a peculiar hamartomatous proliferation of smooth muscle seen exclusively in women (13,15,17,20, 29,39). The lesions affect the lung as well as axial lymphatics and lymph nodes in the chest, abdomen, and retroperitoneum; soft tissue lymphangiomyomas and renal angiomyolipomas are also associated with this condition. The lung lesion occurs sporadically or may be seen in a small percentage of women with tuberous sclerosis. The histologic features in these two settings are identical (15). Affected women are generally in their reproductive years (20 to 50), although postmenopausal patients (many of whom are taking exogenous hormones) are occasionally affected (38). Patients present with interstitial or obstructive lung disease, often punctuated by a history of recurrent pneumothoraces. Over time they develop progressive hyperinflation radiographically,

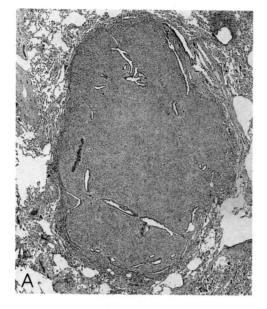

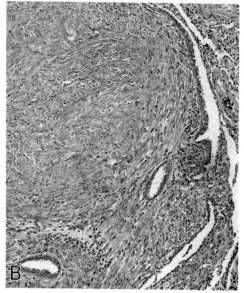

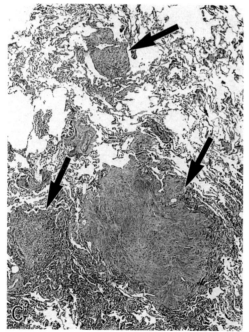

Figure 20-4
BENIGN METASTASIZING LEIOMYOMA
There are discrete well-circumscribed nodules
(A) composed of benign-appearing smooth muscle
cells (B) with increased collagen toward the centers
of the nodules. Alveolar spaces lined by metaplastic
epithelium are seen both within the nodule and at
the edge. Some cases (C) have miliary nodules
(arrows) that arise as tiny interstitial nodules of
smooth muscle.

associated with increasing interstitial infiltrates
that correspond to the deposition of smooth muscle seen grossly and histologically (17). Pulmonary function tests show obstruction and
marked decrease in diffusing capacity. High resolution computerized tomography (CT) shows
the nearly pathognomonic change of diffuse well-
demarcated cysts in the lung parenchyma (35).

Grossly, the lungs may suggest emphysema in
early cases. More advanced cases show diffuse

cystic changes with large cystic spaces lined
by bundles of muscle tissue and resemble
honeycombing.

Histologically, LAM is a multifocal proliferation of immature-appearing smooth muscle cells
in the interstitium, often associated with cystic
spaces, situated subpleurally or along bronchovascular bundles (fig. 20-6). The smooth muscle
proliferation typically is seen as focal fusiform
thickening in walls of cystic spaces, with no

357

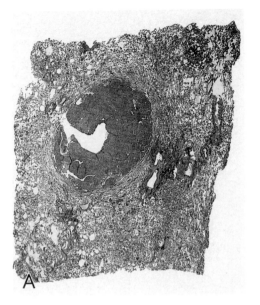

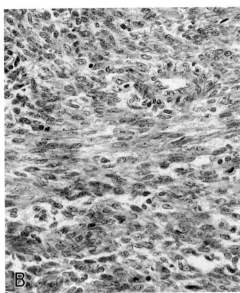

Figure 20-5
BENIGN METASTASIZING LEIOMYOMA
This case was associated with cystic change including some thin-walled cysts (not shown). The nodule in A shows early cystic change. Cytologically, this case shows features of a low-grade leiomyosarcoma with increased cellularity (B) and mild to moderate nuclear atypia with mitotic figures (C, arrow).

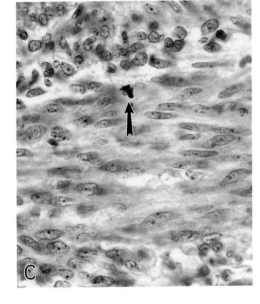

associated scarring. The surrounding lung tissue may have hemosiderin-filled macrophages. Subpleural cysts may rupture and cause a pneumothorax.

Histologically, immunohistochemically, and ultrastructurally the cells of LAM show smooth muscle differentiation although they are often somewhat shorter and contain less cytoplasm than fully differentiated smooth muscle cells (15, 17,19,20,29,38). The nuclei are oval and have distinct nucleoli. The cytoplasm is often pale. The cells proliferate as spindled or polygonal cells, often with lymphatic-like spaces between them. They share many features with the muscle cells of angiomyolipomas and both are probably hamartomatous (19). Unlike normal smooth muscle, the cells in LAM are HMB-45 positive (19). Affected lymph nodes show replacement of lymph node parenchyma by smooth muscle identical to that in the lung, and evaluation of lymphatics adjacent to lymph nodes shows similar changes.

The distinction of LAM from benign metastasizing leiomyoma is generally easy. LAM is associated with cystic spaces with bundles of smooth muscle

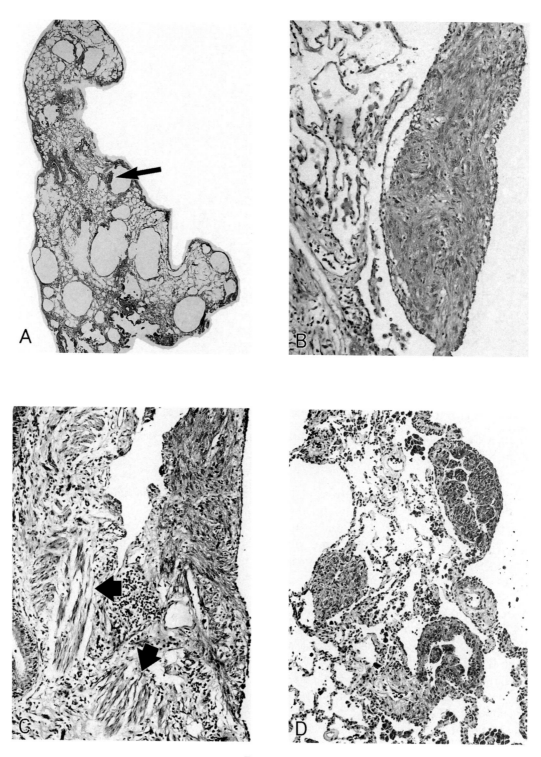

Figure 20-6
LYMPHANGIOLEIOMYOMATOSIS

Lymphangioleiomyomatosis is characterized by multiple holes ("cysts") in the lung parenchyma (A). The holes have fascicles of smooth muscle in their wall (A, arrow and B). The smooth muscle proliferation of lymphangioleiomyomatosis is somewhat more disorganized and immature appearing than that of normal smooth muscle. Normal peribronchiolar smooth muscle (C, arrows) is compared with the proliferation in lymphangioleiomyomatosis (C, upper right). In some cases, the bundles of smooth muscle are more polygonal and may have clefts with polypoid configurations protruding into them (D).

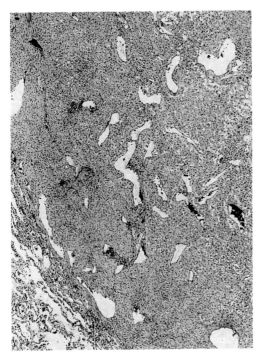 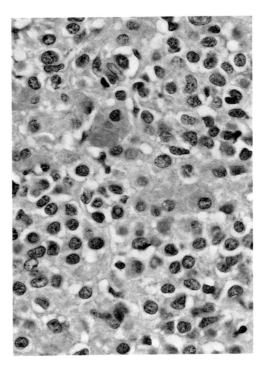

Figure 20-7
GLOMANGIOMA OF THE LUNG

Left: This cellular pulmonary glomangioma shows ectatic thin-walled vascular spaces surrounded by a uniform population of polygonal cells.

Right: The cells, which stained uniformly positive with smooth muscle actin, have round, regular, and somewhat hyperchromatic nuclei.

in the wall without the formation of gross nodules. Benign metastasizing leiomyoma, on the other hand, is associated with nodules and without cystic spaces in the lung parenchyma, although cystic change may occur within the nodules themselves.

The prognosis is variable. In early studies (20) most patients died of pulmonary insufficiency within 10 years. In a more recent review by Taylor et al. (39), 78 percent of the patients (25 of 32) were alive 10 years after disease onset. For the survivors, the median time of survival since the onset was 9.4 years whereas the mean survival time for the entire group was 8.5 years (39). These data suggest individual differences in severity among cases of LAM in terms of survival, prognosis, and rate of disease progression.

There have been a number of cases of LAM that appear to be exacerbated by estrogen, either endogenous or exogenous in origin (39). It has been suggested that measuring estrogen and progesterone receptor status of the tissue is use-

ful. Others find this not prognostically significant (15,39).

Taylor et al. (39) consider oophorectomy a second-line therapy in patients with progressive disease. This group does not recommend tamoxifen therapy and thought that in some patients it might even have a deleterious effect. They recommend a trial of progesterone therapy for at least 1 year.

Glomus Tumors

Glomus tumors (*glomangiomas*) are vascular tumors with stromal cells showing features of smooth muscle differentiation (2,25). They occur at a variety of sites, and the lung and large airways are occasionally affected (fig. 20-7). In the 1991 review by Garcia-Prats (25), there were six cases in the trachea and three in the lung. The light microscopic, immunohistochemical, and ultrastructural features of these tumors are identical to glomus tumors at other sites (2,11, 23,25,26,30).

SKELETAL MUSCLE TUMORS

Rhabdomyoma

Rhabdomyomas of the lung are not well documented. Rhabdomyomatous change in the lung may be seen alone or in association with congenital cystic adenomatoid malformations (see chapter 2) (50,54).

Rhabdomyosarcoma

Rhabdomyosarcomas of the lung are rare and occur in children and adults. Rhabdomyosarcomas in children are solid or multicystic masses involving the lung and sometimes the chest wall. Other sarcomatous elements are often present and most rhabdomyosarcomas in children are included with pleuropulmonary blastomas (chapter 21).

Rhabdomyosarcomas in adults are slightly more common than those in children (49). In 1984, 20 adult cases were found in a review by Avagnina et al (49). Most patients are in the fifth and sixth decades, with a slight male predominance (51). The tumors are large solid masses that may involve more than one lobe and invade bronchovascular structures (49,52,53). The treatment is resection. Prognostic data are limited because of the rarity of the tumors, although aggressive local growth and metastases are documented (53).

The morphologic findings of pulmonary rhabdomyosarcomas are similar to rhabdomyosarcomas at other sites (52a). Rhabdomyosarcomatous differentiation can also be seen in pulmonary artery sarcomas, malignant nerve sheath tumors, pleuropulmonary blastomas, and carcinosarcomas. Metastatic rhabdomyosarcoma should also be excluded.

VASCULAR TUMORS AND RELATED CONDITIONS

Vascular Malformations

Vascular malformations of the lung are rarely encountered by pathologists, since they are often diagnosed radiographically. When vascular malformations are large or multiple, they become clinically significant, as in Osler-Weber-Rendu syndrome (62,113). The gross and histologic features of vascular malformations of the lung are similar to those at other sites. Elastic tissue stains may be helpful in highlighting the abnormal vasculature. Pleural and parenchymal scarring may be associated with markedly thickened and abnormal vessels that may be misinterpreted as vascular malformations of the lung.

Hemangioma/Hemangiomatosis

Hemangiomas of the lung are rare (59,67,89, 113). They may be endobronchial or parenchymal in location, and histologically both cavernous and capillary types are described. They should be distinguished from vascular malformations (113). Hemangiomas are resected for treatment of symptomatic lesions or for diagnosis.

Hemangiomatosis has been associated with two general patterns of pulmonary disease: pulmonary hypertension and interstitial lung disease. The latter may or may not be associated with extrapulmonary hemangiomatous lesions.

Hemangiomatosis of the lung associated with pulmonary hypertension is called *pulmonary capillary hemangiomatosis* (fig. 20-8) (66,71,78, 102,106-108). Most cases are sporadic although Langleben et al. (77) described a familial case. Pulmonary capillary hemangiomatosis may clinically mimic either plexogenic arteriopathy or pulmonary veno-occlusive disease. Histologically, there is an interstitial proliferation of thin-walled, capillary-sized vessels that involve alveolar walls, vessels, and airways. Vascular involvement is thought to lead to vascular occlusion and secondary pulmonary hypertension. The proliferating vessels are cytologically benign, and the differential diagnosis primarily includes chronic venous hypertension with marked passive congestion, changes associated with venous infarction, and pulmonary veno-occlusive disease. The prognosis is poor. Most cases are diagnosed at autopsy (106).

Pulmonary hemangiomatosis has also been applied to a subset of patients presenting with hemoptysis and clinical evidence of interstitial lung disease (93,105). These patients may have pleural effusions (93) and extrapulmonary involvement of the mediastinum and pericardium (105). Histologically, there is a proliferation of cavernous vascular structures along bronchovascular bundles, in the septa and pleura, and at extrapulmonary sites. The clinical and histologic findings overlap with diffuse pulmonary

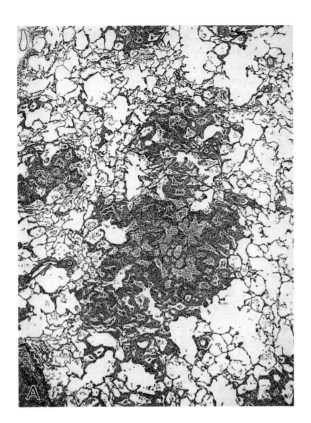

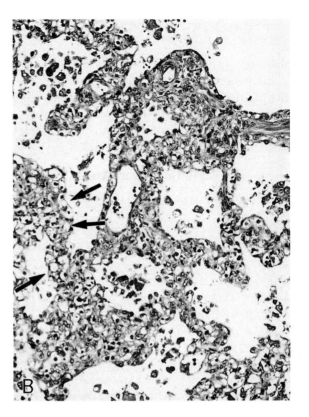

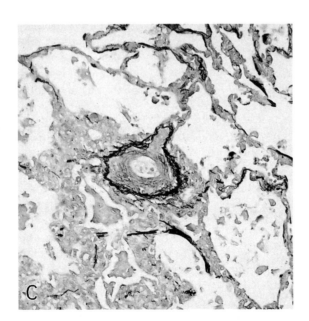

Figure 20-8

PULMONARY CAPILLARY HEMANGIOMATOSIS WITH PULMONARY HYPERTENSION

There is a patchy interstitial widening (A) due to proliferation of thin-walled capillaries in the alveolar walls (B, arrows). Secondary intimal thickening in a pulmonary vein is present (C, elastic tissue stain) indicative of secondary veno-occlusive disease and associated pulmonary hypertension.

lymphangiomatosis (described below); distinguishing between the two may be difficult, and based solely on the presence of red blood cells in the vascular spaces, a notoriously unreliable finding for separating hemangiomatous from lymphangiomatous lesions. The prognosis is poor. White (111) has reported some response to interferon therapy.

Lymphatic Lesions

Lymphatic lesions of the lung can be divided into lymphangiectasis, localized solitary lymphangiomas, and diffuse pulmonary lymphangiomatosis. All are rare, and the distinction between them is not always straightforward. For the interested reader, the classification system of abnormalities of the lymphatics by Hilliard et al. (72) is recommended.

Diffuse pulmonary lymphangiectasis is discussed in chapter 2.

Localized solitary lymphangiomas of the lung are rare, and only a few cases have been reported (73,75,82,116). Children and adults are affected. The reported cases have been associated with mass lesions and symptoms related to the local effects of the mass. The gross and histologic features are similar to lymphangiomas at other sites: anastomosing cavernous spaces, lymphoid follicles, and variable amounts of smooth muscle in the thick fibrous septa (fig. 20-9). The differential diagnosis includes hemangioma and alveolar adenoma. The treatment is excision, and the prognosis is favorable.

Some lymphangiomatous proliferations may affect one lobe diffusely along its lymphatic routes and not affect intervening normal lung tissue. Such lesions represent forms intermediate between localized solitary lymphangioma and diffuse pulmonary lymphangiomatosis.

Diffuse pulmonary lymphangiomatosis is a peculiar condition in which there is a diffuse proliferation of abnormal anastomosing lymphatic structures along the normal lymphatic routes of the lungs (57,61,76,99,100). Extrapulmonary involvement, particularly of mediastinal structures, is common. Diffuse pulmonary lymphangiomatosis has often been confused with lymphangiectasis and in some reports it is difficult to determine which condition is being described. The majority of affected patients are children, although adults into the fourth decade have been reported (99,100). Both sexes are affected. The patients present with respiratory distress or dyspnea; hemoptysis is also common. Chest radiographs show interstitial lung disease, and CT scans confirm the presence of prominent septal lines and bronchovascular thickening corresponding to the pathologic findings.

Grossly and histologically, there is a proliferation of abnormal anastomosing lymphatic channels in the septa, pleura, and along bronchovascular bundles, with normal intervening lung tissue (fig. 20-10). The spaces are generally cavernous, although capillary proliferations can be seen. Some cases have scattered smooth muscle bundles associated with the lymphatic channels. The smooth muscle cells are parallel in orientation and more closely resemble normal smooth muscle than those seen in lymphangioleiomyomatosis. Lymphoid follicles are not seen. Some of the vascular spaces may contain red blood cells, and hemosiderin may be found in the adjacent interstitium. Fresh and old hemorrhage correspond to the hemoptysis that is a common clinical manifestation. Dilated lymphatics involving airways probably predispose to mucosal ulceration and bleeding.

The differential diagnosis includes diffuse pulmonary hemangiomatosis, diffuse pulmonary lymphangiectasis, lymphangioleiomyomatosis, interstitial emphysema, Kaposi sarcoma, and angiosarcoma.

Most patients have progressive disease. In the few cases reported, approximately half the patients died, particularly young children. There is no proven therapy.

Epithelioid Hemangioendothelioma

Epithelioid hemangioendothelioma is the current preferred term for a tumor in the lung that had previously been called an *intravascular bronchoalveolar tumor* (IVBAT) (2,109,110,113). Epithelioid hemangioendotheliomas of the lung are low-grade sclerosing angiosarcomas that typically present with multiple nodules in young women (55,63,64,110,113,115). They also occur in the bone, soft tissue, liver (where they have been called sclerosing cholangiocarcinomas), and other sites (109,110).

The clinical features of epithelioid hemangioendothelioma involving the lung are distinctive (2,64,113,115). Women, within a broad age range,

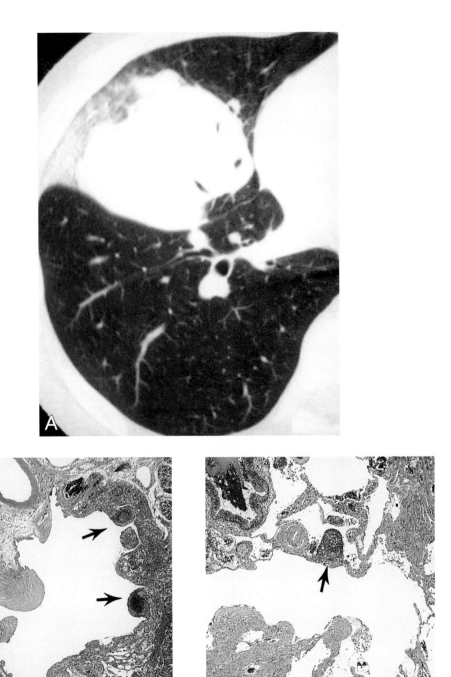

Figure 20-9
LYMPHANGIOMA

This solitary pulmonary mass (A) was resected and showed typical features of a lymphangioma (B,C), with gaping lymphatic vascular spaces and thick fibrous septa containing lymphoid tissue (arrows). The lymphoid tissue in B (arrows) is part of an involved peribronchial lymph node. (Courtesy of Dr. Kaoru Hamada, Nara, Japan.)

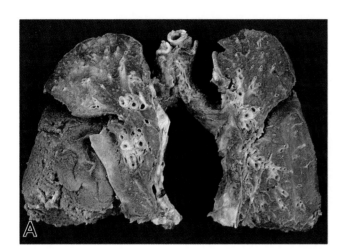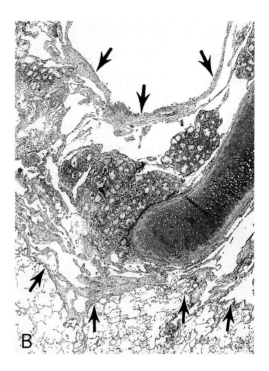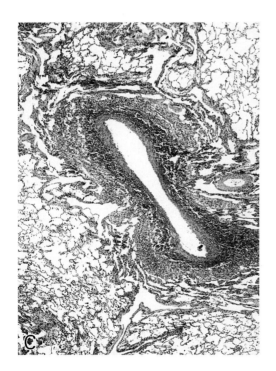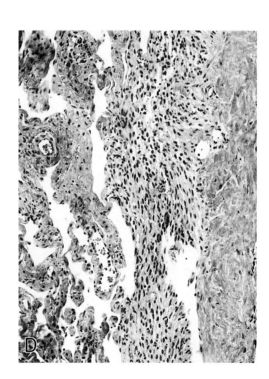

Figure 20-10
DIFFUSE PULMONARY LYMPHANGIOMATOSIS

The lungs at autopsy showed a diffuse thickening and prominence of bronchovascular bundles due to the proliferation of anastomosing lymphatic channels (A). Anastomosing dilated lymphatic spaces permeate the wall of a bronchus (B, arrows) and surround a large pulmonary vein (C). The lymphatic spaces are lined by endothelial cells with fibrous septa (D, left) and (in some cases) there are focal bundles of spindle cells (D, right) which show features of smooth muscle cells.

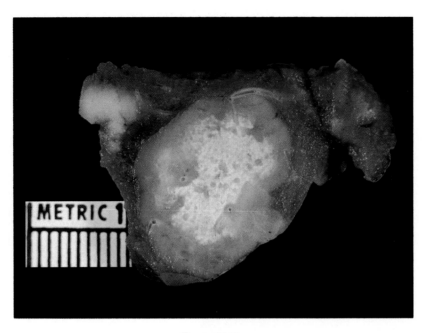

Figure 20-11
EPITHELIOID HEMANGIOENDOTHELIOMA
This resected nodule of epithelioid hemangioma of the lung shows a discrete nodule with central chalky necrosis and a rim of viable tissue with a chondroid appearance.

are primarily affected (4 to 1). Children as young as 7 years have been described (92); over 50 percent of the patients are under age 40. Patients generally have only mild symptoms of cough or dyspnea; some are asymptomatic. Chest radiographs typically show multiple, noncalcified, bilateral nodules up to 2 cm in diameter; most are less than 1 cm. Yousem and Hochholzer (115) have reported unusual intrathoracic presentations, including mediastinal involvement and diffuse pleural thickening, mimicking a malignant mesothelioma. Some patients have concomitant multifocal disease (involving liver, bone, or soft tissue); in such cases lung involvement is considered metastatic, but a multicentric origin has also been suggested (84).

Grossly, epithelioid hemangioendotheliomas of the lung are discrete, circumscribed, firm, gray-white translucent nodules that resemble cartilage (fig. 20-11). They may have a central opaque zone, which can be calcified.

Histologically, there are circumscribed, pale, eosinophilic nodules with central hyalinization or coagulative necrosis that may resemble amyloid or cartilage (fig. 20-12). The periphery of the nodules is more cellular, and balls of cells in a myxohyaline or myxochondroid matrix are seen extending into alveolar spaces, bronchioles, vessels, and lymphatics (115). The cells are most often cytologically bland, polygonal, and eosinophilic with round nuclei and uniform small to moderately sized nucleoli. They occasionally contain sharp single cytoplasmic vacuoles thought to represent vascular lumen differentiation: these may be appreciated in cytologic preparations (fig. 20-13). Some cases show moderate cytologic atypia, necrosis, and numerous mitotic figures (fig. 20-14). In such cases, distinguishing epithelioid hemangioendothelioma from epithelioid angiosarcoma and some poorly differentiated carcinomas may not be straightforward.

The histology in the pleura varies somewhat, and one may see only a moderately cellular spindle cell proliferation (fig. 20-14) or dense hyalinized nodules.

Immunohistochemical and ultrastructural studies show that the proliferating cells are endothelial cells (fig. 20-15) (55,63,64,110). They are factor VIII positive and generally cytokeratin negative. Vimentin stains are also positive. Electron microscopy shows a long-spaced collagenous stroma with cells containing abundant

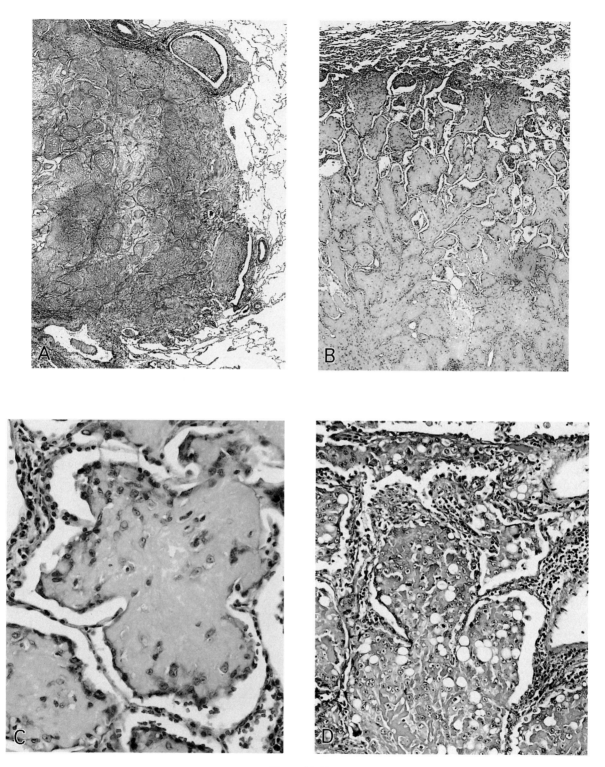

Figure 20-12
EPITHELIOID HEMANGIOENDOTHELIOMA

These cases illustrate the typical discrete well-circumscribed nature of the nodules which grow by extension into adjacent airspaces including bronchioles (A,B). The center of the nodules may show fibrinoid change (A) or a hyaline chondroid appearance (B). The cells are generally bland and embedded in hyaline matrix with prominence of the nuclei at the periphery (C), or, particularly, at the edge of nodules. The intra-alveolar buds are more cellular and may contain numerous sharp vacuoles (D).

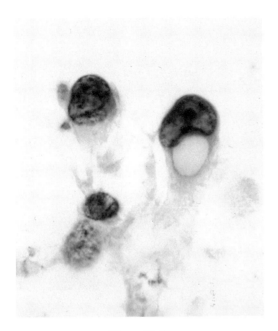

Figure 20-13

EPITHELIOID HEMANGIOENDOTHELIOMA

This fine needle aspirate shows cells with moderately atypical nuclei, one of which contains a clear, sharply demarcated cytoplasmic vacuole.

Table 20-2

EPITHELIOID HEMANGIOENDOTHELIOMA*

Original Diagnoses Submitted
Benign, nonneoplastic
Old granulomatous disease
Organizing infarct
Organizing alveolar proteinosis
Amyloid nodules
Deciduosis
Hamartoma
Fibrous histiocytoma
Chemodectoma
Mesothelioma
Adenocarcinoma
Primary BAC
Cylindromatous
Metastatic tumors
Salivary gland, thyroid, breast, ovary, unknown
Chondro(myxo)sarcoma
Leiomyosarcoma
Angiosarcoma

*Modified from reference 64.

intermediate filaments and Weibel-Palade bodies (63). Occasional cells have single large vacuoles, and are surrounded by an incomplete basement membrane; occasional desmosomal attachments are seen (63).

The histology of epithelioid hemangioendothelioma in the lung is unique, although the unusual features encompass a large differential diagnosis. Table 20-2 shows the diagnoses initially considered in the series of Dail et al. (64) and highlights the variety of lesions that may be considered, including a primary elsewhere with metastasis to the lung.

There is no known treatment for epithelioid hemangioendothelioma. The prognosis is variable: some cases progress very slowly, with survival of 20 years or more, whereas others rapidly lead to death in respiratory failure as the lung is progressively replaced by neoplastic tissue (64,110).

Kaposi Sarcoma

Kaposi sarcoma of the lung generally occurs in the setting of disseminated disease (2,81,91, 101); rarely, the lung is the initial site of presentation (91). Pulmonary involvement can be seen in all clinical forms of Kaposi sarcoma and occurs in up to 25 percent of patients with acquired immunodeficiency syndrome (AIDS) who have evidence of Kaposi sarcoma at extrapulmonary sites (85). Most patients with pulmonary Kaposi sarcoma are symptomatic, although clinically silent pulmonary involvement has been described (69). Symptoms include cough, dyspnea, wheezing, fever, and hemoptysis (85). Chest radiographs show combinations of bilateral alveolar, interstitial, and nodular infiltrates (as large as 3 cm in diameter) (65,97) with pleural effusions present in up to 30 percent of patients. Parenchymal lesions, bronchial lesions, or both are seen. Of the 24 cases described by Naidich et al. (83), 15 were primarily parenchymal, and 9 were primarily bronchial but concurrent involvement with both types is common. The violaceous bronchial plaques are sufficiently characteristic that an experienced bronchoscopist can make a clinical diagnosis without biopsy in patients who already have a diagnosis of Kaposi sarcoma. Biopsies are avoided by some bronchoscopists because of the risk of bleeding.

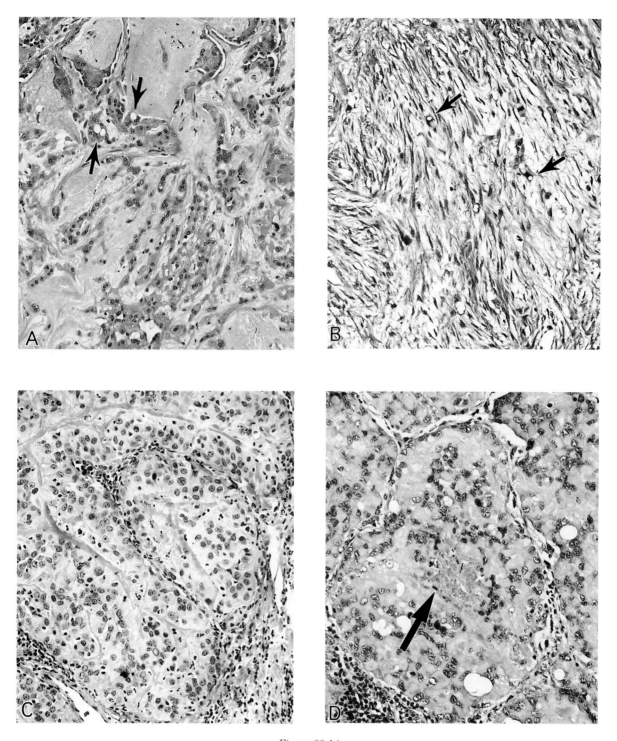

Figure 20-14
EPITHELIOID HEMANGIOENDOTHELIOMA

Some of the histologic variations of epithelioid hemangioendothelioma are illustrated.

A: An epithelioid appearance with cords of endothelial cells in a hyaline stroma. Some cells have cytoplasmic vacuoles (arrows).

B: Epithelioid hemangioendothelioma growing in the pleura with spindle cells in a myxoid stroma. Occasional cells with sharp cytoplasmic vacuoles are apparent (arrows).

C: Cellular nodules with moderate nuclear atypia. Such a case could mimic large cell carcinoma.

D: Moderately atypical nuclei set in a hyaline stroma with necrosis in the center of the nodule (arrow).

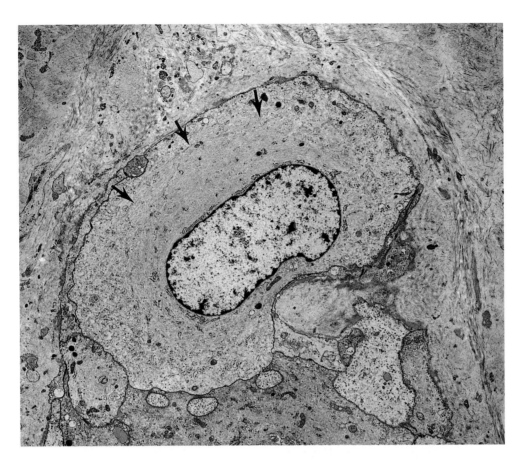

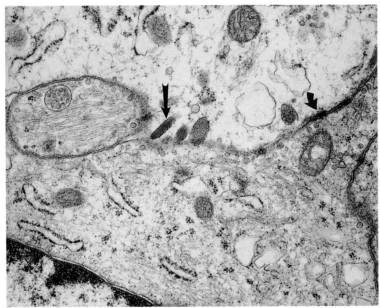

Figure 20-15
EPITHELIOID HEMANGIOENDOTHELIOMA

Ultrastructural features include cells with abundant cytoplasmic intermediate filaments (top, arrows), poorly formed intercellular attachments (bottom, curved arrow), and Weibel-Palade bodies (bottom, straight arrow). (Courtesy of Dr. Sam Hammar, Bremerton, WA.)

Grossly and microscopically, the lesions of Kaposi sarcoma are hemorrhagic nodules found along the lymphatic routes (figs. 20-16–20-18). Mural infiltration of vessels and airways is common; the latter accounts for the characteristic lesions seen at bronchoscopy which can be biopsied to confirm pulmonary involvement (68, 70). The histologic findings are similar to Kaposi sarcoma at other sites in the body. There is a proliferation of spindle cells with intercellular clefts, extravasation of red blood cells, scattered hemosiderin, cytoplasmic eosinophilic bodies, ectasia of surrounding vascular spaces, and prominent plasma cells in the surrounding tissues. Early cases may manifest as peribronchial or perivascular fibrous tissue thickening with increased spindle cells, hemosiderin, and plasma cells.

The differential diagnosis of pulmonary Kaposi sarcoma includes angiosarcoma, diffuse pulmonary lymphangiomatosis and hemangiomatosis, lymphangioleiomyomatosis, and the granulation tissue proliferation seen in organizing pneumonias and organizing diffuse alveolar damage. Angiosarcomas tend to be more nodular (grossly and histologically), have more cytologic atypia, and are associated with occlusion of pulmonary arteries; patients lack the risk factors for Kaposi sarcoma. In cases of pulmonary Kaposi sarcoma in AIDS, concomitant infections should always be sought.

Pulmonary Angiosarcoma

Pulmonary angiosarcoma of the lung is exceedingly rare (2,86,87,98). The few reported cases are of single or multiple mass lesions associated with dyspnea or hemoptysis. In some cases, the distinction between primary angiosarcoma and *metastatic angiosarcoma* is arbitrary (112). Most cases of angiosarcoma in the lung represent metastatic disease, although the lung may be the site of initial presentation (88,112,113). In a review of 15 cases by Patel and Ryu (88), the median age was 45 years (range, 5 to 71 years), and the most common symptom was hemoptysis. Some cases mimic a fulminant alveolar hemorrhage syndrome (94,98). Chest radiographs show multiple nodules or, less commonly, diffuse alveolar infiltrates identical to those seen in an alveolar hemorrhage syndrome. Primary sites of angiosarcoma metastatic to the lung are

heart, pericardium, breast, liver, spleen, kidney, adrenal, bone, and brain (88,112).

Grossly, primary and metastatic angiosarcomas are hemorrhagic nodules involving the lung or pleura, with variable amounts of hemorrhage into the surrounding lung tissue (figs. 20-19, 20-20). The histologic findings are similar to angiosarcomas at other sites with atypical endothelial cells forming variably sized vascular channels and occasional solid spindle or epithelioid cell nodules. The distinctive features in the lung include intra-arterial and periarteriolar involvement, and extensive recent and old hemorrhage.

The differential diagnosis includes Kaposi sarcoma, diffuse pulmonary lymphangiomatosis and hemangiomatosis, pulmonary capillary hemangiomatosis, nodules of metastatic pulmonary artery sarcoma, primary and metastatic spindle cell carcinomas, and, in the case of epithelioid angiosarcoma, primary and metastatic carcinomas.

Pulmonary Artery and Vein Sarcomas

Pulmonary artery and pulmonary vein sarcomas are rare, although the pulmonary artery or its branches are affected more often than the pulmonary vein. There are only a few reports of pulmonary vein sarcomas (74,103).

Sarcomas of the pulmonary arteries show a slight predilection for women; most patients present in the fourth to sixth decades, although there is a broad age range and children are also affected (56,58,60,79,90,96). Symptoms may be insidious and mimic pulmonary emboli; in the review by Bleisch (58), symptoms had been present for a median of 10 months, with a range of 1 to 262 months. Signs and symptoms include dyspnea, systolic murmur, chest pain, cyanosis, cough, edema, hemoptysis, and syncopy. Chest radiographs show abnormalities of the heart or lungs, but specialized studies, such as angiography, are usually needed for definitive visualization. Embolic metastases in the peripheral lung tissue may produce multiple nodular infiltrates simulating pulmonary emboli.

Grossly, the lesions are myxoid or fleshy, sometimes polypoid, masses that involve the pulmonary trunk or its main branches (fig. 20-21). In most cases the tumor is restricted to the vessel lumen or wall, although some cases show

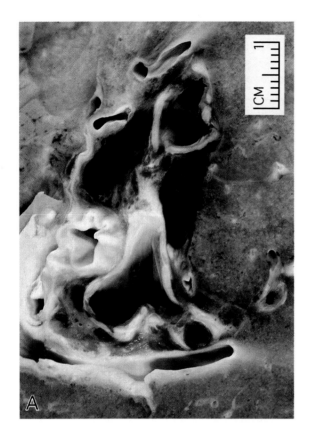
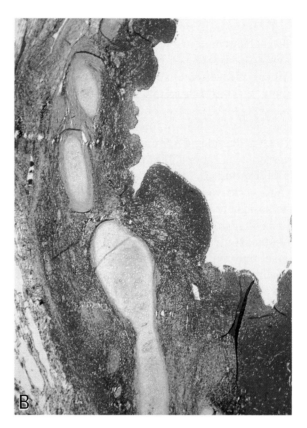
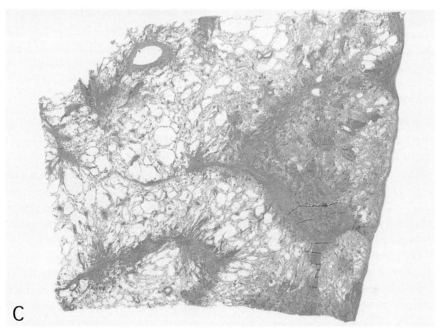

Figure 20-16
KAPOSI SARCOMA

Bronchial involvement at autopsy is seen as dark hemorrhagic tumor tissue involving the bronchial mucosa (A) and permeating the bronchial wall (B). Peripheral lung involvement shows hemorrhagic infiltrates along septa with stellate extension into the surrounding alveoli (C).

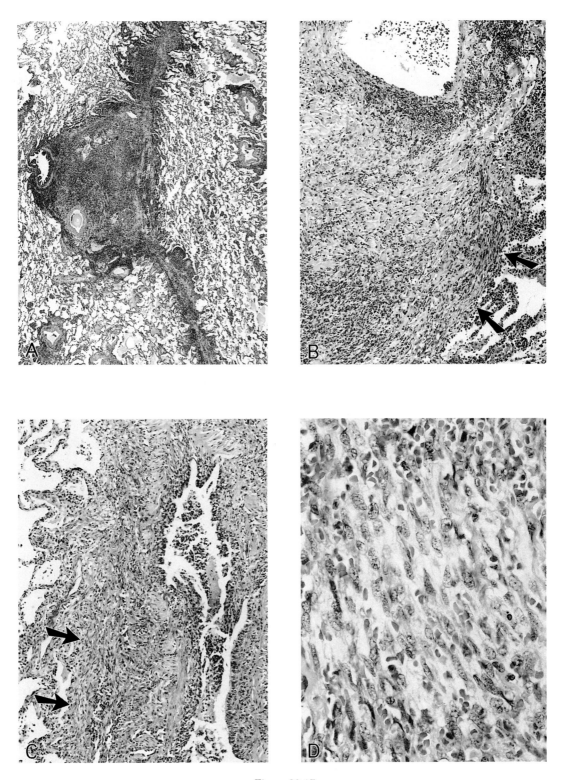

Figure 20-17
KAPOSI SARCOMA

The tumor shows infiltration around a bronchovascular bundle (A, center) with some separation between the bronchiole and pulmonary artery. There is also extension along a septum (top and bottom). B and C show infiltration of a pulmonary artery and bronchiole, respectively. The typical fascicles of spindle cells of Kaposi sarcoma can be seen (C, arrows and D).

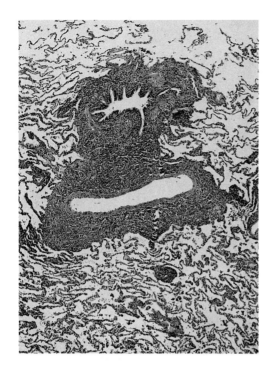

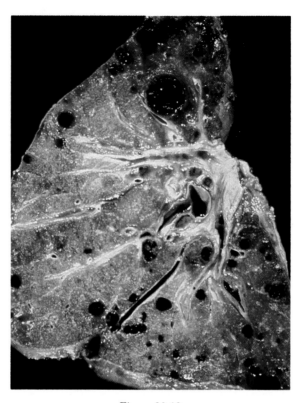

Figure 20-19
METASTATIC ANGIOSARCOMA

Metastatic angiosarcoma is seen as multiple hemorrhagic nodules.

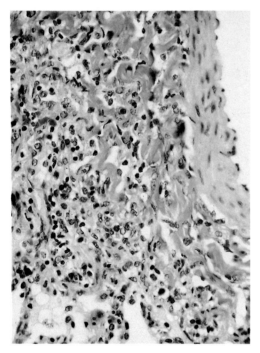

Figure 20-18
KAPOSI SARCOMA

Top: Early involvement of a bronchovascular bundle by Kaposi sarcoma is seen as thickening of the periarterial and peribronchiolar connective tissue.

Bottom: The thickening is due to an infiltrate of nondescript spindle cells and plasma cells. While the low-power appearance is distinctive, definitive confirmation of Kaposi sarcoma was made on the basis of typical fascicles of spindle cells in other fields.

extravascular extension into adjacent structures (such as bronchi) or metastasis to the peripheral lung or, less commonly, outside the thorax.

Some cases manifest primarily as lumenal masses, whereas others are primarily mural; combinations of the two also occur. Histologically, a variety of patterns and mixtures thereof are seen (fig. 20-22). Sarcomatous patterns include undifferentiated sarcoma, myxoid sarcoma, osteosarcoma, malignant fibrous histiocytoma, fibrosarcoma, rhabdomyosarcoma, chondrosarcoma, and angiosarcoma (56,58,60, 66a,113). In some cases there are foci of dense fibrosis alternating with the sarcomatous stroma, and in others the sarcomatous tissue grows over an organized thrombus. The neoplastic cells may have an epithelioid character. Metastatic spread to the more distal vasculature produces a distinctive histology: the vessels are occluded by spindle cells which permeate the vessel wall to produce a perivascular infiltrate.

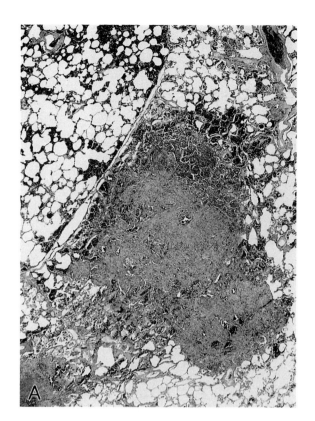

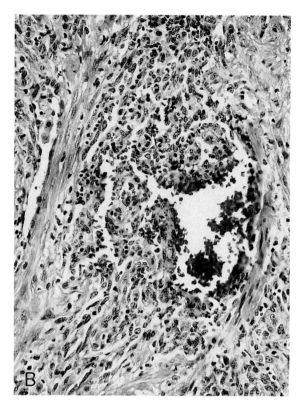

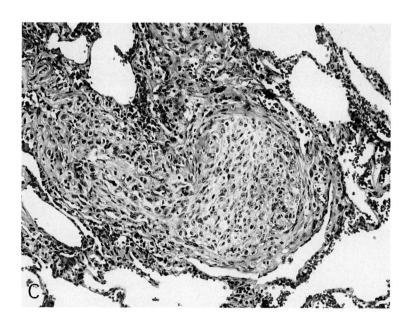

Figure 20-20

METASTATIC ANGIOSARCOMA

There is a hemorrhagic nodule centering on an obliterated pulmonary artery branch in the center of the field (A). The atypical spindle cells form primitive vascular spaces containing red blood cells (B). In another field, neoplastic spindle cells fill a small pulmonary artery (C).

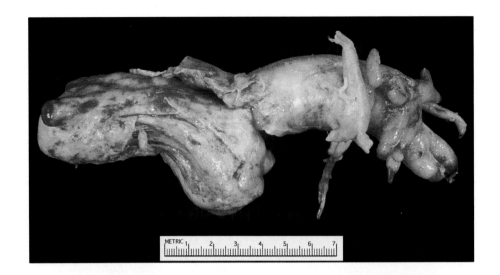

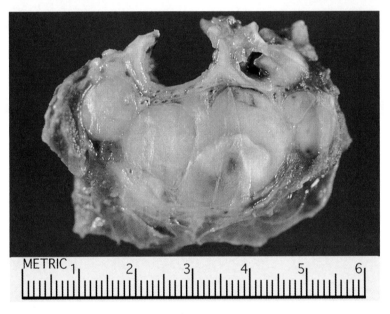

Figure 20-21
PULMONARY ARTERY SARCOMA
Top: A resected tumor thrombus is seen as a neoplastic cast of the right and left pulmonary artery.
Bottom: In another case, the tumor is seen in cross section filling the large branches of the pulmonary artery adjacent to the bronchus.

The pattern may be similar to that seen in some spindle cell carcinomas with vascular invasion. The degree of fresh hemorrhage that typifies metastatic angiosarcomas is usually lacking.

Immunohistochemical findings vary with the histologic pattern (60,79,90). The following stains have been reported to be positive in pulmonary artery sarcomas: vimentin, actin, desmin, S-100 protein, Leu-7, alpha-1-anti-trypsin, alpha-1-antichymotrypsin, and lyso-zyme; negative are myoglobin, cytokeratin, epithelial membrane antigen, and factor VIII.

Ultrastructurally, the cells have features of fibroblasts, histiocyte-like cells, and myofibro-blasts (56,90). Some show chondroid differentia-tion (79). The multiple cell types occasionally encountered have lead to the suggestion of an origin from pluripotential mesenchymal cells (90).

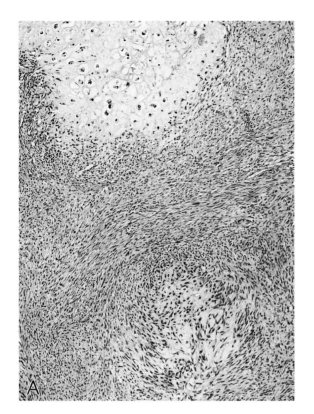
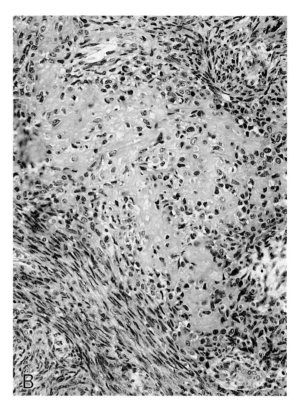
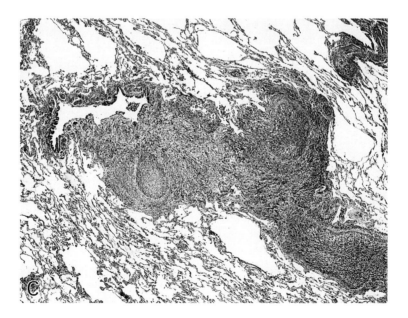

Figure 20-22
PULMONARY ARTERY SARCOMA
Histologic variation of pulmonary artery sarcoma is illustrated by the presence, all in one case, of chondrosarcomatous tissue (A, top), osteosarcomatous tissue with osteoid production (B), and spindle cell sarcoma growing within and around small pulmonary arteries in a peripheral metastasis from the main mass (C).

The differential diagnosis of sarcomas of the pulmonary artery is limited because the gross and radiographic findings are virtually diagnostic. Nevertheless, the possibility of metastatic sarcomas (e.g., angiosarcoma) and carcinomas (e.g., renal cell carcinoma) should be considered as well as spindle cell carcinoma of the lung with vascular invasion.

The treatment is resection. In early studies, most cases were diagnosed only at autopsy; more recent series have included patients undergoing curative resections. In the 16 cases reported by Burke and Virmani (60), curative resection was attempted in 10, and 3 of the patients were alive at 12, 25, and 120 months.

Hemangiopericytoma

Hemangiopericytomas of the lung are similar to their soft tissue counterparts (2,80,95,113, 114). Most patients are in the fifth or sixth decade of life (range, 10 to 73 years) (95). There is an equal sex incidence. Hemoptysis and chest pain are the most common symptoms. Approximately half the patients are asymptomatic; an abnormality is discovered on a routine chest radiograph (95). A solitary mass lesion is the most common finding, although Yousem (114) reported two cases with multiple nodules in one lobe. Invasion of the extrapulmonary structures can be seen radiographically or at surgery (114). Grossly, the tumors are fleshy masses up to 16 cm in diameter. Hemorrhage and necrosis may be seen (fig. 20-23A). An endobronchial component may be present. The histologic findings are similar to hemangiopericytomas at other sites (fig. 20-23B,C).

The treatment of hemangiopericytoma of the lung is resection. As is the case of soft tissue hemangiopericytomas, the prognosis is difficult to predict solely on the basis of histology. Yousem and Hochholzer (114) regarded all cases of hemangiopericytoma of the lung as potentially malignant, and thought that specific clues to aggressive behavior included a size greater than 8 cm, pleural or bronchial invasion, tumor giant cells, greater than 3 mitotic figures per 10 high-power fields, and tumor necrosis. None of these features by itself was predictive in an individual case. Of the 13 patients followed in Yousem's series, 8 were alive without evidence of disease

(at 2 to 168 months): 2 of these relapsed after the initial surgery, one was treated by radiation and one with further surgery; 4 were dead of disease; and 1 died of unrelated causes.

NEUROGENIC TUMORS

Neurilemmoma and Neurofibroma

Neurilemmomas and neurofibromas are rare primary tumors in the lung (2,118,119,126,129, 133,135,140,142,143,147) and account for about 0.2 percent of all lung tumors in the series of Roviaro (140). According to Bartley and Arean (118), neurofibromas are about three times as common as neurilemmomas. Both children (as young as 5 years) and adults are affected (129). Most patients do not have von Recklinghausen disease. Neurofibromas are more frequent in men, whereas neurilemmomas are more frequent in women. Most patients are asymptomatic, except for those whose endobronchial lesions cause obstructive symptoms. O'Donahue et al. (138) described a case of multifocal neurofibroma associated with hypoxia from vascular shunting within the tumor nodules.

Most neurilemmomas and neurofibromas of the lung are solitary nodules; they can attain a size of 8 cm. Unger et al. (147) reported on a patient with von Recklinghausen disease with multiple neurilemmomas involving the submucosa, muscularis, and adventitia of multiple bronchi. Grossly, histologically, immunohistochemically, and ultrastructurally these tumors are similar to their extrapulmonary counterparts (fig. 20-24). The treatment is resection, and the prognosis is excellent.

Neuroma and Ganglioneuroma

Mucosal neuromas and ganglioneuromas may also involve the lung as part of hereditary syndromes (121) or isolated findings (fig. 20-25).

Malignant Nerve Sheath Tumors

Malignant nerve sheath tumors (*malignant schwannoma, neurofibrosarcoma*) represent pathologic curiosities in the lung and very few cases have been reported (128a,128b,136,140). They tend to be larger than their benign counterparts. Grossly, histologically, immunohistochemically,

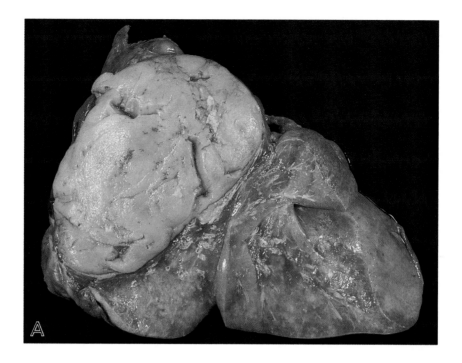

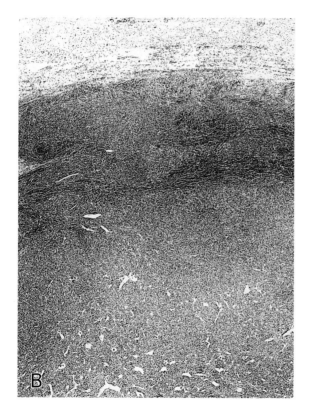

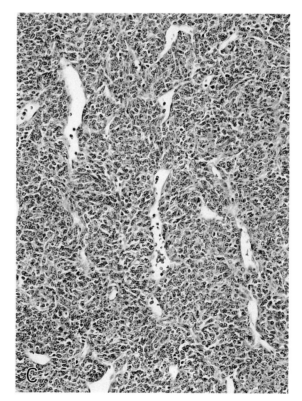

Figure 20-23
HEMANGIOPERICYTOMA OF THE LUNG

This surgically resected pulmonary hemangiopericytoma shows the typical circumscribed fleshy appearance of a sarcoma with focal necrosis (A). The tumor is well demarcated from the surrounding lung tissue. Another case shows sharp demarcation from the lung histologically (B) and the typical cellular appearance of a malignant hemangiopericytoma (C).

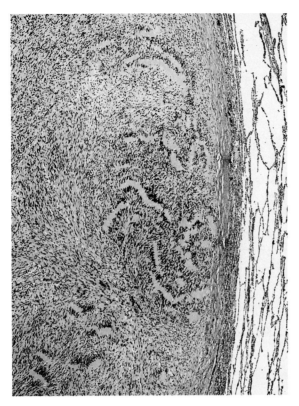

Figure 20-24
NEURILEMMOMA
This solitary encapsulated pulmonary neurilemmoma shows the classic Verocay bodies.

and ultrastructurally these tumors are similar to their extrapulmonary counterparts, and diagnostic criteria are the same as those at other sites.

Malignant Psammomatous Melanotic Schwannoma

A malignant psammomatous melanotic schwannoma of the bronchus (fig. 20-26) was reported by Rowlands et al. (141).

Neuroblastoma and Ganglioneuroblastoma

Neuroblastomas and ganglioneuroblastomas (including primitive neuroectodermal tumors) also represent pathologic curiosities in the lung, and very few cases have been reported. Cooney (123) described a 47-year-old man with a primary pulmonary ganglioneuroblastoma (see chapter 17).

Meningioma

Meningioma of the lung may be seen as a primary tumor (122,125,127,130,131,139,146) or as a metastasis from an intracranial lesion that may or may not have been clinically evident (117,124,131,134,137,144,145) at the time the metastasis was identified.

Most patients with metastatic meningiomas have a history of intracranial meningioma, although the interval from diagnosis of the lesion in the brain to the recognition of metastasis may be many years (131). Whenever a diagnosis of primary meningioma of the lung is considered, the possibility of an occult intracranial primary should be excluded. Some unresected, histologically benign intracranial meningiomas have metastasized (fig. 20-27), and the term *benign metastasizing meningioma* has been applied (134,137,144). The lung lesions in such cases are also histologically benign. Atypical and malignant intracranial meningiomas can also metastasize to the lung.

Less than a dozen primary pulmonary meningiomas have been reported (122,125,127,130, 131,139,146,147). All have been in adults, mostly women, with an average age of 55 to 60 years and a range of 19 to 74 years. The tumors were asymptomatic and were discovered as incidental solitary radiographic nodules or incidental autopsy findings. The largest was 6 cm (125) but most were less than 3 cm in diameter. Unger (147) described an incidental pulmonary meningioma in a patient with a history of von Recklinghausen disease and multiple pulmonary neurilemmomas; since there had been prior surgery for an intracranial meningioma, the lesion may have been metastatic.

The gross, histologic (fig. 20-28), immunohistochemical, and ultrastructural features of primary pulmonary meningioma are similar to intracranial meningioma. None of the reported tumors showed histologic features of malignancy.

A relationship has been postulated between primary pulmonary meningiomas and the microscopic clusters of arachnoidal-type cells commonly found in the lung that are called minute pulmonary meningothelial nodules (originally called minute pulmonary chemodectomas [132]) (122,125,127,128,130,131,139). The cells comprising these nodules share many features with

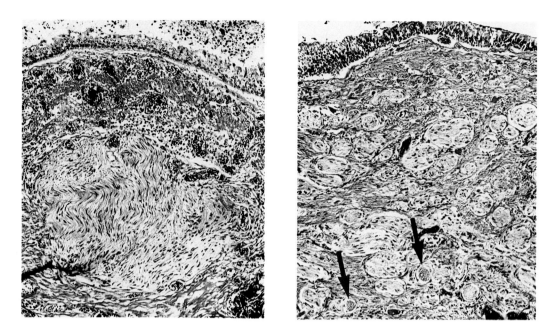

Figure 20-25
BRONCHIAL NEUROMA AND GANGLIONEUROMA

Left: Autopsy lung tissue in a patient with multiple endocrine neoplasia (MEN) type 2 shows a submucosal neuroma involving a large airway. (Courtesy of Dr. J. A. Carney, Rochester, MN.)

Right: This ganglioneuromatous proliferation presented as multiple nodules in a patient with a history of Wilms tumor and islet cell tumor of the pancreas. Neuromatous tissue surrounds the ganglion cells (arrows). A specific syndrome could not be proven in this case. (Courtesy of Dr. Andrew Churg, Vancouver, BC.)

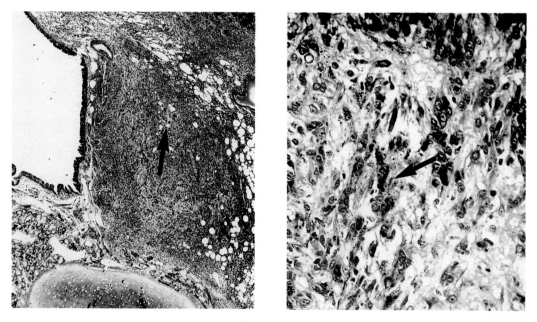

Figure 20-26
MALIGNANT PSAMMOMATOUS MELANOTIC SCHWANNOMA

Left: Tumor tissue around a large airway shows cellular nodules with clusters of psammoma bodies (arrow) and the presence of mature fatty tissue (right).

Right: Cytologically, moderately atypical cells are present. Some cells contain dark granular melanin pigment (arrow). (Courtesy of Dr. J. A. Carney, Rochester, MN.)

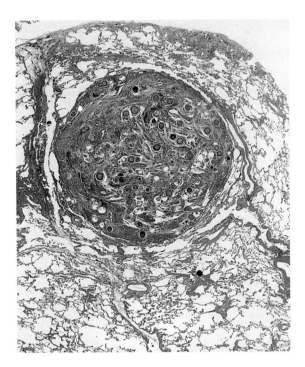

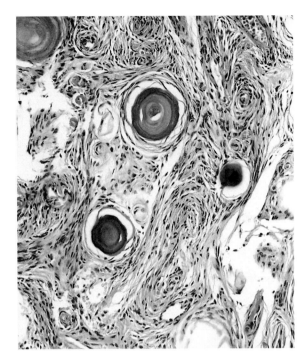

Figure 20-27
METASTATIC MENINGIOMA
A patient known to have a large asymptomatic intracerebral meningioma underwent lobectomy for adenocarcinoma. Multiple nodules (up to 0.7 cm in diameter) of typical benign-appearing meningioma were in the lobe and interpreted as metastases.

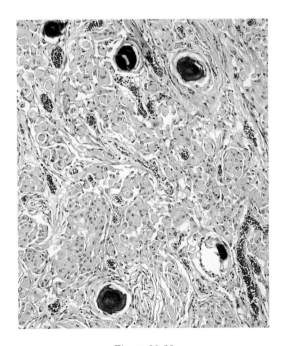

Figure 20-28
PRIMARY PULMONARY MENINGIOMA
This primary pulmonary meningioma shows typical features of a benign meningotheliomatous meningioma with psammoma bodies. (Courtesy of E. M. Drilcek, Vienna, Austria.)

meningioma cells, and are probably the cell of origin of primary pulmonary meningioma.

CARTILAGINOUS TUMORS OF THE LUNG

Chondroma

Chondromas of the lung are rare (148,153a, 161a,162). They may be parenchymal or involve the cartilaginous airways.

Endobronchial tumors are associated with obstructive symptoms. Parenchymal tumors are usually asymptomatic. Many of the reported cases have occurred in women with Carney triad; the presence of a pulmonary chondroma in a young woman should lead to consideration of this triad (multiple gastric smooth muscle tumors, chondromatous tumors of the lung, and extra-adrenal paragangliomas) (149,151,159,160). With Carney triad, single or multiple pulmonary chondromas may be found. Some isolated chondromas do occur over the age of 50 (153a,161a).

Chondromas are well circumscribed and may shell out (fig. 20-29). The tumors are lobulated

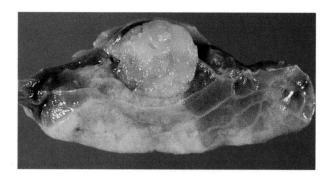

Figure 20-29
PULMONARY CHONDROMA IN CARNEY TRIAD
There is a small, well-circumscribed, gray-white cartilaginous nodule without lobulation. (Courtesy of Dr. P. W. Johnston, Aberdeen, Scotland.)

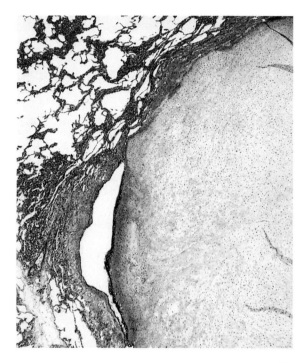
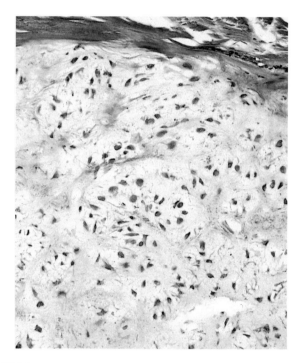

Figure 20-30
PULMONARY CHONDROMA IN CARNEY TRIAD
Left: The sharply circumscribed chondromatous nodule involves a small bronchiole.
Right: Cytologically, stellate cells are set in a myxochondroid matrix.

and gritty on cut section due to calcification, or soft and gelatinous due to cystic degeneration.

Histologically, chondromas are composed of benign cartilaginous tissue (fig. 20-30). In Carney triad, there may be a myxoid stroma with stellate cells, mature cartilage, and even metaplas-tic bone with vascular adipose tissue (149). Chondromas may be moderately cellular and include occasional binucleate cells, but mitotic figures are not seen, and there is often maturation at the edge of the lobules where the mature cartilage and bone are found. Chondromas lack

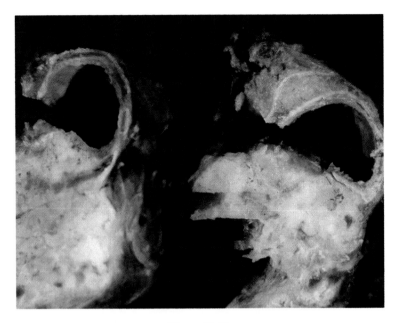

Figure 20-31
TRACHEAL CHONDROSARCOMA
This surgical resection specimen from the trachea shows a large cartilaginous nodule attached to tracheal cartilage. The tumor is grossly typical of chondrosarcoma.

the heterogeneous mesenchymal components and the epithelial-lined clefts seen in hamartomas (chapter 18). Some are covered by bronchiolar epithelium, suggesting proximity to, or origin from, a small bronchus.

The differential diagnosis of pulmonary chondroma includes hamartoma, primary and metastatic chondrosarcoma, carcinosarcomas with cartilage, and epithelioid hemangioendothelioma with a myxochondroid stroma.

Single lesions are resected for diagnosis, and the prognosis is excellent. When multiple lesions are present, as in Carney triad, a conservative approach is reasonable once the diagnosis is established (158). Tumors that grow or cause symptoms should be resected.

Chondroblastoma

Primary chondroblastoma of the lung is not well described. An example involving a bronchus is illustrated in Tumors of the Lower Respiratory Tract, Second Series (150). *Metastatic chondroblastoma* to the lung is, however, well described, although rare (155,157). Lung metastases may be encountered concurrent with, or subsequent to, the recognition of the bone lesion. Histologi-

cally, chondroblastomas that metastasize to the lung are identical to those that do not metastasize, and the histologic appearance of the metastases is similar.

Chondrosarcoma

Primary chondrosarcoma of the lung is rare (152a,153,154,163-166). Hayashi (153) found 16 cases in a 1993 review: 7 men and 9 women, with a mean age of 55 years. The tumors were divided roughly equally between those associated with the major bronchi and those in the lung parenchyma. Most patients have nonspecific symptoms: cough, dyspnea, or chest pain. Tumors associated with bronchial obstruction tend to present earlier than parenchymal tumors.

The gross and histologic findings of primary pulmonary chondrosarcoma are similar to chondrosarcomas at other sites (figs. 20-31, 20-32). As at other sites, it may be difficult to distinguish benign from malignant cartilaginous tumors. The parenchymal tumors tend to be larger than those involving bronchi. A tendency for pulmonary artery invasion in the latter is an unfavorable prognostic finding (153). Sun et al. (164) described an

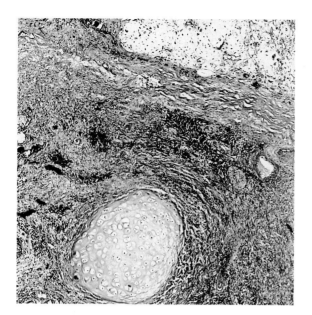 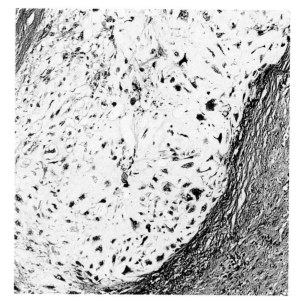

Figure 20-32
CHONDROSARCOMA OF THE LUNG
Left: The chondrosarcomatous nodules (upper right) can be compared with the normal bronchial cartilage (lower left)
Right: The tumor shows features of a grade 2 chondrosarcoma with moderate cytologic atypia.

unusual case with multiple recurrences involving multiple segmental bronchi.

The differential diagnosis of primary chondrosarcoma of the lung includes metastatic chondrosarcoma, chondroma, epithelioid hemangioendothelioma, pleuropulmonary blastoma with chondrosarcomatous foci (see fig. 21-17), carcinosarcoma, primary and metastatic carcinomas with chondroid features, and mesothelioma with chondrosarcomatous differentiation.

The treatment is resection. Most chondrosarcomas are slow-growing tumors that recur locally, and extrathoracic metastases are unusual. In Hayashi's review (153), 10 cases were treated surgically and only 3 died of their tumor.

Mesenchymal chondrosarcoma of the lung has been rarely reported (156,161). Such a tumor in a young child should also raise the possibility of pleuropulmonary blastoma (see chapter 21).

Myxoid chondrosarcoma may present as a lung metastasis. D'Ambrosia (152) reported two patients with solitary metastasis of myxoid chondrosarcoma that predated the discovery of the primary soft tissue neoplasms by 2 years and 10 years. Myxoid features may also be seen in primary chondrosarcoma of the lung.

OSTEOGENIC TUMORS

Metaplastic Bone

Metaplastic bone is the most common cause of histologically benign bone in the lung; it is often an incidental finding. Metaplastic bone may arise in dystrophic calcification, but it is also seen in sites of localized or diffuse lung fibrosis, either as single or multiple nodules or as dendriform ossification (168,169,171–173). Intra-alveolar nodules of metaplastic bone are one of the classic findings in chronic passive congestion, especially in mitral stenosis. In many cases the cause of metaplastic bone in the lung is not apparent. It may also be found in the stroma of a variety of tumors as an incidental finding.

Metaplastic bone may be grossly apparent or an incidental microscopic finding. The bone is of the mature woven type. Fatty marrow, with or without hematopoietic elements, may accompany it.

Osteosarcoma

Osteosarcoma of the lung is rare and less than 10 cases have been reported (167,170,174). Before a diagnosis of primary osteosarcoma of the lung is made, the following should be excluded:

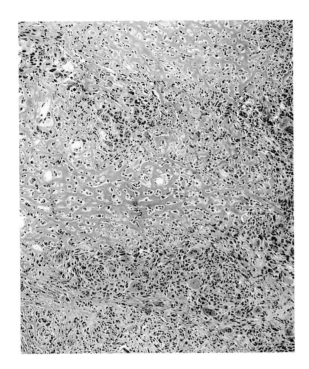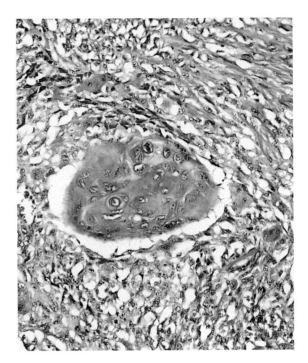

Figure 20-33
OSTEOSARCOMATOUS DIFFERENTIATION IN CARCINOSARCOMA
Left: This case was initially classified as a primary osteosarcoma of the lung with spindle cell sarcomatous stroma and abundant osteoid production.
Right: Fortuitously, while performing special stains, microscopic foci of unequivocal squamous carcinoma were identified, and the case was reclassified as a carcinosarcoma with a dominant osteosarcomatous component.

metastatic osteosarcoma and other metastatic tumors with bone production (e.g., uterine endometrial carcinosarcoma), primary osteosarcoma of the chest wall with secondary invasion of the lung, osteosarcomatous mesothelioma (175) involving the lung, carcinosarcoma with an inconspicuous epithelial component (fig. 20-33) (167, 170), and pulmonary artery sarcoma with osteosarcomatous differentiation.

Cases of primary osteosarcoma of the lung have been reviewed by Colby et al. (167) and Loose et al. (170). All the patients were adults, with an age range of 35 to 83 years. There is a roughly equal sex incidence. Most patients are symptomatic with cough, dyspnea, chest pain, hemoptysis, or history of pneumonia. The tumors are large, solitary, well-circumscribed central or peripheral masses up to 16 cm in greatest dimension.

The gross and histologic findings of primary osteosarcoma of the lung are similar to osteosarcomas at other sites. The defining feature is the presence of neoplastic bone or osteoid, although at other sites, other elements such as a chondro-

sarcoma and malignant fibrous histiocytoma may be very prominent.

The treatment is resection. The prognosis is poor, although there are a few long term survivors.

FATTY TUMORS

Lipomas

Lipomas of the lung are uncommon: less than 100 have been reported. Most are endobronchial (fig. 20-34) and produce signs and symptoms of obstruction (176,176a,177a,178,179,182,184, 186,187a,189,190). Men are more frequently affected. Because of their fatty composition, CT scans may strongly suggest a diagnosis of endobronchial lipoma (181,183).

Lipomas of the peripheral lung are rare, and less than 10 cases have been reported; all were in men (177). In a review by Hirata (177), the largest parenchymal lipoma was nearly 8 cm in greatest dimension; 6 of the 7 patients had symptoms, usually cough or chest pain.

The gross and histologic findings of endobronchial and peripheral lipomas of the lung are similar to lipomas at other sites. Endobronchial lesions usually involve proximal lobar and segmental bronchi. These lipomas may not be well circumscribed and appear to blend with the adjacent submucosal tissues of the bronchi (fig. 20-35). Fibrosis, inflammatory changes, lymphoid tissue, cartilage, and other mesenchymal elements may be present (190). Matsuba et al. (182) have described an endobronchial lipoma with features of an atypical lipoma. The presence of lobules of fatty tissue, epithelial-lined clefts, and chondromyxoid matrix should suggest a hamartoma. Some hamartomas may have a disproportionate amount of fatty tissue (185). Metaplastic fat in the visceral pleura is common in fibrotic lung diseases, and it should not be confused with a subpleural lipoma.

The treatment of lipoma of the lung is resection, and when this is accomplished, the prognosis is excellent. In the case of endobronchial lipomas, a conservative approach is warranted, and many cases are successfully resected bronchoscopically.

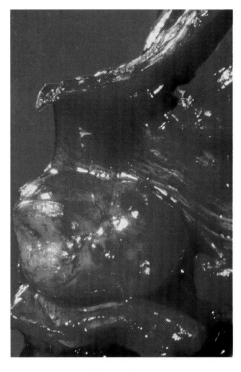

Figure 20-34
ENDOBRONCHIAL LIPOMA
There is a smooth endobronchial polypoid mass composed of yellow fatty tissue.

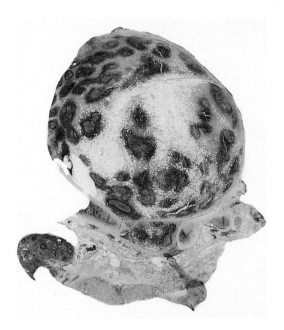
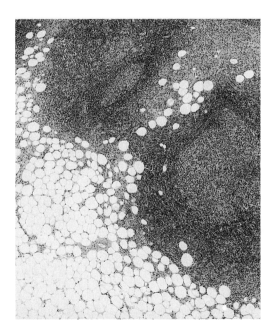

Figure 20-35
ENDOBRONCHIAL LIPOMA
This endobronchial lipoma was associated with recurrent obstructive pneumonia. The resection specimen showed an endobronchial mass (left) composed of fat and fibrous tissue with marked lymphoid hyperplasia (right). The case was arbitrarily classified as a lipoma despite the fact that fibrous tissue and lymphoid tissue were also prominent.

Liposarcomas

Liposarcomas primary in the lung are extremely rare: less than ten cases have been reported (180,187,188). Males and females are equally affected, with a reported age range of 9 to 59 years. The gross, histologic, and ultrastructural (180) features are similar to liposarcomas at other sites.

The differential diagnosis includes lipoma, carcinosarcomas with a prominent liposarcomatous component, metastatic liposarcoma and tumors with liposarcomatous differentiation

(e.g., uterine carcinosarcoma), and, in infants and young children, pleuropulmonary blastoma with liposarcomatous differentiation.

The treatment is resection if this can be accomplished. So few cases have been reported that the prognosis cannot be accurately determined.

ALVEOLAR SOFT PART SARCOMA

There are isolated reports of alveolar soft part sarcoma involving the pulmonary vein (192) and lung parenchyma (191).

REFERENCES

1. Cameron EW. Primary sarcoma of the lung. Thorax 1975;30:516–20.
2. Gal AA, Marchevsky AM, Koss MN. Unusual tumors of the lung. In: Marchevsky AM, ed. Surgical pathology of lung neoplasms. New York: Marcel Dekker, 1990:325–88.
3. Gebauer C. The postoperative prognosis of primary pulmonary sarcomas. A review with a comparison between the histological forms and the other primary endothoracal sarcomas based on 474 cases. Scand J Thor Cardiovasc Surg 1982;16:91–7.
4. _____. Primary pulmonary sarcomas: etiology, clinical assessment and prognosis with a comparison to pulmonary carcinomas—a review of 41 cases and 394 other cases of the literature. Jpn J Surg 1982;12:148–59.
5. Guccion JG, Rosen SH. Bronchopulmonary leiomyosarcoma and fibrosarcoma. A study of 32 cases and review of the literature. Cancer 1972;30:836–47.
6. Hurt R. Benign tumours of the bronchus and trachea, 1951-1981. Ann R Coll Surg Engl 1984;66:22–6.
7. Martini N, Hajdu SI, Beattie EJ Jr. Primary sarcoma of the lung. J Thorac Cardiovasc Surg 1971;61:33–8.
8. Nascimento AG, Unni KK, Bernatz PE. Sarcomas of the lung. Mayo Clin Proc 1982;57:355–9.
9. Salminen S, Halttunen P, Miettinen M, Mattila S. Benign mesenchymal tumours of the lung including sclerosing haemangiomas. Annales Chirurgiae et Gynaecologiae 1990;79:85–91.
10. Tomashefski JF Jr. Benign endobronchial mesenchymal tumors. Am J Surg Pathol 1982;6:531–40.

Smooth Muscle Tumors

11. Alt B, Huffer WE, Belchis DA. A vascular lesion with smooth muscle differentiation presenting as a coin lesion in the lung: glomus tumor versus hemangiopericytoma. Am J Clin Pathol 1983;80:765–71.
12. Archambeaud-Mouveroux F, Bourcereau J, Fressinaud C, Bourras P. Bronchial leiomyoma: report of a case successfully treated by endoscopic neodymiumyttrium aluminum garnet laser. J Thorac Cardiovasc Surg 1988;95:536-8.
13. Banner AS, Carrington CB, Emory WB, et al. Efficacy of oophorectomy in lymphangioleiomyomatosis and benign metastasizing leiomyoma. N Engl J Med 1981;305:204–9.
14. Beluffi G, Bertolotti P, Mietta A, Manara G, Luisetti M. Primary leiomyosarcoma of the lung in a girl. Pediatr Radiol 1986;16:240–4.
15. Bonin M, Myers J, Roche P, Colby T. Pulmonary lymphangiomyomatosis (LAM): an immunohistochemical analysis of 22 cases. Mod Pathol 1992;5:112A.
16. Canzonieri V, Blandamura S, Zanella A, Capitanio G. Uterine benign-appearing smooth muscle tumor metastatic to the lungs: a case report. Tumori 1990;76:513–6.
17. Carrington CB, Cugell DW, Gaensler EA, et al. Lymphangioleiomyomatosis. Physiologic-pathologic-radiologic correlations. Am Rev Respir Dis 1977;116:977–95.
18. Chadwick EG, Connor EJ, Hanson IC, et al. Tumors of smooth-muscle origin in HIV-infected children. JAMA 1990;263:3182–4.
19. Chan JK, Tsang WY, Pau MY, Tang MC, Pang SW, Fletcher CD. Lymphangiomyomatosis and angiomyolipoma: closely related entities characterized by hamartomatous proliferation of HMB-45-positive smooth muscle. Histopathology 1993;22:445–55.
20. Corrin B, Liebow AA, Friedman PJ. Pulmonary lymphangiomyomatosis. A review. Am J Pathol 1975;79:348–82.
21. Dail DH, Hammer SP. Pulmonary pathology. New York: Springer-Verlag, 1988:924–6.
22. Evans AJ, Wiltshaw E, Kochanowski SJ, Macfarlane A, Sears RT. Metastasizing leiomyoma of the uterus and hormonal manipulations. Case report. Br J Obstet Gynaecol 1986;93:646–8.
23. Fabich DR, Hafez GR. Glomangioma of the trachea. Cancer 1980;45:2337–41.

24. Gal AA, Brooks JS, Pietra GG. Leiomyomatous neoplasms of the lung: a clinical, histologic, and immunohistochemical study. Mod Pathol 1989;2:209–15.

25. Garcia-Prats MD, Sotelo-Rodriguez MT, Ballestin C, et al. Glomus tumour of the trachea: report of a case with microscopic, ultrastructural and immunohistochemical examination and review of the literature. Histopathology 1991;19:459–64.

26. Heard BE, Dewar A, Firmin RK, Lennox SC. One very rare and one new tracheal tumour found by electron microscopy: glomus tumour and acinic cell tumour resembling carcinoid tumours by light microscopy. Thorax 1982;37:97–103.

27. Horstmann JP, Pietra GG, Harman JA, Cole NG, Grinspan S. Spontaneous regression of pulmonary leiomyomas during pregnancy. Cancer 1977;39:314–21.

28. Jimenez JF, Uthman EO, Townsend JW, Gloster ES, Seibert JJ. Primary bronchopulmonary leiomyosarcoma in childhood. Arch Pathol Lab Med 1986;110:348–51.

29. Kane PB, Lane BP, Cordice JW, Greenberg GM. Ultrastructure of the proliferating cells in pulmonary lymphangiomyomatosis. Arch Pathol Lab Med 1978;102:618–22.

30. Kim YI, Kim JH, Suh JS, Ham EK, Suh KP. Glomus tumor of the trachea. Cancer 1989;64:881–6.

31. Lillo-Gil R, Albrechtsson U, Jakobsson B. Pulmonary leiomyosarcoma appearing as a cyst. Report of one case and review of the literature. Thorac Cardiovasc Surg 1985;33:250–2.

32. Lipton JH, Fong TC, Burgess KR. Miliary pattern as presentation of leiomyomatosis of the lung. Chest 1987;91:781–2.

33. McGinnis M, Jacobs G, el-Naggar A, Redline RW. Congenital peribronchial myofibroblastic tumor (so-called congenital leiomyosarcoma). A distinct neonatal lung lesion associated with nonimmune hydrops fetalis. Mod Pathol 1993;6:487–92.

34. Morgan PG, Ball J. Pulmonary leiomyosarcomas. Br J Dis Chest 1980;74:245–52.

35. Müller NL, Chiles C, Kullnig P. Pulmonary lymphangiomyomatosis: correlation of CT with radiographic and functional findings. Radiology 1990;175:335–9.

36. Naresh KN, Pai SA, Vyas JJ, Soman CS. Leiomyoma of the bronchus: a case report. Histopathology 1993;22:288–9.

37. Orlowski TM, Stasiak K, Kolodziej J. Leiomyoma of the lung. J Thorac Cardiovasc Surg 1978;76:257–61.

38. Sinclair W, Wright JL, Churg A. Lymphangioleiomyomatosis presenting in a postmenopausal woman. Thorax 1985;40:475–6.

39. Taylor JR, Ryu J, Colby TV, Raffin TA. Lymphangioleiomyomatosis: clinical course in 32 patients. N Engl J Med 1990;323:1254–60.

40. Taylor TL, Miller DR. Leiomyoma of the bronchus. J Thorac Cardiovasc Surg 1969;57:284–8.

41. Uyama T, Monden Y, Harada K, Sumitomo M, Kimura S. Pulmonary leiomyomatosis showing endobronchial extension and giant cyst formation. Chest 1988;94:644–6.

42. Vera-Roman JM, Sobonya RE, Gomez-Garcia JL, Sanz-Bondia JR, Paris-Romeu F. Leiomyoma of the lung. Literature review and case report. Cancer 1983;52:936–41.

43. Wick MR, Scheithauer BW, Piehler JM, Pairolero PC. Primary pulmonary leiomyosarcomas. A light and electron microscopic study. Arch Pathol Lab Med 1982;106:510–4.

44. White SH, Ibrahim NB, Forrester-Wood CP, Jeyasingham K. Leiomyomas of the lower respiratory tract. Thorax 1985;40:306–11.

45. Winkler TR, Burr LH, Robinson CL. Benign metastasizing leiomyoma. Ann Thorac Surg 1987;43:100–1.

46. Wolff M, Silva F, Kaye G. Pulmonary metastases (with admixed epithelial elements) from smooth muscle neoplasms. Report of nine cases, including three males. Am J Surg Pathol 1979;3:325–42.

47. Yamada H, Katoh O, Yamaguchi T, Natsuaki M, Itoh T. Intrabronchial leiomyoma treated by localized resection via bronchotomy and bronchoplasty. Chest 1987;91:283–5.

48. Yellin A, Rosenman Y, Lieberman Y. Review of smooth muscle tumours of the lower respiratory tract. Br J Dis Chest 1984;78:337–51.

Skeletal Muscle Tumors

49. Avagnina A, Elsner B, De Marco L, Bracco AN, Nazar J, Pavlovsky H. Pulmonary rhabdomyosarcoma with isolated small bowel metastasis. A report of a case with immunohistochemical and ultrastructural studies. Cancer 1984;53:1948–51.

50. Chen MF, Onerheim R, Wang NS, Hüttner I. Rhabdomyomatosis of newborn lung: a case report with immunohistochemical and electron microscopic characterization of striated muscle cells in the lung. Pediatr Pathol 1991;11:123–9.

51. Conquest HF, Thornton JL, Massie JR, Coxe JW. Primary pulmonary rhabdomyosarcoma. Ann Surg 1965;161:688–92.

52. Eriksson A, Thunell M, Lundqvist G. Pendulating endobronchial rhabdomyosarcoma with fatal asphyxia. Thorax 1982;37:390–1.

52a. Gal AA, Marchevsky AM, Koss MN. Unusual tumors of the lung. In: Marchevsky AM, ed. Surgical pathology of lung neoplasms. New York: Marcel Dekker, 1990:325–88.

53. Lee SH, Rengachary SS, Paramesh J. Primary pulmonary rhabdomyosarcoma: a case report and review of the literature. Hum Pathol 1981;12:92–5.

54. Vilanova JR, Burgos-Bretones J, Aguirre JM, Rivera-Pomar JM. Rhabdomyomatous dysplasia of lung and congenital diaphragmatic hernia. J Pediatr Surg 1983;18:201–3.

Vascular Tumors

55. Azumi N, Churg A. Intravascular and sclerosing bronchioloalveolar tumor. A pulmonary sarcoma of probable vascular origin. Am J Surg Pathol 1981;5:587–96.

56. Baker PB, Goodwin RA. Pulmonary artery sarcomas. A review and report of a case. Arch Pathol Lab Med 1985;109:35–9.

57. Bhatti MA, Ferrante JW, Gielchinsky I, Norman JC. Pleuropulmonary and skeletal lymphangiomatosis with chylothorax and chylopericardium. Ann Thorac Surg 1985;40:398–401.

58. Bleisch VR, Kraus FT. Polypoid sarcoma of the pulmonary trunk: analysis of the literature and report of a case with leptomeric organelles and ultrastructural features of rhabdomyosarcoma. Cancer 1980;46:314–24.

59. Bowyer JJ, Sheppard M. Capillary haemangioma presenting as a lung pseudocyst. Arch Dis Child 1990;65:1162–4.

60. Burke AP, Virmani R. Sarcomas of the great vessels. A clinicopathologic study. Cancer 1993;71:1761–73.

61. Carlson KC, Parnassus WN, Klatt EC. Thoracic lymphangiomatosis. Arch Pathol Lab Med 1987;111:475–7.

62. Clements BS, Warner JO, Shinebourne EA. Congenital bronchopulmonary vascular malformations: clinical application of a simple anatomical approach in 25 cases. Thorax 1987;42:409–16.

63. Corrin B, Harrison WJ, Wright DH. The so-called intravascular bronchioloalveolar tumour of lung (low-grade sclerosing angiosarcoma): presentation with extrapulmonary deposits. Diagn Histopathol 1983;6:229–37.

64. Dail DH, Liebow AA, Gmelich JT, et al. Intravascular, bronchiolar, and alveolar tumor of the lung (IVBAT). An analysis of twenty cases of a peculiar sclerosing endothelial tumor. Cancer 1983;51:452–64.

65. Davis SD, Henschke CI, Chamides BK, Westcott JL. Intrathoracic Kaposi sarcoma in AIDS patients: radiographic-pathologic correlation. Radiology 1987;163:495–500.

66. Faber CN, Yousem SA, Dauber JH, Griffith BP, Hardesty RL, Paradis IL. Pulmonary capillary hemangiomatosis. A report of three cases and a review of the literature. Am Rev Respir Dis 1989;140:808–13.

66a. Gal AA, Marchevsky AM, Koss MN. Unusual tumors of the lung. In: Marchevsky AM, ed. Surgical pathology of lung neoplasms. New York: Marcel Dekker, 1990:325–88.

67. Galliani CA, Beatty JF, Grosfeld JL. Cavernous hemangioma of the lung in an infant. Pediatr Pathol 1992;12:105–11.

68. Hamm PG, Judson MA, Aranda CP. Diagnosis of pulmonary Kaposi's sarcoma with fiberoptic bronchoscopy and endobronchial biopsy. A report of five cases. Cancer 1987;59:807–10.

69. Hanno R, Owen LG, Callen JP. Kaposi's sarcoma with extensive silent internal involvement. Int J Dermatol 1979;18:718–21.

70. Hanson PJ, Harcourt-Webster JN, Gazzard BG, Collins JV. Fibreoptic bronchoscopy in diagnosis of bronchopulmonary Kaposi's sarcoma. Thorax 1987;42:269–71.

71. Heath D, Reid R. Invasive pulmonary haemangiomatosis. Br J Dis Chest 1985;79:284–94.

72. Hilliard RI, McKendry JB, Phillips MJ. Congenital abnormalities of the lymphatic system: a new clinical classification. Pediatrics 1990;86:988–94.

73. Holden WE, Morris JF, Antonovic R, Gill TH, Kessler S. Adult intrapulmonary and mediastinal lymphangioma causing haemoptysis. Thorax 1987;42:635–6.

74. Kaiser LR, Urmacher C. Primary sarcoma of the superior pulmonary vein. Cancer 1990;66:789–95.

75. Karmazin N, Panitch HB, Balsara RK, Faerber EN, de Chadarevian JP. De novo circumscribed pulmonary lobar cystic lymphatic anomaly in a young boy. A possible sequela of bronchopulmonary dysplasia. Chest 1989;95:1162–3.

76. Kelso JM, Kerr DJ, Lie JT, Sachs MI, O'Connell EJ. Unusual diffuse pulmonary lymphatic proliferation in a young boy. Chest 1991;100:556–60.

77. Langleben D, Heneghan JM, Batten AP, et al. Familial pulmonary capillary hemangiomatosis resulting in primary pulmonary hypertension. Ann Intern Med 1988;109:106–9.

78. Magee F, Wright JL, Kay JM, Peretz D, Donevan R, Churg A. Pulmonary capillary hemangiomatosis. Am Rev Respir Dis 1985;132:922–5.

79. McGlennen RC, Manivel JC, Stanley SJ, Slater DL, Wick MR, Dehner LP. Pulmonary artery trunk sarcoma: a clinicopathologic, ultrastructural, and immunohistochemical study of four cases. Mod Pathol 1989;2:486–94.

80. Meade JB, Whitwell F, Bickford BJ, Waddington JK. Primary haemangiopericytoma of lung. Thorax 1974;29:1–15.

81. Meduri GU, Stover DE, Lee M, Myskowski PL, Caravelli JF, Zaman MB. Pulmonary Kaposi's sarcoma in the acquired immune deficiency syndrome. Clinical, radiographic, and pathologic manifestations. Am J Med 1986;81:11–8.

82. Milovic I, Oluic D. Lymphangioma of the lung associated with respiratory distress in a neonate. Pediatr Radiol 1992;22:156.

83. Naidich DP, Tarras M, Garay SM, Birnbaum B, Rybak BJ, Schinella R. Kaposi's sarcoma. CT-radiographic correlation. Chest 1989;96:723–8.

84. Nerlich A, Berndt R, Schleicher E. Differential basement membrane composition in multiple epithelioid haemangioendotheliomas of liver and lung. Histopathology 1991;18:303–7.

85. Ognibene FP, Shelhamer JH. Kaposi's sarcoma. Clin Chest Med 1988;9:459–65.

86. Ott RA, Eugene J, Kollin J, Kanas RJ, Conston DE, Chi JC. Primary pulmonary angiosarcoma associated with multiple synchronous neoplasms. J Surg Oncol 1987;35:269–6.

87. Palvio DH, Paulsen SM, Henneberg EW. Primary angiosarcoma of the lung presenting as intractable hemoptysis. Thorac Cardiovasc Surg 1987;35:105–7.

88. Patel AM, Ryu JH. Angiosarcoma in the lung. Chest 1993;103:1531–5.

89. Paul KP, Börner C, Müller KM, Vogt-Moykopf I. Capillary hemangioma of the right main bronchus treated by sleeve resection in infancy. Am Rev Respir Dis 1991;143:876–9.

90. Paulsen SM, Egeblad K. Sarcoma of the pulmonary artery. A light and electron microscopic study. J Submicrosc Cytol 1983;15:811–21.

91. Purdy LJ, Colby TV, Yousem SA, Battifora H. Pulmonary Kaposi's sarcoma. Premortem histologic diagnosis. Am J Surg Pathol 1986;10:301–11.

92. Rock MJ, Kaufman RA, Lobe TE, Hensley SD, Moss ML. Epithelioid hemangioendothelioma of the lung (intravascular bronchioloalveolar tumor) in a young girl. Pediatr Pulmonol 1991;11:181–6.

93. Rowen M, Thompson JR, Williamson RA, Wood BJ. Diffuse pulmonary hemangiomatosis. Radiology 1978;127:445–51.

94. Segal SL, Lenchner GS, Cichelli AV, Promisloff RA, Hofman WI, Baiocchi GA. Angiosarcoma presenting as diffuse alveolar hemorrhage. Chest 1988;94:214–8.

95. Shin MS, Ho KJ. Primary hemangiopericytoma of lung: radiography and pathology. AJR Am J Roentgenol 1979;133:1077–83.

96. Shmookler BM, Marsh HB, Roberts WC. Primary sarcoma of the pulmonary trunk and/or right or left main pulmonary artery—a rare cause of obstruction to right ventricular outflow. Report on two patients and analysis of 35 previously described patients. Am J Med 1977;63:263–72.

97. Sivit CJ, Schwartz AM, Rockoff SD. Kaposi's sarcoma of the lung in AIDS: radiologic-pathologic analysis. AJR Am J Roentgenol 1987;148:25–8.

98. Spragg RG, Wolf PL, Haghighi P, Abraham JL, Astarita RW. Angiosarcoma of the lung with fatal pulmonary hemorrhage. Am J Med 1983;74:1072–6.

99. Swank DW, Hepper NGG, Folkert KE, Colby TV. Intrathoracic lymphangiomatosis mimicking lymphangioleiomyomatosis in a young woman. Mayo Clin Proc 1989;64:1264–8.

100. Tazelaar HD, Kerr D, Yousem SA, Saldana MJ, Langston C, Colby TV. Diffuse pulmonary lymphangiomatosis. Hum Pathol. In press.

101. Templeton AC. Studies in Kaposi's sarcoma. Postmortem findings and disease patterns in women. Cancer 1972;30:854–67.

102. Tron V, Magee F, Wright JL, Colby T, Churg A. Pulmonary capillary hemangiomatosis. Hum Pathol 1986;17:1144–50.

103. Tsutsumi Y, Deng Y. Alveolar soft part sarcoma of the pulmonary vein. Acta Pathol Jpn 1991;41:771–7.

104. Verbeken E, Beyls J, Moerman P, Knockaert D, Goddeeris P, Lauweryns JM. Lung metastasis of malignant epithelioid hemangioendothelioma mimicking a primary intravascular bronchioalveolar tumor. A histologic, ultrastructural, and immunohistochemical study. Cancer 1985;55:1741–6.

105. Vevaina JR, Mark EJ. Thoracic hemangiomatosis masquerading as interstitial lung disease. Chest 1988;93:657–9.

106. Wagenaar SS, Mulder JJ, Wagenvoort CA, van den Bosch JM. Pulmonary capillary haemangiomatosis diagnosed during life. Histopathology 1989;14:212–4.

107. Wagenvoort CA, Beetstra A, Spijker J. Capillary haemangiomatosis of the lungs. Histopathology 1978;2:401–6.

108. Whittaker JS, Pickering CA, Heath D, Smith P. Pulmonary capillary haemangiomatosis. Diagn Histopathol 1983;6:77–84.

109. Weiss SW, Enzinger FM. Epithelioid hemangioendothelioma: a vascular tumor often mistaken for a carcinoma. Cancer 1982;50:970–81.

110. _____, Ishak KG, Dail DH, Sweet DE, Enzinger FM. Epithelioid hemangioendothelioma and related lesions. Semin Diagn Pathol 1986;3:259–87.

111. White CW, Wolf SJ, Korones DN, Sondheimer HM, Tosi MF, Yu A. Treatment of childhood angiomatous diseases with recombinant interferon alfa-2a. J Pediatr 1991;118:559–66.

112. Yousem SA. Angiosarcoma presenting in the lung. Arch Pathol Lab Med 1986;110:112–5.

113. _____. Pulmonary vascular neoplasia. Prog Surg Pathol 1989;10:27–62.

114. _____, Hochholzer L. Primary pulmonary hemangiopericytoma. Cancer 1987;59:549–55.

115. _____, Hochholzer L. Unusual thoracic manifestations of epithelioid hemangioendothelioma. Arch Pathol Lab Med 1987;111:459–63.

116. Zimmermann H, Habenicht R. Kongenitales lymphangiom der lunge. Z Kinderchir 1989;44:111–4.

Neurogenic Tumors

117. Aumann JL, Van den Bosch JM, Elbers JR, Wagenaar SJ. Metastatic meningioma of the lung. Thorax 1986;41:487–8.

118. Bartley TD, Arean VM. Intrapulmonary neurogenic tumors. J Thorac Cardiovasc Surg 1965;50:114–23.

119. Bosch X, Ramirez J, Font J, et al. Primary intrapulmonary benign schwannoma. A case with ultrastructural and immunohistochemical confirmation. Eur Respir J 1990;3:234–7.

120. Carney JA. Psammomatous melanotic schwannoma. A distinctive, heritable tumor with special associations, including cardiac myxoma and the Cushing syndrome. Am J Surg Pathol 1990;14:206–22.

121. _____, Sizemore GW, Hayles AB. Multiple endocrine neoplasia, Type 2b. Pathobiol Ann 1978;8:105–53.

122. Chumas JC, Lorelle CA. Pulmonary meningioma. A light- and electron microscopic study. Am J Surg Pathol 1982;6:795–801.

123. Cooney TP. Primary pulmonary ganglioneuroblastoma in an adult: maturation, involution and the immune response. Histopathology 1981;5:451–63.

124. Dastur KJ, Raji MR, Smith WI Jr. Pulmonary metastasis from intraspinal meningioma. AJNR Am J Neuroradiol 1984;5:483–4.

125. Drlicek M, Grisold W, Lorber J, Hackl H, Wuketich S, Jellinger K. Pulmonary meningioma. Immunohistochemical and ultrastructural features. Am J Surg Pathol 1991;15:455–9.

126. Feldhaus RJ, Anene C, Bogard P. A rare endobronchial neurilemmoma (Schwannoma). Chest 1989;95:461–2.

127. Flynn SD, Yousem SA. Pulmonary meningiomas: a report of two cases. Hum Pathol 1991;22:469–74.

128. Gaffey MJ, Mills SE, Askin FB. Minute pulmonary meningothelial-like nodules. A clinicopathologic study of so-called minute pulmonary chemodectoma. Am J Surg Pathol 1988;12:167–75.

128a. Gebauer C. The postoperative prognosis of primary pulmonary sarcomas. A review with a comparison between the histological forms and the other primary endothoracal sarcomas based on 474 cases. Scand J Thor Cardiovasc Surg 1982;16:91–7.

128b. _____. Primary pulmonary sarcomas: etiology, clinical assessment and prognosis with a comparison to pulmonary carcinomas—a review of 41 cases and 394 other cases of the literature. Jpn J Surg 1982;12:148–59.

129. Imaizumi M, Takahashi T, Niimi T, Uchida T, Abe T, Fukatsu T. A case of primary intrapulmonary neurilemoma and review of the literature. Jpn J Surg 1989;19:740–6.

130. Kemnitz P, Spormann H, Heinrich P. Meningioma of lung: first report with light and electron microscopic findings. Ultrastruct Pathol 1982;3:359–65.

131. Kodama K, Doi O, Higashiyama M, Horai T, Tateishi R, Nakagawa H. Primary and metastatic pulmonary meningioma. Cancer 1991;67:1412–7.

132. Korn D, Bensch K, Liebow AA, Castleman B. Multiple minute pulmonary tumors resembling chemodectomas. Am J Pathol 1960;37:641–72.

133. Malik SK, Behera D, Kalra S, Dhaliwal RS, Banerjee CK. Intrabronchial schwannoma. Scand J Thor Cardiovasc Surg 1987;21:281–2.

134. Miller DC, Ojemann RG, Proppe KH, McGinnis BD, Grillo HC. Benign metastasizing meningioma. A case report. J Neurosurg 1985;62:763–6.

135. Muhrer KH, Fischer HP. Primary pulmonary neurilemoma. Thorac Cardiovasc Surg 1983;31:313–6.
136. Neilson DB. Primary intrapulmonary neurogenic sarcoma. J Pathol 1958;76:419–30.
137. Ng TH, Wong MP, Chan KW. Benign metastasizing meningioma. Clin Neurol Neurosurg 1990;92:152–4.
138. O'Donohue WJ Jr, Edland J, Mohiuddin SM, Schultz RD. Multiple pulmonary neurofibromas with hypoxemia. Occurrence due to pulmonary arteriovenous shunts within the tumors. Arch Intern Med 1986;146:1618–9.
139. Robinson PG. Pulmonary meningioma. Report of a case with electron microscopic and immunohistochemical findings. Am J Clin Pathol 1992;97:814–7.
140. Roviaro G, Montorsi M, Varoli F, Binda R, Cecchetto A. Primary pulmonary tumours of neurogenic origin. Thorax 1983;38:942–5.
141. Rowlands D, Edwards C, Collins F. Malignant melanotic schwannoma of the bronchus. J Clin Pathol 1987;40:1449–55.

142. Rutledge JN, Harolds JA. Intratracheal neurofibroma. South Med J 1983;76:1063–5.
143. Shirakusa T, Takada S, Yamazaki S, et al. Intrabronchial neurilemmoma—review of cases in Japan. Thorac Cardiovasc Surg 1989;37:388–90.
144. Som PM, Sacher M, Strenger SW, Biller HF, Malis LI. Benign metastasizing meningiomas. AJNR Am J Neuroradiol 1987;8:127–30.
145. Stoller JK, Kavuru M, Mehta AC, Weinstein CE, Estes ML, Gephardt GN. Intracranial meningioma metastatic to the lung. Cleve Clin J Med 1987;54:521–7.
146. Strimlan CV, Golembiewski RS, Celko DA, Fino GJ. Primary pulmonary meningioma. Surg Neurol 1988;29:410–3.
147. Unger PD, Geller GA, Anderson PJ. Pulmonary lesions in a patient with neurofibromatosis. Arch Pathol Lab Med 1984;108:654–7.

Cartilaginous Tumors

148. Carney JA. The triad of gastric epithelioid leiomyosarcoma, functioning extra-adrenal paraganglioma, and pulmonary chondroma. Cancer 1979;43:374–82.
149. _____. The triad of gastric epithelioid leiomyosarcoma, pulmonary chondroma, and functioning extra-adrenal paraganglioma: a five-year review. Surgical Rounds 1983;62:159–69.
150. Carter D, Eggleston JC. Tumors of the lower respiratory tract. Atlas of Tumor Pathology, 2nd Series, Fascicle 17. Washington, D.C.: Armed Forces Institute of Pathology, 1980:239–40.
151. Dajee AM, Dajee H, Hinrichs S, Lillington G. Pulmonary chondroma, extra-adrenal paraganglioma, and gastric leiomyosarcoma: Carney's triad. J Thorac Cardiovasc Surg 1982;84:377–81.
152. D'Ambrosio FG, Shiu MH, Brennan MF. Intrapulmonary presentation of extraskeletal myxoid chondrosarcoma of the extremity. Report of two cases. Cancer 1986;58:1144–8.
152a. Gal AA, Marchevsky AM, Koss MN. Unusual tumors of the lung. In: Marchevsky AM, ed. Surgical pathology of lung neoplasms. New York: Marcel Dekker, 1990:325–88.
153. Hayashi T, Tsuda N, Iseki M, Kishikawa M, Shinozaki T, Hasumoto M. Primary chondrosarcoma of the lung. A clinicopathologic study. Cancer 1993;72:69–74.
153a. Hurt R. Benign tumours of the bronchus and trachea, 1951-1981. Ann R Coll Surg Engl 1984;66:22–6.
154. Jazy FK, Cormier WJ, Panke TW, Shehata WM, Amongero FJ. Primary chondrosarcoma of the lung. A report of two cases. Clin Oncol 1984;10:273–9.
155. Kunze E, Graewe T, Peitsch E. Histology and biology of metastatic chondroblastoma. Report of a case with a review of the literature. Path Res Pract 1987;182:113–23.
156. Kurotaki H, Tateoka H, Takeuchi M, Yagihashi S, Kamata Y, Nagai K. Primary mesenchymal chondrosarcoma of the lung. A case report with immunohistochemical and ultrastructural studies. Acta Pathol Jpn 1992;42:364–71.

157. Kyriakos M, Land VJ, Penning HL, Parker SG. Metastatic chondroblastoma. Report of a fatal case with a review of the literature on atypical, aggressive, and malignant chondroblastoma. Cancer 1985;55:1770–89.
158. Margulies KB, Sheps SG. Carney's triad: guidelines for management. Mayo Clin Proc 1988;63:496–502.
159. McLaughlin SJ, Dodge EA, Ashworth J, Connors J. Carney's triad. Aust N Z J Surg 1988;58:679–81.
160. Raafat F, Salman WD, Roberts K, Ingram L, Rees R, Mann JR. Carney's triad: gastric leiomyosarcoma, pulmonary chondroma and extra-adrenal paraganglioma in young females. Histopathology 1986;10:1325–33.
161. Rocca M, Vanel D, Couanet D, Caillaud JM, Brugière L. Chondrosarcome mésenchymateux pulmonaire chez l'enfant. Rapport de deux cas et revue de la littérature. J Radiol 1988;69:329–32.
161a. Salminen S, Halttunen P, Miettinen M, Mattila S. Benign mesenchymal tumours of the lung including sclerosing haemangiomas. Annales Chirurgiae et Gynaecologiae 1990;79:85–91.
162. Shermeta DW, Carter D, Haller JA Jr. Chondroma of the bronchus in childhood: a case report illustrating problems in diagnosis and management. J Pediatr Surg 1975;10:545–8.
163. Stanfield BL, Powers CN, Desch CE, Brooks JW, Frable WJ. Fine-needle aspiration cytology of an unusual primary lung tumor, chondrosarcoma: case report. Diagn Cytopathol 1991;7:423–6.
164. Sun CC, Kroll M, Miller JE. Primary chondrosarcoma of the lung. Cancer 1982;50:1864–6.
165. Watanabe A, Ito M, Nomura F, Saka H, Sakai S, Shimokata K. Primary chondrosarcoma of the lung—a case report with immunohistochemical study. Jpn J Med 1990;29:616–9.
166. Yellin A, Schwartz L, Hersho E, Lieberman Y. Chondrosarcoma of the bronchus. Chest 1983;84:224–6.

Osteogenic Tumors

167. Colby TV, Bilbao JE, Battifora H, Unni KK. Primary osteosarcoma of the lung. A reappraisal following immunohistologic study. Arch Pathol Lab Med 1989;113:1147–50.

168. Daugavietis HE, Mautner LS. Disseminated nodular pulmonary ossification with mitral stenosis. Arch Pathol 1957;63:7–12.

169. Joines RW, Roggli VL. Dendriform pulmonary ossification. Report of two cases with unique findings. Am J Clin Pathol 1989;91:398–402.

170. Loose JH, el-Naggar AK, Ro JY, Huang WL, McMurtrey MJ, Ayala AG. Primary osteosarcoma of the lung. Report of two cases and review of the literature. J Thorac Cardiovasc Surg 1990;100:867–73.

171. Müller KM, Friemann J, Stichnoth E. Dendriform pulmonary ossification. Pathol Res Pract 1980;168:163–72.

172. Ndimbie OK, Williams CR, Lee MW. Dendriform pulmonary ossification. Arch Pathol Lab Med 1987;111:1062–4.

173. Popelka CG, Kleinerman J. Diffuse pulmonary ossification. Arch Intern Med 1977;137:523–5.

174. Stark P, Smith DC, Watkins GE, Chun KE. Primary intrathoracic extraosseous osteogenic sarcoma: report of three cases. Radiology 1990;174:725–6.

175. Yousem SA, Hochholzer L. Malignant mesotheliomas with osseous and cartilaginous differentiation. Arch Pathol Lab Med 1987;111:62–6.

Fatty Tumors

176. Dogan R, Ünlü M, GÜngen Y, Moldibi B. Endobronchial lipoma. Thorac Cardiovasc Surg 1988;36:241–3.

176a. Gal AA, Marchevsky AM, Koss MN. Unusual tumors of the lung. In: Marchevsky AM, ed. Surgical pathology of lung neoplasms. New York: Marcel Dekker, 1990:325–88.

177. Hirata T, Reshad K, Itoi K, Muro K, Akiyama J. Lipomas of the peripheral lung—a case report and review of the literature. Thorac Cardiovasc Surg 1989;37:385–7.

177a. Hurt R. Benign tumours of the bronchus and trachea, 1951-1981. Ann R Coll Surg Engl 1984;66:22–6.

178. Iannicello CM, Shoenut JP, Sharma GP, McGoey JS. Endobronchial lipoma: report of three cases. Can J Surg 1987;30:430–1.

179. Jones EL, Lucey JJ, Taylor AB. Intrapulmonary lipoma associated with multiple pulmonary hamartomas. Br J Surg 1973;60:75–8.

180. LaGrange AM, Servais B, Wurtz A, et al. Liposarcome lipoblastique du poumon etude ultrastructurale d'un cas. Ann Pathol 1988;8:152–4.

181. Mata JM, Cáceres J, Ferrer J, Gómez E, Castañer F, Velayos A. Endobronchial lipoma: CT diagnosis. J Comput Assist Tomogr 1991;15:750–1.

182. Matsuba K, Saito T, Ando K, Shirakusa T. Atypical lipoma of the lung. Thorax 1991;46:685.

183. Mendelsohn SL, Fagelman D, Zwanger-Mendelsohn S. Endobronchial lipoma demonstrated by CT. Radiology 1983;148:790.

184. Ovil Y, Schachner A, Schujman E, Spitzer SA, Levy MJ. Benign endobronchial lipoma masquerading as recurrent pneumonia. Eur J Respir Dis 1982;63:481–3.

185. Palvio D, Egeblad K, Paulsen SM. Atypical lipomatous hamartoma of the lung. Virchows Arch [A] 1985;405:253–61.

186. Remigio PA, De La Cruz M. Endobronchial lipoma. N Y State J Med 1988;88:550–1.

187. Ruiz-Palomo F, Calleja JL, Fogue L. Primary liposarcoma of the lung in a young woman. Thorax 1990;45:908.

187a. Salminen S, Halttunen P, Miettinen M, Mattila S. Benign mesenchymal tumours of the lung including sclerosing haemangiomas. Annales Chirurgiae et Gynaecologiae 1990;79:85–91.

188. Sawamura K, Hashimoto T, Nanjo S, et al. Primary liposarcoma of the lung: report of a case. J Surg Oncol 1982;19:243–6.

189. Schraufnagel DE, Morin JE, Wang NS. Endobronchial lipoma. Chest 1979;75:97–9.

190. Tomashefski JF Jr. Benign endobronchial mesenchymal tumors. Am J Surg Pathol 1982;6:531–40.

Soft Part Sarcomas

191. Sonobe H, Ro JY, Macay B, Ordóñez NG, Rundell MM, Ayala AG. Pulmonary alveolar soft-part sarcoma. Int J Surg Pathol 1994;2:57–62.

192. Tsutsumi Y, Deng Y. Alveolar soft part sarcoma of the pulmonary vein. Acta Pathol Jpn 1991;41:771–7.

21

MIXED EPITHELIAL AND MESENCHYMAL TUMORS

PULMONARY BLASTOMA

Pulmonary blastomas are a family of tumors in which the glands or mesenchyme composing the neoplasm are primitive or embryonal in appearance (36). In particular, the glycogen-rich, nonciliated tubules and embryonic stroma resemble that of fetal lung between 10 and 16 weeks' gestation.

The term pulmonary blastoma was initially used to describe a neoplasm consisting of both malignant embryonic-appearing glands and fetal type stroma (3,4,13,37). However, in 1982, Kradin and associates (22) described a "pulmonary blastoma...lacking sarcomatous features (pulmonary endodermal tumor resembling fetal lung)," a tumor whose neoplastic component consisted solely of fetal type glands. This tumor was subsequently given a variety of names: *pulmonary adenocarcinoma of fetal type, well-differentiated adenocarcinoma simulating fetal lung tubules* (20), and *pulmonary endodermal tumor resembling fetal lung* (22,27,31). We prefer the term *well-differentiated fetal adenocarcinoma* (21), which emphasizes not only the resemblance of this adenocarcinoma to fetal lung tubules but its well-differentiated appearance, but we will also use the term pulmonary endodermal tumor (22). Although it is not uniformly accepted that these tumors are simply epithelial variants of blastomas, we and others favor a histogenetic linkage, based in part on the finding of composite tumors showing broad areas of purely epithelial appearance with other, separate areas of biphasic appearance (21).

There are also neoplasms composed solely of primitive malignant stroma, without neoplastic epithelium. These tumors have been classified under the broad category of blastoma because of the embryonic appearance of the malignant stromal cells, but they appear to be clinically, pathologically, and histogenetically distinct from the tumors described above. The term *cystic and pleuropulmonary blastomas of childhood* may be used to describe them (9,15a,26).

Well-Differentiated Fetal Adenocarcinoma (Pulmonary Endodermal Tumor)

Definition. This tumor is composed of neoplastic glands whose glycogen-rich, nonciliated tubules resemble those of fetal lung between 10 and 16 weeks' gestation. The accompanying mesenchyme is histologically benign in appearance (21,22). Other terms include pulmonary adenocarcinoma of fetal type, well-differentiated adenocarcinoma simulating fetal lung tubules (20), and pulmonary endodermal tumor resembling fetal lung (22,27,31).

Clinical Features. Well-differentiated fetal adenocarcinomas are rare tumors, about equal in frequency to biphasic blastomas. Men and women are equally affected (21). Despite the embryonic histologic appearance of these tumors, they have not been reported in children under the age of 10 years (Table 21-1) (21). In fact, the mean and median ages of patients are in the fourth decade (21). Not only are they neoplasms of adults, but approximately 80 percent of patients are smokers (21,31).

Up to 57 percent of patients are asymptomatic (21). The most frequent symptoms are fever, cough, chest pain, and hemoptysis (21,31). These tumors are less likely to provoke symptoms than biphasic pulmonary blastomas, probably because they are smaller at presentation (Table 21-1) (21). This in turn may reflect a difference in biologic growth between the two tumors.

Well-differentiated fetal adenocarcinomas typically present as solitary peripheral or mid-lung masses, with a slight tendency to favor the upper lobes. Adenopathy and pleural effusion are rare or absent.

Gross Findings. The lesions are solitary, well-demarcated but unencapsulated, pulmonary masses that range in size from 1 to 10 cm (mean, 4.5 cm) (21). When multiple masses occur, one is usually dominant with satellite lesions (fig. 21-1). The cut surface is bulging and white, tan, or brown with areas of cystic breakdown and hemorrhage (fig. 21-1). The tumors are

Table 21-1

DIFFERENTIAL DIAGNOSTIC FEATURES
OF PULMONARY BLASTOMAS BY HISTOLOGIC SUBTYPE*

Features	WDFA**	Biphasic Blastoma	Pleuropulmonary Blastoma
Clinical			
% patients <10 years old	0	8	91
Smoker	often	often	no
Location	lung	lung	lung, pleura, mediastinum
Average size (cm)	4.5	10.1	NA[†]
Asymptomatic	often	occasional	rare
Prognosis	good	poor	poor
Pathologic			
Malignant epithelium/malignant stroma	+/–[‡]	+/+	–/+
Morules present	86%	43%	0%
Chromogranin positivity	frequent	frequent	never

*From references 9,21,26.
**WDFA = well-differentiated fetal adenocarcinoma.
[†]NA = not available.
[‡]+ = present; – = absent.

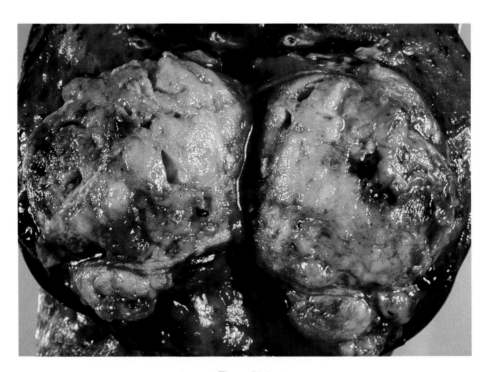

Figure 21-1

PULMONARY BLASTOMA

The cut section of this lung mass shows a peripheral, bulging, fleshy tumor with areas of necrosis, hemorrhage, and early cavitation. The neoplasm is well circumscribed but shows a satellite nodule in one area.

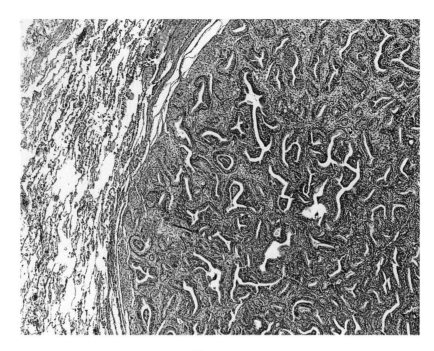

Figure 21-2
WELL-DIFFERENTIATED FETAL ADENOCARCINOMA
Low-power microscopic view showing relatively sharp circumscription from surrounding lung. Note the characteristic branching tubules and scant stroma.

subpleural in approximately 85 percent of cases; a polypoid intrabronchial component may be found in some cases, but this is infrequent.

Microscopic Findings. At low magnification, the tumor is usually well circumscribed and consists of a mass of branching tubules (fig. 21-2). Sometimes a cribriform pattern is prominent (fig. 21-3). The tubules are lined by pseudo-stratified, nonciliated columnar cells, with clear or lightly eosinophilic cytoplasm (figs. 21-4–21-6). The nuclei of these cells are oval or round and usually show little hyperchromasia or pleomorphism (figs. 21-4–21-6); only rarely is there cytologic atypia in the form of large multinucleated cells (41). The cells often have subnuclear and supranuclear cytoplasmic vacuoles, producing a distinctive endometrioid appearance (fig. 21-5). In addition, there may be cords, ribbons, or solid epithelial nests with a basal palisade pattern or containing minute rosette-like glands (21). Between 86 and 100 percent of cases show morules: solid balls of cells with ample eosinophilic cytoplasm at the bases of well-ordered glands (figs. 21-4, 21-6) (21,31,31a). About 50 percent of morules have optically clear nuclei (fig. 21-6), an

abnormality that has been seen in gestational endometrium and endometrial adenocarcinomas (31a,34b). If a malignant stromal component is absent, the combination of glands and morules may resemble adenoacanthoma of the uterus (fig. 21-6).

The clear cytoplasm of the neoplastic glands is due to abundant glycogen, readily demonstrated in periodic acid–Schiff (PAS) stains. There may be small amounts of mucin within the glandular lumens, but intracellular mucin is unusual. Argyrophilic granules can sometimes be found within scattered glandular and, particularly, morular cells.

Both mitoses and necrosis are frequently present. The former does not appear to be of prognostic importance. The stroma of well-differentiated fetal adenocarcinoma is typically scant and is composed of benign spindled myofibroblastic cells (figs. 21-4, 21-6) (20–22,27,31).

Rarely, there may be composite tumors consisting of broad areas resembling well-differentiated fetal adenocarcinoma with foci showing a biphasic pattern, or vice versa (21). Their existence suggests that the two tumors are histogenetically linked. In

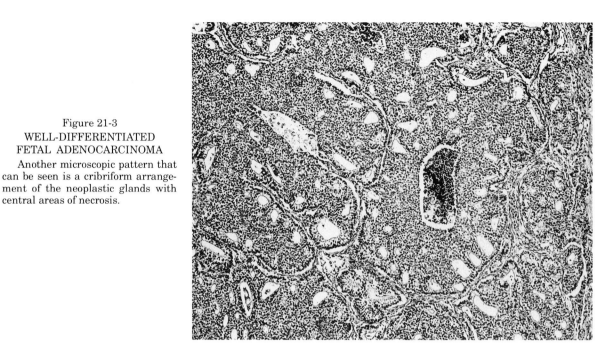

Figure 21-3
WELL-DIFFERENTIATED
FETAL ADENOCARCINOMA
Another microscopic pattern that can be seen is a cribriform arrangement of the neoplastic glands with central areas of necrosis.

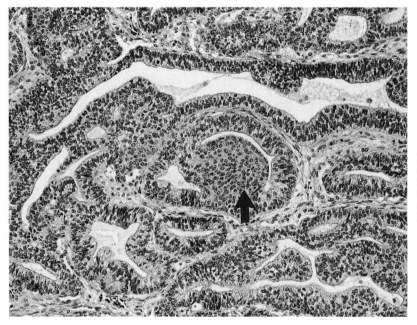

Figure 21-4
WELL-DIFFERENTIATED
FETAL ADENOCARCINOMA
The neoplastic glands are typically lined by pseudostratified columnar epithelium with uniform, oval nuclei and focally clear cytoplasm. Note morule (arrow), consisting of a solid nest of cells beneath the glandular epithelium, and the scant benign stroma.

addition, there are rare cases with a combination of well-differentiated fetal adenocarcinoma and yolk sac tumor (see fig. 23-33) (35).

Immunohistochemical Findings. Well-differentiated fetal adenocarcinomas frequently show neuroendocrine differentiation. In particular, chromogranin and neuron-specific enolase are present in a few glandular epithelial cells and more abundantly in morules (64 to 72 percent of cases) (21). A number of specific amine and polypeptide hormones can also be identified in the cytoplasm of these cells; these include calcitonin and gastrin-releasing peptide, bombesin, leucine enkephalin and methionine enkephalin, synaptophysin, somatostatin, and serotonin (fig. 21-7) (20,21,27, 31). Morules also stain with antibody to N-CAM

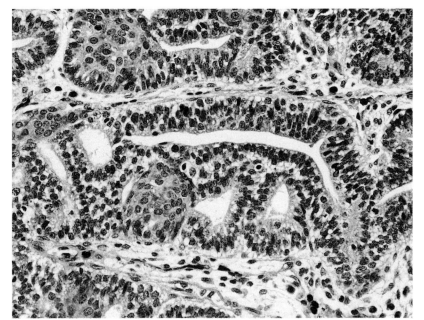

Figure 21-5
WELL-DIFFERENTIATED
FETAL ADENOCARCINOMA
The complex arrangement of
glands and the presence of subnuclear
and supranuclear vacuoles in their
lining cells are features that produce
an appearance reminiscent of endometrial adenocarcinoma.

Figure 21-6
WELL-DIFFERENTIATED
FETAL ADENOCARCINOMA
Morules (arrow) are typically located
at the base of the neoplastic glands, and
often show optically clear nuclei, as
demonstrated in this view.

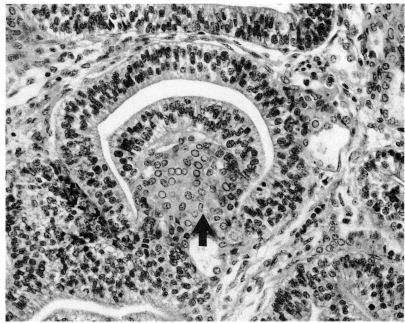

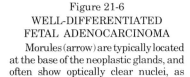

(Shimosato Y, personal communication, 1993).
The optically clear nuclei stain for biotin, much
as do the optically clear nuclei of gestational
endometrium and endometrial adenocarcinomas and adenoacanthomas (31a,34b). The suggestion has been made that the morules resemble neuroepithelial bodies, based on their
histologic appearance and staining for neuroendocrine markers (8).

The malignant embryonic epithelium also
stains with antibodies to cytokeratin, carcinoembryonic antigen, epithelial membrane antigen, and on occasion, alpha-fetoprotein (21,30,31).
Both Clara cell antigen and surfactant apoprotein
are expressed in the epithelial cells and particularly in morules (fig. 21-8) (31,41). These findings
mimic those in developing fetal lung tubules,
which show differentiation towards Clara cells

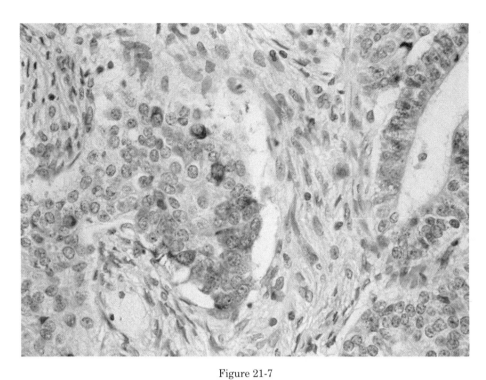

Figure 21-7
PULMONARY BLASTOMA: IMMUNOHISTOCHEMISTRY
A solid nest of morular cells is decorated by antibody to somatostatin. (Courtesy of Dr. Y. Shimosato, Tokyo, Japan.)

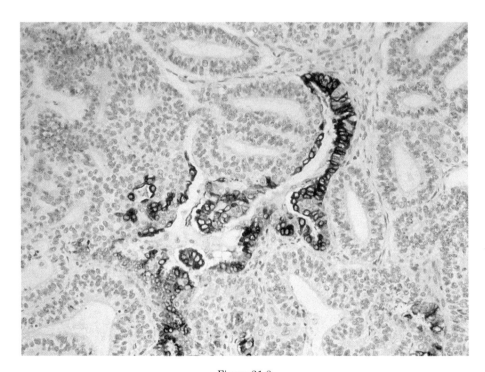

Figure 21-8
PULMONARY BLASTOMA: IMMUNOHISTOCHEMISTRY
Antibody to surfactant apoprotein (PE-10) strongly stains some glands in this pulmonary blastoma. (Courtesy of Dr. Y. Shimosato, Tokyo, Japan.)

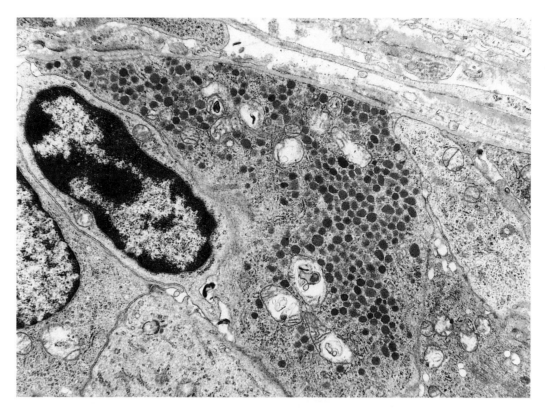

Figure 21-9
WELL-DIFFERENTIATED FETAL ADENOCARCINOMA: ELECTRON MICROSCOPY
An epithelial cell demonstrating numerous dense core granules typical of neuroendocrine differentiation. (Fig. 12 from Nakatani Y, Dickersin GR, Mark EJ. Pulmonary endodermal tumor resembling fetal lung: a clinicopathologic study of five cases with immunohistochemical and ultrastructural characterization. Hum Pathol 1990;21:1097–107.)

beginning at 13 weeks of gestation and towards type 2 pneumocytes at 22 weeks (12,41). Stromal cells of well-differentiated fetal adenocarcinomas show vimentin and muscle-specific actin.

Ultrastructural Findings. The neoplastic glands have a distinct basal lamina, apical junctional complexes, glycogen free spaces, and microvilli on the apical surface of lining cells. Neuroendocrine cells containing typical dense core granules are seen within glands and morules (fig. 21-9) (31). Electron microscopy has led to an intriguing interpretation of the histogenesis of morules. In addition to well-demarcated basal lamina and intercellular desmosomal junctions, there may be areas of differentiating alveolar-like structures lined by cells that contain lamellar inclusions, suggestive of type 2 cells (fig. 21-10) (31). The optically clear areas in morular nuclei consist of intranuclear aggregates of fine filaments or fibrils measuring 7 to 10 nm in diameter. Some of these cells also contain cytoplasmic clusters of spherical bodies of undetermined nature.

The spindle stromal cells surrounding the glands have typical myofibroblastic features, including well-developed rough endoplasmic reticulum, peripheral cytoplasmic filaments forming dense bodies, pinocytotic vesicles, and an investing basal lamina.

Differential Diagnosis. The clinical and microscopic differential diagnosis of well-differentiated fetal adenocarcinoma and other forms of pulmonary blastoma are summarized in Table 21-1. Well-differentiated fetal adenocarcinoma is most easily confused with clear cell adenocarcinoma of lung (fig. 21-11). Some of the cases reported by

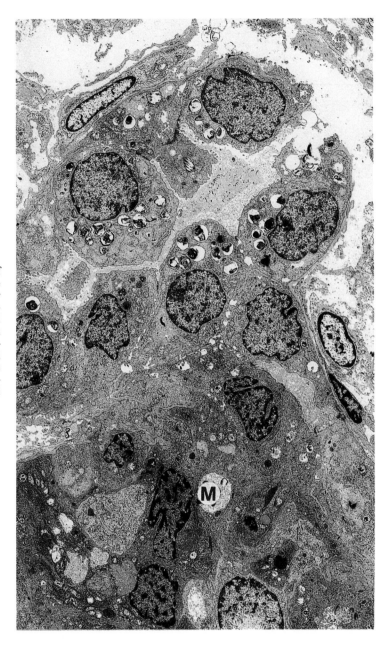

Figure 21-10
WELL -DIFFERENTIATED
FETAL ADENOCARCINOMA:
ELECTRON MICROSCOPY

Low-power electron micrograph of morule (M). At the margin of the morule, the tumor cells show transition to an alveolar structure lined by cells with round osmiophilic laminated cytoplasmic inclusions typical of type 2 pneumocytes. (Fig. 10 from Nakatani Y, Dickersin GR, Mark EJ. Pulmonary endodermal tumor resembling fetal lung: a clinicopathologic study of five cases with immunohistochemical and ultrastructural characterization. Hum Pathol 1990;21:1097–107.)

Kodama and associates (20) as well-differentiated adenocarcinoma simulating fetal lung tissues may be clear cell adenocarcinoma (Y. Nakatani, personal communication, 1993). The nuclear uniformity, endometrioid appearance of the neoplastic glands, presence of morules, periglandular investing sheath of myofibroblasts, and chromogranin reactivity of well-differentiated fetal adenocarcinoma are distinguishing features. Carcinoid tumors also show well-or-

dered glandular epithelium, intraluminal mucin, and chromogranin deposits. Still, the clear glandular epithelium associated with abundant glycogen, the morules, and the relative paucity of chromogranin-positive cells in well-differentiated fetal adenocarcinomas are not typical of carcinoid tumors.

Spread and Metastases. Well-differentiated fetal adenocarcinomas recur in about 30 percent of cases, but the recurrences are usually in ipsilateral

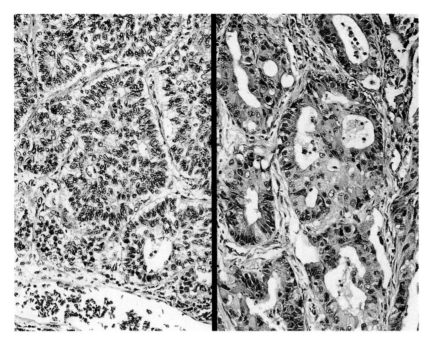

Figure 21-11
ADENOCARCINOMA OF
LUNG WITH FOCAL
CLEAR CELL CHANGES
Adenocarcinomas may show clear
cell cytoplasmic changes (left panel),
but they usually demonstrate significantly more nuclear and cytologic atypia than well-differentiated fetal adenocarcinoma, as seen in the right
panel from the same tumor. Compare
with well-differentiated fetal adenocarcinoma, figures 21-4–21-6.

or contralateral lung (21). Invasion of the chest wall and metastasis to hilar, periaortic, and mediastinal lymph nodes and brain also occur in fatal cases.

Treatment. The primary treatment is surgical excision. Combination chemotherapy, used for local or distant metastasis, may be of palliative benefit, but there are no rigorous or prospective studies of its efficacy (21).

Prognosis. Initially the prognosis seemed poor, with a 56 percent mortality (20); however, these studies may have included adult type clear cell adenocarcinomas. Using more stringent diagnostic criteria and greater numbers of cases, subsequent series have shown the prognosis to be very good, significantly better than for biphasic blastomas (21,31). In particular, in the largest study to date, tumor-associated mortality was only 10 to 14 percent (mean/median follow-up, 97/95 months) (21). This low mortality may reflect both the tendency of this neoplasm to recur in lung where it can be easily resected and a fundamental difference in biologic aggressiveness from biphasic blastoma.

Ominous prognostic factors include metastasis upon presentation, thoracic lymphadenopathy in the chest X ray, and tumor recurrence during the clinical course (21).

Biphasic Pulmonary Blastoma

Definition. Biphasic pulmonary blastoma is a tumor composed of malignant glands and malignant mesenchyme that are primitive or embryonal in appearance (36).

Clinical Features. Pulmonary blastomas are rare, comprising 0.25 to 0.5 percent of all primary malignant lung tumors (13,19). Males and females are equally affected (21). Most are smokers. Over 80 percent of patients are symptomatic: cough, chest pain, dyspnea, and hemoptysis are the most frequent symptoms (21). Patients range in age from the first to the eighth decade of life, with a mean and median age in the fourth decade (21).

On chest X ray, biphasic blastomas usually appear as large, solitary peripheral masses, with a tendency to favor the upper lobes. Adenopathy is infrequent, but pleural effusion occurs in almost 50 percent of cases.

Bronchoscopic and needle biopsies yield a correct or suggestive diagnosis in only one third of the cases in which they are attempted. This low yield probably results from both the histologic resemblance of the tumor to other neoplasms and the problem of small sample size in a lesion with complex histologic features.

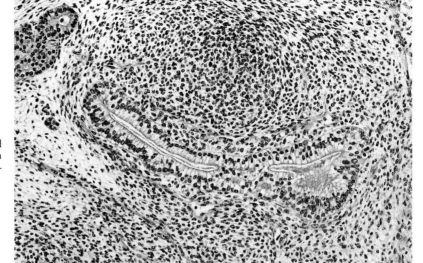

Figure 21-12
PULMONARY BLASTOMA,
BIPHASIC TYPE
Note the centrally placed gland
lined by cells with clear cytoplasm
and surrounded by condensed, embryonic stroma.

Gross Findings. Biphasic blastomas have a similar gross appearance to well-differentiated fetal adenocarcinoma (fig. 21-1). They typically appear as solitary, peripheral pulmonary masses with a pale, fleshy appearance. Areas of cystic breakdown and hemorrhage are common. They differ from well-differentiated fetal adenocarcinomas by their generally larger size: they range from 2 to 27 cm in diameter (average, 10 cm).

Microscopic Findings. In virtually all cases, the characteristic endometrioid glands are seen in the epithelial component, but not as extensively as in well-differentiated fetal adenocarcinoma (fig. 21-12). Most tumors have solid cords, ribbons, or nests of epithelial cells, sometimes with a basaloid pattern. Sheets of poorly differentiated cells with clear cytoplasm may be present. The solid epithelial nests often appear to fade into the malignant stroma and may be difficult to distinguish from it. Morules are less common than in well-differentiated fetal adenocarcinoma, occurring in less than 50 percent of cases (21). Foci of squamous pearl formation can be found, albeit infrequently (13,19,41).

Biphasic blastomas, by definition, have an embryonic or blastematous stroma (fig. 21-12). The stromal cells are usually small, oval, and spindled (fig. 21-12); they are occasionally pleomorphic (fig. 21-13). They lie in a myxoid matrix and tend to condense around the neoplastic glands (fig. 21-12). Small foci of adult type spindle cell sarcoma (most commonly with a fascicular or storiform pattern) are present in up to 83 percent of cases. Foci of immature striated muscle and cartilage are each seen in about 25 percent of cases, while osseous differentiation is found in about 5 percent (fig. 21-14) (13,21). Short fascicles of fetal type smooth muscle have been described in a number of cases (41).

Rare cases of biphasic blastoma have components of yolk sac tumor (see fig. 23-33) (35).

Immunohistochemical Findings. The endometrioid glands and morules of biphasic blastomas have the same antigens as well-differentiated fetal adenocarcinoma and the stromal cells of both are positive for vimentin and muscle-specific actin. Biphasic blastomas demonstrate desmin and myoglobin or S-100 protein when there is, respectively, striated muscle or cartilage. Vimentin and keratin are usually restricted to mesenchymal and epithelial tissues, respectively (21), but one study found vimentin in glands and focal staining for immunoreactive keratin in stromal cells (41).

Differential Diagnosis. Biphasic pulmonary blastomas are compared with other forms of blastomas in Table 21-1. Carcinosarcomas are easily distinguished by using the World Health Organization (WHO) definition for this tumor in lung. Pulmonary carcinosarcomas demonstrate

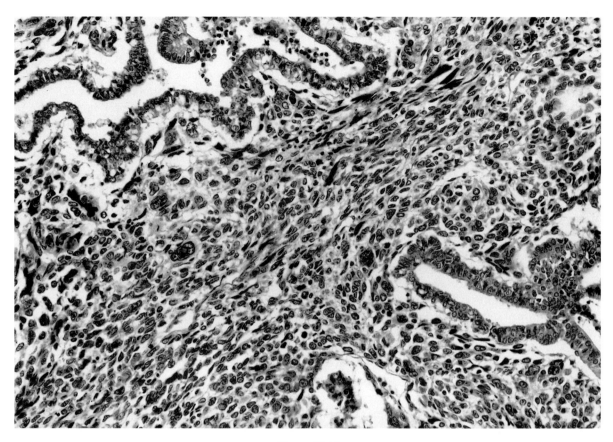

Figure 21-13
PULMONARY BLASTOMA, BIPHASIC TYPE
Pleomorphism in the form of giant and hyperchromatic spindle cells is present in the embryonic stroma of this tumor.

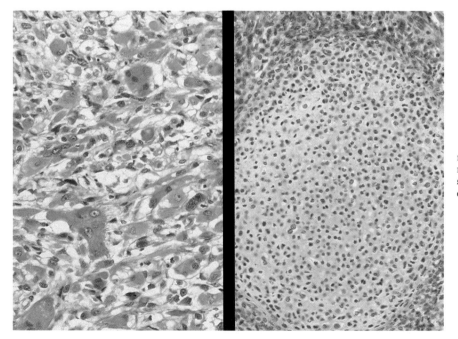

Figure 21-14
PULMONARY BLASTOMA,
BIPHASIC TYPE

Sheets of neoplastic striated muscle (left) and islands of immature cartilage (right) are each seen in the stroma in 25 percent of biphasic blastomas.

a mixture of sarcoma and carcinoma of adult type, without the fetal endometrioid glands or embryonic stroma typical of biphasic blastomas. Metastatic sarcomas may appear biphasic due to the entrapment of bronchoalveolar elements of the lung, but the glandular epithelium is benign.

Spread and Metastases. Biphasic blastomas recur in 43 percent of cases, most commonly in hilar and mediastinal lymph nodes, lung and pleura, chest wall and diaphragm, and brain (21). Less commonly, metastases occur in the liver, extrathoracic lymph nodes, heart, and soft tissue of the extremities.

Prognosis. Patients with biphasic blastoma have as poor a survival as those with common lung carcinomas (13,21). While there are individual reports of long-term tumor-free survival (15), two thirds of patients with biphasic tumors die within 2 years of diagnosis, 16 percent survive 5 years, and only 8 percent survive 10 years (13,21). Prognosis is partly dependent on the stage of the tumor, with stage 1 blastomas having a 5-year survival of about 25 percent (21). Other ominous prognostic factors include an initial diameter greater than 5 cm and tumor recurrence during the clinical course.

Cystic and Pleuropulmonary Blastomas of Childhood

Definition. Most blastomas in children are significantly different from those in adults: they are composed of a malignant, embryonic-appearing mesenchyme, with either no epithelial component or with a non-neoplastic, presumably entrapped, epithelium. The tumors are therefore sarcomas rather than biphasic neoplasms, but they are described in this chapter for purposes of comparison with the other forms of blastoma.

Childhood blastomas span a gross and microscopic spectrum of disease. At one end are thin-walled intrapulmonary cysts, with an underlying cambium layer of embryonic and rhabdomyosarcomatous mesenchyme, which may be termed *cystic blastoma.* These tumors are also known as *pulmonary sarcomas arising in mesenchymal cystic hamartoma, embryonal sarcoma,* and *pulmonary rhabdomyosarcoma arising in congenital cystic adenomatoid malformation or bronchogenic cyst* (5,16,23,34a). At the other end of the spectrum are solid masses of malignant mesenchyme of embryonic (or blastematous) ap-

pearance involving the mediastinum and pleura as well as lung, and termed *pleuropulmonary blastoma* (9,15a,26). Probably many of the biphasic blastomas of lung previously reported in children fall into this tumor category (2).

Clinical Features. Predominantly cystic lesions usually occur in children 1 to 9 years of age. The patients may be asymptomatic or they may have croup, pneumonia, fever, shortness of breath, or rarely, severe dyspnea secondary to pneumothorax (16,34a). Radiographically, a single or multiloculated, peripheral cystic lesion is present, and is often noted some time before the diagnosis is made.

Pleuropulmonary blastomas are largely solid, multilobulated masses that occur as often in mediastinum or pleura as in lung. The patients range from 30 months to 12 years of age, but many are less than 3 years old (15a). They typically have a nonproductive cough, fever, or chest pain of days to weeks duration (9,12,15a,26).

Gross Findings. Cystic tumors are single or multiloculated, involve one or more lobes, and may have nodular, thickened walls (fig. 21-15). Pleuropulmonary blastomas are multilobulated, white or gray, red, and yellow, predominantly solid masses that measure 8 to 23 cm in diameter and weigh 160 to 1100 g (fig. 21-16). Occasionally, they may show a cystic component (15a).

Microscopic Findings. Histologically, cystic tumors consist of one or multiple spaces lined by benign alveolar or ciliated columnar epithelial cells, beneath which is a layer of primitive oval and spindled rhabdomyoblasts in a loose to dense fibrovascular stroma (fig. 21-17). The nodular areas of thickening in the gross specimen are composed of embryonic, oval to stellate cells (39).

Pleuropulmonary blastomas also consist of embryonic or blastemal stromal cells, but frequently there are foci of anaplastic and pleomorphic mesenchymal cells with numerous mitoses (figs. 21-18, 21-19). The stroma often contains alternating bands of compact and loose cells arranged in a myxoid matrix (fig. 21-20). Foci of cells with eosinophilic cytoplasm suggestive of rhabdomyoblasts are common, although cross-striations are hard to find. Spindle cells resembling fascicles of smooth muscle can also be seen on occasion. Malignant cartilage is found in about 25 percent of cases and fat may be seen rarely (fig. 21-21).

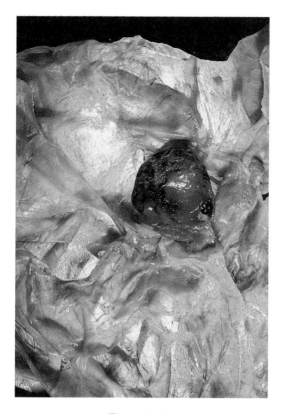

Figure 21-15
CYSTIC PULMONARY BLASTOMA OF CHILDHOOD
    This thin-walled multiloculated cyst from the lung of a
2-year-old boy has a central, hemorrhagic, 2-cm polypoid
nodule. (Fig. 16-57B from Stocker J. The respiratory tract.
In Stocker J, Dehner L, eds. Pediatric pathology. Philadelphia: JB Lippincott, 1992:559.)

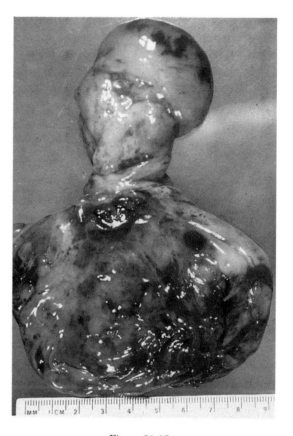

Figure 21-16
PLEUROPULMONARY BLASTOMA OF CHILDHOOD
    This hemorrhagic and focally necrotic solid mass was
resected from the pleura of a 1-year-old boy. (Fig. 16-56A from
Stocker J. The respiratory tract. In Stocker J, Dehner L, eds.
Pediatric pathology. Philadelphia: JB Lippincott, 1992:559.)

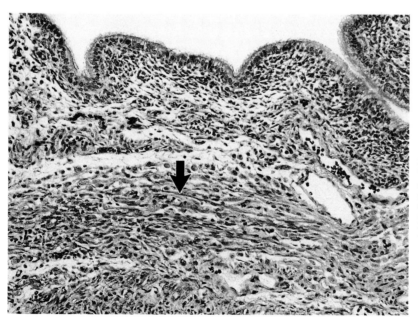

Figure 21-17
CYSTIC PULMONARY BLASTOMA
OF CHILDHOOD
    The cyst is lined by ciliated colum-
nar epithelium, beneath which is a
"cambium" layer of rhabdomyoblasts
including a deeper layer of strap cells
(arrow). (Fig. 16-57D from Stocker J.
The respiratory tract. In Stocker J,
Dehner L, eds. Pediatric pathology.
Philadelphia: JB Lippincott, 1992:559.)

407

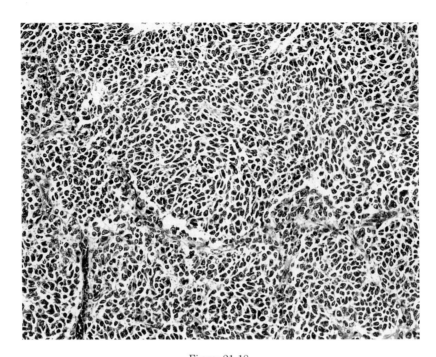

Figure 21-18
PLEUROPULMONARY BLASTOMA OF CHILDHOOD
This microscopic view shows the typical malignant stromal cells with scant cytoplasm. (Courtesy of COL J.T. Stocker, Washington, DC.)

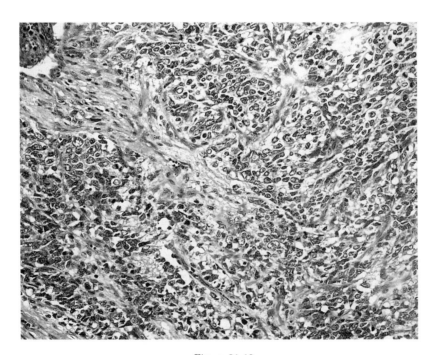

Figure 21-19
PLEUROPULMONARY BLASTOMA OF CHILDHOOD
Anaplasia may be pronounced in the malignant stroma of these tumors. Numerous mitoses were found at higher magnification. (Courtesy of COL J.T. Stocker, Washington, DC.)

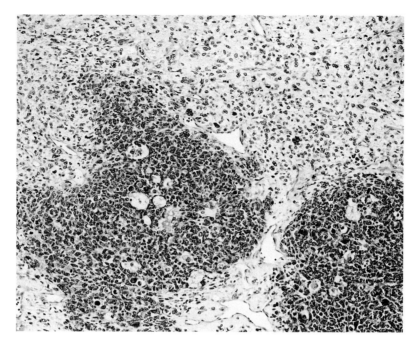

Figure 21-20
PLEUROPULMONARY BLASTOMA OF CHILDHOOD
The stroma of this tumor shows a typical feature of pleuropulmonary blastomas, namely alternating foci of compact cells and loose cells arranged in a myxoid matrix.

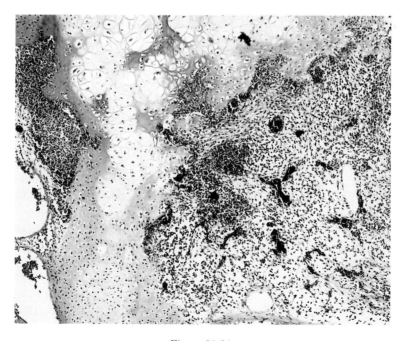

Figure 21-21
PLEUROPULMONARY BLASTOMA OF CHILDHOOD
Islands of malignant cartilage lie within a malignant myxoid stroma. (Courtesy of COL J.T. Stocker, Washington, DC)

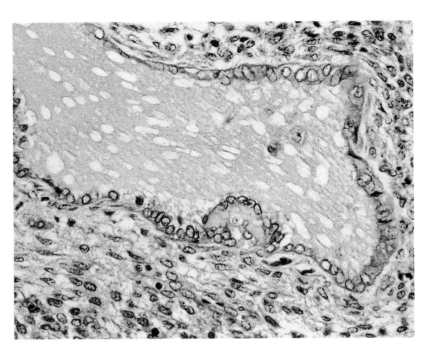

Figure 21-22
PLEUROPULMONARY
BLASTOMA OF CHILDHOOD
A gland is present surrounded by an embryonic stroma. However, unlike biphasic pulmonary blastomas, the epithelium is believed to be entrapped and derived from bronchioloalveolar or mesothelial cells. (Courtesy of Dr. J. Manivel, Minneapolis, MN.)

Cysts or smaller glandular spaces can be present in pleuropulmonary blastomas (fig. 21-22). As in cystic blastomas, they usually have a lining of histologically benign epithelial cells which are probably entrapped bronchiolar, alveolar, or mesothelial cells.

Immunohistochemical Findings. Immunohistochemical staining is seen in the blastema, and especially among pleomorphic giant cells, with antibodies to vimentin, alpha-1-antitrypsin, and alpha-1-antichymotrypsin. Rhabdomyosarcomatous cells are decorated by antibodies to desmin and myoglobin, while chondroid elements stain for S-100 protein. No reactivity is seen in the malignant stroma of these tumors for carcinoembryonic antigen, alpha-fetoprotein, epithelial membrane antigen, or cytokeratin, although the latter two antigens may be found in the benign entrapped epithelial components (9,26).

Ultrastructural Findings. The blastematous cells have large oval nuclei and prominent reticulated nucleoli. There are numerous polysomes in the cytoplasm; other organelles are scant. Cells with the characteristic features of fibroblasts, myofibroblasts, histiocyte-like cells, striated muscle, or chondroid differentiation may be present (9,15a,26).

Differential Diagnosis. The differential diagnoses among common forms of pulmonary blastomas are summarized in Table 21-1. Askin tumor can involve lung or mediastinum and may be difficult to distinguish from pleuropulmonary blastoma. The presence of embryonic-appearing tissue in the latter is diagnostic, but the distinction can be further aided by finding malignant striated muscle or cartilage. Cystic blastomas can resemble congenital cystic adenomatoid malformations, but they lack the mucogenic cells, mature cartilage, and the fibromuscular wall of the latter.

Spread and Metastasis. Lesions at either end of the spectrum can recur or metastasize. However, younger patients with intrapulmonary, thin-walled cystic lesions are more likely to have surgically resectable tumors than those with solid pleural and pulmonary-based lesions. Fatal pleuropulmonary blastomas show massive local recurrence, particularly in the mediastinum, and bilateral pulmonary metastases and spread to such distant sites as brain, spinal cord, skull, and skeletal muscle. Histologically, distant metastases always consist of malignant mesenchyme that resembles the primary neoplasm. No epithelial component is seen.

Prognosis. Long-term survival is 25 to 50 percent for children with solid lesions to over 50 percent for patients with thin-walled cystic lesions (16,26,34a).

CARCINOSARCOMAS OF THE LUNG

Definition. According to the WHO, pulmonary carcinosarcomas are tumors consisting of an admixture of malignant epithelial and mesenchymal elements of the type ordinarily seen in malignancies of adults, i.e., well-defined carcinomas and sarcomas similar to those seen in soft tissues (36). Because of the difficulty in distinguishing these rare tumors from the far more common spindle cell carcinomas of lung (1,18), the WHO added the corollary that pulmonary carcinosarcomas should show differentiation of the mesenchymal component into specific heterologous tissues, such as neoplastic bone, cartilage, and striated muscle, by light microscopy. We adhere to this definition, which has the advantage of being eminently usable at the light microscopic level. Spindle cell carcinomas with sarcomatoid stroma but no heterologous elements are discussed in chapter 11.

Recently, immunohistochemistry and electron microscopy have been used as additional methods of demonstrating differentiated mesenchymal elements (1,17,18). These techniques have led some to propose that carcinosarcoma and spindle cell carcinoma lie on a continuum of differentiation and to suggest unifying terms such as *carcinoma with a sarcomatoid element* or *pulmonary carcinoma with sarcoma-like lesion* to describe all of these tumors (17,18). Nappi and Wick (32) have suggested the terms *monophasic sarcomatoid carcinoma* as a synonym for spindle cell carcinoma and *biphasic sarcomatoid carcinoma* as a synonym for carcinosarcoma.

Clinical Features. Much of the available clinical information about pulmonary carcinosarcoma is based on cases that do not show heterologous sarcomatous elements and that therefore do not fit the WHO definition. Nevertheless, this broader group of patients has many clinical findings in common with the subset whose tumors do meet the definition.

Men are affected far more frequently than women (1,17,18,25,29,33,38,42). Over 90 percent of patients are between 50 and 80 years of age. There is a strong association with smoking (11).

The chest roentgenogram usually shows a well-demarcated lobulated mass. Approximately 75 to 80 percent of cases occur in the upper lobes.

A single tumor with extensive pleural involvement has also been reported (33).

Moore (29) suggested that carcinosarcomas be divided into two clinicopathologic groups on the basis of the location of the tumor in lung: a solid parenchymal type and a central or endobronchial lesion. The solid parenchymal type typically presents as a peripheral, often large mass in lung. It may be asymptomatic in early stages, but it shows a tendency to invade mediastinum, pleura, and chest wall, producing chest pain (17, 38). About one third of carcinosarcomas that meet the WHO criteria fit in this category. By contrast, central or endobronchial tumors are often pedunculated with limited or moderate extension into surrounding lung, involve lobar and segmental bronchi, and frequently present with symptoms such as cough, fever, dyspnea, and hemoptysis because they obstruct an airway (25,29). Two thirds of tumors present in this manner.

Sputum samples are rarely diagnostic (10,11, 38,42). Bronchoscopy yields a diagnosis of malignancy in 40 to 66 percent of cases in which it is attempted (10,11,25,38,42). Transthoracic fine needle aspiration can be used to identify more peripheral tumors; at least four cases have been diagnosed by this technique (7,11). However, bronchoscopy and fine needle aspiration may be inaccurate because they produce fragments of tissue that are too small or necrotic to show both components of the neoplasm (25). Fatal hemorrhage has been reported following bronchoscopic biopsy (25).

Gross Findings. Carcinosarcomas are usually gray-white, with red-brown areas of hemorrhage and yellow zones of necrosis. Peripheral tumors are solitary and well circumscribed (fig. 21-23), while central tumors are largely endobronchial and polypoid or may be parenchymal with an intrabronchial component (fig. 21-24) (25,42). Tumors that meet the WHO criteria measure between 2 and 9 cm, with a mean diameter of 5 cm (1,17,18,25,29,33,38,42).

Microscopic Findings. By definition, these tumors are biphasic and composed of an intimate admixture of carcinomatous and sarcomatous elements. The demarcation between the microscopic phases may be sharp or focally ill-defined. The most frequent epithelial component is squamous cell carcinoma (figs. 21-25, 21-26). Most commonly, areas of spindle cell sarcoma are present in association with foci of osteosarcoma,

411

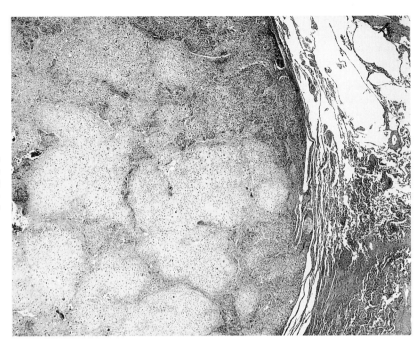

Figure 21-23
PULMONARY
CARCINOSARCOMA
Low magnification view of this peripheral tumor shows the good circumscription that can be seen in this type of neoplasm. Note the pale lobular masses of cartilage composing the bulk of the tumor.

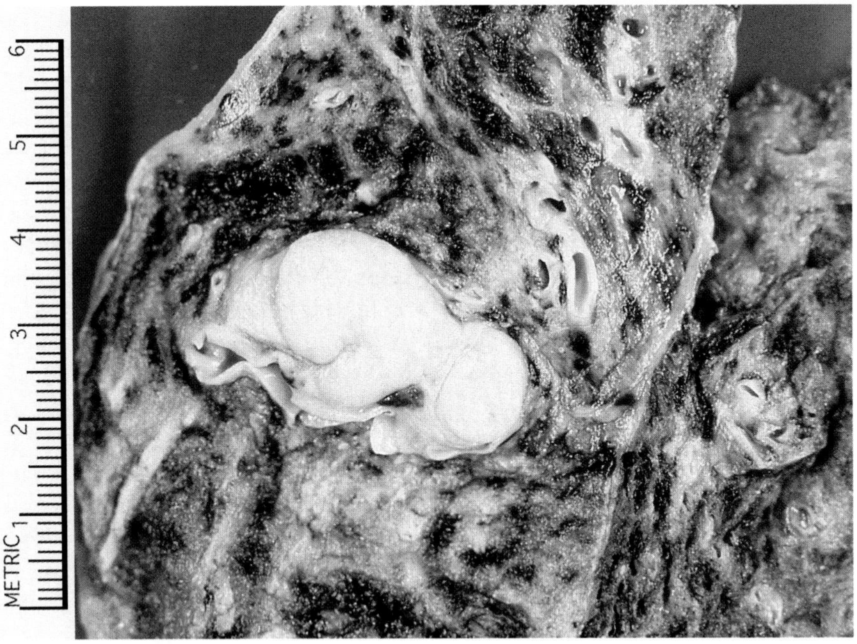

Figure 21-24
PULMONARY
CARCINOSARCOMA
This cream-colored, lobulated tumor presented as a largely endobronchial lesion involving a lobar bronchus. The collapsed pulmonary artery lies adjacent to the mass. (Courtesy of Dr. R. Sobonya, Tucson, AZ.)

chondrosarcoma, or rhabdomyosarcoma (figs. 21-25, 21-26). These differentiated stromal elements are found in almost equal frequency, and diverse combinations of them can be seen in a given case (29,42). The malignant stroma often forms the bulk of the tumor, and only small foci of carcinoma may be seen (25).

Immunohistochemical Findings and Differential Diagnosis. The current WHO definition of carcinosarcoma was proposed before there was systematic application of immunohistochemical staining to these tumors. The use of these staining procedures may be helpful in marginal cases in which there is doubt about the

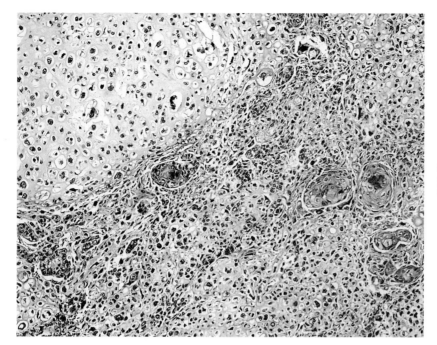

Figure 21-25
PULMONARY
CARCINOSARCOMA
Islands of squamous cell carcinoma showing typical squamous pearls lie at the margin of broad sheets of malignant cartilage in this tumor.

Figure 21-26
PULMONARY CARCINOSARCOMA
High magnification of tumor shown in figure 21-25. Two squamous pearls are surrounded by lobules of malignant cartilage.

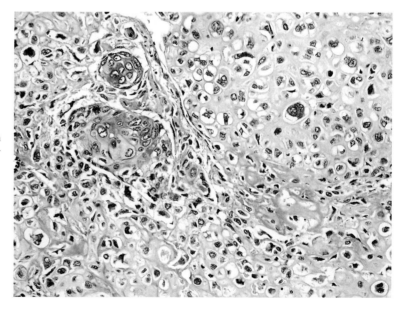

presence of heterologous stromal elements (32). More important, they may aid in identifying the spindle cells of a biphasic tumor as epithelial in phenotype, as occurs in spindle cell carcinoma (17,18,34,40). The problem of distinguishing carcinoma with a focal or extensive spindle cell component from carcinosarcoma is a major one in lung. Not only are carcinomas with spindling of tumor cells more frequent than carcinosarcomas (or other sarcomas) (32), but all of the major

histologic subtypes of nonsmall cell carcinoma can occasionally show either focal or extensive spindling of neoplastic cells (see chapters 11,12,15) (figs. 20-33, 21-27, 21-28). It is for this reason that the WHO definition of carcinosarcoma emphasizes the presence of heterologous differentiation.

Immunohistochemical staining may play a role in establishing the diagnosis of carcinosarcoma in instances where differentiation is poor at the light microscopic level. Stains for S-100 protein or desmin

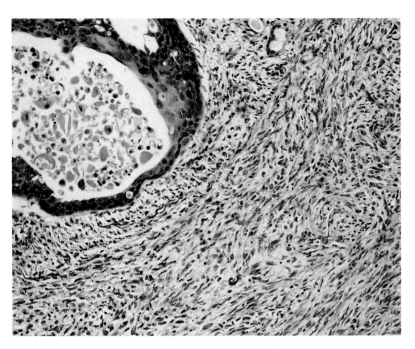

Figure 21-27
SPINDLE CELL
CARCINOMA OF LUNG
An island of squamous cell carcinoma is surrounded by malignant spindle cells. The tumor initially suggested the possibility of carcinosarcoma, but no definitive sarcomatous differentiation was seen, and antibodies to keratin supported an epithelial phenotype for the spindle cells.

can be used to support mesenchymal differentiation. Vimentin is typically present in the mesenchymal component but is of no diagnostic aid.

Interpretation of the immunohistochemical staining pattern of biphasic tumors can be difficult. In particular, reliance on the demonstration of a single antigen or class of antigens, such as keratin, to establish the spindle cell component as epithelial can produce problems. For example, keratin antigenicity can be diminished or lost after formalin fixation and paraffin embedding. Some epithelial tumors with a spindle cell phenotype may also express keratin poorly. In one study, only 9 of 12 "sarcomatoid" carcinomas of lung were keratin positive; the remaining three stained with antibody to EMA (34). There are also reports in which the epithelial component of carcinosarcoma failed to stain for keratin but stained for CEA (17,18). Thus, it is best to perform immunohistochemical stains against a battery of epithelial markers, including a cocktail of cytokeratins of different molecular weights, EMA, and CEA in doubtful cases (fig. 21-29) (18). Antigen retrieval techniques may be necessary in some cases. Electron microscopy with search for desmosomes, keratohyaline granules, or glandular differentiation in the spindle cells can also be employed and correlates well with the immunohistochemical results (17,18).

Not only may the spindle cells of a carcinoma fail to stain for keratin, but it is now clear that a variety of undoubted mesenchymal neoplasms, such as smooth muscle and neural tumors, may focally express keratin (24, 28). At the same time, the spindle cell component of biphasic tumors showing heterologous elements (and therefore, by definition, carcinosarcoma) rarely expresses keratin (10,32). The expression of keratin by the stromal component of carcinosarcomas has been used to link them and spindle cell carcinomas in a continuum of disease in which each is viewed as merely a part of a histologic spectrum (10, 17,18,32). In this regard, Cupples and Wright (10) argue that the presence of epithelial and mesenchymal intermediate filaments reflects the direction of cellular differentiation rather than the cell of origin. Nappi and Wick (32) classify both spindle cell carcinomas and carcinosarcomas as sarcomatoid carcinomas, either monophasic or biphasic, depending on whether a committed heterologous element is absent or present. We agree with this bipartite classification but we continue to prefer the terms spindle cell carcinoma and carcinosarcoma, based on their established use in published reports. A simplified differential diagnostic schema for carcinosarcomas and spindle cell carcinomas is presented in Table 21-2.

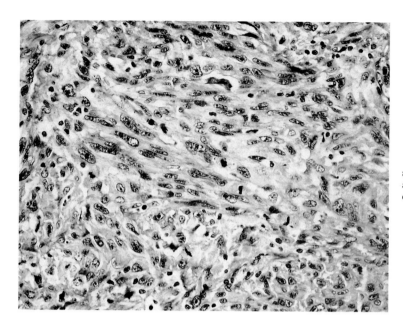

Figure 21-28
SPINDLE CELL
CARCINOMA OF LUNG
The oval and spindle cells of this tumor were strongly decorated with antibodies to keratin and epithelial membrane antigen, supporting a diagnosis of spindle cell carcinoma.

Table 21-2

DIFFERENTIAL DIAGNOSIS OF PULMONARY CARCINOSARCOMA AND SPINDLE CELL CARCINOMA

	Keratin in Epithelium/ Stroma	Heterologous Elements*
Carcinosarcoma	+ / − (usually) to +	+
Spindle cell carcinoma	+ / − to + (usually)	−

*Cartilage, striated muscle, bone, fat, neural tissue, etc. seen by light microscopy or supported by immunohistochemistry.

Biphasic pulmonary blastomas are easily distinguished by the finding of stroma or tubules of embryonic or fetal appearance. These tumors often show neuroendocrine differentiation as well.

Metastatic sarcomas in lung, particularly slow-growing ones, may entrap bronchoalveolar structures, producing a biphasic microscopic appearance. Still, the glandular elements in these instances are cytologically benign, rather than malignant, as would be the case with carcinosarcomas.

Spread and Metastasis. Peripheral carcinosarcomas readily invade the pleura and chest wall, while central tumors extend into mediastinum. The tumors often recur, most commonly in lung. The most frequent metastatic sites are hilar and mediastinal lymph nodes but metastases also occur in spinal cord, adrenal glands, and brain. The metastases can contain both histologic components of the primary tumor or only one (usually epithelial).

Treatment and Prognosis. Surgical resection, usually pneumonectomy or lobectomy, is both diagnostic and the initial treatment in many cases. Ludwigsen (25), in reporting a series of endobronchial tumors, noted that 91 percent of tumors could be resected with a potential for cure, a frequency double that of squamous cell carcinomas of lung. However, while some consider endobronchial tumors to have a more favorable prognosis (25), others note that they have no better outcome than peripheral neoplasms (6,11). Davis and associates (11) suggested that clinical or pathologic staging might be a good method for establishing prognosis. Ishida and colleagues (18) concluded that the presence of definitive sarcomatous differentiation was associated with a poor prognosis.

If there is uncertainty regarding factors determining prognosis, there is general agreement that the outcome of pulmonary carcinosarcoma is poor (11). The average postoperative survival of patients is 9 months and fewer than 10 percent survive 2 years (14). Cabarcos and associates (7), in reviewing previously published reports, noted that only 27 percent of patients survived more than 6 months.

415

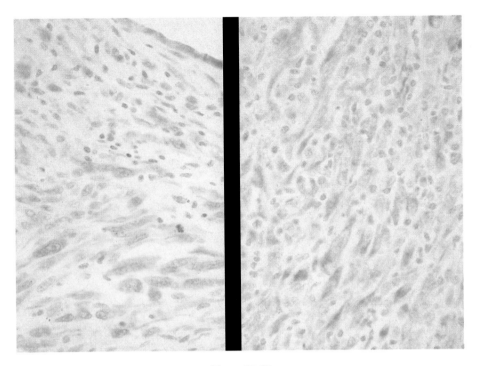

Figure 21-29
SPINDLE CELL CARCINOMA OF LUNG: IMMUNOHISTOCHEMISTRY
Immunohistochemical stains for both keratin (left panel) and vimentin (right panel) diffusely decorate the spindle cells of the carcinoma.

REFERENCES

1. Addis BJ, Corrin B. Pulmonary blastoma, carcinosarcoma, and spindle-cell carcinoma: an immunohistochemical study of keratin intermediate filaments. J Pathol 1985;147:291–301.

2. Ashworth TG. Pulmonary blastomas: a true congenital neoplasm. Histopathology 1983;7:585–94.

3. Barnard W. Embryoma of the lung. Thorax 1952;7:229–301.

4. Barnett N, Barnard W. Some unusual thoracic tumors. Br J Surg 1945; 32:447–57.

5. Becroft D, Jagusch M. Pulmonary sarcoma arising in mesenchymal cystic hamartomas [Abstract]. Pediatr Pathol 1987;7:478.

6. Bull JC Jr, Grimes OF. Pulmonary carcinosarcoma. Chest 1974;65:9–12.

7. Cabarcos A, Gomez Dorronsoro M, Lobo Beristain JL. Pulmonary carcinosarcoma: a case study and review of the literature. Br J Dis Chest 1985;79:83–94.

8. Chejfec G, Cosnow I, Gould, NS, Husain AN, Gould VE. Pulmonary blastoma with neuroendocrine differentiation in cell morules resembling neuroepithelial bodies. Histopathology 1990;17:353–8.

9. Cohen M, Emms M, Kaschula R. Childhood pulmonary blastoma: a pleuropulmonary variant of the adult-type pulmonary blastoma. Pediatr Pathol 1991;11:737–49.

10. Cupples J, Wright J. An immunohistochemical comparison of primary lung carcinosarcoma and sarcoma. Pathol Res Pract 1990;186:326–9.

11. Davis MP, Eagan RT, Weiland LH, Pairolero PC. Carcinosarcoma of the lung: Mayo Clinic experience and response to chemotherapy. Mayo Clin Proc 1984; 59:598–603.

12. Dehner L. Tumors and tumor-like lesions of the lung and chest wall in childhood: clinical and pathologic review. In: Stocker J, Dehner L, eds. Pediatric pathology. Philadelphia: JB Lippincott, 1992:232.

13. Francis D, Jacobsen M. Pulmonary blastoma: Curr Top Pathol 1983;73:265–94.

14. Gebauer C. The postoperative prognosis of primary pulmonary sarcomas. A review with a comparison between the histological forms and the other primary endothoracic sarcomas based on 474 cases. J Thorac Cardiovasc Surg 1982;16:91–7.

15. Gibbons JR, McKeown F, Field TW. Pulmonary blastoma with hilar lymph node metastases: survival for 24 years. Cancer 1981;47:152–5.

15a. Hachitanda Y, Aoyama C, Sato JK, Shimada H. Pleuropulmonary blastoma in childhood. A tumor of divergent differentiation. Am J Surg Pathol 1993;17:382–91.

16. Hedlund GL, Bisset GS III, Bove KE. Malignant neoplasms arising in cystic hamartomas of the lung in childhood. Radiology 1989;173:77–9.

17. Humphrey PA, Scroggs MW, Roggli VL, Shelburne JD. Pulmonary carcinomas with a sarcomatoid element: an immunocytochemical and ultrastructural analysis. Hum Pathol 1988;19:155–65.

18. Ishida T, Tateishi M, Kaneko S, et al. Carcinosarcoma and spindle cell sarcoma of the lung. Clinicopathologic and immunohistochemical studies. J Thorac Cardiovasc Surg 1990;100:844–52.

19. Jacobsen M, Francis D. Pulmonary blastoma. A clinicopathologic study of eleven cases. Acta Path Microbiol Scand [A] 1980;88:151–60.

20. Kodama T, Shimosato Y, Watanabe S, et al. Six cases of well differentiated adenocarcinoma simulating fetal lung tissues in pseudoglandular stage: comparison with pulmonary blastoma. Am J Surg Pathol 1984;8:725–44.

21. Koss MN, Hochholzer L, O'Leary T. Pulmonary blastomas. 1991;67:2368–81.

22. Kradin RL, Young RH, Dickersin GR, Kirkham SE, Mark EJ. Pulmonary blastoma with argyrophil cells lacking sarcomatous features (pulmonary endodermal tumor resembling fetal lung). Am J Surg Pathol 1982;6:165–72.

23. Krous HF, Sexauer CL. Embryonal rhabdomyosarcoma arising within a congenital bronchogenic cyst in a child. J Pediatr Surg 1981;16:506–8.

24. Litzky LA, Brooks JJ. Cytokeratin immunoreactivity in malignant fibrous histiocytoma and spindle cell tumors: comparison between frozen and paraffin-embedded tissues. Mod Pathol 1992;5:30–4.

25. Ludwigsen E. Endobronchial carcinosarcoma. A case with osteosarcoma of pulmonary invasive part, and a review with respect to prognosis. Virchows Arch [A] 1977;373:293–302.

26. Manivel JC, Priest JR, Watterson J, et al. Pleuropulmonary blastoma. The so-called pulmonary blastoma of childhood. Cancer 1988;62:1516–26.

27. Manning JT Jr, Ordonez NG, Rosenberg HS, Walker WE. Pulmonary endodermal tumor resembling fetal lung. Report of a case with immunohistochemical studies. Arch Pathol Lab Med 1985;109:48–50.

28. Miettinen M, Rapola J. Immunohistochemical spectrum of rhabdomyosarcoma and rhabdomyosarcoma-like tumors. Expression of cytokeratin and the 68-kD neurofilament protein. Am J Surg Pathol 1989;13:120–32.

29. Moore T. Carcinosarcoma of the lung. Surgery 1961;50:886–93.

30. Muller-Hermelink HK, Kaiserling E. Pulmonary adenocarcinoma of fetal-type: alternating differentiation argues in favor of a common endodermal stem cell. Virchows Arch [A] 1986;409:195–210.

31. Nakatani Y, Dickersin GR, Mark EJ. Pulmonary endodermal tumor resembling fetal lung: a clinicopathologic study of five cases with immunohistochemical and ultrastructural characterization. Hum Pathol 1990;21:1097–107.

31a. _____, Kitamura H, Inayama Y, Ogawa N. Pulmonary endodermal tumor resembling fetal lung. The optically clear nucleus is rich in biotin. Am J Surg Pathol 1994;18:637–42.

32. Nappi O, Wick MR. Sarcomatoid neoplasms of the respiratory tract. Semin Diagn Pathol 1993;10:137–47.

33. Prive L, Tellem M, Meranze D, Chodoff R. Carcinosarcoma of the lung. Arch Pathol 1961;72:351–7.

34. Ro JY, Chen JL, Lee JS, Sahin AA, Ordonez NG, Ayala AG. Sarcomatoid carcinoma of the lung. Immunohistochemical and ultrastructural studies of 14 cases. Cancer 1992;69:376–86.

34a. Senac MO Jr, Wood BP, Isaacs H, Weller M. Pulmonary blastoma: a rare childhood malignancy. Radiology 1991;179:743–6.

34b. Sickel JZ, di Sant'Agnese A. Anomalous immunostaining of "optically clear" nuclei in gestational endometrium. A potential pitfall in the diagnosis of pregnancy-related herpesvirus infection. Arch Pathol Lab Med 1994;118:831–3.

35. Siegel RJ, Bueso-Ramos C, Cohen C, Koss M. Pulmonary blastoma with germ cell (yolk sac) differentiation: report of two cases. Mod Pathol 1991;4:566–70.

36. Sobin LH, Yesner R. Histological typing of lung tumours. International Histological Classification of Tumours, No. 1. 2nd ed. Geneva: World Health Organization. 1981:19–20.

37. Spencer H. Pulmonary blastomas. J Pathol Bacteriol 1961;82:161–5.

38. Stackhouse EM, Harrison EG Jr, Ellis FH Jr. Primary mixed malignancies of lung: carcinosarcoma and blastoma. J Thorac Cardiovasc Surg 1969;57:385–99.

39. Stocker J. The respiratory tract. In: Stocker J, Dehner L, eds. Pediatric pathology. Philadelphia: JB Lippincott, 1992:559.

40. Suster S, Huszar M, Herczeg E. Spindle cell squamous carcinoma of the lung. Immunocytochemical and ultrastructural study of a case. Histopathology 1987;11:871–8.

41. Yousem SA, Wick MR, Randhawa P, Manivel JC. Pulmonary blastoma. An immunohistochemical analysis with comparison with fetal lung in its pseudoglandular stage. Am J Clin Pathol 1990;93:167–75.

42. Zimmerman KG, Sobonya RE, Payne CM. Histochemical and ultrastructural features of an unusual pulmonary carcinosarcoma. Hum Pathol 1981;12:1046–51.

❖ ❖ ❖

22

LYMPHORETICULAR DISORDERS

Lymphoreticular disorders commonly involve the lung, particularly in patients with systemic disease. The lung may also be the site of presentation and the only site initially involved. Lymphomatoid granulomatosis, a controversial disorder whose histogenesis and precise characterization are still under debate, is considered a lymphoproliferative disorder in this Fascicle.

At the cytologic level, the lymphoreticular processes discussed in this section are identical to their nodal counterparts, although the histologic features are distinct and often unique because of the anatomy of the lung. Understanding the histologic appearance, clinical behavior, and immunologic features of pulmonary lymphoreticular disorders requires knowledge of the pulmonary lymphatics and lymphoid tissue. Except as otherwise noted, the terms used in this section are essentially those of the National Cancer Institute (NCI) working formulation for the classification of non-Hodgkin lymphomas (Table 22-1) (75).

Primary lymphomas of the lung are rare and comprise approximately 0.3 percent of all primary pulmonary neoplasms (70). Among primary lymphomas, low-grade small lymphocytic lymphomas are the most common (Table 22-1), comprising 50 to 90 percent of cases (22,56,61, 87); angiocentric immunoproliferative lesions/ lymphomatoid granulomatosis are the next most common; and large cell lymphomas are third, comprising 6 to 20 percent of primary pulmonary lymphomas (87).

HISTOLOGIC DIAGNOSIS OF LYMPHORETICULAR INFILTRATES IN THE LUNG

The diagnosis of lymphoreticular infiltrates in the lung depends on whether a primary diagnosis is being made or a relapse in the lung is being confirmed. A primary diagnosis usually requires an open lung (or thoracoscopic) biopsy or larger specimen. Occasionally, a transbronchial biopsy is sufficient, particularly when supported by immunohistochemical or similar studies on cells retrieved from concomitant bronchoalveolar lavage. However, for the diagnosis of angiocentric

Table 22-1

NCI WORKING FORMULATION CLASSIFICATION FOR NON-HODGKIN LYMPHOMAS*

Subtype of Lymphoma	Proportion of Primary Lung Lymphomas
Low Grade	
Small lymphocytic (+/- plasmacytoid)	Most common
Follicular small cleaved cell	Rare
Follicular mixed small cleaved and large cell	Rare
Intermediate Grade	
Follicular large cell	Rare
Diffuse small cleaved cell	Rare
Diffuse mixed small and large cell	Second most common; includes many cases of AIL/LYG
Diffuse large cell	Uncommon; includes some cases of AIL/LYG
High Grade	
Large cell, immunoblastic	Uncommon
Lymphoblastic	Very rare
Small noncleaved cell	Very rare

*Modified from reference 58.

419

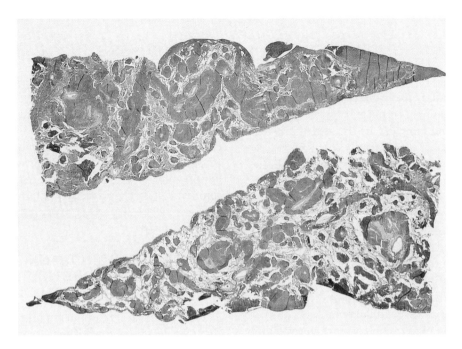

Figure 22-1
LYMPHATIC DISTRIBUTION
This small lymphocytic lymphoma presenting as diffuse lung disease shows exquisite outlining of the lymphatic routes by a dense infiltrate of small lymphocytes. The infiltrate involves the pleura, septa, and bronchovascular bundles with relative sparing of the intervening alveoli.

immunoproliferative and related lesions, a larger sample is usually necessary. Large rather than small nodules should be sampled and several lesions should be retrieved if possible.

The situation is different for patients already diagnosed. In these cases, small specimens, such as may be retrieved by transbronchial biopsy, fine needle aspiration, and other cytologic preparations, or closed pleural biopsy may be sufficient. Many patients in this situation are on chemotherapy, and the possibility of infection is also of concern.

Cavitation, occurring either in primary or secondary lymphomas of the lung, may result in secondary invasion by opportunistic organisms such as *Aspergillus*, which may mask the lymphoid process.

LYMPHATICS AND LYMPHOID TISSUE OF THE LUNG

The anatomy of the pulmonary lymphatics is shown in figure 2-6. The lymphatics are normally inconspicuous slit-like channels around bronchovascular bundles, and in the septa and pleura. In pathologic conditions, like lymphangitic carcinoma, the lymphatics become more

obvious. With lymphoreticular infiltrates, the lymphatic channels themselves are usually inconspicuous, although the cellular infiltrates show the same distribution as the lymphatic channels (fig. 22-1): i.e., a lymphatic distribution ("lymphatic tracking") (15,16).

Lymphoid tissue is not prominent in normal human lung, although it is present in many other mammalian species (for example, rabbits and rats) (77). In inflammatory and lymphoproliferative states, the amount of lymphoid tissue is increased and its distribution becomes apparent. In reactive states, there is a proliferation of lymphoid follicles along lymphatic routes (figs. 22-2, 22-3), particularly airways (so-called follicular bronchiolitis or follicular bronchitis) (14,104); this tissue has been termed bronchus-associated lymphoid tissue (BALT) (5). BALT is a subset of mucosa-associated lymphoid tissue (MALT), found in the gastrointestinal tract and other sites (5,14,38,53). BALT is apparent in 10 percent of normal fetuses and infants, but is much more prominent in infants with an identifiable antigenic stimulant such as infection (35).

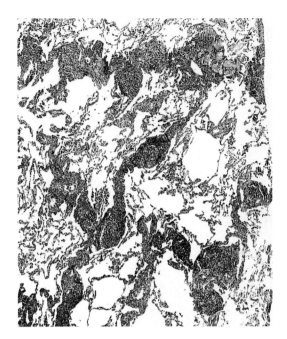

Figure 22-2
DIFFUSE LYMPHOID HYPERPLASIA
IN RHEUMATOID ARTHRITIS
There is a proliferation of germinal centers along inter-lobular septa. The intervening alveoli show minor changes.

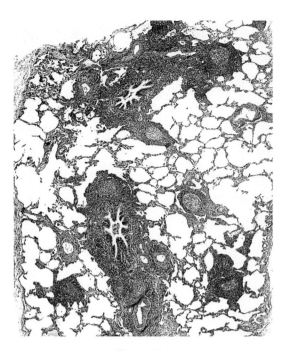

Figure 22-3
FOLLICULAR BRONCHIOLITIS
There is a proliferation of germinal centers along bronchioles, with minor changes in the alveolar walls.

Lymphoid follicles in the septa and pleura are also part of BALT, although technically they are not distributed along airways.

The epithelium overlying the lymphoid nodules of BALT is specialized lymphoepithelium that is somewhat flattened, has decreased numbers of goblet and ciliated cells, increased numbers of cells bearing microvilli, and an infiltration of lymphocytes, especially CD4 (OKT4, Leu-3a)-positive T cells. The epithelium appears to be specialized for antigen transport and presentation.

MALT is part of the immune system that responds to antigens presenting at mucosal surfaces (5,38,53). Histologically, MALT shows an organization of the lymphoid tissue into reactive follicles with prominent marginal zones, epithelial infiltration of the overlying epithelium, and a zone of plasma cells below the epithelial surface (38). The lymphoid follicles comprising MALT include both T cells and B cells, the latter often organized into reactive germinal centers. Memory B cells are generated, and are primarily positive for IgA but also IgG and IgM. These cells have the capacity to circulate and "home" back to the lung or another MALT site.

Lymphomas of MALT have been the subject of a number of recent studies, most notably those of Isaacson and colleagues (38,42,43). These lymphomas share many of the features of MALT itself: low-grade B-cell MALT lymphomas have a histologic spectrum and heterogeneity similar to that of MALT such as a tendency of cells to infiltrate epithelium (lymphoepithelial lesions) and for the circulating neoplastic cells to "home" to the site of origin or other MALT sites. This last feature may in part explain the relatively indolent behavior that characterizes most of these lymphomas.

The histologic heterogeneity of these low-grade B-cell lymphomas and the difficulty in classifying them reflect the normal features of MALT (38): the presence of numerous follicles (which may be reactive or neoplastic) with a cuff of marginal cells (centrocyte-like cells), mucosal infiltration by the lymphoid cells, plasmacytoid differentiation, plasma cells, and variable numbers of transformed cells and immunoblasts. The follicles are often scattered throughout the tumor and may be infiltrated and overrun (follicular colonization) by neoplastic (centrocyte-like) cells (43).

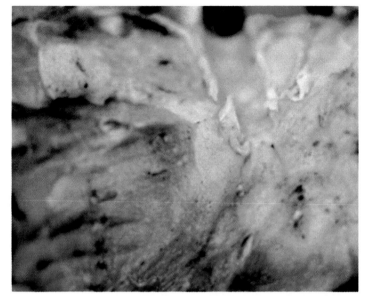

Figure 22-4
PSEUDOLYMPHOMA
There is a circumscribed focus of consolidation involving the lung parenchyma which shows some retraction due to scarring within the lesion.

BENIGN/HYPERPLASTIC DISORDERS

Pseudolymphoma
(Nodular Lymphoid Hyperplasia)

Definition. A pulmonary pseudolymphoma is a radiographically localized (occasionally multifocal) mass or infiltrate composed predominantly of lymphoid tissue that is histologically polymorphous and immunologically polyclonal (14,53). The recognition and immunologic characterization of low-grade extranodal lymphomas at many sites, including the lung, has led to a reclassification of most of the lesions previously classified as pseudolymphomas. In the 1960s and 1970s, close to 90 percent of pulmonary mass lesions composed predominantly of small lymphocytes were interpreted as pseudolymphomas; 10 percent or less are now interpreted as such. Some even question the very existence of pseudolymphomas (1,61), although there are occasional cases that appear to fulfill the criteria.

Clinical Features. Patients with pseudolymphoma are adults in the third to eighth decade of life (14,51,53). A small percent have a history of autoimmune disease such as Sjögren syndrome, lupus erythematosus, and others. A polyclonal hypergammaglobulinemia may be seen. At least 50 percent of patients are asymptomatic and have a solitary mass on chest radiograph. Less commonly, localized infiltrates or multiple nodules are

identified. When lesions are multifocal, low-grade lymphoma is a strong possibility.

Gross Findings. The nodules of pseudolymphoma are rarely over 5 cm in diameter (56). They are firm, white-tan, and may have central scarring and retraction (fig. 22-4).

Microscopic Findings. Pseudolymphomas are heterogeneous cellular lesions with prominent lymphoid tissue, usually with germinal centers (fig. 22-5). Surrounding the follicles is a dense lymphoplasmacytic infiltrate, often with Russell bodies, and variable amounts of scarring, especially near the center of the lesion. Histiocytes, some with epithelioid features and granuloma-forming tendencies, are often present. Giant cells are seen in about one third of the cases. Necrosis and amyloid are rare. Secondary changes, including increased alveolar macrophages, type 2 cell metaplasia, and foci of organizing pneumonia (which may be extensive) may also be seen.

Immunohistochemical Findings. Immunohistochemical studies of pseudolymphoma show a polyclonal population of B lymphocytes and plasma cells and a variable number of T lymphocytes (14,53,56).

Differential Diagnosis. The differential diagnosis primarily includes low-grade B-cell lymphomas of BALT, which can show virtually all of the features of pseudolymphoma including reactive follicles, plasma cells, fibrosis, giant cells, and granulomas. For any lymphoid nodule in

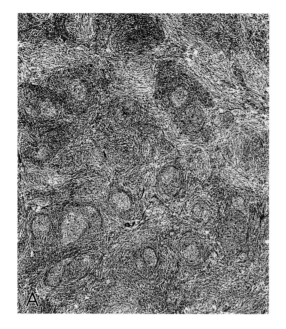

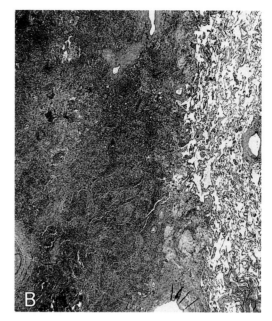

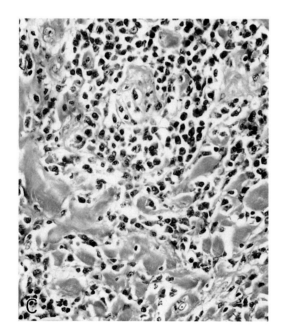

Figure 22-5
PSEUDOLYMPHOMA
A: The center of this lesion shows thick fibrous septa surrounding a polymorphous infiltrate including numerous germinal centers.
B: The edge of the lesion is sharply circumscribed and does not show extension along lymphatic routes.
C: Cytologically, the lesion is composed of a mixed population of lymphocytes and plasma cells.

which the differential diagnosis includes pseudolymphoma and low-grade non-Hodgkin lymphoma, the primary emphasis should be on excluding a lymphoma. Immunohistochemical studies are dependent on sampling, and a monoclonal cell population may be inconspicuous and focal. Plasma cells in lymphomas may be monoclonal or polyclonal; when polyclonal, attention should be focused on the clusters of lympho-

cytes in the mantle layer of the follicles in peribronchial, peribronchiolar, and perivascular locations. Frozen section immunofluorescence and molecular genetic studies are often necessary to confirm a monoclonal population. B-cell gene rearrangements may be sought when immunohistochemical studies are inconclusive. A diagnosis of pseudolymphoma should always remain suspect, and a lymphoma may subsequently be diagnosed.

Treatment and Prognosis. The treatment of localized pseudolymphoma is resection with a margin of normal tissue. Resection may not be possible in rare multifocal cases. Koss (56) found that 10 to 15 percent of cases recurred. All patients with pseudolymphomas should be carefully followed for the development of low-grade lymphoma, either as a result of "transformation" of the pseudolymphoma (53,56) or lack of identification of lymphoma at initial diagnosis.

The prognosis of pseudolymphoma is excellent. Although recurrences are occasionally seen and a few cases ultimately are proven to be lymphomas, no patients in Koss's series died.

Lymphocytic Interstitial Pneumonia and Diffuse Lymphoid Hyperplasia

Definition. Originally, lymphocytic interstitial pneumonia (LIP) was defined as a condition with widespread, dense lymphoplasmacytic infiltrates of such degree as to produce signs and symptoms of interstitial lung disease (63,64). Histologically, the infiltrates were "exquisitely interstitial," prominently surrounding bronchioles, and involving interlobular septa with a few "small" germinal centers "focally" (63). Based on these descriptions and the serum protein data in some of Liebow's 1973 cases (64) which suggested a monoclonal protein was present, we believe many of the original cases of LIP were actually diffuse low-grade lymphomas of the lung. Cases now classified as LIP range from dense, diffuse, polymorphous and polyclonal interstitial lymphoplasmacytic infiltrates to cases in which there is a marked proliferation of germinal centers along lymphatic routes (bronchovascular bundles, pulmonary veins, septa, and pleura) (14,53,54). There is considerable overlap between these two patterns, and the term diffuse lymphoid hyperplasia (DLH) is descriptively appropriate for the latter. Currently in the literature, LIP includes the entire spectrum.

Clinical Features. Patients with LIP have evidence of interstitial lung disease clinically, radiographically, or functionally (14,53,54). LIP is seen in children and adults; some patients have congenital or acquired immunodeficiency syndromes (including AIDS). Cough and dyspnea are the most common symptoms; others include fever, weight loss, arthralgias, hemoptysis, and chest pain. Some symptoms are due to

Table 22-2

CONDITIONS ASSOCIATED WITH LYMPHOCYTIC INTERSTITIAL PNEUMONITIS*

Autoimmune Diseases
    Sjögren syndrome
    Primary biliary cirrhosis
    Myasthenia gravis
    Hashimoto thyroiditis
    Pernicious anemia/agammaglobulinemia
    Autoimmune hemolytic anemia
    Systemic lupus erythematosus
    Celiac disease**

Immunodeficiency Syndromes
    Common variable immunodeficiency
    Unexplained childhood immunodeficiency
    Acquired immunodeficiency syndrome

Viral-Associated (Excluding HIV Infection)
    Epstein-Barr infection
    Chronic active hepatitis

Other infections (e.g., pneumocystis, tuberculosis)

Drug-Induced

Allogeneic bone marrow transplantation
    (Graft vs host disease)

Extrinsic allergic alveolitis

Miscellaneous
    Familial

*Modified from reference 53.

the many conditions associated with LIP (Table 22-2). Dysproteinemias occur in most patients; the most common is a polyclonal hypergammaglobulinemia, although hypogammaglobulinemia is also reported. The presence of a monoclonal spike suggests a lymphoma.

Several studies have shown the presence of Epstein-Barr virus (EBV) or human immunodeficiency virus (HIV) in some of the cases of LIP and an etiologic role for these viruses has been suggested (14,53).

Gross Findings. The gross findings of LIP are similar to those of other interstitial pneumonias.

Microscopic Findings. Microscopically, there is a spectrum from dense, diffuse lymphoplasmacytic infiltrates involving most alveolar walls to diffuse lymphoid hyperplasia (DLH) with reactive follicles distributed along lymphatic routes and relative sparing of the intervening alveolar walls (figs. 22-6, 22-7). There is

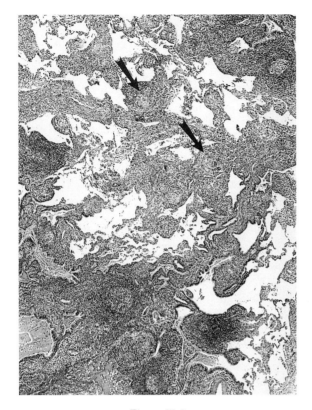

Figure 22-6
LYMPHOCYTIC INTERSTITIAL PNEUMONIA
IN SJÖGREN SYNDROME
This case of LIP shows a dense interstitial infiltrate including germinal centers and a few small granulomas (arrows). The infiltrate includes lymphocytes, mature plasma cells, and histiocytes.

considerable overlap between these, and the most common pattern is probably that of patchy, albeit dense, alveolar septal infiltrates of lymphocytes and plasma cells with scattered lymphoid follicles, many with germinal centers. In either pattern, granulomas, giant cells, and histiocyte clusters may be seen. Alveolar septal fibrosis and, to a lesser extent, honeycombing can be seen. Other secondary changes include increased alveolar macrophages, type 2 cell metaplasia, and foci of organization.

Immunohistochemical Findings. Immunohistochemical studies reveal a polyclonal population of B cells comprising the follicles, with a cuff of T cells (53). A few cases are composed predominantly of T cells (53). In AIDS cases, T cells tend to predominate, particularly CD8 (OKT8, Leu-2a)-positive T cells.

Differential Diagnosis. The differential diagnosis of LIP is extensive since LIP is a histologic reaction pattern seen in a number of clinical conditions (Table 22-2). The differential diagnosis includes diffuse low-grade lymphomas; other interstitial pneumonias with prominent cellular infiltrates, particularly extrinsic allergic alveolitis; and infections, especially from *Pneumocystis* pneumonia.

As with pseudolymphoma, it is important to exclude a low-grade lymphoma of the lung (1). Low-grade lymphomas usually have a dense, monomorphous infiltrate of lymphoid cells along lymphatic routes. Pleural invasion, bronchial cartilage invasion, and lymphoepithelial lesions all favor lymphoma. Granulomas, giant cells, germinal centers, and secondary inflammatory changes in the lung are of no help in the differential diagnosis since they may be seen in LIP as well as lymphomas. When trying to exclude a lymphoma, one should concentrate on the most dense and monomorphous foci of lymphocytes for histologic and immunohistologic evaluation.

The distinction of LIP from extrinsic allergic alveolitis may be difficult. Features that favor the latter include accentuation of peribronchiolar inflammation, foamy alveolar macrophages, and airspace organization (in bronchioles or alveolar ducts).

The interstitial pneumonias that tend to show the densest lymphoplasmacytic infiltrates are extrusive allergic alveolitis and drug reactions. In some instances, these conditions cannot be separated from idiopathic LIP without knowledge of the clinical history. *Pneumocystis carinii* pneumonia may have an exuberant interstitial lymphoplasmacytic reaction and produce the pattern of LIP. In some cases, organisms may be few and difficult to identify.

Treatment and Prognosis. Treatment results and prognosis of LIP have been difficult to evaluate, in part because many cases previously called LIP were actually low-grade lymphomas and in part because the conditions associated with LIP (for example, AIDS) have significant prognostic implications of their own. One third to half of patients with LIP die within 5 years (53,54). Some respond to steroids or immunosuppressive therapy (14,53,54), but these forms of therapy carry their own significant risks and complications. Surprisingly, patients with LIP

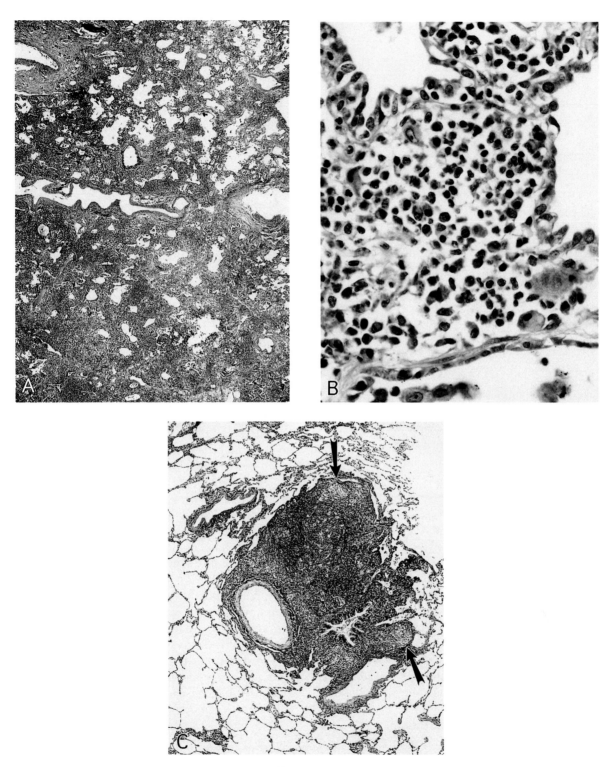

Figure 22-7
LYMPHOCYTIC INTERSTITIAL PNEUMONIA IN AIDS

Two cases of LIP in AIDS show a histologic spectrum from a dense, diffuse, lymphoid infiltrate involving virtually all alveolar walls (A) and composed of a population of lymphocytes and plasma cells (B), to diffuse lymphoid hyperplasia along lymphatic routes with a germinal center around a bronchiole (C) and sparing of adjacent alveoli. In the latter case, a few small granulomas (arrows) were associated with the lymphoid hyperplasia.

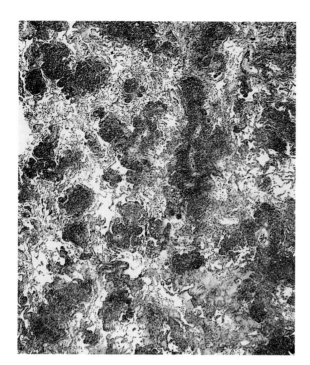 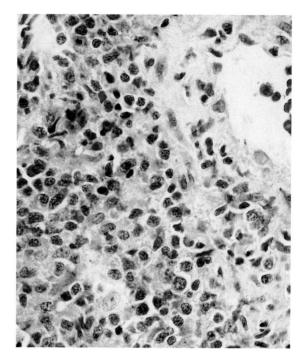

Figure 22-8
ANGIOIMMUNOBLASTIC LYMPHADENOPATHY INVOLVING THE LUNGS
This case of AILD with pulmonary involvement showed the typical lymph node findings of AILD. The lung has dense perivascular lymphoid infiltrates (left) composed of histiocytes, lymphocytes, plasma cells, and immunoblasts which show some predilection to infiltrate vessels (right). Most of these cases are now accepted as variants of T-cell lymphomas (as is this case). Note the similarity to figure 22-23 left.

associated with immunodeficiency syndromes, including AIDS, may respond to steroid therapy (14). In older reports, there was a significant risk of the development of lymphoma (up to 50 percent) in patients with LIP (53), but many of those cases were probably de novo lymphomas (1). Nevertheless, LIP, as defined above, probably carries an approximately 5 percent risk of the development of lymphoma (53), partly owing to the associated conditions (e.g., Sjögren syndrome, AIDS) that themselves carry a significant risk of the development of lymphoma.

Giant Lymph Node Hyperplasia (Castleman Disease)

Giant lymph node hyperplasia (Castleman disease) may occasionally involve the lung parenchyma, although presentation as a hilar mass is much more common. In the original series of Keller et al. (49), 2 of 81 cases were intrapulmonary and 24 presented as hilar masses. Most cases involving the lung and hilum

are of the hyaline vascular type and present as a solitary, often asymptomatic, mass. The lesions are well circumscribed and often have a thick fibrous capsule and septa. The distinctive hyaline vascular change of the germinal centers and interfollicular stroma rich in plasma cells and small vessels are features not seen in other forms of lymphoid hyperplasia in the lung.

Angioimmunoblastic Lymphadenopathy

The initial descriptions of angioimmunoblastic lymphadenopathy (AILD) included a number of patients with pulmonary involvement (31,101). Most cases are now considered variants of T-cell lymphomas (i.e., AILD-like T-cell lymphoma) (58), and pulmonary involvement is thus a manifestation of lymphomatous infiltration of the lung. Histologically, the lung shows interstitial, septal, and perivascular infiltrates (along lymphatic routes) composed of a mixed population of cells including immunoblasts, lymphocytes, plasma cells, and occasional histiocytes (fig. 22-8).

427

LYMPHOMAS PRESENTING IN LUNG

Small Lymphocytic and Lymphoplasmacytoid Lymphomas (Including Low-Grade Lymphomas of BALT)

Malignant lymphomas composed predominantly of small lymphocytes and lymphoplasmacytoid cells are the most common primary lymphomas of the lung (22,53,56,61,87). Most are low-grade B-cell lymphomas of BALT (1,22,53, 61); T-cell small lymphocytic lymphomas are occasionally seen (61). Many cases now classified in this category were previously classified as pseudolymphomas if localized, or LIP if diffuse and bilateral. The recognition of extranodal lymphomas and their immunologic confirmation as clonal proliferations has led to the reclassification of most of these cases as lymphomas (14,15,53,56). In future studies, the separation of low-grade lymphomas of BALT from other small lymphocytic lymphomas of the lung will probably become important.

Clinical Features. Most patients are adults in the sixth decade, although patients as young as 12 have been observed (14,50,53,56,59,61,97). The sex distribution is roughly equal. About half the patients are symptomatic and the rest are identified on the basis of an abnormal chest X ray. Symptoms include cough, dyspnea, hemoptysis, weight loss, chest pain, and occasionally, fever, malaise, and other constitutional symptoms.

Close to 20 percent of patients, usually those with a lymphoplasmacytoid histology, have a monoclonal protein in the serum. Bone marrow involvement at the time of diagnosis is seen in 10 to 20 percent of patients. Waldenström macroglobulinemia with pulmonary or pleural involvement is included in this category. Cases associated with cryoglobulinemia have been reported. Patients with diffuse bilateral infiltrates may have the signs, symptoms, and functional deficits of interstitial lung disease.

In 50 percent of cases the chest X ray shows a localized infiltrate or solitary nodule (14,53,56, 97). Other radiographic presentations include multiple nodules, patchy infiltrates, and diffuse bilateral infiltrates. Cavitation, hilar adenopathy, and pleural effusion are unusual. Five to 10 percent of cases show interstitial lung disease radiographically (56,97).

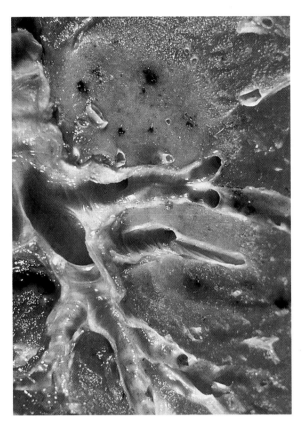

Figure 22-9
SMALL LYMPHOCYTIC LYMPHOMA
This resected nodule shows consolidation of the lung parenchyma by a tan mass which preserves lung architecture and surrounds a segmental bronchus.

Gross Findings. The gross features of localized cases are characteristic: a fleshy, non-necrotic, gray-white mass (typical of lymphoid tissue), showing infiltrative and nondestructive growth with preservation of lung architecture (fig. 22-9) (53,56).

Microscopic Findings. Microscopically, the changes are distinctive (1,14,53,56,59,61,97), and in most cases the diagnosis is apparent at scanning power magnification due to the sheer density and monotony of the lymphoid infiltrate and its predilection for lymphatic routes (lymphatic tracking) in the septa, around veins, in the pleura, and along bronchovascular bundles (figs. 22-10–22-14). The cells form sheets, thick cuffs, and micronodules along these structures; large mass lesions entirely overrun the lung

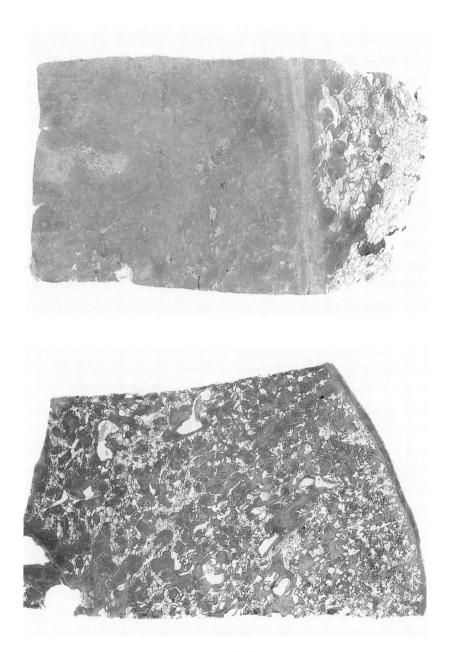

Figure 22-10
SMALL LYMPHOCYTIC LYMPHOMA
This resected localized small lymphocytic lymphoma was composed of sheets of small lymphocytes centrally which track along vessels at the edge of the nodules (top) and form perivascular nodular aggregates in less severely affected regions of the lung (bottom).

architecture centrally, and the lymphatic character of the process may only be apparent at the edge. Invasion of the pleura and bronchial cartilage are uncommon but good evidence for a diagnosis of lymphoma when present.

The cytologic recognition of small lymphocytic and lymphoplasmacytoid lymphomas centers on the identification of monotonous sheets and micronodules of neoplastic cells (fig. 22-13). These foci may be surrounded by germinal centers (fig. 22-14), reactive (polyclonal) lymphoplasmacytic infiltrates, and inflammatory changes in the lung parenchyma. Germinal centers are present in up to 70 percent of cases (53),

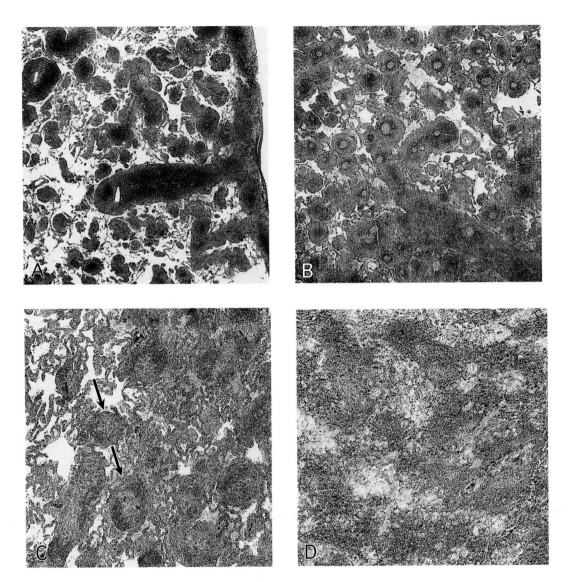

Figure 22-11
SMALL LYMPHOCYTIC LYMPHOMA

These four cases illustrate some of the scanning power appearances of small lymphocytic lymphoma.

A: There is a dense monomorphous infiltrate of small lymphocytes involving the pleura and septa, and surrounding vessels.

B: There is a perivascular infiltrate of lymphoid tissue which includes numerous germinal centers. The cuffs of lymphocytes around the germinal centers were monoclonal whereas the follicles were polyclonal.

C: There is a perivascular and interstitial infiltrate of lymphocytes. The lymphoid nodules appear to have pale germinal centers (arrows) although these were shown to be vessels infiltrated by T cells (see figure 22-12) and the monoclonal population of cells comprised the darker mantle zone around the vessels.

D: Sheets of small lymphocytes are seen in a dense acellular hyaline fibrous stroma.

and may be extremely numerous (fig. 22-11B). Immunologic staining (see below) highlights the extent of reactive cells (polyclonal plasma cells and T cells) that may surround the monomorphous (monoclonal) foci.

Cytologically, these lymphomas are composed primarily of small lymphocytes or plasmacytoid lymphocytes (or plasma cells) with a small number of transformed cells and immunoblasts. Proliferation centers may be difficult to separate from germinal centers, particularly those secondarily infiltrated (colonized) by neoplastic cells. In some cases there is cytologic atypia, with cells resembling those seen in lymphocytic lymphomas

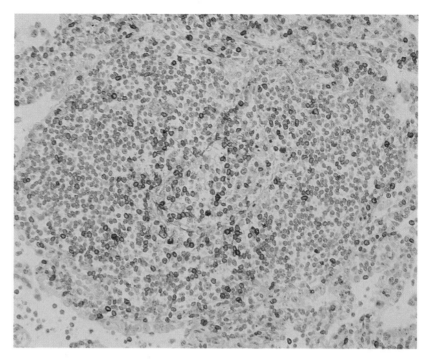

Figure 22-12
SMALL LYMPHOCYTIC LYMPHOMA
A stain for T cells (CD3) shows a vessel infiltrated by CD3-positive cells (center). The clusters of small lymphocytes surrounding the vessel (right and left) showed kappa light chain restriction by frozen section immunohistochemistry. This is the same case as shown in figure 22-11C.

of intermediate differentiation (centrocytic cells). Rarely, there are cases composed of small cleaved cells. The plasma cells are usually polyclonal and found around the foci of lymphoma, but in a small number of cases the plasma cells are monoclonal and the lesions qualify as lymphoplasmacytic lymphomas (fig. 22-13D). The histologic heterogeneity of small lymphocytic lymphomas and lymphoplasmacytic lymphomas parallels that seen in lymphomas of MALT in general, and monocytoid B-cell foci are occasionally seen in low-grade B-cell lymphomas of BALT. Helpful clues to the diagnosis are the identification of lymphoepithelial lesions (fig. 22-15) which are characteristic of, but not specific for (61), lymphomas of MALT, and Dutcher bodies with periodic acid–Schiff (PAS)-positive intranuclear inclusions. Granulomas may also be encountered.

Some cases have increased numbers of large cells, and when they form sheets, the possibility of transformation to a large cell lymphoma should be considered (fig. 22-16).

Immunohistochemical Findings and Molecular Genetics. Immunohistochemical and molecular genetic studies are generally not necessary for a diagnosis, but in some cases they are extremely useful in confirming a monoclonal (lymphomatous) process. Most small lymphocytic lymphomas of the lung are low-grade B-cell tumors, and a monoclonal population can be confirmed with the appropriate techniques. Light chain restriction can sometimes be shown with paraffin section immunostaining in lymphoplasmacytoid lymphomas with cytoplasmic immunoglobulin, but frozen section immunostaining or flow cytometry of fresh material is usually necessary in cases composed predominantly of small lymphocytes. Clonal B-cell gene rearrangements can be confirmed with molecular genetic studies which sometimes prove more sensitive than immunohistochemical and flow cytometric techniques. Among heavy chains, IgM and IgA are found more frequently than IgG.

B-cell antigens commonly expressed by the neoplastic cells include CD20 (B1, L26), CD21

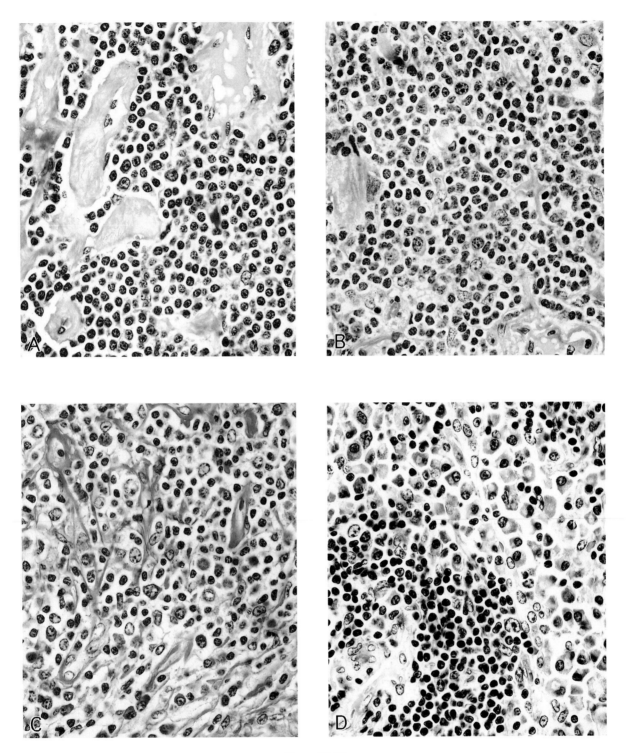

Figure 22-13
CYTOLOGIC SPECTRUM OF SMALL LYMPHOCYTIC LYMPHOMA

These four cases illustrate:
A: Predominantly small lymphocytes with rare large cells and associated dense sclerotic reaction.
B: Plasmacytoid differentiation including immature plasmacytoid forms. Occasional atypical small lymphocytes are also present.
C: Relatively numerous large cells and fine pericapillary sclerosis.
D: A population of lymphocytes and mature plasma cells that both showed the same light chain restriction.

(B2), CD22 (Leu-14), CD35, CD45RA (4KB5), KB61, KB3, and Ki-B3 (53). CD10 (CALLA) and CD5 (Leu-1) are usually not expressed in low-grade lymphomas of BALT.

Polyclonal plasma cells and variable numbers of reactive T cells typically surround the monoclonal B-cell foci. In some cases the T cells overshadow the B cells in number, and they may show vascular infiltration (fig. 22-12). In occasional cases, the plasma cells are monoclonal and have the same light chain restriction as the neoplastic population of lymphocytes (11).

A small number of lymphocytic lymphomas of the lung are composed entirely of T cells (61).

Differential Diagnosis. The differential diagnosis of small lymphocytic and lymphoplasmacytoid lymphomas of the lung includes LIP, pseudolymphoma, leukemic infiltrates (especially chronic lymphocytic leukemia), other lymphomas, and small lymphocytic lymphoma in transformation.

LIP and pseudolymphoma contrast with small lymphocytic lymphoma by their histologic heterogeneity and polyclonal cell population. The diffuse lymphoid hyperplasia (DLH) form of LIP is characterized by a proliferation of histologically normal germinal centers along lymphatic routes;

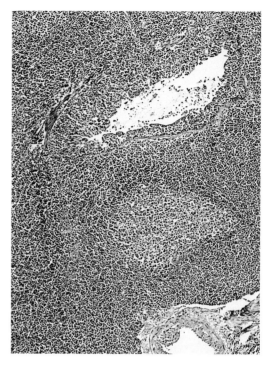

Figure 22-14
SMALL LYMPHOCYTIC LYMPHOMA

This small lymphocytic lymphoma shows peribronchiolar germinal center formation (proven to be polyclonal) as well as a dense monomorphous (monoclonal) infiltrate of small lymphocytes which invades the bronchiole (top).

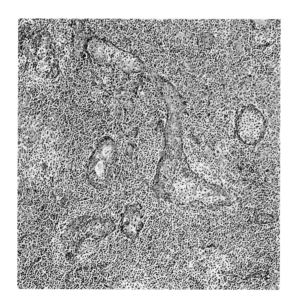 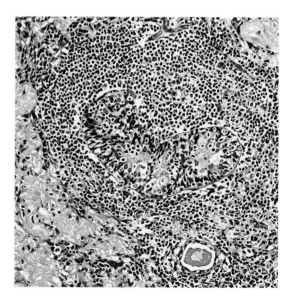

Figure 22-15
LYMPHOEPITHELIAL LESIONS

Left: In this small lymphocytic lymphoma, the lymphoepithelial lesions are seen as pale islands less densely infiltrated by lymphocytes. The epithelial cells are not prominent.

Right: This lymphoepithelial lesion shows an island of recognizable epithelial cells infiltrated by lymphocytes. This lesion was found around a focus of active tuberculosis in a patient with no evidence of lymphoproliferative disease.

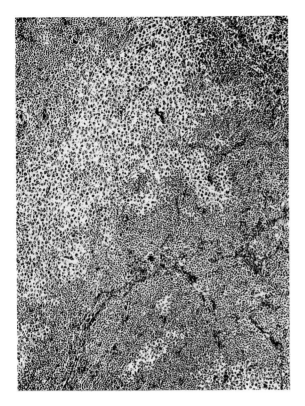

Figure 22-16
SMALL LYMPHOCYTIC LYMPHOMA
IN TRANSFORMATION
This small lymphocytic lymphoma of the lung shows transformation to a diffuse large cell lymphoma, with sheets of large cells (upper left) replacing the small lymphocytes.

the germinal centers lack the dense cuff of lymphocytes and septal infiltration by a uniform population of small lymphocytes that characterizes lymphomas.

Germinal centers, granulomas, giant cells, and fibrosis are all not helpful for diagnosis since they are seen in lymphomas with appreciable frequency. The presence of Dutcher bodies, lymphoepithelial lesions, and pleural and bronchial cartilage invasion favors the diagnosis of lymphoma.

Chronic lymphocytic leukemia may be associated with infiltrates along lymphatic routes that are histologically indistinguishable from small lymphocytic lymphomas.

Treatment and Prognosis. The treatment of choice for localized lesions is resection (14,52, 54), and the prognosis is very good. A small number of cases relapse in the lung, sometimes years or decades later, whereas other cases re-

lapse in other sites of MALT. A small percentage become aggressive systemic lymphomas.

Cases with multiple nodules or diffuse and bilateral involvement may eventually require chemotherapy when they become symptomatic. Sometimes there is dramatic and sustained response to steroid therapy alone whereas other cases may require more aggressive chemotherapy as the disease progresses.

Angiocentric Immunoproliferative Lesions/Angiocentric Lymphomas (Lymphomatoid Granulomatosis/ Polymorphic Reticulosis)

After small lymphocytic lymphomas, the next most common pulmonary lymphomas are the angiocentric lymphomas and related lesions. This group is still thought by some to be in a gray zone between reactive and neoplastic proliferations. Practically speaking, these lesions are clinically and histogenetically closest to lymphomas (14–16,53,55). Lesions described as *lymphomatoid granulomatosis (LYG)* (46,55,65), *polymorphic reticulosis* (25), *benign* and *malignant angiitis* and *granulomatosis* (86), and *angiocentric immunoproliferative lesions (AIL)* (44,66), are all included in this group. The nomenclature is cumbersome, and no one term is universally preferred; as a compromise we call this group AIL/LYG (53), recognizing that many (some would say nearly all) (58) of these lesions are lymphomas. The definition of AIL, according to Liebow's original series (65), is an angiocentric and angiodestructive process of lymphoreticular cells with vascular invasion. It is now clear that other lymphoid lesions may show these changes; nevertheless, AIL/LYG remains a distinctive clinicopathologic group (53). Early studies suggested AIL/LYG was a T-cell proliferative process (66), although recent data suggests that some cases are T-cell–rich, B-cell proliferations in which the B cells are infected by Epstein-Barr virus (36).

Clinical Features. The clinical features of AIL/LYG are compiled from five series, comprising 277 patients, and reviewed by Koss (53). Men predominate 2 to 1. Most patients are diagnosed in the fifth decade; the reported age ranges from 8 to 85 years, but some of the earlier cases in children occurred in patients with immunodeficiency syndromes and might now be classified differently.

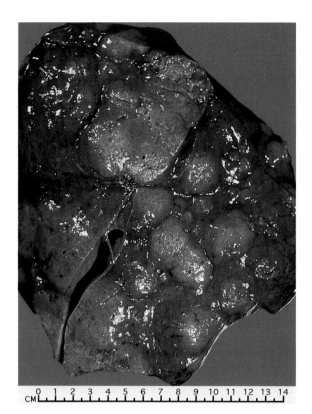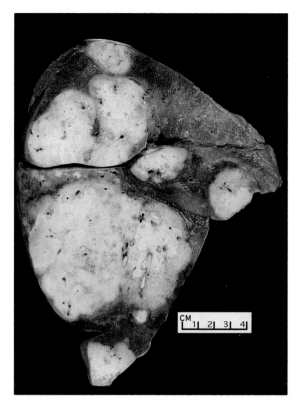

Figure 22-17
FRESH (LEFT) AND FIXED (RIGHT) AUTOPSY LUNG SPECIMENS
SHOWING TYPICAL GROSS FEATURES OF AIL/LYG
Multiple consolidated nodules of fleshy lymphoid tissue replace the lung parenchyma.

AIL/LYG shows a predilection for lung involvement (up to 100 percent of cases in some reports) (53). Pulmonary symptoms include cough, dyspnea, and chest pain. About 10 percent of patients are asymptomatic at the time of diagnosis. The skin and nervous system are also frequently affected. In some patients symptoms of extrapulmonary lesions dominate. This is particularly true of skin involvement, which may precede lung disease by months or years (99). Cutaneous lesions include nodules, ulcers, and maculopapular eruptions. Skin biopsy is diagnostic in only about half of these cases. Central nervous system involvement may be associated with cranial nerve deficits, diplopia, blindness, ataxia, paresthesias, vertigo, headache, or seizures. Peripheral neuropathy occurs in 10 percent of cases. Head and neck involvement, especially nose, sinuses, and nasopharynx, is also relatively common.

Radiographically, bilateral nodules are present in three fourths of the patients. The nodules

may wax and wane spontaneously, and cavitation is relatively common (25 percent). Less common patterns include diffuse interstitial or alveolar infiltrates, localized infiltrates, and solitary nodules. Pleural effusions occur in a small percentage of cases.

Some patients, ultimately diagnosed on the basis of lung biopsy, have a peculiar prolonged history (often a fever of unknown origin) without specific diagnosis; some have undergone multiple skin biopsies, laparotomy with lymph node biopsy, liver biopsy, and even splenectomy without a specific diagnosis.

Involvement of traditional sites of hematologic disease such as lymph nodes, bone marrow, spleen, and liver are relatively unusual but are seen late in the course of AIL/LYG.

Gross Findings. These are characteristic (fig. 22-17) (46,53,55,65). There is nodular consolidation of the lung with nodules up to 10 cm in diameter, often with central necrosis and a rim of viable tissue

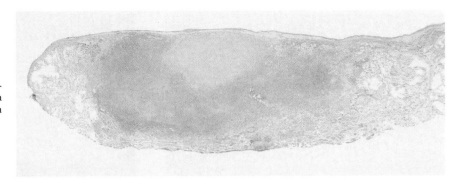

Figure 22-18
AIL/LYG
This small peripheral nodule in a wedge biopsy shows a dense lymphoid infiltrate with central necrosis.

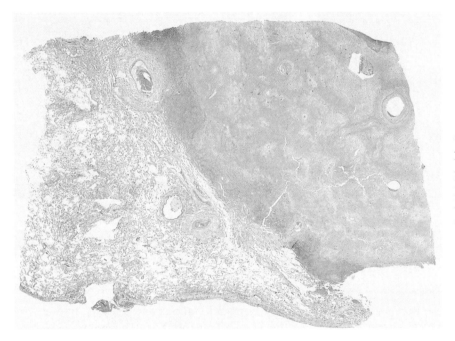

Figure 22-19
AIL/LYG
This whole mount section of a large necrotic nodule of AIL/LYG shows extensive central necrosis with a thin viable rim of lymphoid tissue. Foci of high-grade AIL/LYG were found in the viable lymphoid cells in this case, but they required a search of several blocks.

with a "fish flesh" appearance. Cavitation is common. Necrotic lesions usually do not have the peripheral wedge-shaped appearance of an infarct but appear as tumor nodules with central necrosis.

Microscopic Findings. The microscopic findings of AIL/LYG set this lesion apart from most conventional lymphomas and from other examples of so-called angiitis and granulomatosis of the lung (figs. 22-18–22-26) (14–16,25,44, 46,53,55,65,66). There are nodular as well as more diffuse interstitial infiltrates of lymphoid cells. The nodules and infiltrates tend to be centered on, or adjacent to, the structures along lymphatic routes, particularly bronchovascular bundles. Small perivascular nodules may expand to involve the adjacent alveoli, and there is often a fibrinous exudate at the growing edge of the nodules. As the nodules enlarge, central necrosis and cavitation develop. In the centers of the nodules a large vessel may be present, and infiltrated by lymphoid cells, justifying the descriptive designation angiocentric and angiodestructive (fig. 22-22). A rim of viable cells usually remains around the vessels in the center of the necrotic nodules. The necrosis in these lesions is seen as part of the central necrosis of the nodule rather than infarction secondary to a necrotizing vasculitis (figs. 22-18, 22-19). The cells that infiltrate the vessels show the same cytologic variation and heterogeneity as seen in the parenchymal lymphoid infiltrates (see below), however, high-grade lesions may have vessels infiltrated by a cytologically benign and polymorphous cell population.

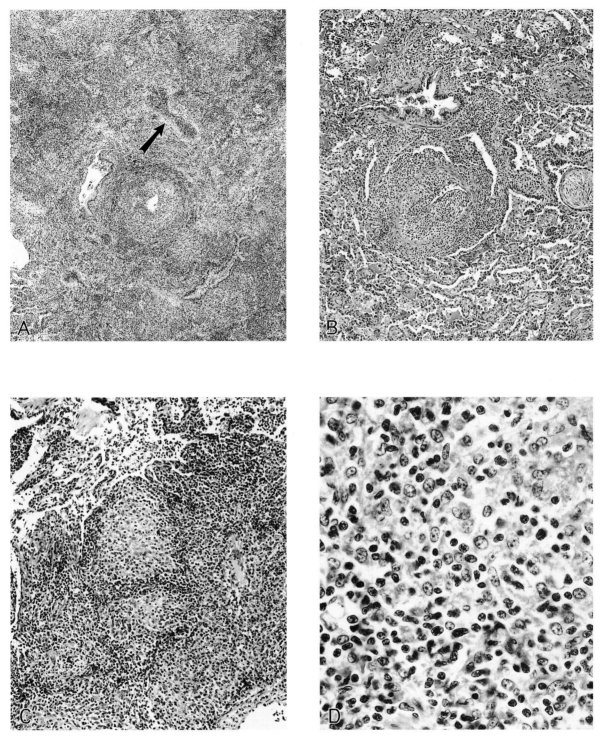

Figure 22-20
LOW-GRADE AIL/LYG

A: A nodule with dense lymphoid infiltrate, vascular invasion (center), and foci of organization (arrow).

B: Another case shows prominent vascular infiltration with surrounding inflammatory changes in the lung including focal airspace organization (right center).

C & D: A third case shows granulomas (C) and a relatively bland cytogenic appearance (D) with many of the larger nuclei belonging to histiocytes.

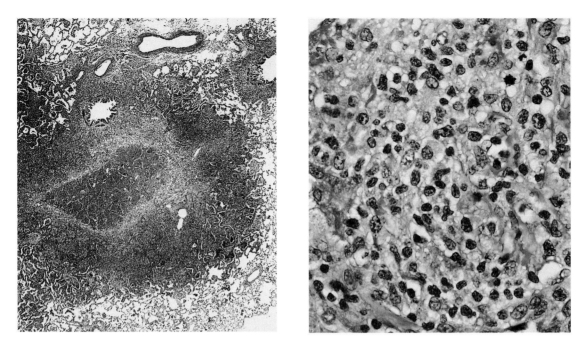

Figure 22-21
HIGH-GRADE AIL/LYG
Left: There is a centrally necrotic lymphoid nodule which (in this field) does not show vascular infiltration.
Right: Cytologically, there are moderate numbers of intermediate-size and large lymphoid cells with some atypia in the small lymphocytes. All the cells in this case stained as T cells with paraffin section immunostaining.

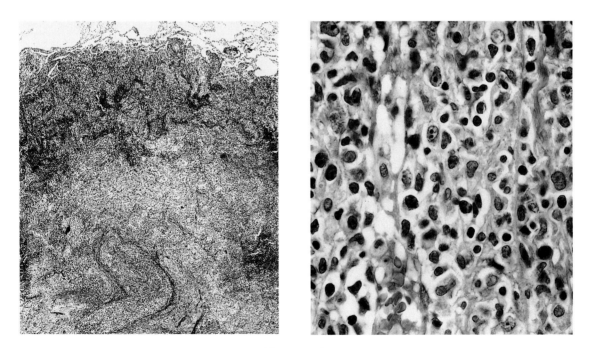

Figure 22-22
HIGH-GRADE AIL/LYG
Left: This centrally necrotic nodule shows prominent vascular infiltration and a rim of viable lymphoid cells.
Right: The vascular infiltrate from another nodule shows numerous atypical large cells. The large cells stained as B cells in this case.

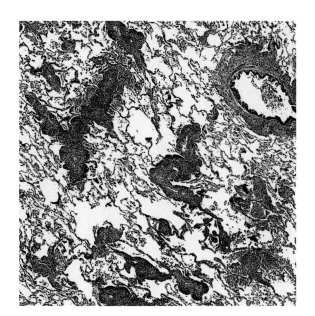

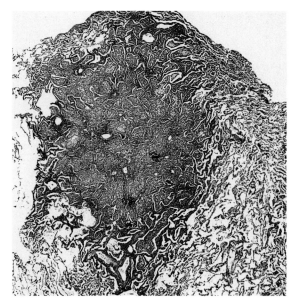

Figure 22-23
HIGH-GRADE AIL/LYG

Left: The field illustrated shows dense perivascular infiltrates and was found adjacent to a large necrotic nodule showing typical features of high-grade AIL/LYG.

Right: An early nodule from another case of high-grade AIL/LYG. There is a prominent fibrinous exudate in the airspaces.

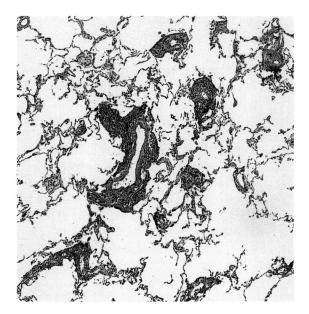

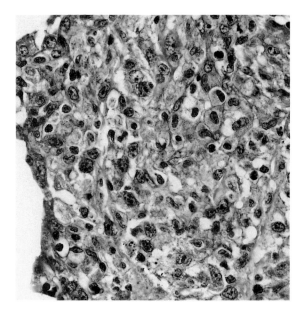

Figure 22-24
HIGH-GRADE AIL/LYG

This case of high-grade AIL/LYG was associated with diffuse radiographic infiltrates and respiratory insufficiency. Nodules were not identified radiographically or histologically. There are diffuse perivascular infiltrates (left) of atypical large lymphoid cells (right). In the absence of identifiable necrotic nodules, some would question inclusion of this case as an example of AIL/LYG.

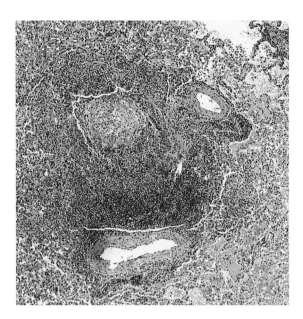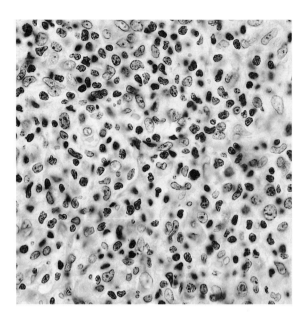

Figure 22-25
BRONCHIOLAR INVOLVEMENT IN AIL/LYG
Left: This case of high-grade AIL/LYG showed relative vascular sparing (in this field) and prominent infiltration of a bronchiole with associated intraluminal organization.
Right: The infiltrate is composed of atypical small and large lymphoid cells.

The cytologic composition of the lesions of AIL/LYG contrast with classic lymphomas: a heterogeneous population of cells in contrast to a monomorphous population (figs. 22-20–22-24). In addition, the cytologic composition commonly varies from field to field, making cytologic assessment difficult and sample dependent. Typically, there are variable numbers of small lymphocytes, plasma cells, histiocytes (occasionally aggregating as epithelioid cell clusters and granulomas), small lymphoid cells with atypical "twisted" nuclei, intermediate-sized lymphoid cells that may be cytologically atypical, large lymphoid cells resembling large cleaved or noncleaved cells or immunoblasts, and rarely, large bizarre lymphoid cells, some of which may resemble Reed-Sternberg cells. The most cytologically atypical foci are usually found in the larger nodules and are composed of clusters of intermediate-sized and large cells, and these foci should be sought for diagnosis and grading (see below). Many fields in a given case may be composed of a cytologically bland ("benign") and mixed infiltrate of small lymphocytes, histiocytes, and plasma cells with a

few intermediate-sized lymphoid cells. Eosinophils and giant cells are occasionally present.

Vascular, and sometimes bronchial or bronchiolar, infiltration (fig. 22-25) is a distinctive histologic feature of these lesions. Infiltration of vessels and airways is usually a secondary phenomenon due to the presence of lymphoid infiltrates along the lymphatic routes adjacent to these structures. In some cases, vessels and airways are simply overrun as the nodules expand. Nevertheless, there are occasional cases with dramatic and preferential vascular involvement.

Depending on the cytologic composition of AIL/LYG, there is a spectrum from low grade to high grade that shows correlation with clinical behavior and response to therapy. Initially, three grades were suggested to encompass this spectrum (44, 66), but two grades, a low grade and high grade, have been found to be easier to apply. Low-grade lesions, which are uncommon, have a polymorphous composition, little cytologic atypia, a small proportion of large cells, a few mitotic figures, and little necrosis. High-grade lesions (angiocentric lymphomas) have cytologic atypia in the lymphoid cells, an increased population of large

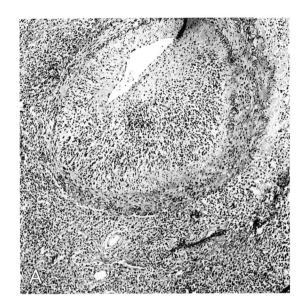
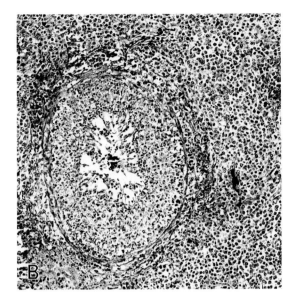
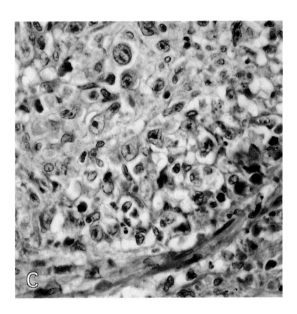

Figure 22-26
"TRANSFORMATION" OF AIL/LYG

In the first biopsy (A), this case of AIL/LYG showed vascular infiltration by lymphocytes and plasma cells without cytologic atypia. There was no response to chemotherapy, and pneumonectomy was eventually required (B,C). The lymphoid infiltrate was composed entirely of large cells with prominent vascular infiltration.

transformed cells, a more monomorphous appearance, and usually extensive necrosis. Most cases fall into the latter category, although in some, the monomorphous foci of large cells may require a careful search. Some high-grade lesions are indistinguishable from other large cell lymphomas (see below).

The lung tissue around the lesions of AIL/LYG commonly shows a mild interstitial infiltrate of lymphocytes and plasma cells; an increase in alveolar macrophages, which may be foamy; metaplasia of type 2 cells; and occasionally, organization with proliferation of fibroblastic tissue in airspaces.

441

Immunohistochemical Findings. Immunohistochemical studies of AIL/LYG show that most of the lymphoid cells are CD4 (OKT4, Leu-3a)-positive T cells: some have a mixture of CD4- and CD8 (OKT8, Leu-2a)-positive T cells and some are composed primarily of CD8-positive T cells (44,53,66,101). In the past, such findings were evidence that AIL/LYG was a T-cell lymphoproliferation, and there are some cases that show gene rearrangements typical of T-cell lymphomas (53,58). Recently, however, Guinee et al. (36) have shown that many cases of typical AIL/LYG are T-cell–rich, B-cell lymphoproliferations with Epstein-Barr virus (EBV) infection of the B cells as well as immunoglobulin gene rearrangements (indicative of clonality of the B cells) in a proportion of the cases; i.e., T-cell–rich, B-cell lymphoma.

Molecular studies of AIL/LYG show an association with EBV in at least half to three fourths of the cases, confirming earlier studies that showed increased titers to EBV antigens in some cases (36,47,53,68). Medeiros et al. (68,69) found that EBV was more likely present in high-grade cases, and particularly in large atypical cells. They suggested that the expansion of the number of EBV-infected cells was associated with the development of a high-grade lesion (angiocentric lymphoma).

Differential Diagnosis. The differential diagnosis for AIL/LYG can be grouped into necrotizing inflammatory/infectious conditions, primary and secondary nonlymphomatous malignancies, small lymphocytic lymphomas/low-grade lymphomas of BALT, large cell lymphomas, Hodgkin disease, and lymphomas secondarily involving the lung.

Some degree of vascular infiltration is common in inflammatory and infectious lesions of the lung. Similarly, any lesion with necrosis may have a surrounding lymphoid reaction. The presence of neutrophils is unusual in AIL/LYG and much more characteristic of an inflammatory/infectious lesion. Granulomatous inflammation is uncommon in AIL/LYG; granulomatous infections typically have non-necrotizing granulomas away from the main lesion, which overshadow the lymphoid tissue. The small necrotic lesions of varicella-zoster virus pneumonia may have a lymphoid reaction prominent enough to raise the possibility of AIL/LYG. Wegener granulomatosis typically has giant cells, microabscesses of neutrophils, and relatively few lymphoid cells. Necrotizing sarcoid granulomatosis is dominated by granulomas with relatively few lymphocytes. Bronchocentric granulomatosis is bronchocentric with numerous eosinophils and relatively few lymphocytes, and often a history of asthma and allergic bronchopulmonary aspergillosis.

Primary and secondary nonlymphomatous malignancies (including carcinomas and sarcomas) may show vascular infiltration and a prominent lymphoid infiltrate. In general, there are larger, more monomorphous, atypical cells with more vesicular nuclei than in AIL/LYG. Immunohistochemistry may prove particularly helpful in these cases, for example, in differentiating a dyscohesive large cell carcinoma or metastatic nasopharyngeal carcinoma from a lymphoma.

Small lymphocytic lymphomas and low-grade lymphomas of BALT are composed primarily of small lymphocytes, have relatively little necrosis and vascular infiltration, and only occasionally produce multiple bilateral nodules. They often have germinal centers and lymphoepithelial lesions, both of which are unusual in AIL/LYG.

AIL/LYG merges with conventional large cell lymphomas at the high-grade end of the spectrum, and differentiation may not be possible in the individual case.

Hodgkin disease of the lung, both primary and secondary, often has extensive vascular infiltration, necrosis with acute inflammation, and a polymorphous lymphoid infiltrate. Nevertheless, there is generally the typical background ("milieu") of Hodgkin disease, classic Reed-Sternberg cells, and often a nodular sclerosing pattern. Immunohistochemistry, particularly CD15 (Leu-M1) and CD30 (Ber-H2), may help confirm a diagnosis of Hodgkin disease.

Secondary non-Hodgkin lymphomas may produce histologic features similar to AIL/LYG. In fact, a T-cell lymphoma that initially presents in the lymph nodes may produce lesions in the lung indistinguishable (and some would say they are the same disease) from AIL/LYG.

Treatment and Prognosis. The treatment and prognosis of AIL/LYG are somewhat controversial (14,46,53,55,66). A conservative approach is reasonable in the minority of cases in which the diagnosis is not certain or in which a solitary nodule has been entirely resected and there is no other evidence of disease. In general, however, most patients have symptoms and widespread disease, and need therapy. High-grade AIL/LYG is treated with aggressive multi-agent chemotherapy; low-grade lesions with single-agent chemotherapy plus steroids (66). Patients with low-grade lesions treated with a relatively nonaggressive regimen have a risk of relapse (66), and it can be argued that aggressive chemotherapy is indicated in all cases. Since most cases of AIL/LYG are high grade, aggressive therapy is usually indicated.

Over the course of the disease, AIL/LYG may progress to involve multiple sites, including traditional lymphoid organs, and show progressive increase in the number of large cells, resulting in the appearance of a conventional monomorphous large cell lymphoma (fig. 22-26) (46). Two explanations for this "evolution" are possible: 1) there is true evolution of a premalignant process or 2) there is transformation of a low-grade lymphoma into a high-grade lymphoma analogous to many B-cell lymphomas.

Large Cell Lymphoma of Lung

The spectrum of large cell lymphomas seen in lymph nodes is also seen in the lung, including large cell anaplastic (Ki-1) lymphoma (12,14, 16,22,56,61). Vascular infiltration is common, and the distinction of some cases from high-grade AIL/LYG is arbitrary. The radiographic features of large cell lymphomas are generally similar to those of AIL/LYG.

Most cases produce mass lesions that may be necrotic and cavitated. The microscopic findings of large cell lymphomas in the lung parallel those in the lymph nodes (figs. 22-27–22-30). There are sheets of large lymphoid cells that may resemble large cleaved cell, large noncleaved cell, immunoblastic, or anaplastic large cell (Ki-1) lymphoma (figs. 22-29, 22-30). A reactive-appearing cellular infiltrate at the lesion edge is common. Necrosis and vascular infiltration may be marked.

Staging and treatment are the same as for similar lesions in the lymph nodes, with the exception of the occasional localized large cell lymphoma of the lung that is cured by resection (14,21). The prognosis is not clear because of the small number of cases studied. By analogy with high-grade AIL/LYG and the few reports available (16,66), response to chemotherapy can be expected in some patients.

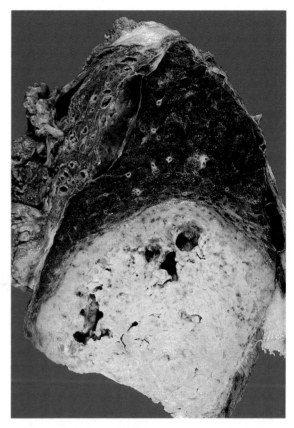

Figure 22-27
PRIMARY LARGE CELL LYMPHOMA
This large solitary mass replaces much of the lower lobe. Histologically, this was a large noncleaved cell lymphoma.

Intravascular Lymphomatosis (Angiotropic Lymphoma)

Intravascular lymphomatosis (IVL) is an uncommon malignant lymphoma in which the tumor cells proliferate within small vessels. Involvement of the skin and central nervous system are best known, but presentation as pulmonary disease is well described (92,103). In virtually all patients, even if their disease appears restricted to the lung, multisystem involvement develops, and at autopsy widespread disease is usually found. The term, intravascular lymphomatosis, is preferred to angiotropic lymphoma because the latter may be confused with angiocentric lymphoma.

The features of pulmonary involvement in IVL are interstitial lung disease with dyspnea,

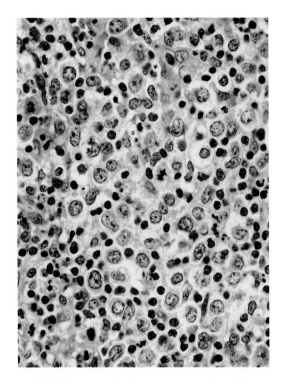

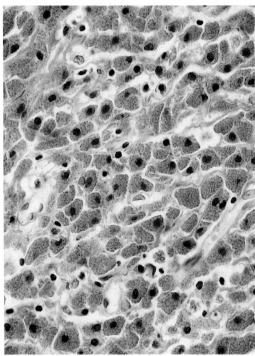

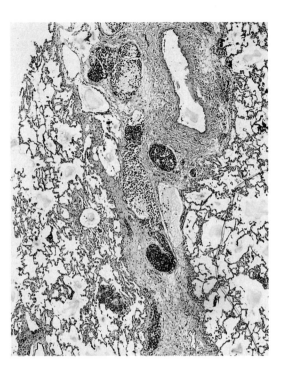

Figure 22-29
ANAPLASTIC LARGE CELL LYMPHOMA
INVOLVING THE LUNG

This case of anaplastic large cell lymphoma, previously reported by Colby et al. (17) as malignant histiocytosis, shows neoplastic cells filling lymphatic spaces, an uncommon finding in lymphoreticular infiltrates of the lung. The cytologic features were typical of anaplastic large cell lymphoma, and the cells were CD30 (Ber-H2) positive.

Figure 22-28
LARGE CELL LYMPHOMA, B-CELL TYPE

Top: This resected solitary mass was composed of numerous large noncleaved cells (proven to be monoclonal B cells) with associated infiltrates of small cells, all of which were T cells.

Bottom: Immunoglobulin production was manifested by scattered nodules of histiocytes containing immunoglobulin crystals.

fever, and diffuse radiographic infiltrates. Snyder et al. (92) reported a case manifesting as pulmonary hypertension.

The resemblance of IVL to interstitial pneumonia is maintained at the histologic level (fig. 22-31). Scanning power evaluation shows hypercellularity of the alveolar walls which is easily mistaken for an inflammatory infiltrate if attention is not paid to the cytologic features of the cells and their location within dilated alveolar capillaries. The capillaries are filled with large lymphoid cells resembling large noncleaved cells. Some of these cells may also be seen in small arterioles and veins. They are noncohesive, in contrast to intravascular clusters of carcinoma cells, and unlike some metastatic carcinomas, IVL does not have prominent thrombosis and intimal proliferation in the involved vessels.

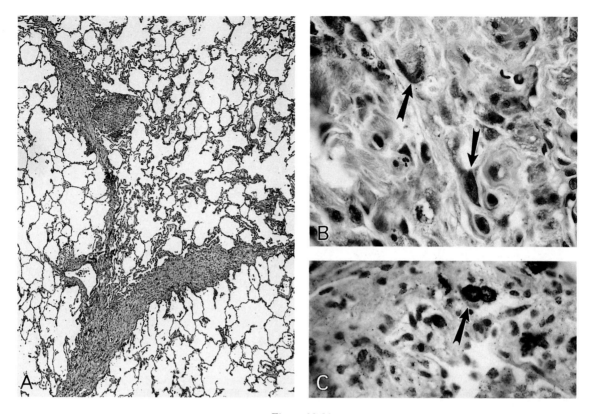

Figure 22-30
ANAPLASTIC LARGE CELL LYMPHOMA PRESENTING WITH RESPIRATORY INSUFFICIENCY
This case, previously reported by Colby et al. (17) as malignant histiocytosis, presented with diffuse pulmonary infiltrates radiographically and respiratory failure. The infiltrates were due to septal and perivascular fibroblastic thickening (A) with a scant infiltrate of bizarre atypical large cells (B, arrows) which were shown to be CD30 (Ber-H2) positive (C, arrow).

A histologic diagnosis is usually possible, although immunohistochemical confirmation is comforting. The cells are CD45 (LCA) positive in contrast to endothelial cells and type 2 cells. In addition, most cases can be further characterized as B-cell tumors, although a few T-cell cases have been described. Pulmonary artery cytology preparations may be useful in confirming the diagnosis in some cases.

IVL should be treated as an aggressive high-grade lymphoma. Some cases, including those presenting in the lung, respond to chemotherapy (103).

Other Non-Hodgkin Lymphomas of the Lung

Subtypes of lymphomas involving the lung other than small lymphocytic lymphomas, AIL/LYG, Hodgkin disease, and large cell lymphomas, are only occasionally seen (figs. 22-32, 22-33).

Primary Pulmonary Hodgkin Disease

Hodgkin disease commonly involves the lung by direct extension from the mediastinum, or as disseminated disease either at presentation or during relapse. In one large series, 13.5 percent of patients with Hodgkin disease had lung involvement at presentation (19). Primary pulmonary Hodgkin disease, without evidence of extrapulmonary involvement, is rare but well documented (106): 61 cases were included in a recent review (79). Women are more frequently affected (2 to 1), with an average age of 33 years for men and 51 years for women. Symptoms include cough, fever, weight loss, dyspnea, fatigue, anorexia, chest pain, and pleuritis. Chest radiographs most commonly show multiple nodules, but single nodules, localized infiltrates, and bilateral reticulonodular shadows are also described. Cavitation may be seen.

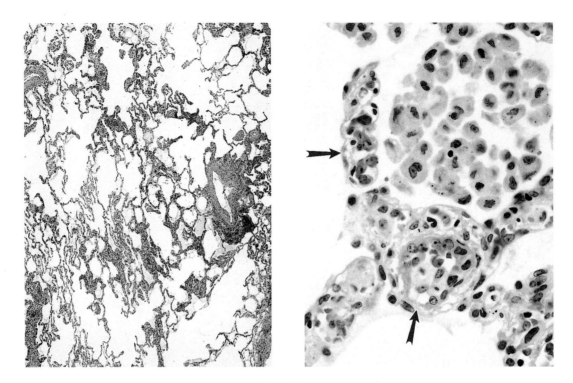

Figure 22-31
INTRAVASCULAR LYMPHOMATOSIS PRESENTING IN THE LUNG
Left: There is patchy interstitial thickening simulating an interstitial pneumonia.
Right: Cytologically, atypical large cells (arrows), proven by paraffin section immunostaining to be B cells, stuff the ectatic alveolar capillaries.

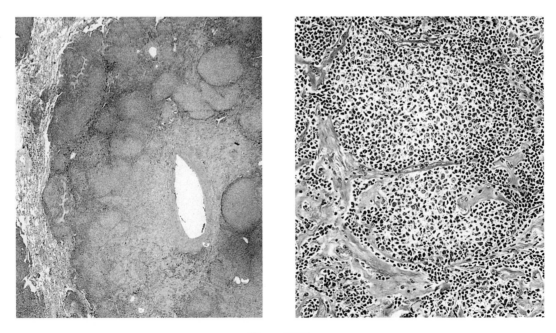

Figure 22-32
FOLLICULAR LYMPHOMA PRESENTING IN THE LUNG
Left: The neoplastic follicles surround a large pulmonary artery and are associated with sclerosis.
Right: The cytologic features are typical of follicular small cleaved cell lymphoma involving lymph nodes.

The histologic findings are similar to Hodgkin disease in the lymph nodes (figs. 22-34–22-36). Nodular sclerosis is the most common subtype, followed by mixed cellularity. Lymphocyte predominant Hodgkin disease may rarely involve the lung (61). Vascular infiltration and necrosis, similar to that seen in AIL/LYG, are common. A lymphatic distribution can be appreciated, with diffuse infiltrates or satellite nodules around larger masses. Some cases have a dramatic granulomatous reaction (fig. 22-36) which may simulate sarcoidosis (24) or a granulomatous infection. As with nodular sclerosing Hodgkin disease of lymph nodes, numerous neutrophils may be found in the centers of some of the nodules.

The immunohistochemical findings, especially positive staining of the large cells by CD15 (Leu-M1) and CD30 (Ber-H2), may be helpful in confirming the diagnosis and excluding other lesions in the differential diagnosis: inflammatory and infectious lesions, other lymphomas, and carcinomas, especially giant cell carcinoma with dyscohesion and tumor giant cells simulating Reed-Sternberg cells and lacunar cells.

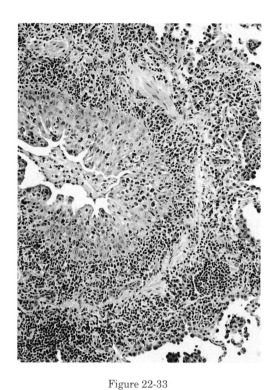

Figure 22-33
EPITHELIOTROPIC T-CELL LYMPHOMA

This peculiar T-cell lymphoma, which presented in the lung, showed a marked propensity to infiltrate airway epithelium (epitheliotropism).

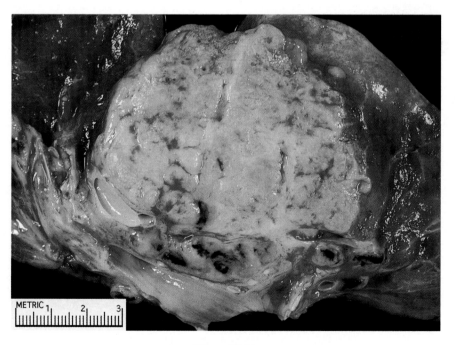

Figure 22-34
PRIMARY PULMONARY HODGKIN DISEASE

This solitary nodule, which was entirely resected, shows a multinodular character due to the nodular sclerosing histology.

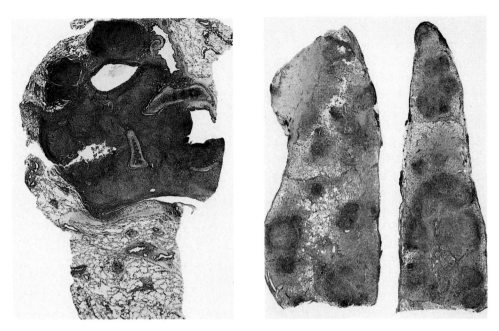

Figure 22-35
PRIMARY PULMONARY HODGKIN DISEASE

Two patterns of pulmonary Hodgkin disease are illustrated.
Left: A localized nodule involves a large bronchus. Vague nodularity typical of nodular sclerosing Hodgkin disease is apparent.
Right: These multiple cellular nodules were centrally necrotic and some contained large numbers of neutrophils, mimicking abscesses.

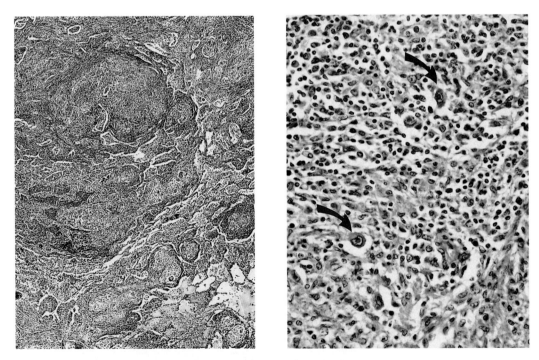

Figure 22-36
PRIMARY PULMONARY HODGKIN DISEASE

Left: This case was associated with a prominent granulomatous reaction. The nodule of Hodgkin disease (upper middle) is surrounded by numerous non-necrotizing granulomas in the lung parenchyma.
Right: Detail of Reed-Sternberg cells (arrows) in the nodule of Hodgkin disease.

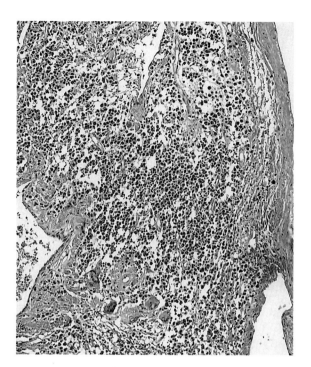 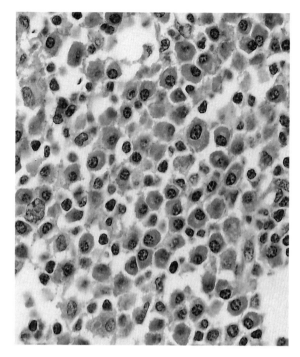

Figure 22-37
PLASMACYTOMA
This primary pulmonary plasmacytoma shows sheets of relatively mature plasma cells and focal giant cell reaction (left, bottom) associated with amyloid deposition.

Plasmacytoma

Plasmacytomas of the lung are extremely rare. They should be distinguished from other lesions with numerous plasma cells including lymphoplasmacytoid and lymphoplasmacytic lymphomas, plasma cell granuloma, the plasma cell variant of giant lymph node hyperplasia, and pulmonary involvement by multiple myeloma.

There is a wide age range (3 to 72 years) with a median of 42 years and an equal sex incidence (45). Pancoast syndrome caused by a plasmacytoma was described by Chen and Padmanabhan (10).

Grossly, plasmacytomas lack specific features. Histologically, there are sheets of plasma cells that vary from entirely normal with "mature" morphology to atypical and immature with prominent nucleoli and an increased nuclear-cytoplasmic ratio (fig. 22-37). A few cases have crystalline inclusions of immunoglobulin, either in the plasma cells or macrophages (48). Amyloid production may be encountered (fig. 22-37).

Primary pulmonary plasmacytomas are sufficiently rare that firm statements regarding their prognosis cannot be made. Some are associated with disseminated disease within a few years of presentation whereas others behave in an entirely benign fashion. Amin (2) reported three cases that disseminated within 3 years of presentation. Roikjaer and Thomsen (84) described a patient with two separate pulmonary plasmacytomas occurring 5 years apart in which there was no evidence of disseminated disease 4 years after the second lesion was resected. In 1993, Joseph et al. (45) compiled 19 cases of primary pulmonary plasmacytoma in the literature. Based on this small number of cases, surgery and radiation therapy seemed to be equally effective forms of treatment. Local recurrences were rare, but overall, the follow-up data available were inadequate. At least three patients developed multiple myeloma.

Mast Cell Tumor

Solitary mast cell tumors of the lung are very rare. The three reported cases were small peripheral nodules that were resected (57). Distinction from mast cell–rich inflammatory pseudotumors may be difficult.

449

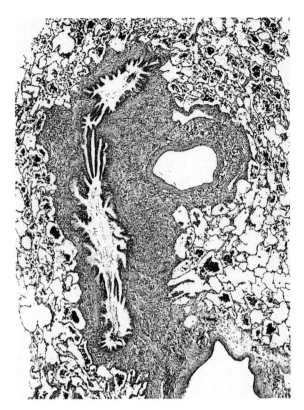

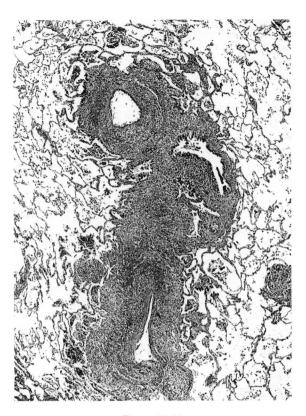

Figure 22-38
HODGKIN DISEASE INVOLVING
THE LUNG AT PRESENTATION
This patient presented with stage IV disease and diffuse pulmonary infiltrates. Lung biopsy shows an infiltrate along bronchovascular structures which cytologically showed features of Hodgkin disease.

Figure 22-39
PULMONARY RELAPSE OF HODGKIN DISEASE
This patient developed relapse of Hodgkin disease restricted to the lung. There are infiltrates along bronchovascular structures which showed cytologic features of Hodgkin disease.

SYSTEMIC LYMPHOPROLIFERATIVE DISORDERS SECONDARILY INVOLVING THE LUNG

Hodgkin Disease and Non-Hodgkin Lymphoma

The lung is frequently involved in disseminated lymphomas (figs. 22-38–22-44). The incidence at autopsy in patients with active disease is 58 percent in patients with Hodgkin disease (18) and 50 percent in those with non-Hodgkin lymphoma (83). The manifestations in such cases vary from clinically insignificant to respiratory failure mimicking a fulminant infection. Radiographically, any combination of nodules or infiltrates can be seen.

The histologic findings similarly vary from incidental focal infiltrates to massive diffuse or nodular infiltrates, usually with a lymphatic distribution. Large nodules may show necrosis or cavitation, and vascular infiltration may be marked. Peripheral T-cell lymphomas with secondary pulmonary involvement may be histologically and immunohistochemically identical to AIL/LYG. Secondary changes are similar to those seen for primary lymphomas including granulomas, obstructive pneumonia, organization, or fibrinous exudation into the airspaces.

Cutaneous T-Cell Lymphomas (Mycosis Fungoides and Sézary Syndrome)

These commonly affect the lung in patients with disseminated disease (21,29,67,71,94). Radiographically, nodules and localized or diffuse infiltrates may be seen. The clinical findings are similar to other secondary lymphomas; some patients have a fulminant course with the adult

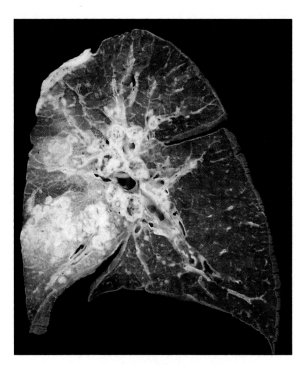

Figure 22-40
HODGKIN DISEASE AT AUTOPSY

This patient with disseminated Hodgkin disease died after showing no response to chemotherapy. Pulmonary involvement is extensive and is seen both as nodular infiltrates (lower left) as well as diffuse infiltrates extending along bronchovascular structures in the upper lobe and posterior lower lobe.

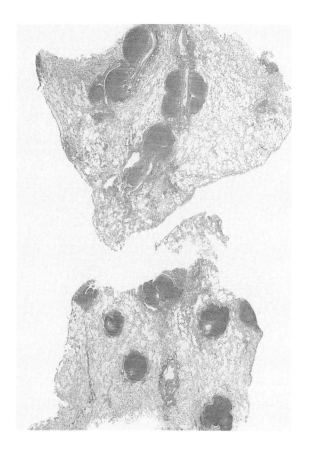

Figure 22-41
PULMONARY RELAPSE OF
LARGE CELL LYMPHOMA

Fulminant pulmonary relapse mimicked an opportunistic infection clinically. The biopsy shows multiple small nodules distributed along vascular structures.

respiratory distress syndrome (29,71). Histologically, there is a dense interstitial infiltrate of atypical cells that generally is most marked along vessels, bronchovascular structures, septa, and pleura (i.e., a lymphatic distribution) (fig. 22-44) (21). Vascular infiltration and necrosis may be seen in larger nodules. A granulomatous reaction is occasionally present. The cytologic spectrum is similar to that in skin and nodes involved by cutaneous T-cell lymphoma.

Malignant Histiocytosis

Malignant histiocytosis has been reported to involve the lung (17). It is now recognized that most, if not all, cases previously labeled malignant histiocytosis represent other lymphomas, particularly anaplastic large cell (Ki-1) lymphoma and T-cell lymphomas (58). Atypical large cells from three of five cases of malignant histiocytosis involving the lung previously reported (17) were found by one of the authors to

stain for CD30 (Ber-H2) (figs. 22-29, 22-30). All three cases showed typical cytologic features of anaplastic large cell lymphoma. Most cases of malignant histiocytosis involving the lung described prior to reclassification showed signs and symptoms of acute interstitial lung disease, including respiratory failure. Close et al. (12) described a case of anaplastic large cell lymphoma mimicking miliary tuberculosis. Histologically, an infiltrate of atypical large lymphoid cells is found along lymphatic routes. Nodules are also seen.

Multiple Myeloma

Pulmonary disease in patients with multiple myeloma is usually due to infection but secondary amyloidosis of the lung (usually the diffuse

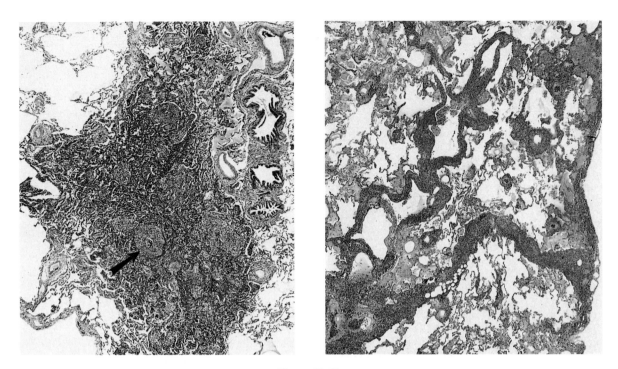

Figure 22-42
PATTERNS OF PULMONARY RELAPSE OF NON-HODGKIN LYMPHOMA
Left: This case of diffuse mixed small cleaved and large cell lymphoma relapsed as multiple nodules which showed vascular infiltration (arrow).
Right: This small lymphocytic lymphoma shows a dense infiltrate of lymphoid cells along septa, around vessels, and in the pleura.

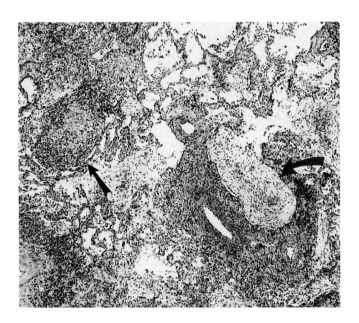

Figure 22-43
DISSEMINATED LYMPHOMA WITH ASSOCIATED INFLAMMATORY CHANGES
Lung biopsy shows a dense lymphoid infiltrate with invasion of vessels (straight arrow) and an associated nonspecific organizing pneumonia including foci of bronchiolitis obliterans with intraluminal granulation tissue polyps (curved arrow).

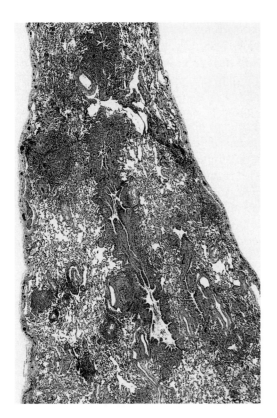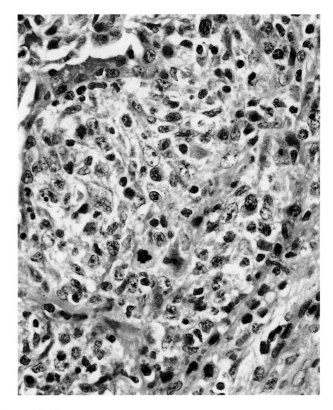

Figure 22-44
DISSEMINATED CUTANEOUS T-CELL LYMPHOMA
This disseminated cutaneous T-cell lymphoma (mycosis fungoides) shows perivascular and peribronchiolar infiltrates (left) composed of a cytologically malignant population of the small and large lymphoid cells (right).

alveolar septal pattern) and neoplastic plasma cell infiltration of the lung are also seen (8,32,33,87-89). The latter usually occurs in the setting of disseminated myeloma (including plasma cell leukemia) and manifests as nodules or infiltrates. Gilchrist et al. (33) described an unusual case of unilateral lung collapse secondary to bronchial mucosal infiltration. The pattern of tissue involvement is similar to other lymphoreticular processes. Crystalline material, similar to that seen in myeloma kidney, has been reported in the lung (8).

Systemic Light Chain Disease

Kijner and Yousem (51) reported a case of systemic light chain disease with bilateral nodular pulmonary infiltrates. Histologically, the nodules were composed of eosinophilic material similar to amyloid but distinguished from it by the

lack of characteristic apple green color with birefringence on Congo red–stained sections and a granular amorphous appearance ultrastructurally rather than the fibrillar pattern of amyloid.

Waldenström Macroglobulinemia

This clinicopathologic syndrome associated with elevated IgM is usually caused by lymphoplasmacytoid lymphomas, including some presenting in the lung or pleura (52,82). Chest radiographic manifestations include masses, infiltrates, and pleural effusions, or combinations of these. Isolated nodules are rare but do occur. The most common symptoms are dyspnea and cough, although approximately 15 percent of patients are asymptomatic (82). The condition is slowly progressive. Histologically, there are lymphoplasmacytoid infiltrates similar to those in other small lymphocytic lymphomas.

453

POST-TRANSPLANT LYMPHOPROLIFERATIVE DISORDERS AND RELATED CONDITIONS

Patients who have undergone organ transplantation and those with immunodeficiency states (including AIDS) are at increased risk for developing lymphoproliferative disorders, many of which are histologically identical to ordinary lymphomas (39,80,81,105). The commonly affected extranodal sites include the lung. Most of these disorders are associated with EBV infection (14). The clinical and radiographic findings vary, and pulmonary involvement may be seen as single or multiple nodules or infiltrates. The histologic spectrum varies from a polymorphous lymphoid population including small lymphocytes, plasma cells, and transformed lymphocytes to monomorphic lesions composed entirely of large cells and indistinguishable from an ordinary large cell lymphoma (fig. 22-45) (80,81,105). Necrosis and vascular invasion may be present. Immunohistochemical studies may show a monoclonal or polyclonal population of cells, and EBV has been demonstrated in the proliferating cells (80,81). The histologic similarities of post-transplant lymphoproliferative disorders to AIL/LYG is apparent, and they both share a common association with EBV. The exact relationship between these two groups of lesions remains to be clarified.

The prognosis for post-transplant lymphoproliferative disorders varies (80,81,105). Some cases, particularly those that are polyclonal and polymorphous in appearance, undergo spontaneous remission with decrease in immunosuppression. Other cases behave in an aggressive fashion and are fatal regardless of all therapeutic manipulations.

LEUKEMIC INFILTRATES INVOLVING THE LUNG

The majority of patients with leukemia and pulmonary disease have something other than leukemia, often an infection, causing the respiratory problems (14,41). Causes of clinically significant infiltrates in leukemics include hemorrhage, heart failure, chemotherapy and radiotherapy reactions, and alveolar proteinosis (14,41). Nevertheless, leukemic infiltration of the lung does occur and may be identified histologically in biopsy material, usually in one of two settings: as a clinically insignificant and incidental finding, and, more rarely, as the cause of clinically significant pulmonary disease.

In patients with active leukemia, lung infiltration is found at autopsy in nearly two thirds of cases, although clinically significant infiltrates are found during life in less than 7 percent (14). In most cases, it is an incidental finding, although severe cases with respiratory failure have been described (14,26,78). Any subtype of acute or chronic leukemia may involve the lung, although such involvement is uncommon. In biopsy material, chronic lymphocytic leukemia is probably the most commonly encountered subtype. In adult T-cell leukemia the incidence of pulmonary leukemic infiltrates may be relatively high, as evidenced by involvement in 13 of 29 patients reported by Yoshioka et al. (102). In approximately half of those patients, a diagnosis of "chronic lung disease" had been present for up to 6 years prior to the diagnosis of leukemia.

Leukemic involvement of the lung is usually seen in patients known to have leukemia. Rarely, the pulmonary disease is the initial manifestation of the leukemia. This occurs in lymphocytic leukemias as well as myeloid leukemias (also known as granulocytic sarcomas), and these cases may show radiographic infiltrates or nodules (14,40,78,85,102).

The radiographic changes include localized or diffuse infiltrates, "recurrent pneumonias," and nodules (7,14,26,40,78,85,102). As with other lymphoreticular infiltrates, leukemic infiltrates follow lymphatic routes and may infiltrate vascular structures (figs. 22-46–22-49). The infiltrates may be sparse and easily overlooked.

Transformation of chronic lymphocytic leukemia (Richter syndrome) may occasionally occur in the lung (91). Another unusual lesion seen in chronic lymphocytic leukemia is preferential bronchiolar involvement producing clinical evidence of airflow obstructive disease and simulating asthma (78).

Three peculiar reactions have been identified in patients with acute leukemia who develop acute pulmonary disease, in addition to those conditions already mentioned (14). These include pulmonary leukostasis, leukemic cell lysis pneumopathy, and hyperleukocytic reaction. In pulmonary leukostasis, the vessels are occluded by blast cell aggregates; this usually occurs in

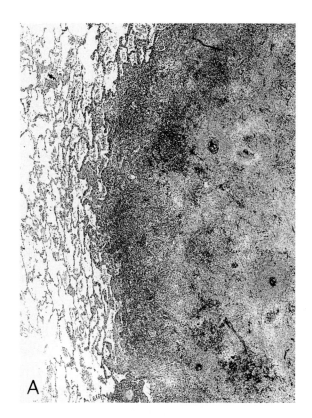

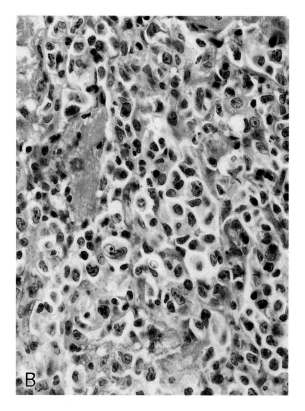

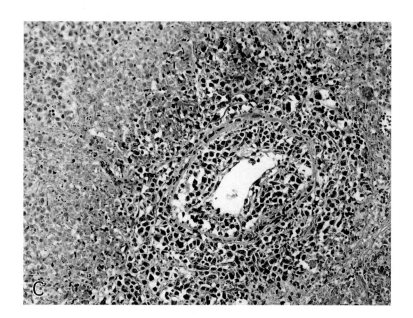

Figure 22-45
POST-TRANSPLANT LYMPHOPROLIFERATIVE DISORDER PRESENTING IN THE LUNG

A,B: A centrally necrotic nodule with rim of viable cells (A) composed of a heterogeneous cell population including atypical large cells (B).

C: A centrally necrotic nodule in which the remaining islands of viable atypical large cells show prominent vascular infiltration.

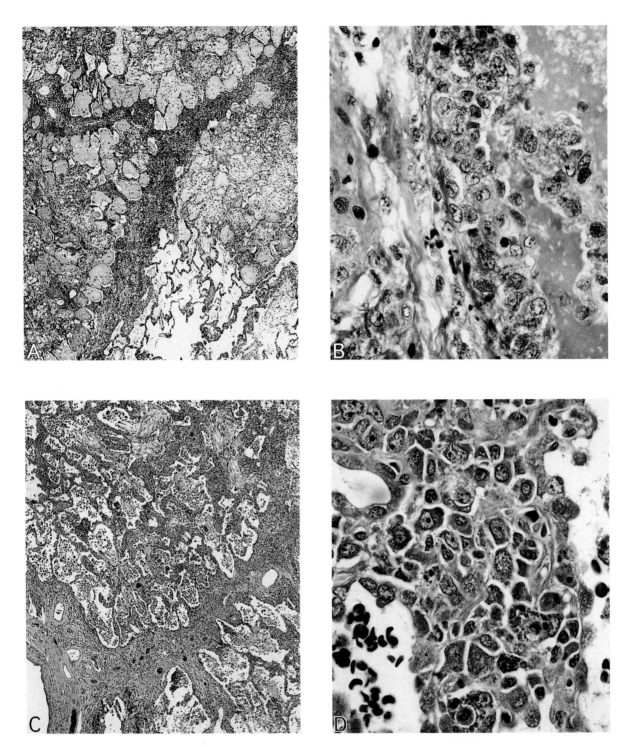

Figure 22-46
ACUTE MYELOID LEUKEMIA IN THE LUNG

A,B: A septa (A) is infiltrated by blast cells (B) in a patient with acute myeloid leukemia and high blast counts in the peripheral blood. The alveoli show diffuse alveolar damage.

C,D: This case presented in the lung. A septal infiltrate of leukemic cells (C, lower right) was associated with surrounding inflammatory changes and airspace organization. Cytologically, the cells (D) show features of promyelocytes with large vesicular nuclei, prominent nucleoli, and abundant eosinophilic cytoplasm which were positive with the chloroacetate esterase stain. A similar case showing peribronchiolar infiltration is illustrated in figure 22-47.

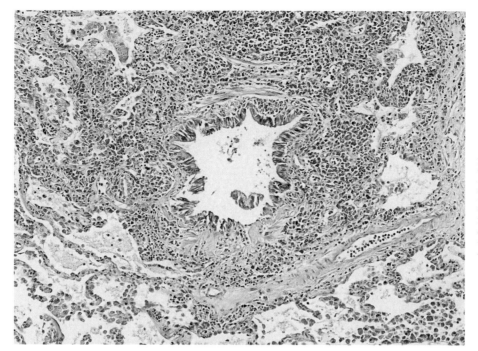

Figure 22-47
ACUTE MYELOID
LEUKEMIA
PRESENTING AS
LUNG INFILTRATES
This case was origi-
nally misinterpreted as
vasculitis because the neoplastic cell showed vascular infiltration. This field
shows a peribronchiolar
infiltrate of immature myeloid cells that stain red
with the chloroacetate esterase stain.

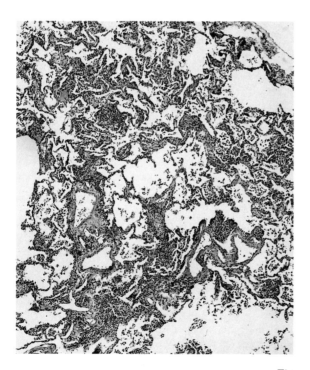

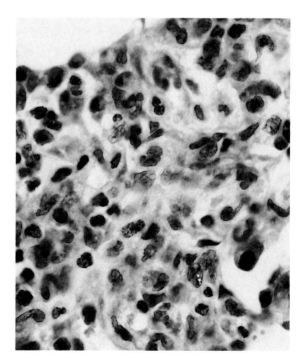

Figure 22-48
ACUTE MYELOMONOCYTIC LEUKEMIA INVOLVING THE LUNG AT PRESENTATION
Left: Interstitial infiltrates mimic an interstitial pneumonia.
Right: Cytologically, cells with atypical folded and complex nuclei characteristic of myelomonocytic leukemia are present.
The bone marrow biopsy in this case showed similar cells.

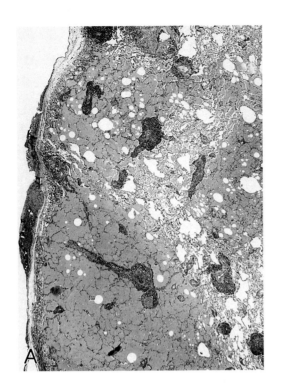

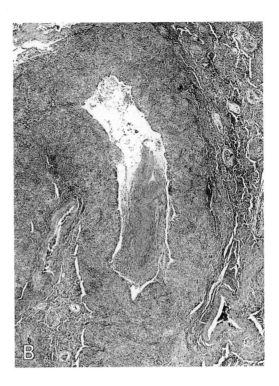

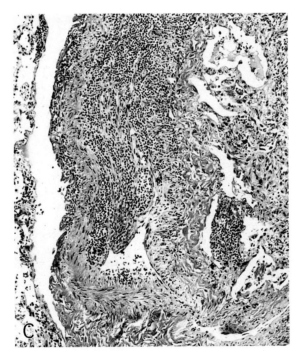

Figure 22-49

CHRONIC LYMPHOCYTIC LEUKEMIA AFFECTING THE LUNG

Three different patterns of leukemic involvement are illustrated.

A: Perivascular leukemic infiltrates found incidentally in a patient with *Aspergillus* involving numerous airways. Proteinaceous edema fluid is present in the airspaces.

B: Dense bronchiolar infiltrates of CLL caused airflow obstruction in this case.

C: Vascular involvement by CLL from the edge of a nodule resected from a patient known to have CLL. The nodular lesion was an infarct which resulted from vascular occlusion by leukemic cells, an extremely unusual finding with leukemic infiltrates.

patients with peripheral white cell counts greater than 200,000/μL. Leukemic cell lysis pneumopathy is seen within days of the onset of chemotherapy in patients with high peripheral blast counts (generally over 200,000/μL) and is associated with diffuse pulmonary infiltrates and severe hypoxemia. Histologic changes include pulmonary capillary congestion by blast cell aggregates, small infarcts, alveolar hemorrhage, interstitial edema, and diffuse alveolar damage. The hyperleukocytic reaction is seen when there is a rapid increase in peripheral blast cell counts, usually greater than 245,000/μL. Patients develop acute respiratory distress and have blast cells in the small vessels, with microhemorrhages and intra-alveolar edema.

Myelofibrosis

Myelofibrosis (*agnogenic myeloid metaplasia*) is associated with progressive bone marrow fibrosis and extramedullary hematopoiesis at a variety of sites, particularly the spleen and liver (3,34). The lung and pleura are occasionally involved. Extramedullary hematopoiesis may produce pleural nodules, pulmonary nodules, or infiltrates. In some cases, pulmonary involvement is associated with progressive and, ultimately fatal interstitial pulmonary fibrosis (3). The aggregates of extramedullary hematopoietic cells follow lymphatic routes, and are often accompanied by variable amounts of fibrous tissue (fig. 22-50). The infiltrates may be diffuse or nodular, and chloroacetate esterase stains may be helpful in recognizing the immature myeloid cells. In some cases the fibrosis overshadows the hematopoietic cells and produces signs and symptoms of fibrosing interstitial lung or pleural disease.

PLEURAL INVOLVEMENT IN LYMPHORETICULAR DISORDERS

Pulmonary lymphoreticular infiltrates commonly involve the pleura as part of their lymphatic distribution. In some cases, pleural involvement and effusions are the dominant clinical manifestation and overshadow the lung disease. Practically any of the lymphoreticular diseases discussed in this section may manifest primarily as pleural rather than pulmonary parenchymal disease. In such cases, closed pleural

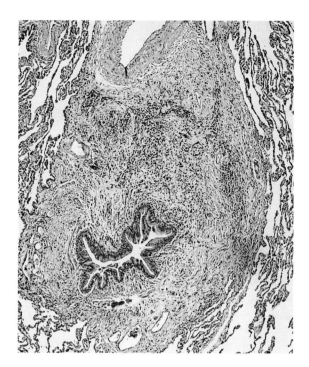

Figure 22-50
PULMONARY INVOLVEMENT IN MYELOFIBROSIS

This patient had a long history of myelofibrosis and slowly progressive interstitial lung disease. The interstitial lung disease was caused by patchy scarring secondary to infiltrates of hematopoietic cells and associated fibrosis, which in this field, are causing peribronchiolar fibrosis. Most of the dark staining cells (upper center) are myeloid precursors that are staining positively with the chloroacetate esterase stain.

biopsy and pleural effusion cytology may allow for a diagnosis, particularly in patients already known to have a lymphoreticular malignancy.

PULMONARY HISTIOCYTOSIS X

Pulmonary histiocytosis X (HX), also known as *Langerhans cell granulomatosis* or *pulmonary eosinophilic granuloma*, is a condition associated with a proliferation of Langerhans or HX cells (62,96). Most patients with pulmonary HX have disease limited to the lung; only a small proportion have extrapulmonary involvement or a systemic disorder.

Pulmonary HX is typically seen in smokers in the third and fourth decades of life, although there is a broad age range (16,23,30,37,93,96). Women are affected three times more often than men. Over 90 percent of the patients are smokers, and cigarette smoking is probably involved in the pathogenesis. Symptoms include dyspnea, cough, chest pain, sputum production, fever, weight loss, and malaise. Close to 20 percent of patients are asymptomatic and found to have an abnormal chest radiograph; a lesser proportion present with a pneumothorax. Chest radiographs show bilateral reticular or reticulonodular infiltrates, sometimes with cystic changes or honeycombing, and often with sparing of the costophrenic angles. High resolution computerized tomography (CT) scans may be virtually diagnostic based on the predilection of the cysts and nodules for the upper lung zones (73,96).

HX cells may be recovered in bronchoalveolar lavage fluid of patients with active disease, and greater than 5 percent in such preparations is considered diagnostic of pulmonary HX in the appropriate clinical setting (37). However, cigarette smokers without pulmonary HX have increased HX cells as well (8).

Grossly, the lung tissue may show cysts, honeycombing, and nodules that may be as large as 2 cm in diameter (the majority are less than 5 mm in diameter) (20,96). The histologic findings (fig. 22-51) depend on the stage of the lesions, which are multiple and scattered throughout the lung tissue, sometimes with a large amount of intervening normal lung tissue (6,20,23,28,30,96). Early lesions are characterized by cellular infiltrates along alveolar ducts or bronchioles. These infiltrates expand to form cellular nodules which may be solid or centrally cavitated. The cellular nodules then become fibrotic centrally and ultimately entirely fibrotic. This late or healed stage of HX typically produces stellate scars in the centrilobular regions.

The cellular infiltrates of pulmonary HX are characterized by HX cells, eosinophils, pigmented alveolar macrophages, lymphocytes, and occasionally, a few neutrophils. HX cells have pale cytoplasm with indistinct cytoplasmic margins (in contrast to the denser, eosinophilic, tan-brown cytoplasm of alveolar macrophages), delicate nuclei with prominent nuclear folds, and small nucleoli. In highly cellular lesions, mitotic figures may be numerous suggesting a malignant tumor, particularly a lymphoma. HX cells

stain for S-100 protein in paraffin sections (96, 97) and CD1 (OKT6, Leu-6) in frozen sections or fresh preparations (6,28). Ultrastructurally, there are distinctive granules called Birbeck granules (4,23,37,96).

Most cases of pulmonary HX are diagnosed by open lung biopsy, however, approximately 20 percent of transbronchial biopsies show the nodular lesions or portions thereof. The combination of the characteristic CT findings and HX cells in bronchoalveolar lavage fluid should decrease the number of cases requiring open biopsy.

The differential diagnosis of pulmonary HX depends on the histologic stage. Active cellular lesions with little fibrosis may mimic a lymphoma. When eosinophils are numerous, eosinophilic pneumonia is a consideration, although eosinophilic pneumonia typically is associated with airspace consolidation, whereas the infiltrates of pulmonary HX are primarily nodular and interstitial with less impressive airspace filling. The pleural reaction to pneumothorax, eosinophilic pleuritis, may result in a proliferation of mesothelial cells and eosinophils that mimics pulmonary HX. The fibrotic lesions of pulmonary HX resemble fibrosing interstitial pneumonia. The discrete stellate shape and centrilobular distribution help separate pulmonary HX from usual interstitial pneumonia. Some cases of pulmonary HX have large numbers of pulmonary alveolar macrophages in adjacent airspaces and mimic desquamative interstitial pneumonia. When lung biopsy findings are equivocal, immunohistochemical stains for S-100 protein, electron microscopy, and correlation with the CT and bronchoalveolar lavage findings may be helpful in establishing a diagnosis (95). Also, alveolar macrophages are PAS positive and HX cells are not.

Management of pulmonary HX includes cessation of smoking, and steroid therapy for symptomatic patients. In most patients, including those who continue to smoke, the lesions burn out and leave inactive fibrous scars. The prognosis is favorable and less than 20 percent of patients develop progressive fibrotic lung disease and respiratory failure (20,30,37,93,96).

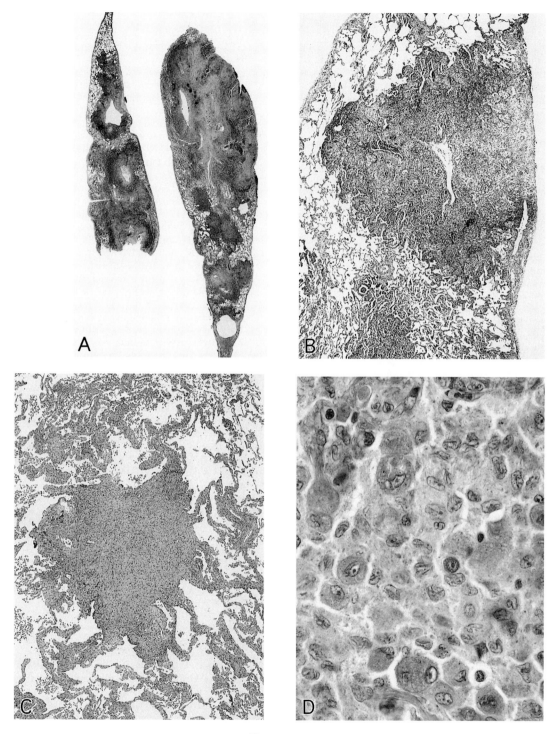

Figure 22-51
PULMONARY HISTIOCYTOSIS X

A,B: The nodules of HX may or may not have central cavitation.

C: As the lesions age, they become more fibrotic and commonly assume a stellate character with surrounding emphysematous change. HX cells are found in cellular nodules and sometimes at the periphery of fibrotic nodules.

D: HX cells have delicate complex folded nuclei and pale inconspicuous cytoplasm that lacks prominent cell borders. The cytoplasm contrasts with the dense eosinophilic cytoplasm of pulmonary alveolar macrophages, which is well demarcated and often contains fine tan-brown pigment, characteristic of cigarette smokers.

REFERENCES

1. Addis BJ, Hyjek E, Isaacson PG. Primary pulmonary lymphoma: a re-appraisal of its histogenesis and its relationship to pseudolymphoma and lymphoid interstitial pneumonia. Histopathology 1988;13:1–17.

2. Amin R. Extramedullary plasmacytoma of the lung. Cancer 1985;56:152–6.

3. Asakura S, Colby TV. Two cases of agnogenic myeloid metaplasia with extramedullary hematopoiesis and fibrosis in the lung. Chest 1994;105:1866–8.

4. Basset F, Soler P, Jaurand MC, Bignon J. Ultrastructural examination of broncho-alveolar lavage for diagnosis of pulmonary histiocytosis X: preliminary report on 4 cases. Thorax 1977;32:303–6.

5. Bienenstock J, Befus D. Gut- and bronchus-associated lymphoid tissue. Am J Anat 1984;170:437–45.

6. Cagle PT, Mattioli CA, Truong LD, Greenberg SD. Immunohistochemical diagnosis of pulmonary eosinophilic granuloma on lung biopsy. Chest 1988;94:1133–7.

7. Callahan M, Wall S, Askin F, Delaney D, Koller C, Orringer EP. Granulocytic sarcoma presenting as pulmonary nodules and lymphadenopathy. Cancer 1987;60:1902–4.

8. Casolaro MA, Bernaudin JF, Saltini C, Ferrans VJ, Crystal RG. Accumulation of Langerhans' cells on the epithelial surface of the lower respiratory tract in normal subjects in association with cigarette smoking. Am Rev Respir Dis 1988;137:406–11.

9. Chejfec G, Natarelli J, Gould VE. Myeloma lung—a previously unreported complication of multiple myeloma. Hum Pathol 1983;14:558–61.

10. Chen KT, Padmanabhan A. Pancoast syndrome caused by extramedullary plasmacytoma. J Surg Oncol 1983;24:117–8.

11. Chetty R, Close PM, Timme AH, Willcox PA, Forder MD. Primary biphasic lymphoplasmacytic lymphoma of the lung. A mucosa-associated lymphoid tissue lymphoma with compartmentalization of plasma cells in the lung and lymph nodes. Cancer 1992;69:1124–9.

12. Close PM, Macrae MB, Hammond JM, et al. Anaplastic large-cell Ki-1 lymphoma. Pulmonary presentation mimicking miliary tuberculosis. Am J Clin Pathol 1993;99:631–6.

13. Colby TV. Critical commentary to "pulmonary involvement by mycosis fungoides." Pathol Res Pract 1993;189:598–600.

14. _____. Lymphoproliferative diseases. In: Dail, DH, Hammar SA, eds. Pulmonary pathology. 2nd ed. New York: Springer-Verlag, 1994:1097–122.

15. _____, Carrington CB. Pulmonary lymphomas: current concepts. Hum Pathol 1983;14:884–7.

16. _____, Carrington CB. Pulmonary lymphomas simulating lymphomatoid granulomatosis. Am J Surg Pathol 1982;6:19–32.

17. _____, Carrington CB, Mark GJ. Pulmonary involvement in malignant histiocytosis. A clinicopathologic spectrum. Am J Surg Pathol 1981;5:61–73.

18. _____, Hoppe RT, Warnke RA. Hodgkin's disease at autopsy: 1972-1977. Cancer 1981;47:1852–62.

19. _____, Hoppe RT, Warnke RA. Hodgkin's disease: a clinicopathologic study of 659 cases. Cancer 1981;49:1848–58.

20. _____, Lombard C. Histiocytosis X in the lung. Hum Pathol 1983;14:847–56.

21. _____, Yousem SA. Pulmonary lymphoid neoplasms. Semin Diagn Pathol 1985;2:183–96.

22. Cordier JF, Chailleux E, Lauque D, et al. Primary pulmonary lymphomas. A clinical study of 70 cases in nonimmunocompromised patients. Chest 1993;103:201–8.

23. Corrin B, Basset F. A review of histiocytosis X with particular reference to eosinophilic granuloma of the lung. Invest Cell Pathol 1979;2:137–46.

24. Daly PA, O'Briain DS, Robinson I, Guckian M, Prichard JS. Hodgkin's disease with a granulomatous pulmonary presentation mimicking sarcoidosis. Thorax 1988;43:407–9.

25. DeRemee RA, Weiland LH, McDonald TJ. Polymorphic reticulosis, lymphomatoid granulomatosis. Two diseases or one? Mayo Clin Proc 1978;53:634–40.

26. Dugdale DC, Salness TA, Knight L, Charan NB. Endobronchial granulocytic sarcoma causing acute respiratory failure in acute myelogenous leukemia. Am Rev Respir Dis 1987;136:1248–50.

27. Ferry JA, Harris NL, Picker LJ, et al. Intravascular lymphomatosis (malignant angioendotheliomatosis). A B cell neoplasm expressing surface homing receptors. Mod Pathol 1988;1:444–52.

28. Flint A, Lloyd RV, Colby TV, Wilson BW. Pulmonary histiocytosis X. Immunoperoxidase staining for HLA-DR antigen and S100 protein. Arch Pathol Lab Med 1986;110:930–3.

29. Foster GH, Eichenhorn MS, Van Slyck EJ. The Sézary syndrome with rapid pulmonary dissemination. Cancer 1985;56:1197–8.

30. Friedman PJ, Liebow AA, Sokoloff J. Eosinophilic granuloma of the lung. Clinical aspects of primary histiocytosis in the adult. Medicine (Baltimore) 1981;60:385–96.

31. Frizzera G, Moran EM, Rappaport H. Angio-immunoblastic lymphadenopathy. Diagnosis and clinical course. Am J Med 1975;59:803–18.

32. Garewal H, Durie BG. Aggressive phase of multiple myeloma with pulmonary plasma cell infiltrates. JAMA 1982;248:1875–6.

33. Gilchrist D, Chan CK, LaRoye GJ, Messner HA, Curtis JE. Bronchial mucosal infiltration and unilateral lung collapse: an unusual complication of multiple myeloma. Am J Med 1988;85:74–1.

34. Glew RH, Haese WH, McIntyre PA. Myeloid metaplasia with myelofibrosis. Clinical spectrum of extramedullary hematopoiesis and tumor formation. Johns Hopkins Med J 1973;132:253–70.

35. Gould SJ, Isaacson PG. Bronchus-associated lymphoid tissue (BALT) in human fetal and infant lung. J Pathol 1993;169:229–34.

36. Guinee DG, Jaffe E, Kingma D, et al. Pulmonary lymphomatoid granulomatosis: evidence for a proliferation of Epstein-Barr virus infected B lymphocytes with a prominent T cell component and vasculitis. Am J Surg Pathol 1994;18:753–64.

37. Hance AJ, Cadranel J, Soler P, Basset F. Pulmonary and extrapulmonary Langerhans' cell granulomatosis (histiocytosis X). Semin Respir Med 1988;9:349–68.

38. Harris NL. Extranodal lymphoid infiltrates and mucosa-associated lymphoid tissue (MALT). A unifying concept. Am J Surg Pathol 1991;15:879–84.

39. Heitzman ER. Pulmonary neoplastic and lymphoproliferative disease in AIDS: a review. Radiology 1990;177:347–51.

40. Hicklin GA, Drevyanko TF. Primary granulocytic sarcoma presenting with pleural and pulmonary involvement. Chest 1988;94:655–6.

41. Hildebrand FL Jr, Rosenow EC III, Habermann TM, Tazelaar HD. Pulmonary complications of leukemia. Chest 1990;98:1233–9.

42. Isaacson PG, Spencer J. Malignant lymphoma of mucosa-associated lymphoid tissue. Histopathology 1987;11:445–62.

43. _____, Wotherspoon AC, Pan L. Follicular colonization in B-cell lymphoma of mucosa-associated lymphoid tissue. Am J Surg Pathol 1991;15:819–28.

44. Jaffe ES, Lipford EH Jr, Margolick JB, et al. Lymphomatoid granulomatosis and angiocentric lymphoma: a spectrum of post-thymic T-cell proliferations. Semin Respir Med 1993;10:167–72.

45. Joseph G, Pandit M, Korfhage L. Primary pulmonary plasmacytoma. Cancer 1993;71:721–4.

46. Katzenstein AL, Carrington CB, Liebow AA. Lymphomatoid granulomatosis. A clinicopathologic study of 152 cases. Cancer 1979;43:360–73.

47. _____, Peiper SC. Detection of Ebstein-Barr virus genomes in lymphomatoid granulomatosis: analysis of 29 cases by the polymerase chain reaction technique. Mod Pathol 1990;3:435–41.

48. Kazzaz B, Dewar A, Corrin B. An unusual pulmonary plasmacytoma. Histopathology 1992;21:285–7.

49. Keller AR, Hochholzer L, Castleman B. Hyaline-vascular and plasma-cell types of giant lymph node hyperplasia of the mediastinum and other locations. Cancer 1972;29:670–83.

50. Kennedy JL, Nathwani BN, Burke JS, Hill LR, Rappaport H. Pulmonary lymphomas and other pulmonary lymphoid lesions. A clinicopathologic and immunologic study of 64 patients. Cancer 1985;56:539–52.

51. Kijner CH, Yousem SA. Systemic light chain deposition disease presenting as multiple pulmonary nodules. A case report and review of the literature. Am J Surg Pathol 1988;12:405–13.

52. Kobayashi H, Ii K, Hizawa K, Maeda T. Two cases of pulmonary Waldenström's macroglobulinemia. Chest 1985;88:297–9.

53. Koss M. Pulmonary lymphoproliferative disorders. In: Churg A, Katzenstein AL, eds. The lung. Philadelphia: Williams & Wilkins, 1993. In press.

54. _____, Hochholzer L, Langloss JM, Wehunt WD, Lazarus AA. Lymphoid interstitial pneumonia: clinicopathological and immunopathological findings in 18 cases. Pathology 1987;19:178–85.

55. _____, Hochholzer L, Langloss JM, Wehunt WD, Lazarus AA, Nichols PW. Lymphomatoid granulomatosis: a clinicopathologic study of 42 patients. Pathology 1986;18:283–8.

56. _____, Hochholzer L, Nichols PW, Wehunt WD, Lazarus AA. Primary non-Hodgkin's lymphoma and pseudolymphoma of lung: a study of 161 patients. Hum Pathol 1983;14:1024–38.

57. Kudo H, Morinaga S, Shimosato Y, et al. Solitary mast cell tumor of the lung. Cancer 1988;61:2089–94.

58. Lennert K, Feller AC. Histopathology of non-Hodgkin's lymphomas (based on the updated Kiel classification). 2nd ed. Springer-Verlag, 1990;24–25,243,260.

59. L'Hoste RJ Jr, Filippa DA, Lieberman PH, Bretsky S. Primary pulmonary lymphomas. A clinicopathologic analysis of 36 cases. Cancer 1984;54:1397–406.

60. Li G, Hansmann ML. Lymphocyte predominant Hodgkin's disease of nodular subtype combined with pulmonary lymphoid infiltration and hypogammaglobulinaemia. Virchows Arch [A] 1989;415:481–7.

61. _____, Hansmann ML, Zwingers T, Lennert K. Primary lymphomas of the lung: morphological, immunohistochemical, and clinical features. Histopathology 1990;16:519–31.

62. Lichtenstein L. Histiocytosis X: integration of eosinophilic granuloma of bone, "Letterer-Siwe disease," and "Schüller-Christian disease" as related manifestations of a single nosologic entity. Arch Pathol 1953;56:84–102.

63. Liebow AA. New concepts and entities in pulmonary disease. In: Liebow AA, Smith DE, eds. The lung, by 25 authors. Baltimore: Williams & Wilkins, 1968:332–65.

64. _____, Carrington CB. Diffuse pulmonary lymphoreticular infiltrations associated with dysproteinemia. Med Clin North Am 1973;57:809–43.

65. Liebow AA, Carrington CR, Friedman PJ. Lymphomatoid granulomatosis. Hum Pathol 1972;3:457–558.

66. Lipford EH Jr, Margolick JB, Longo DL, Fauci AS, Jaffe ES. Angiocentric immunoproliferative lesions: a clinicopathologic spectrum of post-thymic T-cell proliferations. Blood 1988;72:1674–81.

67. Marglin SI, Soulen RL, Blank N, Castellino RA. Mycosis fungoides. Radiographic manifestations of extracutaneous intrathoracic involvement. Radiology 1979;130:35–7.

68. Medeiros LJ, Jaffe ES, Chen YY, Weiss LM. Localization of Epstein-Barr viral genomes in angiocentric immunoproliferative lesions. Am J Surg Pathol 1992;16:439–47.

69. _____, Peiper SC, Elwood L, Yano T, Raffeld M, Jaffe ES. Angiocentric immunoproliferative lesions: a molecular analysis of eight cases. Hum Pathol 1991;22:1150–7.

70. Miller DL, Allen MS. Rare pulmonary neoplasms. Mayo Clin Proc 1993;68:492–8.

71. Miller KS, Sahn SA. Mycosis fungoides presenting as ARDS and diagnosed by bronchoalveolar lavage. Radiographic and pathologic pulmonary manifestations. Chest 1986;89:312–4.

72. Morinaga S, Watanabe H, Gemma A, et al. Plasmacytoma of the lung associated with nodular deposits of immunoglobulin. Am J Surg Pathol 1987;11:989–95.

73. Müller NL, Miller RR. Computed tomography of chronic diffuse infiltrative lung disease (Parts I and II). Am Rev Respir Dis 1990;142:1206–15,1440–8.

74. Neil GA, Lukie BE, Cockcroft DW, Murphy F. Lymphocytic interstitial pneumonia and abdominal lymphoma complicating celiac sprue. J Clin Gastroenterol 1986;8:282–5.

75. The Non-Hodgkin's Lymphoma Pathologic Classification Project National Cancer Institute sponsored study of classifications of non-Hodgkin's lymphomas. Summary and description of a Working Formulation for clinical usage. Cancer 1982;49:2112–35.

76. Okura T, Tanaka R, Shibata H, Kukita H. Adult T-cell leukemia with a solitary lung mass. Chest 1992;101:1471–2.

463

77. Pabst R, Gehrke I. Is the bronchus-associated lymphoid tissue (BALT) an integral structure of the lung in normal mammals, including humans? Am J Respir Cell Mol Biol 1990;3:131–5.

78. Palosaari DE, Colby TV. Bronchiolocentric chronic lymphocytic leukemia. Cancer 1986;58:1695–8.

79. Radin AI. Primary pulmonary Hodgkin's disease. Cancer 1990;65:550–63.

80. Randhawa PS, Yousem SA. Epstein-Barr virus associated lymphoproliferative disease in a heart-lung allograft. Demonstration of host origin by restriction fragment length polymorphism analysis. Transplantation 1990;49:126–30.

81. _____, Yousem SA, Paradis IL, Dauber JA, Griffith BP, Locker J. The clinical spectrum, pathology, and clonal analysis of EBV associated lymphoproliferative disorders in heart-lung transplant recipients. Am J Clin Pathol 1989;92:177–85.

82. Rausch PG, Herion JC. Pulmonary manifestations of Waldenström macroglobulinemia. Am J Hematol 1980;9:201–9.

83. Risdall R, Hoppe RT, Warnke R. Non-Hodgkin's lymphoma: a study of the evolution of the disease based upon 92 autopsied cases. Cancer 1979;44:529–42.

84. Roikjaer O, Thomsen JK. Plasmacytoma of the lung. A case report describing two tumors of different immunologic type in a single patient. Cancer 1986;58:2671–4.

85. Rollins SD, Colby TV. Lung biopsy in chronic lymphocytic leukemia. Arch Pathol Lab Med 1988;112:607–11.

86. Saldana MJ, Patchefsky AS, Israel HI, Atkinson GW. Pulmonary angiitis and granulomatosis. The relationship between histological features, organ involvement, and response to treatment. Hum Pathol 1977;8:391–409.

87. Salhany KE, Pietra GG. Extranodal lymphoid disorders. Am J Clin Pathol 1993;99:472–85.

88. Scully RE, Mark EJ, McNeely BU. Case records of the Massachusetts General Hospital. Weekly clinicopathological exercises. Case 17-1984. New Engl J Med 1984;310:1103–12.

89. _____, Mark EJ, McNeely WF, McNeely BU. Case records of the Massachusetts General Hospital. Weekly clinicopathologic exercises. Case 20-1987. New Engl J Med 1987;316:1259–67.

90. Sekulich M, Pandola G, Simon T. A solitary pulmonary mass in multiple myeloma. Dis Chest 1969;48:100–3.

91. Snyder LS, Cherwitz DL, Dykoski RK, Rice KL. Endobronchial Richter's syndrome. A rare manifestation of chronic lymphocytic leukemia. Am Rev Respir Dis 1988;138:980–3.

92. _____, Harmon KR, Estensen RD. Intravascular lymphomatosis (malignant angioendotheliomatosis) presenting as pulmonary hypertension. Chest 1989;96:1199–200.

93. Soler P, Kambouchner M, Valeyre D, Hance AJ. Pulmonary Langerhans' cell granulomatosis (histiocytosis X). Annu Rev Med 1992;43:105–15.

94. Stokar LM, Vonderheid EC, Abell E, Diamond LW, Rosen SE, Goldwein MI. Clinical manifestations of intrathoracic cutaneous T-cell lymphoma. Cancer 1985;56:2694–702.

95. Swensen SJ, Aughenbaugh GL, Douglas WW, Myers JL. High-resolution CT of the lungs: findings in various pulmonary diseases. AJR Am J Roentgenol 1992;158:971–9.

96. Travis WD, Borok Z, Roum JH. Pulmonary Langerhans' cell granulomatosis (histiocytosis X). A clinicopathologic study of 48 cases. Am J Surg Pathol 1993;17:971–86.

97. Turner RR, Colby TV, Doggett RS. Well-differentiated lymphocytic lymphoma. A study of 47 patients with primary manifestation in the lung. Cancer 1984;54:2088–96.

98. Webber D, Tron V, Askin F, Churg A. S-100 staining in the diagnosis of eosinophilic granuloma of lung. Am J Clin Pathol 1985;84:447–53.

99. Weis JW, Winter MW, Phyliky RL, Banks PM. Peripheral T-cell lymphomas: histologic, immunohistologic, and clinical characterization. Mayo Clin Proc 1986;61:411–26.

101. Weiss LM, Yousem SA, Warnke RA. Non-Hodgkin's lymphomas of the lung. A study of 19 cases emphasizing the utility of frozen section immunologic studies in differential diagnosis. Am J Surg Pathol 1985;9:480–90.

100. Weisenburger D, Armitage D, Dick F. Immunoblastic lymphadenopathy with pulmonary infiltrates, hypocomplementemia, and vasculitis. Am J Med 1977;63:849–54.

102. Yoshioka R, Yamaguchi K, Yoshinaga T, Takatsuki K. Pulmonary complications in patients with adult T-cell leukemia. Cancer 1985;55:2491–4.

103. Yousem SA, Colby TV. Intravascular lymphomatosis presenting in the lung. Cancer 1990;65:349–53.

104. _____, Colby TV, Carrington CB. Follicular bronchitis/bronchiolitis. Hum Pathol 1985;16:700–6.

105. _____, Randhawa P, Locker J, et al. Post-transplant lymphoproliferative disorders in heart-lung transplant recipients. Hum Pathol 1987;20:361–9.

106. _____, Weiss LM, Colby TV. Primary pulmonary Hodgkin's disease. A clinicopathologic study of 15 cases. Cancer 1986;57:1217–24.

❖ ❖ ❖

23

MISCELLANEOUS TUMORS AND
TUMORS OF UNCERTAIN HISTOGENESIS

SCLEROSING HEMANGIOMA OF LUNG

Definition. Sclerosing hemangioma of the lung is an unusual benign tumor originally described by Liebow and Hubbell in 1956 (62). Its peculiar histologic features often present a diagnostic challenge and have led to extensive speculation about the histogenesis. Liebow coined the term "sclerosing hemangioma" because he thought that the prominent vascular lakes or hemorrhagic areas were actually vascular spaces. Various terms have been used for these tumors including *postinflammatory pseudotumor, histiocytoma, fibroxanthoma,* and *papillary pneumocytoma.*

Clinical Features. More than 80 percent of patients with sclerosing hemangioma are female (53,62,95). The average age is 44 years (range, 15 to 83 years). Most patients are asymptomatic and the tumor is detected on a routine chest X ray. Symptoms include cough, chest pain, a history of "colds," and hemoptysis. Radiographically, sclerosing hemangioma appears as a solitary, circumscribed mass that is occasionally calcified.

Gross Findings. The typical gross appearance of sclerosing hemangioma is a circumscribed, round or oval mass averaging 2.8 cm in size (range, 0.4 to 8.0 cm) (fig. 23-1) (53,62). The cut surface reveals a gray-red mass which may have mottled yellow areas. These tumors are usually located within the lung parenchyma, however, they may occasionally extend into interlobar fissures or adhere to adjacent structures such as the pericardium. Almost half of the cases occur in the lower lobes. Rarely, sclerosing hemangiomas may be multiple (51,79).

Microscopic Findings. Four major histologic patterns occur: solid (fig. 23-2), papillary (fig. 23-3), sclerotic (fig. 23-3, left), and hemorrhagic (fig. 23-4). In over 90 percent of cases, at least three of these patterns are present and more than one pattern is present in all cases. The epithelioid round cells are uniform and bland-appearing, with round to oval nuclei, distinct cytoplasmic borders, and fine chromatin with inconspicuous nucleoli (fig. 23-2). Tumor cells with clear cytoplasm may be found in a small

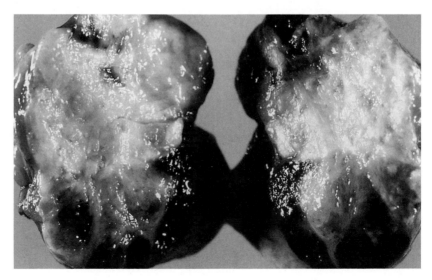

Figure 23-1
SCLEROSING HEMANGIOMA: GROSS FEATURES
This 4 by 3 cm mass is circumscribed, but not encapsulated, with a predominantly tan and yellow but focally red hemorrhagic cut surface.

465

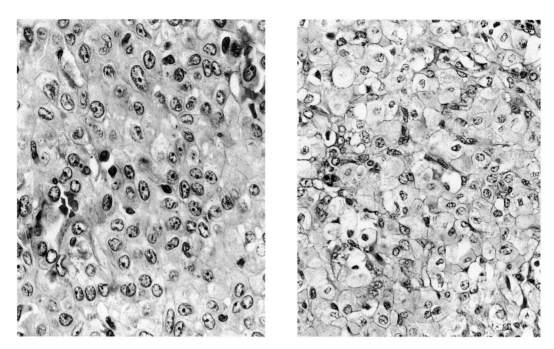

Figure 23-2
SCLEROSING HEMANGIOMA: MICROSCOPIC FEATURES
Left: The round to oval epithelioid cells have eosinophilic cytoplasm and sharp cytoplasmic borders. The nuclei are uniform and bland with vesicular chromatin and frequent nucleoli.
Right: Many of these epithelioid cells have clear cytoplasm. The nuclei are uniform, and nucleoli are inconspicuous or absent.

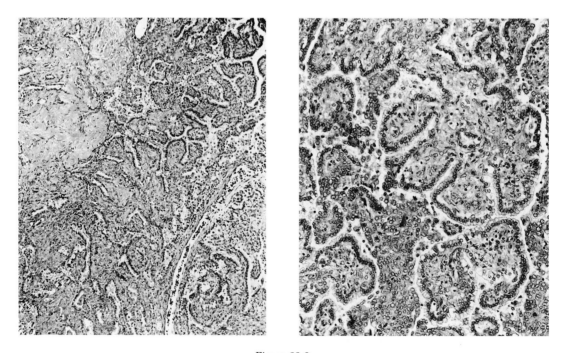

Figure 23-3
SCLEROSING HEMANGIOMA: MICROSCOPIC FEATURES
Left: Both sclerotic (upper left) and papillary patterns are present in this field.
Right: These papillary projections contain epithelioid tumor cells within the cores and have a prominent cuboidal epithelial lining along the surface.

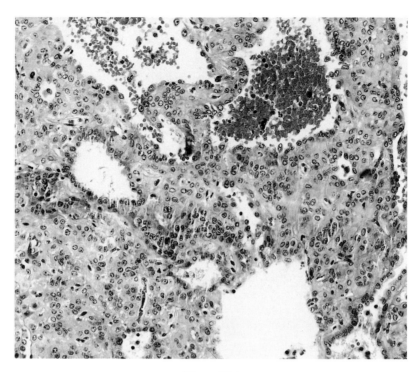

Figure 23-4
SCLEROSING HEMANGIOMA: MICROSCOPIC FEATURES
Collections of red blood cells within the lumens of these cystic spaces give a hemorrhagic or vascular appearance. Cuboidal epithelial cells line the cystic spaces that are present within the solid proliferation of epithelioid tumor cells.

percentage of cases (fig. 23-2, right). Cells lining the surface of the papillary structures are cuboidal or large, with voluminous eosinophilic cytoplasm and prominent nuclei that may have intranuclear cytoplasmic inclusions. In addition, a variety of associated histologic features may be observed including cholesterol clefts (fig. 23-5), chronic inflammation, xanthoma cells, hemosiderin, calcification, laminated scroll-like whorls (fig. 23-6), necrosis, and mature fat. Mast cells may be numerous (fig. 23-7). Rarely, lymph node metastases may occur (fig. 23-8) (101).

Cytology. The results of fine needle aspiration cytology in two cases of sclerosing hemangioma have been reported (15,106). One case was initially mistaken for bronchioloalveolar carcinoma while the other was correctly diagnosed. The characteristic "blood spaces" surrounded by bland polygonal tumor cells is a helpful clue to the diagnosis (fig. 23-9).

Immunohistochemical Findings. For many years, the origin of sclerosing hemangioma was obscure, with numerous studies supporting widely varied hypotheses including endothelial,

mesothelial, epithelial, and mesenchymal origins (5,47,54,74,75,91,112). Neoplastic, hamartomatous, and reactive etiologies have been proposed. Most immunohistochemical and ultrastructural data support the concept that sclerosing hemangioma is an epithelial neoplasm derived from type 2 pneumocytes and bronchiolar epithelial cells (91,112). Sclerosing hemangioma stains for a variety of antibodies against epithelial markers including surfactant apoprotein, cytokeratin, epithelial membrane antigen, carcinoembryonic antigen, and Clara cell antigen (91,112). One difficulty in interpreting these stains is that the surface cells lining the papillary structures tend to stain well with these epithelial antibodies while the epithelioid cells of the solid areas do not. The cytoplasm of the surface cells and their intranuclear cytoplasmic inclusions stain for surfactant apoprotein (fig. 23-10).

Ultrastructural Findings. An epithelial origin has been supported by electron microscopy, which reveals a microvillus-like folding of the cell membrane, lamellar inclusions similar to those seen in type 2 pneumocytes, and desmosomes (41,45,69).

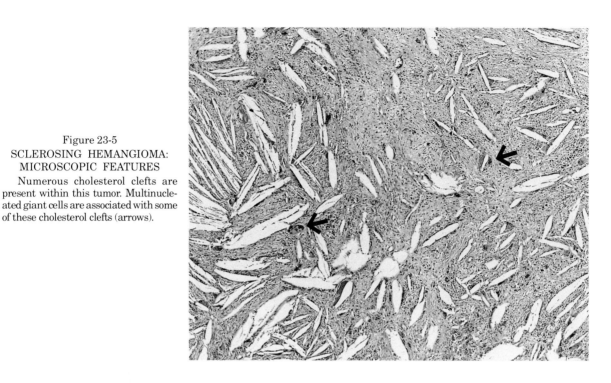

Figure 23-5
SCLEROSING HEMANGIOMA:
MICROSCOPIC FEATURES
Numerous cholesterol clefts are present within this tumor. Multinucleated giant cells are associated with some of these cholesterol clefts (arrows).

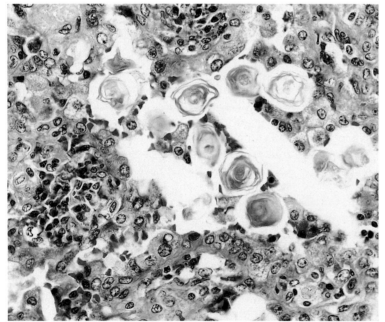

Figure 23-6
SCLEROSING HEMANGIOMA:
MICROSCOPIC FEATURES
These scroll-like whorls stain positively with surfactant apoprotein and resemble the lamellar bodies seen by ultrastructure in type 2 pneumocytes.

Differential Diagnosis. The differential diagnosis includes inflammatory pseudotumor, benign clear cell "sugar" tumor, carcinoid, and papillary carcinomas such as bronchioloalveolar carcinoma or metastatic thyroid or renal carcinoma. Inflammatory pseudotumor lacks the distinct epithelioid cells, papillary growth, and vascular spaces of sclerosing hemangioma but consists primarily of a mass of inflammatory and fibrous tissue. Benign clear cell tumor cells have clear, glycogen-rich cytoplasm and delicate vascular spaces that are thin-walled and sinusoidal; this contrasts with the more irregular vascular spaces of sclerosing hemangioma. Electron microscopy

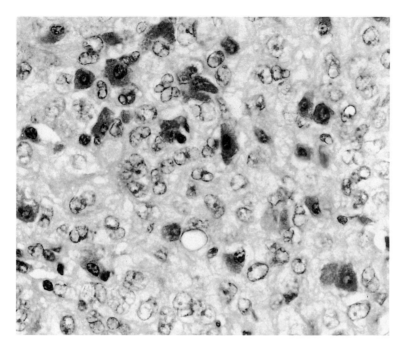

Figure 23-7
SCLEROSING HEMANGIOMA:
MICROSCOPIC FEATURES
The dark staining cells are mast cells, which are numerous within this tumor. (Alcian blue stain)

Figure 23-8
SCLEROSING HEMANGIOMA
INVOLVING
HILAR LYMPH NODE:
MICROSCOPIC FEATURES
This tumor metastasized to a hilar lymph node. Histologically, the tumor in the lymph node was identical to that seen in the lung.

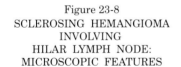
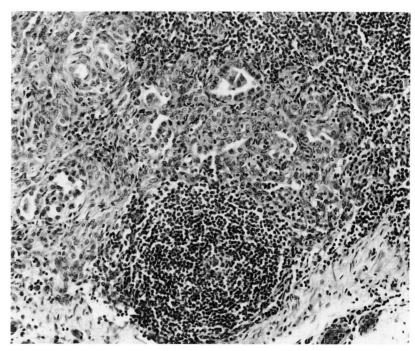

of clear cell tumors shows abundant membrane-bound glycogen; the presence of glycogen can also be confirmed by positive staining with periodic acid–Schiff (PAS) which is removed by diastase digestion. Sclerosing hemangioma differs from papillary carcinomas by the presence of the distinct round cells within the papillary stalks as well as the characteristic solid, hemorrhagic, or sclerotic patterns. Metastatic renal cell carcinoma may have tumor cells with clear cytoplasm that resemble sclerosing hemangioma; however, renal cell carcinoma often shows malignant cytologic features, and generally lacks the distinct varied patterns seen in sclerosing hemangioma.

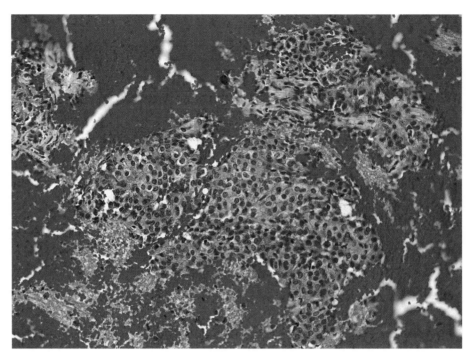

Figure 23-9
SCLEROSING HEMANGIOMA: FINE NEEDLE ASPIRATION CYTOLOGY
Clusters of uniform cells with abundant eosinophilic cytoplasm and sharp intracytoplasmic borders are surrounded by abundant hemorrhage. The nuclei are uniform, round to oval, and have evenly dispersed chromatin with occasional faint nucleoli.

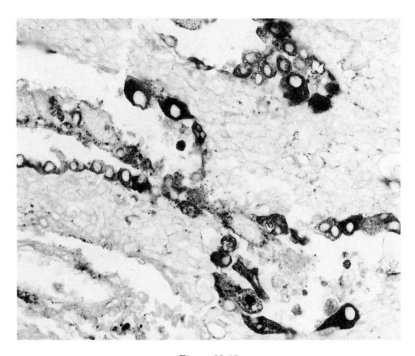

Figure 23-10
SCLEROSING HEMANGIOMA: IMMUNOHISTOCHEMICAL FEATURES
These reactive type 2 pneumocytes lined the surface of a papillary focus and stained with an antibody to surfactant apoprotein. (Courtesy of Dr. R.I. Linnoila, Bethesda, MD.)

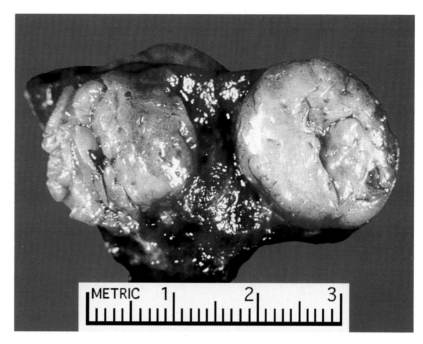

Figure 23-11
CLEAR CELL TUMOR: GROSS APPEARANCE
This tumor is circumscribed with a yellow-tan solid cut surface. (Courtesy of Dr. Anthony A. Gal, Atlanta, GA.)

Sclerosing hemangiomas lack the organoid, trabecular, rosette, or spindle cell histologic patterns of carcinoid tumors and do not have neuroendocrine features by immunohistochemistry or electron microscopy.

Treatment and Prognosis. The prognosis for patients with sclerosing hemangioma is excellent and surgical excision is curative.

CLEAR CELL TUMOR

Definition. Clear cell (sugar) tumors of the lung are rare tumors composed of cells with clear or eosinophilic cytoplasm that contains abundant glycogen. The histogenesis is uncertain but it has been proposed that clear cell tumors have an origin related to Kulchitsky cells (8), nonciliated bronchiolar (Clara) cells (6), smooth muscle (46), or pericytic cells (46,61).

Clinical Features. There is a slight female predominance in the reported cases (16 females, 11 males) (33). The median age is 51 years (range, 8 to 67 years) (33). Clear cell tumors are characteristically discovered incidentally on chest X ray in an asymptomatic patient. Virtually all cases occur in the lung, although one was reported in the trachea (60).

Gross Findings. Clear cell tumors are usually small, with a median size of 2.0 cm (range, 1.0 to 6.5 cm). The tumors appear as small, nodular, red-tan masses which shell out from the surrounding lung parenchyma (33). The cut surface is uniform without evidence of necrosis or hemorrhage, with rare exception (fig. 23-11) (33,90).

Microscopic Findings. The tumors histologically appear as circumscribed, but not encapsulated, nodules of cells consisting of abundant clear to eosinophilic, granular cytoplasm (fig. 23-12) (30,61). Typically, there is little connective tissue stroma. Due to the abundant glycogen, there is strong diastase-sensitive cytoplasmic staining with PAS. Thin-walled blood vessels without a muscular coat are prominent (fig. 23-13). Hyaline changes are sometimes encountered in the vessel walls. Extracellular amorphous eosinophilic material may be prominent (fig. 23-14) and may be associated with calcification, which can be psammomatous.

The cells tend to be round to oval with distinct cellular borders and may be elongated or spindle shaped. Large cells that have granules radiating from the nucleus in a linear fashion are called "spider cells"; rounded or polygonal cells with

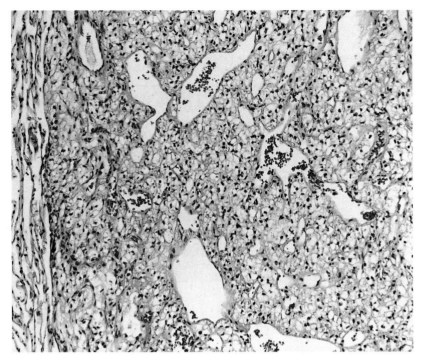

Figure 23-12
CLEAR CELL TUMOR:
HISTOLOGY
This tumor is circumscribed but not encapsulated and compresses the adjacent lung parenchyma (left). There are multiple thin-walled vascular spaces lined by endothelium without a muscular layer. The tumor cells have abundant clear cytoplasm.

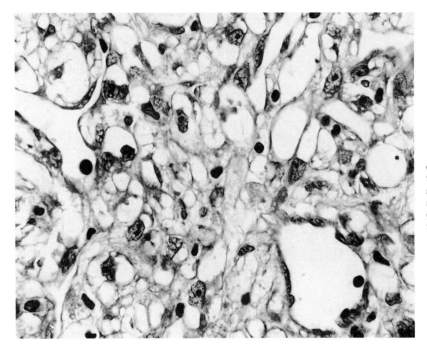

Figure 23-13
CLEAR CELL TUMOR:
HISTOLOGY
The tumors cells have abundant clear cytoplasm and are mostly round to oval with a few that are spindle shaped. The nuclei range from a small size with dense chromatin to larger ones with distinct nuclear membranes, vesicular chromatin, and nucleoli.

homogeneous acidophilic cytoplasm are called "neuroid cells." Finely granular brown lipochrome pigment may be found in the tumor cells. Multinucleated cells are seen in most tumors and, rarely, may be prominent (61).

The nuclei vary in size, but have prominent nuclear membranes (fig. 23-13). Nucleoli may be prominent. Mitoses are usually absent. Necrosis is rare and may be associated with malignant behavior (90).

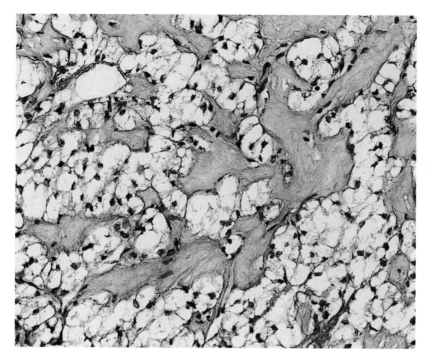

Figure 23-14
CLEAR CELL TUMOR:
HISTOLOGY
A dense hyaline stroma is present
between these clear tumor cells.

Cytology. Although one clear cell tumor was analyzed by fine needle aspiration cytology, the diagnosis was based on a surgical biopsy specimen rather than on the cytology specimen (77). It is difficult to distinguish clear cell tumor from clear cell carcinoma by cytology alone.

Immunohistochemical Findings. Most clear cell tumors stain strongly for HMB-45, HMB-50, and cathepsin B, and are focally reactive with S-100 protein (33,35,84). Some stain positively with neuron-specific enolase, synaptophysin, HAM-56, and CD57 (Leu-7) (33,34).

Ultrastructural Findings. Clear cell tumors have abundant cytoplasmic glycogen which is both free and membrane bound (8,30,46,90). Some (46), but not all (30), investigators have found the membrane-bound glycogen to have a rosette-like appearance. This distribution has been compared to that seen in the type II glycogenosis (Pompe disease) (8). Basement membrane material often surrounds the tumor cells. Intracytoplasmic filaments may be present. The plasma membrane may have pinocytotic vesicles and plaque-like densities (30,46).

Neurosecretory granules measuring 70 to 150 μm have been observed in 2 to 5 percent of cells (8,33,34). These granules may be melanosomes (34,84).

Differential Diagnosis. Clear cell tumors of the lung must be distinguished from clear cell carcinoma, either primary in the lung or metastatic from other sites such as the kidney. The prominent cytoplasmic glycogen is a distinguishing feature usually not seen in clear cell carcinoma. Glycogen can be appreciated by light microscopy with PAS staining or by electron microscopy. Many renal cell carcinomas contain lipid rather than glycogen (33). The tendency for clear cell tumors to stain with HMB-45 but not keratin also distinguishes them from clear cell carcinoma (34). Since HMB-45 also stains the smooth muscle of angiomyolipomas of the kidney and lymphangioleiomyomatosis, it has been suggested that clear cell tumors are smooth muscle in origin. Most clear cell carcinomas have vessels with a muscular wall in contrast to clear cell tumors.

Other diagnostic considerations include carcinoid tumor, granular cell tumor, oncocytoma, acinic cell tumor, and metastatic clear cell sarcoma. While the cells of these tumors may contain clear cytoplasm, they lack the prominent cytoplasmic glycogen, ectatic vascular spaces without a muscle layer in the wall, and positive staining for HMB-45 (except for clear cell sarcoma) (35).

Treatment and Prognosis. Virtually all clear cell tumors are cured by surgical excision.

There is only one reported tumor that metastasized to the liver and peritoneum 10 years after initial surgical resection; death occurred 17 years after diagnosis (89). Since this was the largest tumor ever reported (4.5 cm) and the only one ever known to show columnar cells and necrosis (90), this case should not be used to make generalizations regarding the behavior of other clear cell tumors (21).

MINUTE PULMONARY MENINGOTHELIAL-LIKE NODULES ("MINUTE PULMONARY CHEMODECTOMAS")

Definition. Minute pulmonary meningothelial-like nodules, previously known as minute pulmonary chemodectomas, are relatively common, perivenular, millimeter-sized, interstitial nodular proliferations of small, oval- to spindle-shaped cells arranged in a "zellenballen" nesting pattern. The origin and nature of these lesions has been the subject of much debate, with theories including an origin from chemoreceptors or paraganglia (56), mesothelial hamartomas of pleural origin (19), and muscle cells (103). Recent studies indicate that the cells in these lesions are similar to those of meningiomas, thus the term, minute pulmonary meningothelial-like nodules (16,32,58). The older term, chemodectoma, has led to confusion in the literature since it has also been used for pulmonary neoplasms thought to be paragangliomas (39).

The function of these lesions is not known. They may represent chemoreceptors, similar to the tumors of the glomus jugulare which are located in the adventitia of the bulb of the jugular vein (48,56), but this has not been proven. An association with thromboemboli has led to the consideration that pulmonary minute meningothelial-like nodules might be induced by pulmonary thromboemboli (48). According to this theory, ischemia induced by vascular obstruction causes the "chemodectomas" to develop from precursor chemoreceptor cells in the lung (94).

Clinical Features. Minute pulmonary meningothelial-like nodules are incidental pathologic findings, usually discovered microscopically in surgical or autopsy pulmonary specimens: there are no symptoms. The frequency in autopsy series is estimated at 0.3 to 4 percent (32,48,56,94). With increasing sensitivity of radiologic methods such as thin-section, high resolution computerized tomography, eventually these lesions may be detected by radiographs since they can attain a size of 3 mm.

There is a definite female predominance of 5.4 to 1 (16,32,56). They are found virtually always in adults with a mean age of 58 years (range, 12 to 91 years); most patients are in the sixth decade of life (32). The lesions are associated with thromboembolism in up to 51 percent of cases (48), cardiac disease in 48 percent (32), and malignancy in 28 percent (32). Thromboembolism has been suggested as a potential etiologic factor due to its frequency (94). However, it has been argued that a 51 percent incidence does not exceed that expected in a typical autopsy patient population (32).

Gross Findings. The nodules are 1 to 3 mm in diameter and usually multiple, but in any given specimen only one may be identified depending on the extent of sampling (32). In most cases, they are overlooked on gross exam and are incidental microscopic findings (56). They may be seen as ill-defined grey-white nodules on the pleural surface, bulging above the cut surface (fig. 23-15); are often situated at the septal insertions into the pleura; and are associated with black dust deposits. These lesions may also appear as pale tan nodules within the lung parenchyma most often in a subpleural location (fig. 23-15) (56). They are found most often in the upper lobes although they occur in all lobes of the lung (32).

Microscopic Findings. At low power, multiple minute pulmonary meningothelial-like nodules appear as scattered, circumscribed but ill-defined cellular nodules (fig. 23-16). Histologically, they appear as irregular nodules situated in a perivenular location, often with a cellular expansion of alveolar septal interstitium (fig. 23-17). Smaller lesions consist primarily of cellular nests while larger ones are frequently associated with fibrotic thickening of the interstitium (fig. 23-18), with fibrosis around individual nests. These nodules tend to laterally displace capillaries due to expansive growth within the alveolar septa (32). They consist of round spindle- or oval-shaped cells arranged in nests associated with a delicate network of capillaries, sometimes resembling the zellenballen pattern seen in paragangliomas. The cells frequently approximate the surrounding alveolar spaces

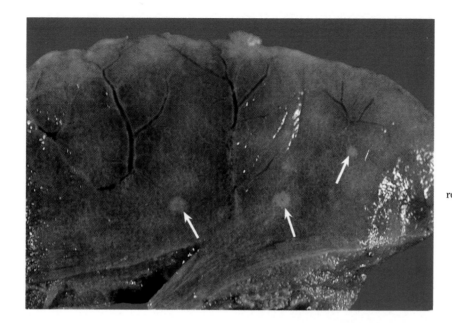

Figure 23-15
MINUTE
MENINGOTHELIAL-LIKE
NODULES: GROSS
APPEARANCE WITH
MULTIPLE LESIONS
Several ill-defined tan nodules (arrows) are seen on the pleural surface.

Figure 23-16
MINUTE MENINGOTHELIAL-LIKE
NODULES: HISTOLOGY
AT SCANNING POWER
Multiple ill-defined nodules are scattered in
the lung parenchyma.

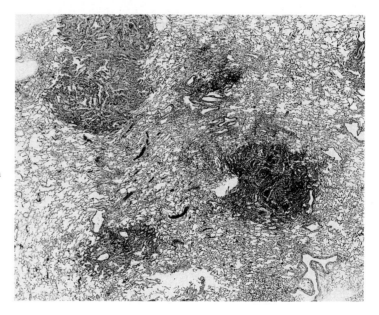

(fig. 23-19). The cytoplasm of the tumor cells is usually eosinophilic, but may be vacuolated or clear (56). The nuclei are uniform, round to oval, with vesicular or finely granular chromatin (fig. 23-20) lacking the salt and pepper nuclear morphology of carcinoid tumorlets. Intranuclear cytoplasmic inclusions may be seen but mitoses are absent. The cells do not stain with argyrophil or argentaffin stains. The adjacent lung may show evidence of thromboembolic or hyaline vascular changes (56).

Immunohistochemical and Ultrastructural Findings. It was the ultrastructural studies of Churg and Warnock (16) and Kuhn and Askin (58) that first indicated that the cells of minute pulmonary meningothelial-like nodules were not related to paraganglia, but actually resembled cells of meningiomas. The cells have prominent interdigitating cytoplasmic processes with a whorling or jigsaw-puzzle pattern, often in a perinuclear location (32). There are numerous interconnecting desmosomes (16,32,58). Nuclei

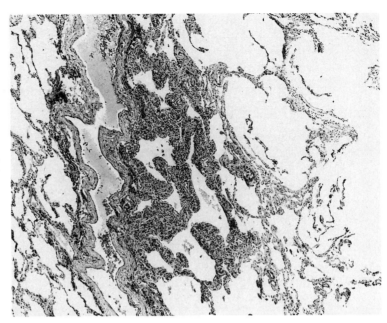

Figure 23-17
MINUTE MENINGOTHELIAL-LIKE
NODULE: HISTOLOGY
This lesion is situated adjacent to a vein
and consists of a cellular interstitial prolif-
eration that expands the alveolar septa.

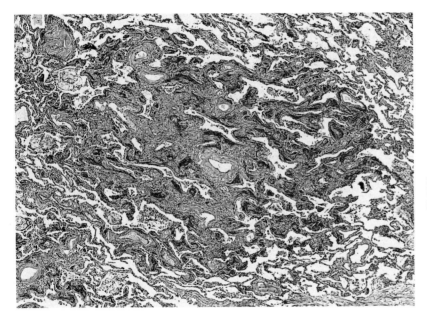

Figure 23-18
MINUTE
MENINGOTHELIAL-LIKE
NODULE: HISTOLOGY
Substantial stromal fibrosis is ad-
mixed with the cellular nests of pro-
liferating cells which tend to be at the
periphery along the airspaces.

are often indented. Neuroendocrine granules are absent (58).

Most minute meningothelial-like nodules stain with epithelial membrane antigen and vimentin, and are negative for cytokeratin, neuron-specific enolase, S-100 protein, and actin (32). Meningiomas also stain for epithelial membrane antigen and vimentin (see chapter 20).

Differential Diagnosis. The differential diagnosis includes carcinoid tumorlets, angiomatoid lesions of pulmonary hypertension,

granulomas, interstitial fibrosis, and metastatic carcinoma (32,56). Carcinoid tumorlets are usually associated with bronchioles rather than venules and although they tend to have an organoid nesting pattern, a whorling zellenballen pattern is not seen. In addition, the cells of carcinoid tumorlets differ from those of minute pulmonary meningothelial-like nodules in that they show neuroendocrine granules by electron microscopy and stain for neuroendocrine immunohistochemical markers such as chromogranin. The

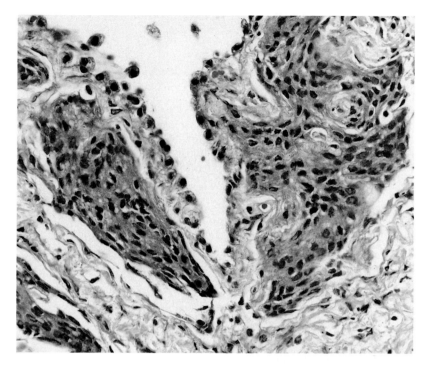

Figure 23-19
MINUTE MENINGOTHELIAL-
LIKE NODULE: HISTOLOGY
These cells are round, oval, or spindle shaped, with an organoid nest or zellenballen arrangement.

Figure 23-20
MINUTE MENINGOTHELIAL-LIKE
NODULE: HISTOLOGY
The cells have a moderate amount of eosinophilic cytoplasm with uniform round to oval nuclei showing vesicular or finely granular chromatin. Some cells show faint nucleoli.

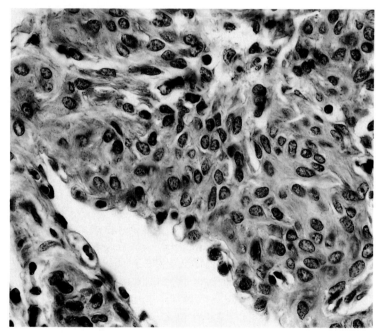

angiomatoid lesions of pulmonary hypertension consist of organoid vascular spaces associated with arterioles, in contrast to the venule-associated whorling nests of proliferating cells in minute meningothelial-like nodules. The epithelioid cells of granulomas may be multinucleated and have more abundant cytoplasm than the cells of minute meningothelial-like nodules. Larger lesions may have significant fibrosis, but differ from interstitial fibrotic disorders by the intermixed nests of meningothelial-like cells. These lesions may also be confused with metastatic carcinoma or paraganglioma, however, the consistent perivenular and interstitial location

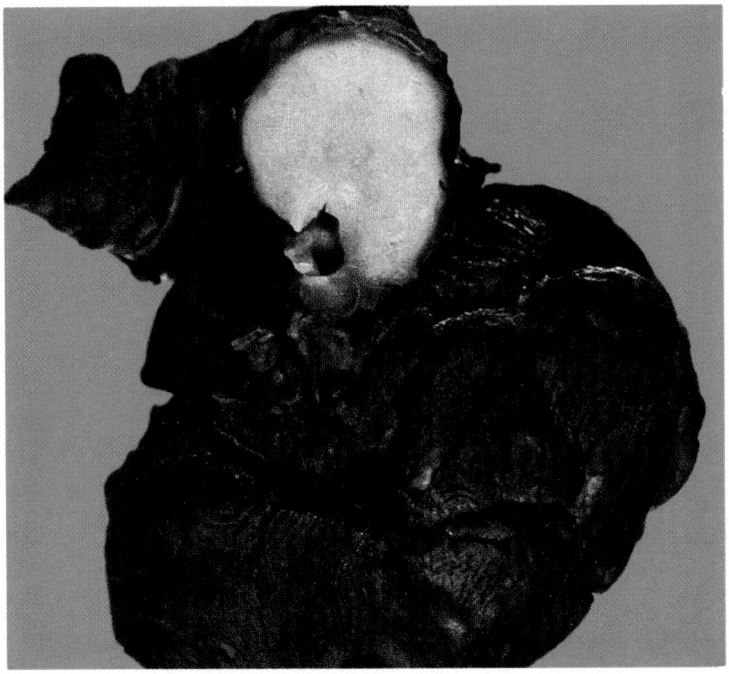

Figure 23-21
GRANULAR CELL TUMOR:
GROSS FEATURES
This tumor is peribronchial, circum-
scribed, and has a tan, solid, cut surface.

without lymphangitic involvement, the bland appearance with a whorling nesting pattern, and the lack of staining with keratin or chromogranin should aid in the correct diagnosis.

Treatment and Prognosis. Since these lesions are incidental findings of no known clinical significance, no therapy is required and there is no adverse impact on survival.

GRANULAR CELL TUMOR

Definition. Granular cell tumors are mesenchymal tumors composed of cells with abundant granular eosinophilic cytoplasm. They were originally described by Abrikossoff in 1926 (1), who thought they were derived from skeletal muscle. Since that time, a variety of cellular origins have been proposed but most studies support the concept that granular cell tumors are of Schwann cell origin. Terminology used for this tumor includes *granular cell myoblastoma* and *Abrikossoff tumor*. They occur most commonly in the tongue, skin, and breast. Two to 6 percent of all granular cell tumors occur in the lung (68,80). Since Kramer (57) described the first granular cell tumor in the bronchus in 1939, only about 100 cases have been reported (24).

Clinical Features. Granular cell tumors of the lung occur equally in men and women (24, 105). The median age is approximately 40 years (range, 8 to 59 years) (24,105). Almost half of the cases are discovered as incidental radiographic or bronchoscopic findings. The most common symptom is cough (53 percent), followed by recurrent obstructive pneumonitis (24 percent), chest pain (24 percent), fever (24 percent), sputum production (24 percent), hemoptysis (22 percent), dyspnea (22 percent), and weight loss (11 percent) (105). Wheezing may also occur (80). Lung abscess and bronchiectasis are infrequent complications (9,111). Chest X rays usually show atelectasis or postobstructive pneumonia, but there may be a coin lesion in an asymptomatic patient (105).

Gross Findings. The tumors range from 0.3 to 6.5 cm in greatest diameter, but most are small, with a median diameter of 1.0 cm (9,24). Granular cell tumors occur in all lobes of the lung, with a relatively equal distribution between the right and left lung, but occasionally they can be found within the interlobar fissures (24). An endobronchial location is seen in over 90 percent of cases and the tumors are often situated near points of bifurcation (fig. 23-21). Endobronchial tumors may have a papillary appearance or the

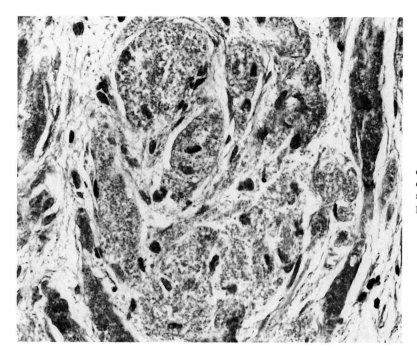

Figure 23-22
GRANULAR CELL TUMOR:
HISTOLOGIC FEATURES
The tumor cells have finely granular cytoplasm that stains with PAS. The nuclei are small and mostly eccentrically situated. A delicate fibrous stroma is present between the tumor cells.

overlying mucosa may be smooth. The tumors may be circumscribed, but are usually locally infiltrative and extend around the bronchial cartilage rings into peribronchial tissues. In less than 10 percent of cases, granular cell tumors occur as peripheral lung lesions without an apparent relationship to a bronchus.

Multicentric endobronchial lesions occur in 4 to 10 percent of pulmonary granular cell tumors (24,105). Occasional cases involve the trachea, thus the term *tracheobronchial granular cell tumor* (23). In approximately 10 percent (range, 4 to 16 percent) of patients, other organs are involved (14,108), such as skin (107), tongue, or esophagus (36,80). Up to 13 percent of granular cell tumors may be associated with a variety of other neoplasms of the lung, kidney, and esophagus (68).

Microscopic Findings. Granular cell tumors are composed of cells with abundant eosinophilic granular cytoplasm that stains with PAS (fig. 23-22). The tumor cells are mostly round to oval, but may be spindle shaped. The cytoplasmic granules are usually fine but are sometimes clumped (fig. 23-23). The nuclei are small and usually situated centrally or paracentrally. The chromatin is finely granular and occasional small nucleoli may be seen. Endobronchial tumors infiltrate the submucosa, distending the

overlying mucosa in a polypoid fashion (fig. 23-24). The tumor cells infiltrate around submucosal glands (fig. 23-25), nerves, and cartilage rings. Squamous metaplasia of the overlying mucosa is common; occasionally, the squamous epithelium may become hyperplastic with the pattern of pseudoepitheliomatous hyperplasia. Hyaline thickening of the subepithelial basement membrane is common (fig. 23-26). Rare examples of lymph node involvement are reported, but this appears to be due to direct extension.

Cytology. In bronchial brushings and washings, the tumor cells are found in clusters or small sheets, but occasionally as single cells (14). The cells are usually round to oval, measuring 20 to 50 μm by 10 to 20 μm, but they may be spindle shaped and measure up to 150 μm by 10 to 20 μm (14). The predominant feature is that of abundant cytoplasm distended with numerous eosinophilic granules. The nuclei are relatively small, centrally or slightly eccentrically situated, oval or round, and vesicular.

Immunohistochemical and Ultrastructural Findings. Granular cell tumors stain with S-100 protein, cathepsin B, myelin-associated protein, myelin-basic protein, and neuron-specific enolase (24,66).

As seen by electron microscopy, the granular cells contain numerous cytoplasmic, osmiophilic,

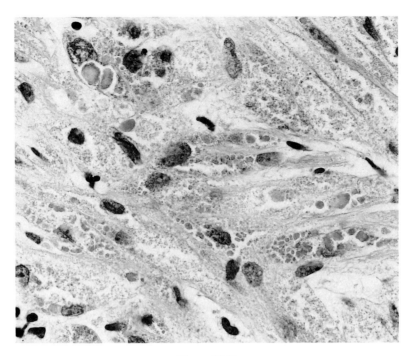

Figure 23-23
GRANULAR CELL TUMOR: HISTOLOGIC FEATURES
The cytoplasm of these tumor cells shows irregular, coarse cytoplasmic globules.

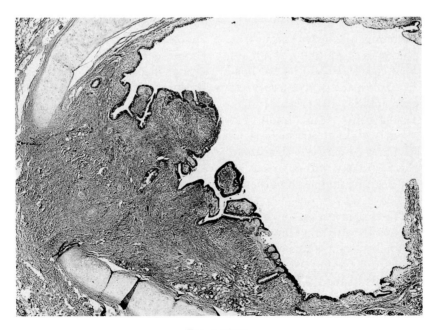

Figure 23-24
GRANULAR CELL TUMOR: LOW-POWER HISTOLOGY
This endobronchial tumor infiltrates the submucosa, extending between the cartilage rings of the bronchus and causes a papillary appearance on the mucosal surface.

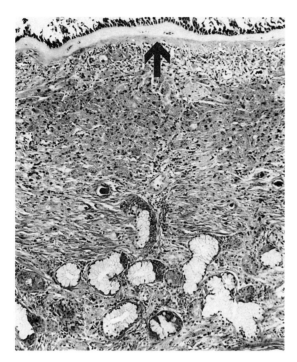

Figure 23-25
GRANULAR CELL TUMOR:
HISTOLOGIC FEATURES
The tumor infiltrates the bronchial submucosa and there is prominent hyaline thickening of the subepithelial basement membrane (arrow).

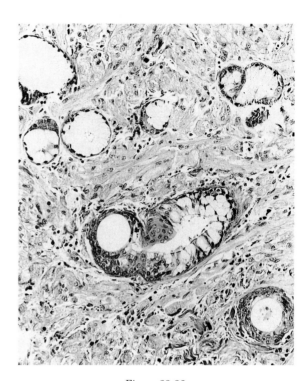

Figure 23-26
GRANULAR CELL TUMOR:
HISTOLOGIC FEATURES
The tumor infiltrates between the submucosal bronchial glands.

membrane-limited granules of varying shapes and sizes. These granules are sometimes regarded as secondary lysosomes (36). Larger granules have a lamellated structure and smaller ones a granular content (4). The cytoplasmic borders are generally smooth with a few short projections and desmosomal attachments (4).

Other Special Techniques. Tissue culture studies have shown active growth of granular cells with a specific in vitro pattern that is different from tumors of fibrohistiocytic and schwannian origin (4). A combination of spindle fibroblastic cells and granular cells is seen and mitotic figures indicate proliferation of the granular tumor cells.

Differential Diagnosis. The differential diagnosis includes oncocytic carcinoid tumors, oncocytoma, acinic cell carcinoma, metastatic neoplasms such as the granular cell variant of renal cell carcinoma, and histiocytic proliferations such as malakoplakia. The abundant eosinophilic granular cytoplasm and small central or paracentral nuclei distinguish these from granular cell tumors. Immunohistochemical staining for S-100 protein, but not for chromogranin and keratin, help distinguish granular cell tumors from carcinoids and carcinomas. The electron microscopic presence of numerous secondary lysosomes rather than mitochondria is different than oncocytomas or oncocytic carcinoids. The lack of epithelial characteristics or neuroendocrine granules distinguishes granular cell tumors from carcinomas and carcinoids, respectively. The histiocytes in malakoplakia may show coarse granules, but are negative for S-100 protein. Malakoplakia also contains abundant chronic inflammation and Michaelis-Gutmann bodies.

Prominent pseudoepitheliomatous hyperplasia associated with granular cell tumors may be confused with squamous cell carcinoma. The presence of the submucosal granular cells is key to the diagnosis. Although malignant granular cell tumors may metastasize to the lungs, a malignant granular cell tumor of the lung with distant metastases has not been reported (86).

Treatment and Prognosis. Lobectomy or pneumonectomy may be necessary if extensive destruction of distal lung parenchyma has occurred. However, if extensive lung destruction has not occurred, local extirpation is recommended (23). This may be achieved by endoscopic biopsy for lesions less than 8 mm, or sleeve resection (23,100). Careful observation may be all that is necessary for asymptomatic tumors, especially multiple endobronchial lesions (86).

Comparative Tumors in Animals. Granular cell tumors occur in animals including dogs, cats, horses, and birds (82). In contrast to other species, these tumors occur only in the lungs of horses (78,81,82,104). The immunohistochemical properties are similar to human pulmonary granular cell tumors: positive staining for S-100 protein, vimentin, and neuron-specific enolase (82).

THYMOMA

Definition. Primary pulmonary thymomas are very rare, with approximately 20 reported cases in the English literature. They present as either intrapulmonary nodules or pleural masses that are histologically identical to thymomas at other sites (29,72). Before the tumor can be regarded as primary in the lung, the presence of a primary mediastinal tumor must be excluded by radiographic studies or surgical inspection.

The origin of intrapulmonary thymomas is not known. Several proposed theories include monodermal differentiation of a pulmonary teratoma, derivation from the ectopic intrapulmonary thymic tissue, and migration of mediastinal thymomas into the lung (110).

Clinical Features. Primary thymomas of the lung can present primarily as an intrapulmonary or pleural mass. There is an equal sex distribution (11 men, 9 women). Of the 10 patients with intrapulmonary tumors, the median age is 55 years (range, 19 to 74 years). Three of these patients presented with myasthenia gravis, and one also had cough and fever. One presented with hemoptysis and the remaining seven were asymptomatic.

The median age for the reported patients with pleural thymomas is 51 years (range, 37 to 71 years) (29,72,83). Patients can present with symptoms of weight loss, chest pain, fever, shortness of breath, or they may be asymptomatic.

Myasthenia gravis has not been observed in association with pleural-based thymomas. Radiographically, pleural thymomas may mimic malignant mesothelioma (72).

Gross Findings. Intrapulmonary thymomas are divided into peripheral and hilar types (110). Most of the hilar tumors occur in the left lung; most of the peripheral thymomas occur in the right lung. The average size of intrapulmonary thymomas is 3 cm (range, 1.7 to 12 cm). Typically, they appear as a circumscribed encapsulated solitary mass. Multiple encapsulated nodules may also be seen. Pleural-based thymomas may present as a diffuse pleural thickening encasing the lung or as a solitary nodular mass. The cut surface is frequently lobulated and may be partially cystic. The tumor is usually tan, soft and fleshy but may be hemorrhagic or white and firm.

Microscopic Findings. Histologically, most intrapulmonary thymomas are well circumscribed and encapsulated; most pleural tumors are unencapsulated and infiltrative. The tumor cells often grow in lobules which are separated by fibrous trabeculae (fig. 23-27). The tumors may be epithelial, lymphocyte predominant, or mixed type. Spindle cell features may also be present. Storiform and hemangiopericytomatous patterns can be seen. The tumors usually compress the adjacent lung parenchyma but do not involve a bronchus. Most intrapulmonary thymomas are encapsulated while most pleural thymomas consist of an infiltrative mass causing pleural thickening.

Immunohistochemical Findings. In paraffin-embedded tissues, the thymic epithelial cells of thymomas stain with epithelial markers such as keratin and the lymphocytes stain with CD45RO (UCHL-1) but not CD20 (L26). Lymphocytes from frozen tissue from intrapulmonary thymomas stain with CD8 (Leu-2a), CD4 (Leu-3a), and CD5 (Leu-3b), but not CD20 and CD21 (29,40). The lymphocytes also stain with CD1a (OKT6) and show nuclear immunoreactivity for terminal deoxynucleotidyl transferase (29).

Ultrastructural Findings. A mixture of epithelial and lymphoid cells are seen with electron microscopy. The thymic epithelial cells show numerous desmosomes and cytoplasmic bundles of wavy intermediate filaments (40).

Differential Diagnosis. The differential diagnosis of primary pleural and intrapulmonary thymomas includes secondary lung involvement

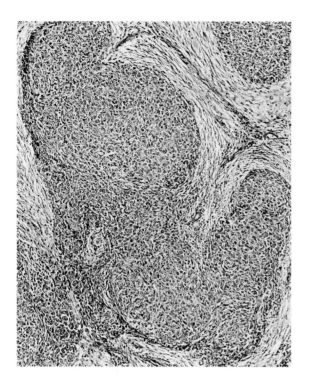 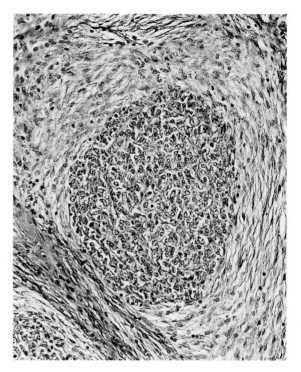

Figure 23-27
PLEURAL THYMOMA: HISTOLOGY
Left: This pleural thymoma shows lobules of predominantly epithelial tumor cells surrounded by fibrous trabeculae.
Right: The nests of tumor cells are separated by a fibrous stroma and consist of an admixture of epithelial and lymphoid cells.

by a mediastinal thymoma, malignant lymphoma, carcinoma, and malignant mesothelioma. Mediastinal thymomas may invade the pleura, lung parenchyma, or large airways and, rarely, they may secondarily involve the lung as a solitary pulmonary mass (25). Malignant lymphomas are not composed of epithelial cells mixed among the lymphoid cells. Carcinomas may have intermixed lymphoid cells but generally show cytologic atypia in contrast to the epithelial cells of thymomas. The tumor cells of malignant mesotheliomas have more abundant eosinophilic cytoplasm, sharper outlines, and less conspicuous lymphoid infiltrates. A trabecular fibrous stroma is unusual in mesothelioma.

Treatment and Prognosis. Due to the rarity of pleural and intrapulmonary thymomas, it has been difficult to establish firm prognostic factors. However, the literature suggests that patients with myasthenia gravis or extensive pleural involvement have a worse prognosis.

MALIGNANT MELANOMA

Definition. Primary malignant melanoma of the lung is very rare, with less than 25 reported cases (49). Criteria for the diagnosis include: 1) junctional change with a "dropping off" or "nesting" of malignant cells containing melanin (melanoma cells) just beneath the bronchial epithelium; 2) invasion of the bronchial epithelium by the melanoma cells in an area where the bronchial epithelium is not ulcerated; 3) a malignant melanoma associated with these epithelial changes; 4) a solitary lung tumor; 5) no past history of excision or fulguration of a cutaneous, mucous membrane, or ocular lesion; and 6) no demonstrable tumor elsewhere at the time of diagnosis (ideally proven ultimately by autopsy) (3,50). The presence of a nevus-like lesion in the bronchial mucosa adjacent to the tumor also supports the diagnosis of primary malignant melanoma (3).

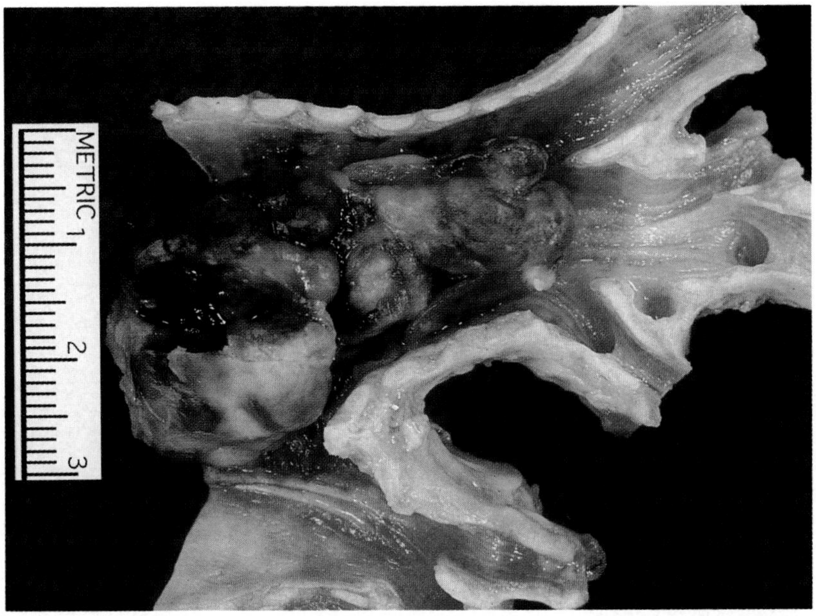

Figure 23-28
MALIGNANT MELANOMA:
GROSS FEATURES
This darkly pigmented endo-
bronchial polypoid mass protrudes
into the proximal bronchial lumen.

Several theories have been postulated to explain pulmonary melanomas, including derivation
from benign melanocytes which migrate with the
pulmonary anlage during embryogenesis; melanocytic metaplasia of bronchial epithelial cells; and
origin from neuroendocrine (Kulchitsky) cells,
which can show melanocytic differentiation.

Clinical Features. Of 18 patients with pulmonary malignant melanoma reviewed by Jennings et
al. (49), 10 were men and 8 were women. All cases
occurred in adults with a median age at diagnosis of
51 years (average, 52 years; range, 29 to 80 years).
Two of the cases involved the trachea.

Gross Findings. The majority of cases are
situated centrally and have an intraluminal endobronchial component (fig. 23-28). In tracheal melanomas, flat lesions have been described (49).

Microscopic Findings. A polypoid endobronchial growth pattern can also be seen microscopically, with ulceration of the overlying bronchial mucosa (fig. 23-29). The tumor may show a
lobular growth pattern and a delicate fibrovascular stroma. The tumor cells have abundant
eosinophilic cytoplasm with varying degrees of
brown granular melanin pigment (fig. 23-30). This
pigment stains positively with the Fontana-Masson stain and negatively with the Prussian blue
stain for iron. The nuclei are medium or large with
dense chromatin. Intranuclear cytoplasmic inclusions can be seen and scattered mitotic figures are

typically present. The tumor spreads in an in situ
or pagetoid fashion in the bronchial mucosa adjacent to the tumor (fig. 23-31). Submucosal nests of
benign-appearing melanocytic cells may resemble a
nevus (fig. 23-32).

**Immunohistochemical and Ultrastruc-
tural Findings.** Melanoma cells stain positively with S-100 protein (fig. 23-29) and HMB-
45 and negatively with epithelial markers such
as keratin. By electron microscopy, the distinguishing feature of the melanoma tumor cells is
the presence of melanosomes.

Differential Diagnosis. Malignant melanoma metastasizes to the lung in 12 percent of
cases; in 20 percent of these cases the patient
presents with an asymptomatic solitary pulmonary nodule (42,98). Metastatic melanoma to the
lung can manifest as a solitary mass, multiple
nodules, an endobronchial mass, or as melanosis
of bronchial mucosa (98). Metastases to the lung
may develop after a long disease-free interval
following removal of a cutaneous primary, reflecting the well-known clinical variability and
unpredictable biologic behavior of malignant
melanoma (11). In situ pagetoid spread in the
mucosa adjacent to a melanoma is evidence of
primary lung involvement. However, since this
phenomenon can also be observed in metastatic
melanoma to the lung (64), it raises doubts about
the specificity of this criteria and emphasizes the

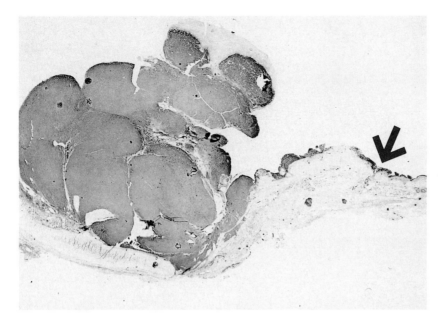

Figure 23-29
MALIGNANT MELANOMA:
HISTOLOGY
This low-power section of an endobronchial malignant melanoma shows polypoid growth into the bronchial lumen. The tumor stains faintly for S-100 protein but the cells showing pagetoid involvement of the adjacent bronchial mucosa stain strongly (arrow).

Figure 23-30
MALIGNANT MELANOMA:
HISTOLOGY
The tumor cells have abundant cytoplasm with varying amounts of brown melanin pigment. The nuclei vary in size but are atypical, with irregular shapes and occasional nucleoli.

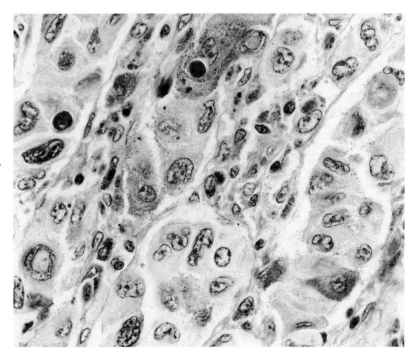

importance of obtaining an accurate history regarding prior pigmented skin lesions.

Of the primary malignant tumors of the lung, the most likely to be confused with malignant melanoma are carcinoid tumors. Carcinoid tumors share the features of nesting pattern, delicate fibrovascular stroma, uniform cytologic features, and may even exhibit pigmentation and melano-cytic differentiation (13). However, carcinoid tumors stain for neuroendocrine immunohistochemical markers and show neuroendocrine granules by electron microscopy. They also stain with argyrophil stains such as Grimelius, while melanomas stain with argentaffin stains such as Fontanna-Masson. The majority of carcinoid tumors stain for keratin in contrast to melanomas.

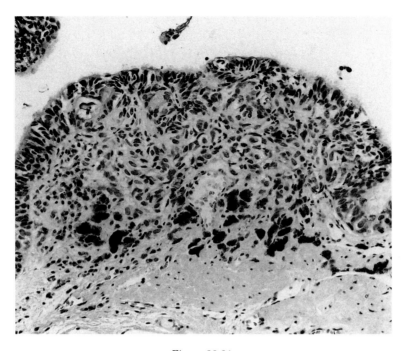

Figure 23-31
MALIGNANT MELANOMA: HISTOLOGY
In the bronchial submucosa and extending into the overlying epithelium adjacent to the tumor are numerous melanocytic cells reminiscent of a nevus.

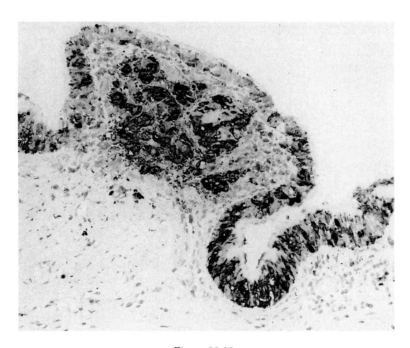

Figure 23-32
MALIGNANT MELANOMA: HISTOLOGY
Both the nests of submucosal cells and the pagetoid cells infiltrating the epithelium stain strongly for S-100 protein.

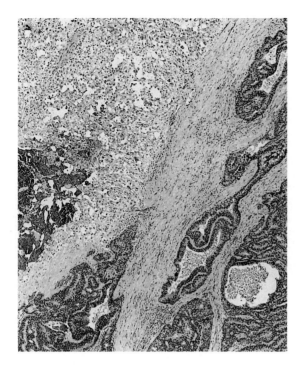 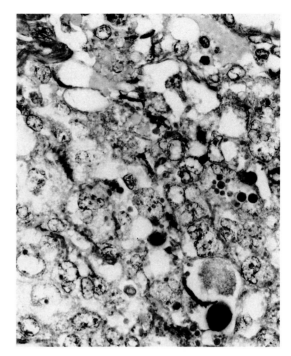

Figure 23-33
COMBINED YOLK SAC TUMOR AND PULMONARY BLASTOMA
Left: This tumor shows a blastoma characterized by glandular formation in an endometrioid arrangement as well as a yolk sac tumor characterized by glandular formations in a papillary and embryoid arrangement.
Right: In the yolk sac tumor component, eosinophilic hyaline globules of alpha-fetoprotein were present.

Focal S-100 protein staining may occur in some carcinoid tumors and both HMB-45 and S-100 may stain melanocytic carcinoid tumors.

Amelanotic melanomas can be confused with large cell carcinoma. However, large cell carcinomas stain for keratin and not HMB-45 and S-100 protein, while epithelial features such as desmosomes are seen with electron microscopy and melanosomes are absent.

Rarely, malignant melanoma is a component of pulmonary blastoma (17). A malignant melanotic schwannoma has also been reported in the lung (see fig. 20-26) (88).

Treatment and Prognosis. The reported cases were treated by either pneumonectomy or lobectomy, or they received no therapy. Eight patients died with tumor after therapy. Of the patients that were alive at the time of publication, two had disease at 12 and 19 months, and six were alive without tumor up to 11 years following surgical resection (49).

GERM CELL TUMORS

Primary germ cell tumors of the lung are very rare, although pulmonary teratomas are well documented. Some cases reported as choriocarcinoma may not be germ cell tumors but nonsmall cell lung carcinomas with giant cell features and ectopic production of human chorionic gonadotropin (hCG). Virtually any of the serum markers for germ cell tumors can be produced by lung carcinomas including alpha-fetoprotein, beta-hCG, alpha-hCG, and placental lactogen (43,70,93). However, no bona fide examples of pure primary embryonal carcinoma or yolk sac tumor are well documented. Two cases of yolk sac tumor arising in the lung were observed as a component of pulmonary blastoma (fig. 23-33) (see chapter 21) (92). It is not clear why teratomas and choriocarcinomas occur in the lung but the existence of primary teratocarcinomas, embryonal carcinomas, or yolk sac tumors remains to be documented.

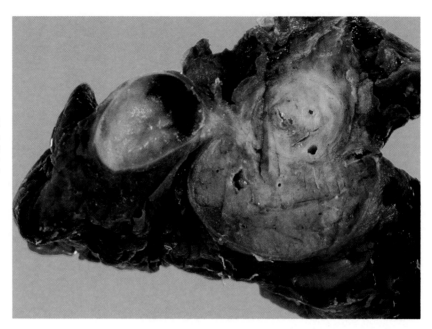

Figure 23-34
PRIMARY
PULMONARY TERATOMA:
GROSS FEATURES
This teratoma consists of a solid and cystic circumscribed mass. (Fig. LUN.9 from Curran RC, Jones EL. Tumours: structure and diagnosis. New York: Oxford University Press, 1991:282.)

Teratoma

Definition. Teratomas can consist of tissues representing all three germ cell layers or manifest as dermoid cysts consisting entirely of ectodermal tissue. To consider a teratoma primary in the lung, the tumor should be entirely intrapulmonary without involvement of the mediastinum or a gonadal or extragonadal primary. Intrapulmonary teratomas are rare, with only 33 published cases (73,99). They are considered to be derived from the third pharyngeal pouch.

Clinical Features. Patients with pulmonary teratomas present most often with chest pain (52 percent), followed by hemoptysis (42 percent) and cough (39 percent) (73). Trichoptysis or expectoration of hair is the most specific symptom and occurs in 13 percent of cases. The majority of cases occur in the second to fourth decades of life (range, 10 months to 68 years). There is a slight female predominance (18 women, 15 men) (73,99).

Radiographically, pulmonary teratomas typically present as a lobulated upper lobe mass which may be calcified and show a peripheral radiolucent area (73).

Gross Findings. Pulmonary teratomas are a median of 6 cm in maximum diameter (range, 2.8 to 30 cm). Two thirds occur in the upper lobes and most of these are in the left upper lobe (73,99). Mature teratomas usually have a large cystic component (fig. 23-34), although they may

be predominantly solid (37). Immature or malignant teratomas tend to be solid. Cysts often contain keratin debris, calcifications, or hair. Continuity with a bronchus can be found in 42 percent of cases and one third of these have an endobronchial component. Bronchiectasis occurs in 16 percent of cases and may delay recognition of the pulmonary tumor (73).

Microscopic Findings. Histologically, most pulmonary teratomas consist of a mixture of tissues derived from all three germ cell layers, although some may be dermoid cysts (figs. 23-35, 23-36). Pancreatic and thymic tissues occur more commonly than in gonadal teratomas. Of the 31 cases reviewed by Morgan et al. (73), 65 percent were benign and 35 percent malignant. Malignant elements generally consist of sarcoma or carcinoma. Immature elements, such as neural tissue, uncommonly occur. Malignant germ cell components such as seminoma, choriocarcinoma, or yolk sac tumor are generally not seen.

Differential Diagnosis. The differential diagnosis includes metastatic teratoma, carcinosarcoma, blastoma, and pleuropulmonary blastoma. Metastatic testicular teratocarcinomas may present as histologically mature teratoma in the lung (7,71). Generally, metastases are multiple and primary teratomas are solitary. Lung metastases can occur in patients with an occult testicular primary teratocarcinoma. This

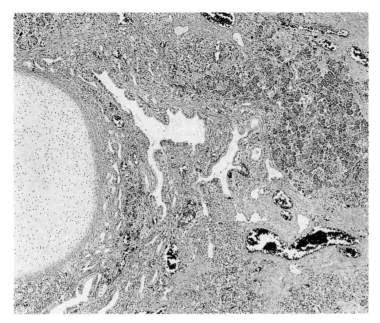

Figure 23-35
PRIMARY
PULMONARY TERATOMA:
HISTOLOGIC FEATURES
This teratoma consists of a mixture of carti-
lage, cystic spaces lined by a glandular epithe-
lium, and pancreatic tissue. (Courtesy of Drs. E.L.
Jones, and R.C. Curran, and Mr. H.I. Miller,
Birmingham, England.)

Figure 23-36
PRIMARY
PULMONARY TERATOMA:
HISTOLOGIC FEATURES
The pancreatic tissue from this teratoma shows
acinar tissue, ducts, and islets of Langerhans.
(Courtesy of Drs. E.L. Jones, and R.C. Curran, and
Mr. H.I. Miller, Birmingham, England.)

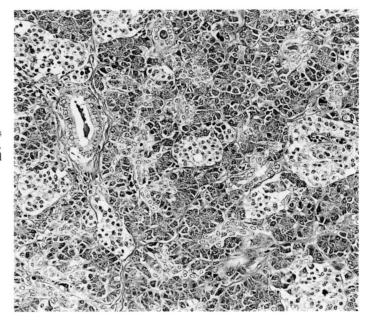

phenomenon has been described as *growing ter-atoma syndrome* (7,18,71). Growing teratoma syndrome occurs in 1.9 percent of patients with residual teratomas. This syndrome is character-ized by a history of a nonseminomatous testicular germ cell tumor, previous radiographic evidence of metastasis with elevated serum gonadotropin levels (alpha-fetoprotein, beta-hCG), reduction in the serum levels to normal following chemo-therapy, and increase in size of the metastasis with normal levels of serum gonadotropins. Al-though most cases occur in the retroperitoneum, approximately 15 cases have been reported in the lung (7,18,71).

While carcinosarcomas, blastomas, and pleuropulmonary blastomas can show heterolo-gous elements such as malignant cartilage, bone, or skeletal muscle, these tissues generally do not recapitulate specific organ structures as seen in teratomas.

Treatment. The optimal therapy is surgical resection. All patients with mature pulmonary teratomas that were resected were cured (73). However, four patients with mature teratomas died of postoperative complications and one patient who refused surgery died of hemoptysis. Four patients with resected malignant pulmonary teratomas were without disease 6 months to 17 years after surgery. While death occurred within 6 months in the remaining seven patients, these patients had either unresectable tumors or did not have surgery (73).

Choriocarcinoma

An estimated 2 percent of all nongestational, extragonadal germ cell tumors occur in the lung (59). Approximately 10 cases of primary pulmonary choriocarcinoma are reported in the English literature (12,22,38,44,52,55,67,85,96,97,102, 113). A smaller number of cases have been reported as a mixture of choriocarcinoma with adenocarcinoma (2), large cell carcinoma (see giant cell carcinoma and pleomorphic carcinoma, chapter 15) (26,31), and small cell carcinoma (43).

Pathologic Features. Grossly, choriocarcinomas tend to be extensively necrotic and hemorrhagic. Histologically, there are two major cell types: the syncytiotrophoblast and the cytotrophoblast. The former consists of large multinucleated giant cells with anaplastic histologic features; the latter consists of medium-sized uniform cells, often with clear cytoplasm. Immunohistochemically, the tumor cells, especially the syncytiotrophoblast, typically stain for alpha or beta subunits of hCG, keratin, and human placental lactogen (85,97).

Several theories have been used to explain the occurrence of choriocarcinoma in the lung: 1) abnormal migration of primordial germ cells during embryonal development (85); 2) metastasis from a gonadal primary, or trophoblastic emboli following molar pregnancies (102); and 3) metaplasia or divergent differentiation of pulmonary epithelial cells (85). The latter theory suggests expression of a fetal gene in a malignancy of somatic origin.

Differential Diagnosis. The differential diagnosis of primary pulmonary choriocarcinoma includes lung carcinoma with choriocarcinomatous foci and metastasis from an extrapulmonary primary. Large cell carcinomas of the lung can have giant cell features and ectopically produce hCG (fig. 23-37) (28,87). Such tumors can resemble choriocarcinoma both clinically and pathologically. Thus it may be difficult to distinguish between choriocarcinoma and giant cell carcinoma. The malignant cells of large cell carcinomas and giant cell carcinomas with ectopic hCG production range in size, rather than being two distinct populations of trophoblasts. The presence of large uninucleate giant cells favors the diagnosis of primary carcinoma of the lung rather than choriocarcinoma. By immunohistochemistry, 84 percent of lung carcinomas stain for beta-hCG (109). Virtually any placental protein can be produced ectopically by lung carcinoma. Analysis of cell lines revealed the presence of hCG or its subunits in 72 percent of nonsmall cell carcinomas, 10 percent of small cell carcinomas, and 75 percent of carcinoid tumors (10).

In most cases, it is not difficult to determine whether a germ cell tumor in the lung is a metastasis. However, on occasion it may be difficult. Usually there are multiple pulmonary tumors; however, a metastatic choriocarcinoma to the lung may form a solitary lung mass (65). Occult germ cell tumors of the testes are also well known (27).

In a young woman, the possibility of trophoblastic emboli at the time of abortion or delivery should be considered. Tanimura et al. (102) described such a case and demonstrated trophoblasts in the pulmonary arteries of 9 of 10 women who died after delivery or abortion.

EPENDYMOMA

Primary ependymoma of the lung is extremely rare: only a single case was reported in a 64-year-old female with a right upper lobe mass (20). Exclusion of a metastasis is essential since the lung is the most common site of extraneural metastasis of central nervous system ependymomas (5 percent of cases) (76). A quiescent cerebral lesion may metastasize to lung up to 12 years after initial diagnosis (63).

The single reported lung tumor consisted of a 2.0 by 1.0 by 0.8 cm circumscribed but unencapsulated mass with a pale gray and lobulated cut surface (20). Histologically, the tumor consisted of spindle- to oval-shaped cells with abundant eosinophilic fibrillary cytoplasm (fig. 23-38). Focally, the tumor cells showed marked pleomorphism and

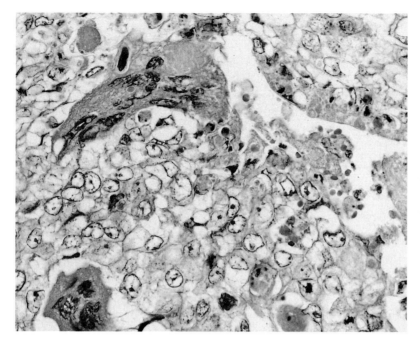

Figure 23-37
GIANT CELL CARCINOMA
WITH CHORIOCARCINOMA-LIKE
FEATURES
This microscopic focus shows a choriocarcinomatous-appearing lesion characterized by tumor cells with giant cell features resembling syncytiotrophoblast admixed with cells similar to cytotrophoblasts. Elsewhere this tumor had the histologic appearance of an ordinary lung carcinoma with large cell and giant cell components. (Fig. 8 from Fishback NF, Travis WD, Moran CA, Guinee DG, McCarthy WF, Koss MN. Pleomorphic (spindle and giant cell) carcinoma of the lung: a clinicopathologic study of 78 cases. Cancer 1994;73:2942.)

Figure 23-38
EPENDYMOMA
The tumor consists of spindle- to oval-shaped cells with abundant eosinophilic fibrillary cytoplasm. The cells are arranged in a perivascular pseudorosette.

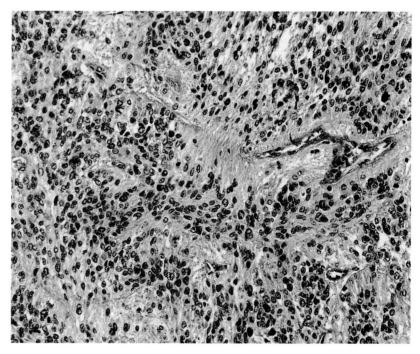

numerous mitotic figures. Nuclei were hyperchromatic with prominent nucleoli. Perivascular pseudorosettes were seen but no true rosettes were identified. Focal calcification was present. The tumor stained strongly for glial fibrillary acidic protein; less strongly for vimentin, Leu-7, and S-100 protein; and focally and weakly for epithelial membrane antigen.

REFERENCES

1. Abrikossoff A. Über Myome, ausgehend von der quergestreiften willkrlichen Muskulatur. Virchows Arch Pathol Anat Physiol Klin Med 1926;260:215–33.
2. Adachi H, Aki T, Yoshida H, Yumoto T, Wakahara H. Combined choriocarcinoma and adenocarcinoma of the lung. Acta Pathol Jpn 1989;39:147–52.
3. Allen MS Jr, Drash EC. Primary melanoma of lung. Cancer 1968;21:154–9.
4. Alvarez-Fernandez E, Carretero-Albinana L. Bronchial granular cell tumor. Presentation of three cases with tissue culture and ultrastructural study. Arch Pathol Lab Med 1987;111:1065–9.
5. _____, Carretero-Albinana L, Menarguez-Palanca J. Sclerosing hemangioma of the lung. An immunohistochemical study of intermediate filaments and endothelial markers. Arch Pathol Lab Med 1989;113:121–4.
6. Andrion A, Mazzucco G, Gugliotta P, Monga G. Benign clear cell (sugar) tumor of the lung. A light microscopic, histochemical, and ultrastructural study with a review of the literature. Cancer 1985;56:2657–63.
7. Basheda SG, Gephardt G, Meeker DP. The growing teratoma syndrome. Chest 1991;100:259–60.
8. Becker NH, Soifer I. Benign clear cell tumor (sugar tumor) of the lung. Cancer 1971;27:712–9.
9. Benson WR. Granular cell tumors (myoblastomas) of the tracheobronchial tree. J Thorac Cardiovasc Surg 1966;52:17–30.
10. Bepler G, Jaques G, Oie HK, Gazdar AF. Human chorionic gonadotropin and related glycoprotein hormones in lung cancer cell lines. Cancer Lett 1991;58:145–50.
11. Blumenfeld D, Berman ML, Kerner H, DiSaia PJ. Unusual metastases from a malignant melanoma. A case report. J Reprod Med 1991;36:688–90.
12. Cacciamani J. Case of choriocarcinoma of the lung. Clin Notes Respir Dis 1971;10:10–1.
13. Cebelin MS. Melanocytic bronchial carcinoid tumor. Cancer 1980;46:1843–8.
14. Chen KT. Cytology of bronchial benign granular-cell tumor. Acta Cytol 1991;35:381–4.
15. Chow LT, Chan SK, Chow WH, Tsui MS. Pulmonary sclerosing hemangioma. Report of a case with diagnosis by fine needle aspiration. Acta Cytol 1992;36:287–92.
16. Churg AM, Warnock ML. So-called minute pulmonary chemodectoma: a tumor not related to paragangliomas. Cancer 1976;37:1759–69.
17. Cohen RE, Weaver MG, Montenegro HD, Abdul-Karim FW. Pulmonary blastoma with malignant melanoma component. Arch Pathol Lab Med 1990;114:1076–8.
18. Coscojuela P, Llauger J, Përez C, Germa J, Castaner E. The growing teratoma syndrome: radiologic findings in four cases. Eur J Radiol 1991;12:138–40.
19. Costero I, Barroso-Moguel R, Martinez-Palomo A. Pleural origin of some of the supposed chemodectoid structures of the lung. Beitr Pathol 1972;146:351–65.
20. Crotty TB, Hooker RP, Swensen SJ, Scheithauer BW, Myers JL. Primary malignant ependymoma of the lung. Mayo Clin Proc 1992;67:373–8.
21. Dail DH. Benign clear cell ('sugar') tumor of lung [Letter]. Arch Pathol Lab Med 1989;113:573–4.
22. Dailey JE, Marcuse PM. Gonadotropin secreting giant cell carcinoma of the lung. Cancer 1969;24:388–96.
23. Daniel TM, Smith RH, Faunce HF, Sylvest VM. Transbronchoscopic versus surgical resection of tracheobronchial granular cell myoblastomas. Suggested approach based on follow-up of all treated cases. J Thorac Cardiovasc Surg 1980;80:898–903.
24. Deavers M, Guinee D, Koss M, Travis W. Granular cell tumors of the lung: clinicopathologic study of 15 cases [Abstract]. Mod Pathol 1993;6:129A.
25. Derow HA, Schlesinger MJ, Persky L. Myasthenia gravis: a clinical and pathological study of a case associated with a primary mediastinal thymoma and a solitary secondary intrapulmonary thymoma. N Engl J Med 1950;243:478–82.
26. Deshpande JR, Kinare SG. Choriocarcinomatous transformation in metastases of an anaplastic lung carcinoma—a case report. Indian J Cancer 1987;24:161–6.
27. Fine G, Smith RW, Pachter MR. Primary extragenital choriocarcinoma in the male subject. Am J Med 1962;32:776–94.
28. Fishback NF, Travis WD, Moran CA, Guinee DG, McCarthy WF, Koss MN. Pleomorphic (spindle and giant cell) carcinomas of the lung: a clinicopathologic study of 78 cases. Cancer 1994;73:2936–45.
29. Fukayama M, Maeda Y, Funata N, et al. Pulmonary and pleural thymoma. Diagnostic application of lymphocyte markers to the thymoma of unusual site. Am J Clin Pathol 1988;89:617–21.
30. Fukuda T, Machinami R, Joshita T, Nagashima K. Benign clear cell tumor of the lung in an 8-year-old girl. Arch Pathol Lab Med 1986;110:664–6.
31. Fusco FD, Rosen SW. Gonadotropin-producing anaplastic large-cell carcinomas of the lung. N Engl J Med 1966;275:507–15.
32. Gaffey MJ, Mills SE, Askin FB. Minute pulmonary meningothelial-like nodules. A clinicopathologic study of so-called minute pulmonary chemodectoma. Am J Surg Pathol 1988;12:167–75.
33. _____, Mills SE, Askin FB, et al. Clear cell tumor of the lung. A clinicopathologic, immunohistochemical, and ultrastructural study of eight cases. Am J Surg Pathol 1990;14:248–59.
34. _____, Mills SE, Zarbo RJ, Weiss LM, Gown AM. Clear cell tumor of the lung. Immunohistochemical and ultrastructural evidence of melanogenesis. Am J Surg Pathol 1991;15:644–53.
35. Gal AA, Koss MN, Hochholzer L, Chejfec G. An immunohistochemical study of benign clear cell ('sugar') tumor of the lung. Arch Pathol Lab Med 1991;115:1034–8.
36. Garancis JC, Komorowski RA, Kuzma JF. Granular cell myoblastoma. Cancer 1970;25:542–50.
37. Gautam HP. Intrapulmonary malignant teratoma. Am Rev Respir Dis 1969;100:863–5.
38. Gerin-Lajoie L. A case of chorioepithelioma of the lung. Am J Obstet Gynecol 1954;68:391.
39. Goodman ML, Laforet EG. Solitary primary chemodectomas of the lung. Chest 1972;61:48–50.
40. Green WR, Pressoir R, Gumbs RV, Warner O, Naab T, Qayumi M. Intrapulmonary thymoma. Arch Pathol Lab Med 1987;111:1074–6.
41. Haas JE, Yunis EJ, Totten RS. Ultrastructure of a sclerosing hemangioma of the lung. Cancer 1972;30:512–8.
42. Harpole DH Jr, Johnson CM, Wolfe WG, George SL, Seigler HF. Analysis of 945 cases of pulmonary metastatic melanoma. J Thorac Cardiovasc Surg 1992;103:743–8.

43. Hattori M, Imura H, Matsukura S, et al. Multiple-hormone producing lung carcinoma. Cancer 1979;43:2429–37.

44. Hayakawa K, Takahashi M, Sasaki K, Kawaoi A, Okano T. Primary choriocarcinoma of the lung: case report of two male subjects. Acta Pathol Jpn 1977;27:123–35.

45. Hill GS, Eggleston JC. Electron microscopic study of so-called pulmonary sclerosing hemangioma. Report of a case suggesting epithelial origin. Cancer 1972;30:1092–106.

46. Hoch WS, Patchefsky AS, Takeda M, Gordon G. Benign clear cell tumor of the lung. An ultrastructural study. Cancer 1974;33:1328–36.

47. Huszar M, Suster S, Herczeg E, Geiger B. Sclerosing hemangioma of the lung. Immunohistochemical demonstration of mesenchymal origin using antibodies to tissue-specific intermediate filaments. Cancer 1986;58:2422–7.

48. Ichinose H, Hewitt RL, Drapanas T. Minute pulmonary chemodectoma. Cancer 1971;28:692–700.

49. Jennings TA, Axiotis CA, Kress Y, Carter D. Primary malignant melanoma of the lower respiratory tract. Report of a case and literature review. Am J Clin Pathol 1990;94:649–55.

50. Jensen OA, Egedorf J. Primary malignant melanoma of the lung. Scand J Respir Dis 1967;48:127–35.

51. Joshi K, Gopinath N, Shankar SK, Kumar R, Chopra P. Multiple sclerosing hemangiomas of the lung. Postgrad Med J 1980;56:50–3.

52. Kalla AH, Voss EC, Reed RJ. Primary choriocarcinoma of the lung. W Va Med J 1980;76:261–3.

53. Katzenstein AL, Gmelich JT, Carrington CB. Sclerosing hemangioma of the lung: a clinicopathologic study of 51 cases. Am J Surg Pathol 1980;4:343–56.

54. _____, Weise DL, Fulling K, Battifora H. So-called sclerosing hemangioma of the lung. Evidence for mesothelial origin. Am J Surg Pathol 1983;7:3–14.

55. Kay S, Reed WG. Chorioepithelioma of the lung in a female infant. Am J Pathol 1953;21:555–61.

56. Korn D, Bensch K, Liebow AA, Castleman B. Multiple minute pulmonary tumors resembling chemodectomas. Am J Pathol 1960;37:641–72.

57. Kramer R. Myoblastoma of the bronchus. Ann Otol Rhinol Laryngol 1939;48:1083–6.

58. Kuhn C, Askin FB. The fine structure of so-called minute pulmonary chemodectomas. Hum Pathol 1975;6:681–91.

59. Kühn MW, Weissbach L. Localization, incidence, diagnosis and treatment of extratesticular germ cell tumors. Urol Int 1985;40:166–72.

60. Küng M, Landa JF, Lubin J. Benign clear cell tumor (sugar tumor) of the trachea. Cancer 1984;54:517–9.

61. Liebow AA, Castleman B. Benign clear cell (sugar) tumors of the lung. Yale J Biol Med 1971;43:213–22.

62. _____, Hubbell DS. Sclerosing hemangioma (histiocytoma, xanthoma) of the lung. Cancer 1956;9:53–75.

63. Lioté HA, Vedrenne C, Schlienger M, Milleron BJ, Akoun GM. Late pleuropulmonary metastases of a cerebral ependymoma. Chest 1988;94:1097–8.

64. Littman CD. Metastatic melanoma mimicking primary bronchial melanoma. Histopathology 1991;18:561–3.

65. Mazur MT. Metastatic gestational choriocarcinoma. Unusual pathologic variant following therapy. Cancer 1989;63:1370–7.

66. _____, Shultz JJ, Myers JL. Granular cell tumor. Immunohistochemical analysis of 21 benign tumors and one malignant tumor. Arch Pathol Lab Med 1990;114:692–6.

67. McLeod DT. Gestational choriocarcinoma presenting as endobronchial carcinoma. Thorax 1988;43:410–1.

68. McSwain GR, Colpitts R, Kreutner A, O'Brien PH, Spicer S. Granular cell myoblastoma. Surg Gynecol Obstet 1980;150:703–10.

69. Mikuz G, Szinicz G, Fischer H. Sclerosing angioma of the lung. Case report and electron microscope investigation. Virchows Arch [A] 1979;385:93–101.

70. Miyake M, Ito M, Mitsuoka A, et al. Alpha-fetoprotein and human chorionic gonadotropin-producing lung cancer. Cancer 1987;59:227–32.

71. Moran CA, Travis WD, Carter D, Koss MN. Metastatic mature teratoma in lung following testicular embryonal carcinoma and teratocarcinoma. Arch Pathol Lab Med 1993;117:641–4.

72. _____, Travis WD, Rosado-de-Christenson M, Koss MN, Rosai J. Thymomas presenting as pleural tumors. Report of eight cases. Am J Surg Pathol 1992;16:138–44.

73. Morgan DE, Sanders C, McElvein RB, Nath H, Alexander CB. Intrapulmonary teratoma: a case report and review of the literature. J Thorac Imaging 1992;7:70–7.

74. Nagata N, Dairaku M, Ishida T, Sueishi K, Tanaka K. Sclerosing hemangioma of the lung. Immunohistochemical characterization of its origin as related to surfactant apoprotein. Cancer 1985;55:116–23.

75. _____, Dairaku M, Sueishi K, Tanaka K. Sclerosing hemangioma of the lung. An epithelial tumor composed of immunohistochemically heterogenous cells. Am J Clin Pathol 1987;88:552–9.

76. Newton HB, Henson J, Walker RW. Extraneural metastases in ependymoma. J Neurooncol 1992;14:135–42.

77. Nguyen GK. Aspiration biopsy cytology of benign clear cell (sugar) tumor of the lung. Acta Cytol 1989;33:511–5.

78. Nickels FA, Brown CM, Breeze RG. Myoblastoma. Equine granular cell tumor. Mod Vet Pract 1980;61:593–6.

79. Noguchi M, Kodama T, Morinaga S, Shimosato Y, Saito T, Tsuboi E. Multiple sclerosing hemangiomas of the lung. Am J Surg Pathol 1986;10:429–35.

80. Oparah SS, Subramanian VA. Granular cell myoblastoma of the bronchus: report of 2 cases and review of the literature. Ann Thorac Surg 1976;22:199–202.

81. Parker GA, Novilla NM, Brown AC, Flor WJ, Stedham MA. Granular cell tumour (myoblastoma) in the lung of a horse. J Comp Pathol 1979;89:421–30.

82. Patnaik AK. Histologic and immunohistochemical studies of granular cell tumors in seven dogs, three cats, one horse, and one bird. Vet Pathol 1993;30:176–85.

83. Payne CB, Morningstar WA, Chester EH. Thymoma of the pleura masquerading as diffuse mesothelioma. Am Rev Respir Dis 1960;94:441–6.

84. Pea M, Bonetti F, Zamboni G, Martignoni G, Fiore-Donati L, Doglioni C. Clear cell tumor and angiomyolipoma [Letter]. Am J Surg Pathol 1991;15:199–201.

85. Pushchak MJ, Farhi DC. Primary choriocarcinoma of the lung. Arch Pathol Lab Med 1987;111:477–9.

86. Redjaee B, Rohatgi PK, Herman MA. Multicentric endobronchial granular cell myoblastoma. Chest 1990;98:945–8.

87. Rosen SW, Becker CE, Schlaff S, Easton J, Gluck MC. Ectopic gonadotropin production before clinical recognition of bronchogenic carcinoma. N Eng J Med 1968;279:640–1.

88. Rowlands D, Edwards C, Collins F. Malignant melanotic schwannoma of the bronchus. J Clin Pathol 1987;40:1449–55.

89. Sale GE, Kulander BG. 'Benign' clear-cell tumor (sugar tumor) of the lung with hepatic metastases ten years after resection of pulmonary primary tumor [Letter]. Arch Pathol Lab Med 1988;112:1177–8.

90. Sale GF, Kulander BG. Benign clear cell tumor of lung with necrosis. Cancer 1976;37:2355–8.

91. Satoh Y, Tsuchiya E, Weng SY, et al. Pulmonary sclerosing hemangioma of the lung. A type II pneumocytoma by immunohistochemical and immunoelectron microscopic studies. Cancer 1989;64:1310–7.

92. Siegel RJ, Bueso-Ramos C, Cohen C, Koss M. Pulmonary blastoma with germ cell (yolk sac) differentiation: report of two cases. Mod Pathol 1991;4:566–70.

93. Skrabanek P, Kirrane J, Powell D. A unifying concept of chorionic gonadotrophin production in malignancy. Invest Cell Pathol 1979;2:75–85.

94. Spain DM. Intrapulmonary chemodectomas in subjects with organizing pulmonary thromboemboli. Am Rev Respir Dis 1967;96:1158–64.

95. Spencer H, Nambu S. Sclerosing haemangiomas of the lung. Histopathology 1986;10:477–87.

96. Sridhar KS, Saldana MJ, Thurer RJ, Beattie EJ. Primary choriocarcinoma of the lung: report of a case treated with intensive multimodality therapy and review of the literature. J Surg Oncol 1989;41:93–7.

97. Sullivan LG. Primary choriocarcinoma of the lung in a man. Arch Pathol Lab Med 1989;113:82–3.

98. Sutton FD Jr, Vestal RE, Creagh CE. Varied presentations of metastatic pulmonary melanoma. Chest 1974;65:415–9.

99. Suzuki Y, Saiga T, Ozeki Y, Koyama A, Homma M, Ohba S. Two cases of intrapulmonary teratoma. Nippon Kyobu Geka Gakkai Zasshi 1993;41:498–502.

100. Symbas PN, Logan WD Jr, Vakil HC. Granular cell myoblastoma of the bronchus. Long-term follow-up after its local resection. Ann Thorac Surg 1970;9:136–42.

101. Tanaka I, Inoue M, Matsui Y, et al. A case of pneumocytoma (so-called sclerosing hemangioma) with lymph node metastasis. Jpn J Clin Oncol 1986;16:77–86.

102. Tanimura A, Natsuyama H, Kawano M, Tanimura Y, Tanaka T, Kitazono M. Primary choriocarcinoma of the lung. Hum Pathol 1985;16:1281–4.

103. Torikata C, Mukai M. So-called minute chemodectoma of the lung. An electron microscopic and immunohistochemical study. Virchows Arch [A] 1990;417:113–8.

104. Turk MA, Breeze RG. Histochemical and ultrastructural features of an equine pulmonary granular cell tumour (myoblastoma). J Comp Pathol 1981;91:471–81.

105. Valenstein SL, Thurer RJ. Granular cell myoblastoma of the bronchus. Case report and literature review. J Thorac Cardiovasc Surg 1978;76:465–8.

106. Wang SE, Nieberg RK. Fine needle aspiration cytology of sclerosing hemangioma of the lung, a mimicker of bronchioloalveolar carcinoma. Acta Cytol 1986;30:51–4.

107. Weitzner S, Oser JF. Granular cell myoblastoma of bronchus. Am Rev Respir Dis 1968;97:923–30.

108. White SW, Gallager RL, Rodman OG. Multiple granular-cell tumors. J Dermatol Surg Oncol 1980;6:57–61.

109. Wilson TS, McDowell EM, McIntire KR, Trump BF. Elaboration of human chorionic gonadotropin by lung tumors: an immunocytochemical study. Arch Pathol Lab Med 1981;105:169–73.

110. Yeoh CB, Ford JM, Lattes R, Wylie RH. Intrapulmonary thymoma. J Thorac Cardiovasc Surg 1966;51:131–6.

111. Young CD, Gay RM. Multiple endobronchial granular cell myoblastomas discovered at bronchoscopy. Hum Pathol 1984;15:193–4.

112. Yousem SA, Wick MR, Singh G, et al. So-called sclerosing hemangiomas of lung. An immunohistochemical study supporting a respiratory epithelial origin. Am J Surg Pathol 1988;12:582–90.

113. Zapatero J, Bellon J, Baamonde C, et al. Primary choriocarcinoma of the lung. Presentation of a case and review of the literature. Scand J Thorac Cardiovasc Surg 1982;16:279–81.

✧✧✧

24
TUMOR-LIKE CONDITIONS

NODULAR PULMONARY AMYLOIDOSIS

Definition. This is a form of isolated or limited amyloidosis characterized by one or multiple intrapulmonary nodules or masses of amyloid. Amyloid consists of extracellular deposits of chemically diverse protein fibrils whose three-dimensional conformation is that of a twisted beta-pleated sheet (12). Recent reviews have stressed the biochemical diversity of amyloid (27,32). Clinically recognizable disease limited to the lungs and pleura occurs. Pulmonary amyloidosis can be divided into several categories (Table 24-1). Of these, nodular parenchymal amyloidosis is particularly likely to be misconstrued as a neoplasm.

Firestone and Joison (11) and Saab et al. (30) provided the first large reviews of nodular pulmonary amyloidosis. By 1988, 134 cases had been described (4).

Clinical Features. When pulmonary amyloidosis occurs as a solitary nodule, it most often presents as an incidental finding in an adult (4,7,14). Multiple nodules and confluent miliary nodules are likely to provoke symptoms including cough, hemoptysis, and pleuritic chest pain (4,15).

The chest X ray shows one or more well-circumscribed mid-lung or peripheral nodules, most often 1 to 4 cm in diameter, which grow slowly over a period of years (10,15,23). The nodule(s) can impinge on bronchi or pleura, and pleural effusion may occur (31,35). Calcification or ossification is more common than cavitation (4,22). The clinical impression, particularly in cases without radiographic calcification, is of a neoplasm (4,7).

About 10 percent of patients have monoclonal proteins in serum or urine (15). Associated diseases include benign monoclonal gammopathy,

Table 24-1

AMYLOIDOSIS OF THE LOWER RESPIRATORY TRACT*

Clinical Type	Biochemical Type
In Generalized Amyloidosis	
Immunocytoma (primary/multiple myeloma)	AL (immunoglobulin light chain)
Reactive systemic (secondary)	AA (serum AA protein)
Heredofamilial	
Familial amyloidotic polyneuropathy	AF (transthyretin or prealbumin)
Familial Mediterranean fever	AA (serum AA protein)
Dialysis associated	Beta-2-microglobulin
Senile cardiac	Thyroxine-binding prealbumin
In Limited Amyloidosis	
Tracheobronchial	Mostly AL
Localized	
Diffuse	
Nodular parenchymal	Mostly AL
Solitary	
Multinodular	
Miliary or confluently nodular	
Diffuse alveolar septal	Mostly AL**
Pleural†	Mostly AL

* Adapted from reference 4.
** From reference 25. Alveolar septal amyloidosis also occurs in the setting of senile cardiac amyloid.
†From reference 17.

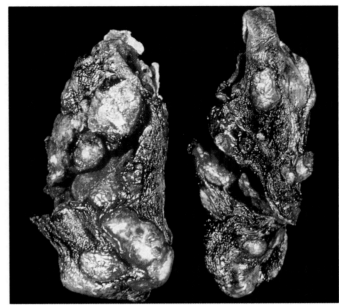

Figure 24-1
NODULAR PARENCHYMAL AMYLOIDOSIS
Bilateral, well-defined masses are present in these lungs at autopsy. (Fig. 2 from Fenoglio C, Pascal RR. Nodular amyloidosis of the lungs. An unusual case associated with chronic lung disease and carcinoma of the bladder. Arch Pathol 1970;90:577–82.)

Table 24-2

LYMPHOID LESIONS AND EPITHELIAL TUMORS IN LUNG ASSOCIATED WITH AMYLOID

Lymphoid Lesions

Nodular hyperplasia of BALT (pseudolymphoma) (21)

Diffuse hyperplasia of BALT (19)

Low-grade B-cell lymphomas of BALT, immunoblastic lymphoma (5,20)

Multiple myeloma

Epithelial Tumors

Carcinoid tumor/neuroendocrine carcinoma (1,2,13)

Small cell carcinoma (8)

Bronchogenic carcinoma with systemic amyloid (29)

Metastatic renal cell carcinoma (8) and neuroendocrine carcinoma

multiple myeloma, lymphoid interstitial pneumonitis (about 10 percent of cases), low-grade B-cell lymphomas of bronchus-associated lymphoid tissue (BALT) and immunoblastic lymphomas (5,7,15,20), and Sjögren syndrome (Table 24-2) (3,18,28).

The diagnosis in most cases is made at thoracotomy or autopsy. Percutaneous needle and transbronchial biopsies have been useful in some instances, but they may also lead to an incorrect diagnosis of malignancy if attention is focused only on atypical epithelial changes (6,9,34).

Gross Findings. Grossly, the lung shows irregular nodules that are waxy, hard, firm or gritty (when calcified), and yellow, gray, tan, or white (figs. 24-1, 24-2) (10,18,30). The nodules range from 0.6 to 15 cm, with an average of 3 cm (15,22).

Microscopic Findings. Irregular nodular masses of amyloid replace the lung parenchyma (fig. 24-3). The amyloid appears as an amorphous sheet of eosinophilic extracellular material, in areas wrapping around vessels (figs. 24-4–24-6). Clusters of small lymphocytes, plasma cells, and multinucleated giant cells occur throughout the amyloid deposits, but the lymphoplasmacytic infiltrate is usually most marked at the margin of the nodular masses (figs. 24-4–24-6). Ossification or calcification often occurs (fig. 24-7). Amyloid is frequently found in the walls of small arteries and veins adjacent to the nodular deposits; on occasion, it may be present in draining lymph nodes. Congo red stains show apple-green birefringence when examined by polarizing microscopy that is usually unaffected by potassium permanganate digestion, a finding indicative of non-AA amyloid (fig. 24-8) (4,7,15,22). Electron microscopy shows nonbranching, hollow-core fibrils measuring 7.5 to 12 nm that are arrayed in a disorderly fashion (fig. 24-9).

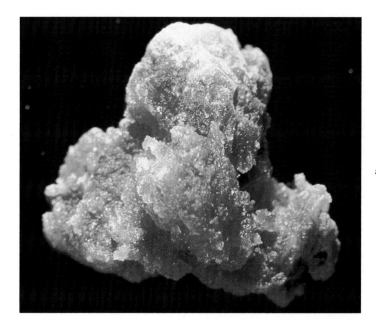

Figure 24-2
NODULAR PARENCHYMAL AMYLOIDOSIS
This nodule of amyloid shells out from the lung
as an irregular, tan, waxy mass.

Figure 24-3
NODULAR PARENCHYMAL
AMYLOID REPLACING
LUNG PARENCHYMA
Low magnification view shows
obliteration of the pulmonary parenchyma (except for residual vessels) by
a solid mass that sends short tendrils
into the contiguous lung.

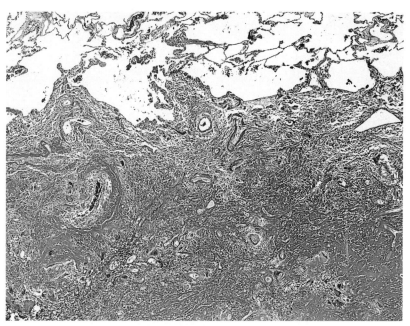

Etiology and Pathogenesis. The association of some cases of nodular amyloidosis with
monoclonal gammopathy, the results of the potassium permanganate reaction, and the finding
of protein identical to the variable region of immunoglobulin light chain in one case suggest that
nodular amyloidosis may be derived from AL
amyloid (7,15,26). It is possible that a local monoclonal proliferation of immunocytes gives rise to
the amyloid nodules (26). In many instances, the
plasma cells adjacent to amyloid nodules appear
to be polytypic, but there are now several documented cases of clonally imbalanced or monoclonal plasma cell or small lymphocytic proliferations in isolated pulmonary amyloidosis (7,15,
18). This theory could also explain the finding of
amyloid in draining lymph nodes.

Differential Diagnosis. Multiple pulmonary nodules composed of amyloid-like material
and containing foreign body giant cells have

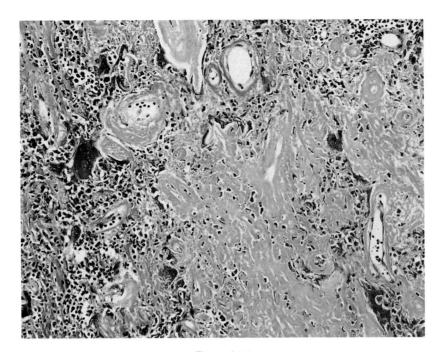

Figure 24-4
NODULAR PARENCHYMAL AMYLOIDOSIS
The amyloid consists of solid masses and bands of amorphous, eosinophilic, extracellular material. A multinucleated giant cell reaction is present, a typical finding in pulmonary amyloidosis.

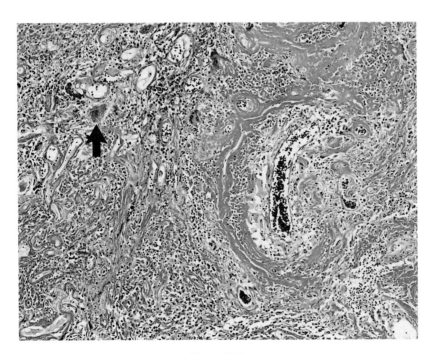

Figure 24-5
NODULAR PARENCHYMAL AMYLOIDOSIS WITH VASCULAR INVOLVEMENT
Amyloid distinctively lines the wall of a large vessel as well as obliterating the contiguous lung. Note the giant cell reaction in the parenchyma (arrow). A diffuse scattering of lymphocytes and plasma cells is present throughout the field.

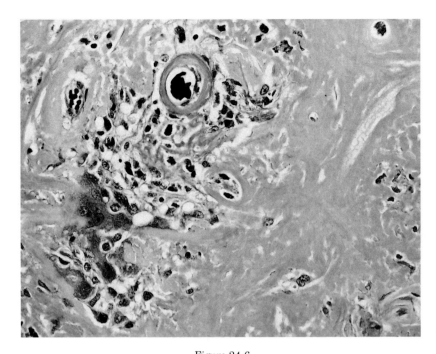

Figure 24-6
NODULAR PARENCHYMAL AMYLOIDOSIS WITH SMALL VESSEL INVOLVEMENT
In this view, the amyloid is present in amorphous masses and concentrically wraps around small vessels. Collections of lymphocytes and plasma cells, and a multinucleated giant cell are also present.

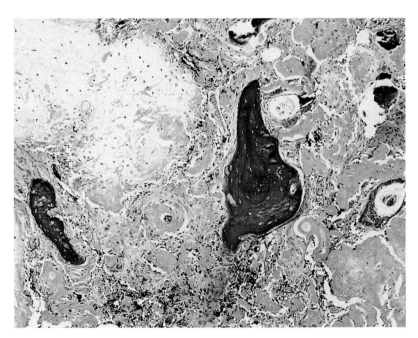

Figure 24-7
NODULAR PARENCHYMAL AMYLOIDOSIS WITH BONE FORMATION
Irregular trabeculae of bone and pale cartilaginous masses are present.

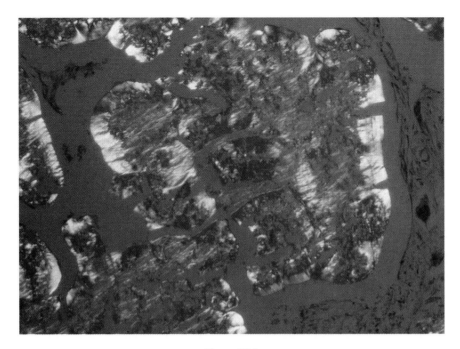

Figure 24-8
NODULAR PARENCHYMAL AMYLOIDOSIS
Congo red stain viewed by polarizing microscopy. The amyloid shows typical apple-green birefringence.

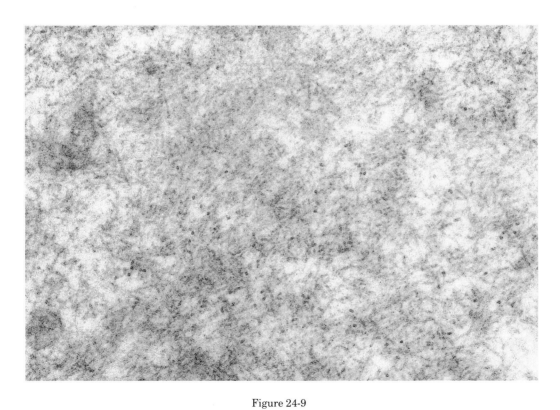

Figure 24-9
ULTRASTRUCTURAL APPEARANCE OF AMYLOID
There are masses of nonbranching fibrils measuring 8 to 10 nm in diameter. The fibrils form no discernible pattern.

been described in a patient with systemic kappa light chain disease (see chapter 22) (16). The kappa light chain deposits showed neither the typical apple-green birefringence nor the fibrillar ultrastructure of amyloid; rather they consisted of granular electron-dense deposits, sometimes with admixed 11- to 14-nm fibrils. In addition, Morinaga and associates (25) described "amyloid-like" masses within a plasmacytoma of lung, but the deposits failed to show either the histochemical or ultrastructural features of amyloid and contained kappa IgG.

Nodular amyloidosis also needs to be distinguished from pulmonary hyalinizing granuloma. The eosinophilic extracellular material in hyalinizing granuloma is lamellar collagen, rather than amyloid, despite initial reports to the contrary.

Amyloid can be present in the stroma of a number of lymphoproliferative disorders (as previously mentioned) and can occur in the stroma of several primary and metastatic neoplasms in lung (Table 24-2). Rare patients with nodular hyperplasia of BALT (pseudolymphoma) of lung and up to 10 percent of patients with diffuse hyperplasia of BALT (lymphocytic interstitial pneumonitis) may have congophilic amyloid deposits associated with the lymphoid proliferation (19,21,33). Amyloid may also infrequently complicate malignant lymphomas and multiple myeloma (less than 3 percent of lymphoplasmacytic lymphomas in one large series of pulmonary lymphomas) (7,20). In these cases, the amyloid is typically microscopic rather than macroscopic and is histologically subordinate to the lymphoid proliferation.

Microscopic amyloid deposits infrequently occur in association with epithelial tumors in lung (Table 24-2). Neuroendocrine tumors such as carcinoid tumors or small cell carcinomas are the foremost examples. One carcinoid tumor showed calcitonin gene-related peptide within both tumor cells and amyloid stroma by immunohistochemical methods (1). Amyloid has also been seen within the stroma of a renal cell carcinoma metastatic to bronchus, an interesting finding in view of the known association of this tumor with stromal deposits of AA amyloid (8). Again, in these cases the amyloid is typically a microscopic rather than macroscopic finding and identification of the neoplasm is the key to diagnosis.

Many conditions, notably epithelioid hemangioendothelioma, small lymphocytic lymphoma, pulmonary hyalinizing granuloma, and healed granulomatous diseases, are associated with hyaline fibrosis resembling amyloid. A hyaline amyloid-like, noncongophilic stroma (due most likely to basement membrane-like material) was reported in a small series of adenosquamous carcinomas (see chapters 6 and 16) (36).

Treatment and Prognosis. For solitary nodules, resection is both diagnostic and curative. There are exceptional reports of numerous and confluent nodules leading to respiratory insufficiency over a 10-year period (22). There does not appear to be effective treatment for such cases.

PULMONARY HYALINIZING GRANULOMA

Definition. These are pulmonary nodules of undetermined etiology that consist of microscopically distinctive, haphazard or whorled arrays of lamellar, keloid-like collagen. Hyalinizing granuloma was initially reported by Engleman and associates in 1977 (40) and an additional 24 cases were studied by Yousem and Hochholzer in 1987 (47). Over 50 cases were compiled by 1988 (43). Hyalinizing granulomas comprise about 2 percent of solitary "granulomas" of lung (46).

Clinical Features. The disease occurs most frequently in adults, with a mean age of about 45 years. Symptoms include cough, dyspnea, chest pain, and, on occasion, hemoptysis. Up to 25 percent of patients are asymptomatic (40,47).

The chest X ray typically shows ill-defined, bilateral pulmonary nodules or masses; however, solitary lesions are found in up to one third of patients (47). About 10 percent of lesions show speckled calcification (47). Cavitation is rare (40,41,44). The radiologic differential diagnosis includes metastatic or primary malignancy or granulomatous disease (43).

The most important associated diseases are sclerosing mediastinitis (16 to 20 percent of cases) and retroperitoneal fibrosis (38–40). They may precede, occur simultaneously with, or, less frequently, appear after the pulmonary lesions (37).

Gross Findings. The lung contains subpleural or intrapulmonary nodules varying from 0.2 to 9.0 cm in diameter (fig. 24-10). They are usually well circumscribed, firm, and have the white to gray

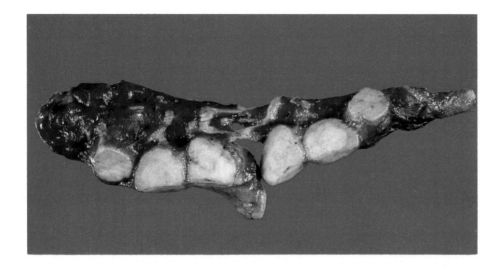

Figure 24-10
PULMONARY HYALINIZING GRANULOMA
The typical gross presentation of this lesion is in the form of multiple, subpleural, white nodules, as demonstrated in this case.

appearance expected of fibrous connective tissue. The nodules or masses are rarely cystic (43).

Microscopic Findings. At low magnification, the lesions appear reasonably well circumscribed (fig. 24-11). The lung parenchyma is replaced by ropy or lamellar hyaline collagen resembling that seen in keloids of the skin. The collagen is characteristically arrayed in a disorderly, whorled or storiform fashion but has a tendency to layer concentrically around small blood vessels (figs. 24-12, 24-13). Large blood vessels entrapped within the hyalinized nodule may be obliterated (fig. 29-14). There is a mild infiltrate of plasma cells and lymphocytes that can be prominent at the margin of the nodules (fig. 24-15). There may be admixed macrophages and a few multinucleated giant cells, neutrophils, or eosinophils. Karyorrhectic nuclei and microcalcification may be seen between the collagen bundles, but broad areas of necrosis are rare. If necrosis is found, the case should be studied for fungal and bacterial organisms (45,47). Non-necrotizing epithelioid granulomas are very unusual. Special stains for acid fast bacilli and fungi are negative. Rarely, hyalinizing lesions microscopically identical to those in lung are also found in other organs such as kidney and tonsil (38,47).

Ultrastructural Findings. It seems likely that the initial reports of congophilia (39,40,45) were due to factitious staining, since neither histologic study of a subsequent large series of cases nor electron microscopic evaluation has confirmed the presence of amyloid (42,47). Rather, electron-dense, compact, homogeneous, amorphous material and swollen collagen fibrils are present (42).

Etiology and Pathogenesis. The etiology and pathogenesis of hyalinizing granuloma are unknown. Possibly, it results from an exaggerated immune and fibrotic reaction to antigens such as *Histoplasma capsulatum* or mycobacteria (37,47). For example, pulmonary hyalinizing granuloma is histologically similar to sclerosing mediastinitis, the two diseases may occur together, and it therefore appears reasonable that they share a common pathogenesis (37,38). Sclerosing mediastinitis can be associated with histoplasmosis or tuberculosis, and some cases are probably an exaggerated immunologic response to these organisms. By analogy, the same may be true for pulmonary hyalinizing granuloma. Rarely, patients have clear evidence of healed histoplasmosis prior to the development of hyalinizing granuloma (38); however, only a few have documented fungal or tuberculous exposure (40,47). No patients are known to have been exposed to methylsergide, another proposed etiologic agent for sclerosing mediastinitis.

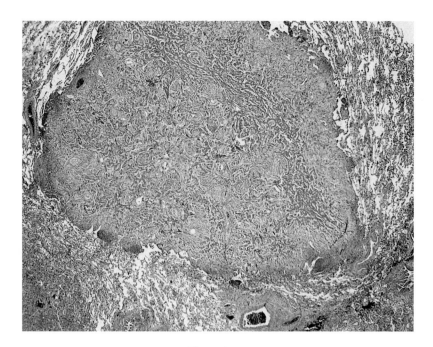

Figure 24-11
LOW MAGNIFICATION MICROSCOPIC VIEW OF PULMONARY HYALINIZING GRANULOMA
The lesion obliterates the underlying lung architecture and appears reasonably well circumscribed. The darker areas at the edge of the lesion are due to a chronic inflammatory infiltrate. (Fig. 1 from Yousem SA, Hocholzer L. Pulmonary hyalinizing granuloma. Am J Clin Pathol 1987;87:1–6.)

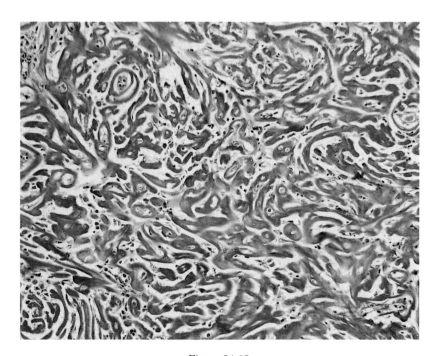

Figure 24-12
PULMONARY HYALINIZING GRANULOMA
This view shows the characteristic ropy or lamellar hyaline collagen arrayed in a whorled or storiform fashion.

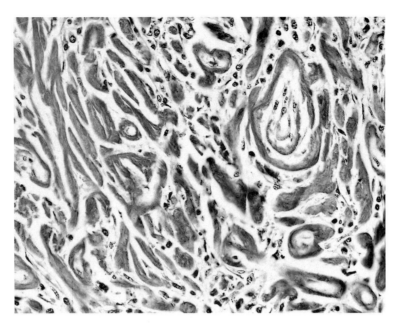

Figure 24-13
PULMONARY HYALINIZING GRANULOMA
Higher magnification view shows the thick collagen bundles that are concentrically layered around small blood vessels, along with a scattering of interspersed mononuclear cells (principally lymphocytes and plasma cells).

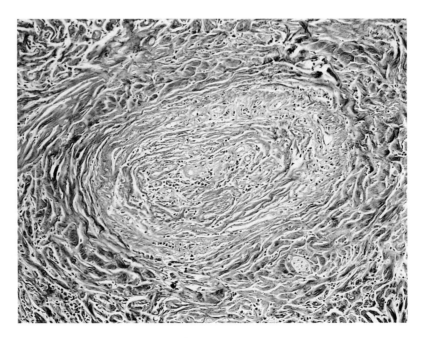

Figure 24-14
LARGE BLOOD VESSEL IN PULMONARY HYALINIZING GRANULOMA
The vascular lumen is obliterated by concentrically arrayed fibrous connective tissue.

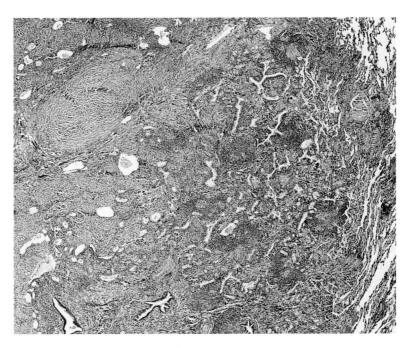

Figure 24-15
MARGIN OF THE NODULE IN PULMONARY HYALINIZING GRANULOMA
There is an intense chronic inflammatory infiltrate of lymphocytes and plasma cells locally infiltrating the interstitium of the adjacent lung.

Up to 60 percent of patients with hyalinizing granuloma have serologic evidence of autoimmunity, such as elevated titers of antinuclear, antismooth muscle, antimicrosomal, and antithyroglobulin antibodies, and rheumatoid factor (39,45,47). Whether autoimmunity is a preexisting and predisposing factor or occurs subsequent to the disease is unclear.

Differential Diagnosis. The differential diagnosis of pulmonary hyalinizing granuloma is shown in Table 24-3. Sclerosed plasma cell granulomas (inflammatory pseudotumors) can be difficult to distinguish, and in fact some cases of hyalinizing granuloma may result from sclerosis of plasma cell granulomas (47). Some differences do exist. Plasma cell granulomas, unlike hyalinizing granulomas, are usually solitary. They show a more diffuse and heavy infiltrate of plasma cells and lymphocytes and tend to lack the lamellar collagen bundles typical of hyalinizing granuloma.

Intrapulmonary fibrous tumor (chapter 19) presents as a solitary subpleural mass or nodule, rather than as multiple nodules of more diverse location. Further, intrapulmonary fibrous tumor, like its counterpart on the pleural surface, shows greater cellularity and a variety of histologic patterns, such as focal storiform or hemangiopericytomatous areas, features not seen in hyalinizing granulomas. Finally, intrapulmonary fibrous tumors lack a lymphoplasmacytic infiltrate.

Nodular amyloidosis may occur as multiple nodules, but hyalinizing granuloma has distinct lamellar collagen bands and fewer giant cells, and is less likely to show metaplastic ossification. Overstaining of a hyalinized lesion with Congo red may sometimes lead to an incorrect diagnosis of amyloid, but hyalinizing granuloma lacks the typical fibrillar substructure of amyloid by electron microscopy.

Infectious granulomas, especially histoplasmosis, may show hyaline collagen bands, but they are generally arrayed in parallel around areas of central necrosis rather than distributed in a haphazard manner as in hyalinizing granuloma. The presence of necrotizing granulomatous inflammation favors infection, as does the finding of

Table 24-3

DIFFERENTIAL DIAGNOSIS OF PULMONARY HYALINIZING GRANULOMA

	Nodular Amyloid	Pulmonary Hyalinizing Granuloma	Plasma Cell Granuloma	Intrapulmonary Fibrous Tumor	Histo-plasmosis
Lamellar collagen	0*	+	+/0	+	+
Lymphoid infiltrate	+	+	+	0	+
Extensive necrosis	occasional	rare	rare	0	+
Congo red affinity	+	0	0	0	0
Single/multiple	+/+	occasional/+	+/rare	+/0	+/+
Necrotizing granuloma	0	0	0	0	+

*0 = absent; + = present.

calcified hilar lymph nodes. Nevertheless, distinction between the two diseases may be difficult and we have seen examples of hyalinizing granuloma in which a small satellite focus of necrotizing granuloma is present, suggesting that *Histoplasma* or some other organism may initiate pulmonary hyalinizing granuloma in some cases.

A number of lymphoid lesions can occasionally produce difficulties in the differential diagnosis. Sclerosing non-Hodgkin lymphoma and nodular sclerosing Hodgkin disease, especially after treatment, may cause particular problems in this regard. Still, Hodgkin disease localized to lung is rare; involvement of the lung usually occurs by direct extension from a mediastinal tumor or, in the case of multiple pulmonary nodules, as a result of dissemination of established systemic disease. Attention to the increased cellularity and cytologic appearance of the lymphoid cells seen in Hodgkin disease and non-Hodgkin lymphoma aids in differential diagnosis.

Treatment and Prognosis. There is no effective therapy, but the prognosis is still very good. Patients have been followed up to 28 years with stable or slowly enlarging nodules. Radiologic progression may sometimes be accompanied by increasing dyspnea. Rarely, coalescent nodules may lead to respiratory insufficiency. Concurrent mediastinal or retroperitoneal sclerosis can result in entrapment of vessels and airways with resultant sequelae (38,40).

PULMONARY MALAKOPLAKIA

Definition. Pulmonary malakoplakia is a chronic inflammatory disorder of uncertain etiology characterized by tumor-like aggregates of benign macrophages containing characteristic intracellular calcified (Michaelis-Gutmann) bodies. Malakoplakia was initially described in, and most commonly affects, the urinary tract, particularly the bladder, in patients with chronic urinary tract infections (48,50,51); nevertheless, it can occur in numerous other sites ranging from tongue to vagina. The lung is a rare site of involvement (48).

Clinical Features. Patients who have pulmonary malakoplakia are adults with some form of compromised immunity or underlying illness. The associated diseases include acquired immunodeficiency syndrome, cardiac transplantation, Hodgkin disease, alcohol abuse, and emaciation. The chest X ray may show a single cavitary or noncavitary mass, or multiple bilateral nodular densities. This appearance may suggest recurrent neoplasm in patients with a history of tumor (50). Malakoplakic masses may also intrude into a bronchial lumen, simulating cancer (fig. 24-16) (49). The diagnosis is made using transbronchial biopsy and needle aspiration (49). Cultures taken at the time of bronchoscopy or autopsy show a variety of bacteria, most often *Rhodococcus equi* or *Escherichia coli* (50,52). Pulmonary malakoplakia may be associated with

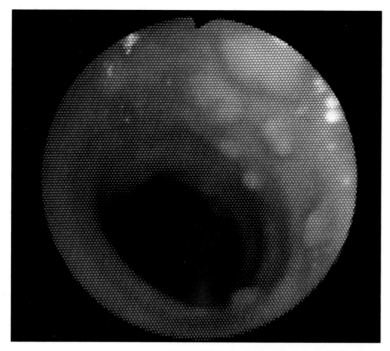

Figure 24-16
PULMONARY MALAKOPLAKIA:
BRONCHOSCOPIC APPEARANCE
As shown here through the bronchoscope, malakoplakia can involve the bronchial mucosa in the form of small nodules.

Figure 24-17
PULMONARY
MALAKOPLAKIA:
GROSS APPEARANCE
The cut surface of the lung shows a cream-colored and red mass that compresses surrounding parenchyma. Satellite areas of pneumonic consolidation are also present.

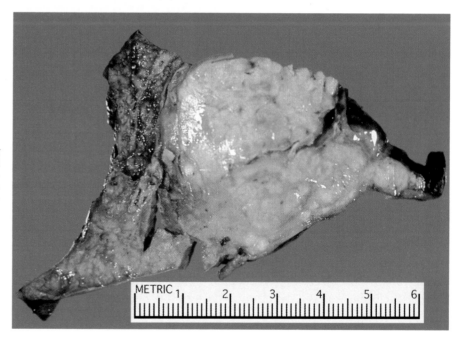

malakoplakia elsewhere in the body, such as bladder and kidney, cerebellum, and perianal region.

Gross and Microscopic Findings. Grossly, the lesions are tan-yellow or gray, well demarcated, and slightly firm to palpation (fig. 24-17). Cavitation may be present. Histologically, the lung architecture is usually effaced by sheets of macrophages (von Hansemann histiocytes) associated with variable numbers of lymphocytes, plasma cells, and neutrophils (fig. 24-18). The inflammatory mass is sometimes ringed by granulation tissue. The macrophages have abundant, coarsely granular cytoplasm (fig. 24-19). The granules vary in size and shape, are periodic

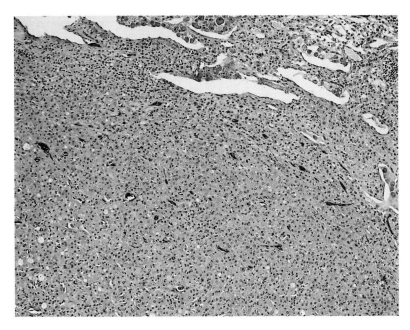

Figure 24-18
PULMONARY MALAKOPLAKIA
A solid mass of pale macrophages obliterates the underlying lung. The border with relatively uninvolved lung is seen on the upper right.

acid–Schiff (PAS) positive, and diastase resistant. A diagnostic finding is the presence of intracellular and extracellular basophilic, laminated calcospherites measuring 5 to 10 mm in diameter: Michaelis-Gutmann bodies (fig. 24-19). The bodies stain for calcium and iron. Bacterial stains usually show intracellular bacterial aggregates.

By electron microscopy, the macrophage granules seen by light microscopy correspond to intracytoplasmic membrane-bound bodies, some of which contain degenerating bacteria (50). Michaelis-Gutmann bodies show concentric laminations of variable electron density (fig. 24-20). Some of the bodies contain radially arrayed crystalline material. Electron microprobe and X ray diffraction analyses show the bodies to consist of iron mixed with calcium and phosphorus as amorphous calcium phosphate and hydroxyapatite (50).

Etiology and Pathogenesis. The underlying defect is currently believed to be an acquired inability to maintain intralysosomal pH, leading to reduced bactericidal activity and accumulation of lysosomes (48). This may in turn be due to reduced carbonic anhydrase activity caused by an as yet unidentified bacterial toxin (48). A

deficiency of the lysosomal enzyme 3',5'-guanosine monophosphate dehydrogenase has been reported (53). How immunosuppression or underlying debilitating disorders might lead to this result is unclear.

Differential Diagnosis. Accumulations of histiocytes with granular cytoplasm can occur in immunosuppressive disorders, particularly acquired immunodeficiency syndrome, as a response to a number of infectious disorders. These include *Mycobacterium avium-intracellulare* complex, *Cryptococcus neoformans,* and *Histoplasma capsulatum.* Acid fast and fungal stains usually exclude these possibilities. Whipple disease occasionally involves the lung, but the histiocytes are more likely to be interstitial in location, lack Michaelis-Gutmann bodies, and show characteristic PAS-positive bacillary inclusions. Endogenous lipid pneumonia may show intra-alveolar foamy macrophages secondary to airway obstruction, but lacks Michaelis-Gutmann bodies and bacteria. Finally, renal cell carcinoma with clear cell features is usually easily dismissed because malakoplakic cells express macrophage markers rather than cytokeratin.

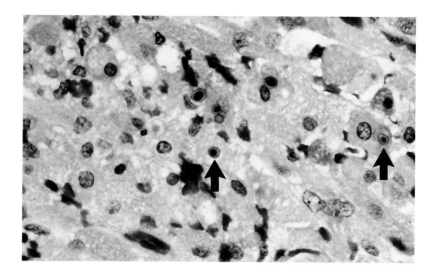

Figure 24-19
PULMONARY MALAKOPLAKIA
A sheet of histiocytes with abundant pale cytoplasm and ill-defined cell borders is present. Concentrically laminated, oval Michaelis-Gutmann bodies are seen within the cytoplasm of some macrophages (arrows).

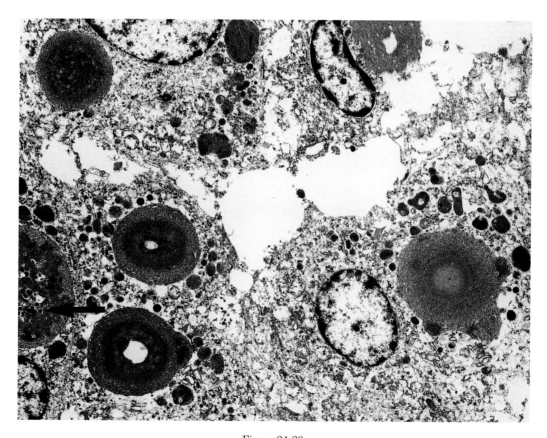

Figure 24-20
ELECTRON MICROSCOPIC APPEARANCE OF PULMONARY MALAKOPLAKIA
This view shows several intracellular laminated electron-dense Michaelis-Gutmann bodies. Structures believed to be degenerated bacteria are present within one of the bodies (arrow).

Treatment and Prognosis. The disease is most often treated with antibiotics. The mortality is high, but it is uncertain whether this is due to underlying disease or associated infection (52).

ROUNDED ATELECTASIS

Definition. Rounded atelectasis is a localized area of subpleural lung collapse associated with visceral pleural fibrosis that radiographically presents as a pulmonary mass. Other synonymous terms include *round atelectasis, folded lung syndrome, shrinking pleuritis with atelectasis, vanishing lung, Blesovsky syndrome,* and *atelectatic pseudotumor.*

Clinical Features. Most patients are asymptomatic adult men (56,58). A history of exposure to asbestos is common (60).

Chest X ray shows a round or oval, pleural-based shadow measuring 2 to 7 cm, forming an acute angle with the pleura (58,59). Most cases are in the posterior aspect of a lower lobe, which usually shows volume loss. Infrequently, bilateral lesions occur or there may be spontaneous resolution (56,57). A frequently present pathognomonic finding is the "comet's tail sign," one or more curvilinear shadows that curl from the hilum towards the inferior pole of the mass (56,61). Computerized axial tomography is a sensitive method for detecting this sign (fig. 24-21). It can also be used to demonstrate visceral or parietal pleural thickening, and sometimes effusion.

Bronchoscopic biopsy is nondiagnostic and fine needle aspiration of limited use in evaluation of the "mass" because a negative result does not exclude malignancy. The diagnosis may be suggested at thoracotomy by the presence of visceral pleural fibrosis corresponding to the area of the lesion (56). The parietal pleura often shows fibrous plaques (58). Wedge resection or lobectomy is usually performed (58).

Gross Findings. The visceral pleura is irregularly thickened, white or gray, and may adhere to parietal pleura (fig. 24-22). The lung beneath the pleural scar shows a corresponding ill-defined area of atelectasis that may contain deeply invaginated folds of visceral pleura up to 2 cm in length (55,58). Typically, the "mass" disappears as it is dissected. Parietal pleural biopsies may show hyaline plaques.

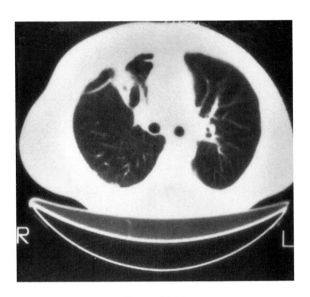

Figure 24-21
ROUNDED ATELECTASIS
This computerized axial tomograph shows the typical appearance. A wedge-shaped peripheral mass is present in the right middle lobe. There are curvilinear strands with a "comet's tail" appearance.

Microscopic Findings. There is microscopic fibrosis of the visceral pleura ranging from hyaline plaque-like lesions to more loose and chronically inflamed fibrous connective tissue. The fibrosis is typically superficial to the pleural elastic lamina, which is often deeply folded and invaginated into the subjacent lung, a finding that can be verified through the use of elastic stains (figs. 24-23–24-25) (58). The subjacent lung shows atelectasis (fig. 24-25). Fibrous connective tissue may extend down the lobular septa from the pleura, producing finger-like projections into the atelectatic alveolar parenchyma. In the cases associated with asbestos exposure (see below), there may be asbestos bodies and interstitial fibrosis (asbestosis).

Etiology and Pathogenesis. At least 65 percent of patients have a definite history of exposure to asbestos, but other causes of chronic pleuritis such as tuberculosis and histoplasmosis, lung infarcts, and congestive heart failure have also been associated with rounded atelectasis.

A pathogenetic theory that is currently in favor is "shrinking pleuritis," wherein localized visceral pleural fibrosis produces subsequent shrinkage and folding of the pleura, resulting in

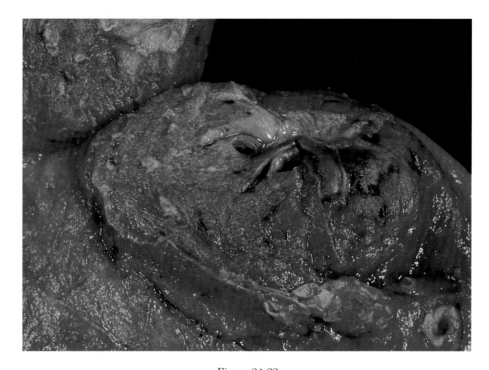

Figure 24-22
ROUNDED ATELECTASIS: GROSS APPEARANCE
The pleural surface is puckered and the underlying lung collapsed in association with an area of anthracotic scarring.

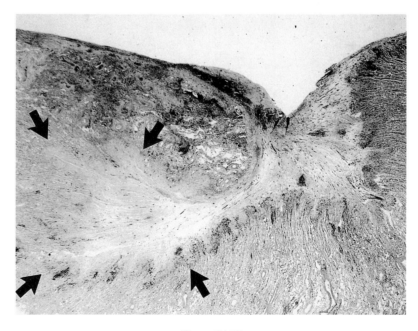

Figure 24-23
ROUNDED ATELECTASIS
A scanning magnification view shows fibrous thickening and invagination (arrows) of visceral pleura. The contiguous lung is atelectatic.

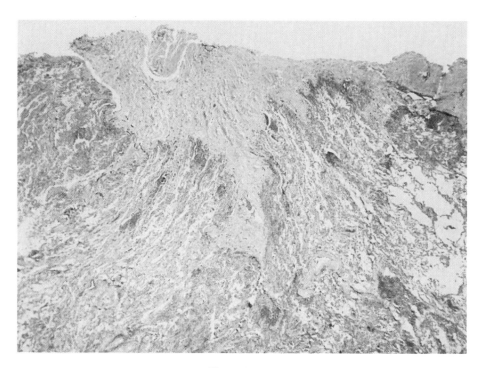

Figure 24-24
ROUNDED ATELECTASIS
Scanning magnification view of thickened, markedly fibrotic visceral pleura in rounded atelectasis. Part of the pleura is invaginated into lung, which is atelectatic.

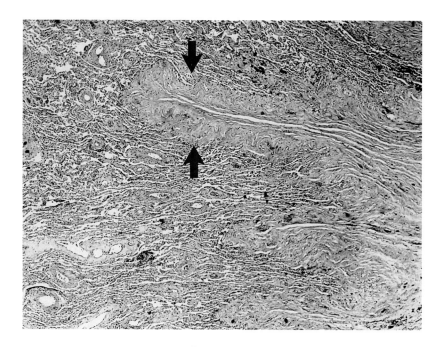

Figure 24-25
ROUNDED ATELECTASIS
The fibrotic visceral pleura is thrown into a series of waves, some of which are deeply invaginated into subjacent lung (arrows). The underlying lung is atelectatic.

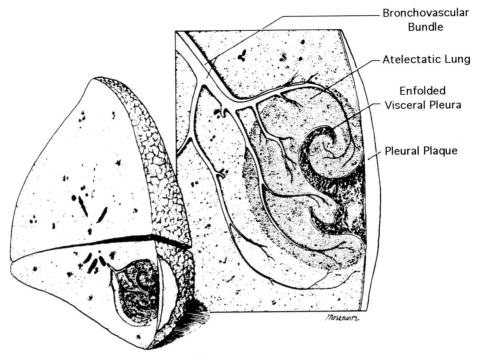

★ Diagrammatic Representation of a Rounded Area of Atelectasis beneath a Pleural Plaque.

Figure 24-26
ROUNDED ATELECTASIS
Schematic drawing showing proposed pathogenesis of the lesion. The fibrotic pleura of a lower lobe enfolds in a spiral manner, entrapping and collapsing subjacent lung. The folding of the lung gives a curvilinear configuration to bronchovascular structures feeding the entrapped parenchyma ("comet's tail sign"). (Fig. 4 from Mark EJ. Case records of the Massachusetts General Hospital. Case 24-1983. N Engl J Med 1983;308:1466–72.)

atelectasis of the underlying lung that assumes a rounded appearance and produces a mass on chest radiographic studies (fig. 24-26) (54).

Differential Diagnosis. The pathologist may be misled by the clinical presumption of lung cancer when a mass lesion occurs in an asbestos worker. The disappearance of the mass under gross dissection is key to the correct diagnosis.

The infolded fibrotic visceral pleura that is a hallmark of rounded atelectasis may suggest an intrapulmonary scar. Elastic stains will show the relationship to visceral pleura.

Treatment and Prognosis. Radiologically diagnosed lesions usually remain stable, but they may increase or spontaneously decrease in size over weeks to months (61). When the diagnosis is made at thoracotomy, decortication appears to be adequate treatment and the involved lung often reinflates. Recurrence is rare after decortication (61).

FOCAL ORGANIZING PNEUMONIA

A subset of patients with idiopathic *bronchiolitis obliterans-organizing pneumonia (BOOP)* present with solitary localized masses that can simulate cancer (63). We have elected to use the term focal organizing pneumonia for these cases. Very likely, some of the cases reported by Ackerman and associates (62) as "localized organized pneumonia" also fit into this category. Patients may have a history of fever, cough, dyspnea, or even hemoptysis. Usually a solitary opacity, sometimes cavitary, occurs in an upper lobe. By definition, the etiology of these cases is unclear.

Pathologically, the lung shows areas of gray-red to light yellow parenchymal consolidation corresponding to the radiographic lesion (62). Microscopically, focal organization by intra-alveolar plugs of fibrous connective tissue (Masson bodies) is found (figs. 24-27, 24-28). Interstitial inflammatory cells,

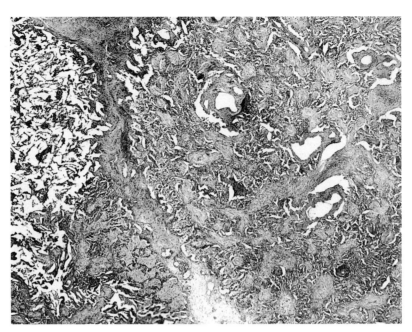

Figure 24-27
FOCAL ORGANIZING
PNEUMONIA
This type of localized consolidation of the lung may appear as a mass lesion in the chest X ray. Note the uninvolved adjacent lung (left).

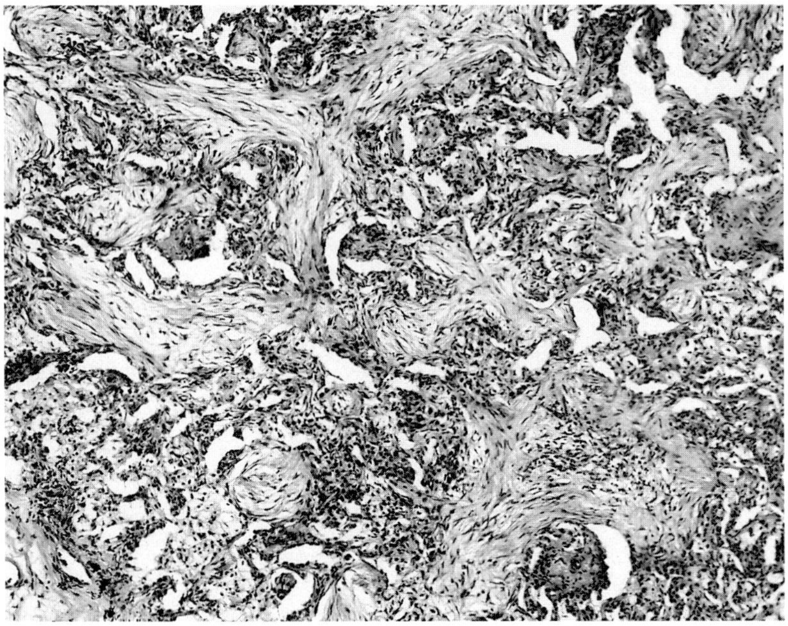

Figure 24-28
FOCAL ORGANIZING
PNEUMONIA
There are intra-alveolar tufts of fibrous connective tissue (Masson bodies). This finding may be seen in organizing pneumonias of infectious origin as well as in idiopathic bronchiolitis obliterans-organizing pneumonia.

usually lymphocytes, are common. Finally, alveolar collections of foamy macrophages due to bronchiolar obstruction may be prominent. When there is extensive central obliteration of the underlying lung architecture, the histology may suggest inflammatory pseudotumor (see figs. 19-2–19-4).

Cytologic studies of localized pneumonias may prove a pitfall for the pathologist. Both sputum cytology (62) and fine needle aspiration specimens may yield remarkably atypical epithelial cells with prominent nuclei and nucleoli, leading to a false diagnosis of cancer.

REFERENCES

Amyloidosis

1. Abe Y, Utsunomiya H, Tsutsumi Y. Atypical carcinoid tumor of the lung with amyloid stroma. Acta Pathol Jpn 1992;42:286–92.
2. Al-Kaisi N, Abdul-Karim FW, Mendelsohn G, Jacobs G. Bronchial carcinoid tumor with amyloid stroma. Arch Pathol Lab Med 1988;112:211–4.
3. Bonner H Jr, Ennis RS, Geelhoed GW, Tarpley TM Jr. Lymphoid infiltration and amyloidosis of lung in Sjogren's syndrome. Arch Pathol 1973;95:42–4.
4. Chen KT. Amyloidosis presenting in the respiratory tract. Pathol Annu 1989;24(Pt 1):253–73.
5. Colby TV, Carrington CB. Pulmonary lymphomas: current concepts. Hum Pathol 1983;14:884–7.
6. Dahlgren SE, Lewenhaupt A, Ovenfors CO. Fine needle biopsy diagnosis in nodular pulmonary amyloidosis. Acta Path Microbiol Scand [A] 1970;78:1–5.
7. Davis CJ, Butchart EG, Gibbs AR. Nodular pulmonary amyloidosis occurring in association with pulmonary lymphoma. Thorax 1991;46:217–8.
8. Dictor M, Hasserius R. Systemic amyloidosis and non-hematologic malignancy in a large autopsy series. Acta Pathol Microbiol Scand [A] 1981;89:411–6.
9. Dyke PC, Demaray MJ, Delavan JW, Rasmussen RA. Pulmonary amyloidoma. Am J Clin Pathol 1974;61:301–5.
10. Fenoglio C, Pascal RR. Nodular amyloidosis of the lungs. An unusual case associated with chronic lung disease and carcinoma of the bladder. Arch Pathol 1970;90:577–82.
11. Firestone FN, Joison J. Amyloidosis. A cause of primary tumors of the lung. J Thorac Cardiovasc Surg 1966;51:292–9.
12. Glenner GG. Amyloid deposits and amyloidosis. The beta-fibrilloses. N Engl J Med 1980;302:1283–92,1333–43.
13. Gordon HW, Miller R Jr, Mittman C. Medullary carcinoma of the lung with amyloid stroma: a counterpart of medullary carcinoma of the thyroid. Hum Pathol 1973;4:431–6.
14. Holmes S, Desai JB, Sapsford RN. Nodular pulmonary amyloidosis: a case report and review of literature. Br J Dis Chest 1988;82:414–7.
15. Hui AN, Koss MN, Hochholzer L, Wehunt WD. Amyloidosis presenting in the lower respiratory tract. Clinicopathologic, radiologic, immunohistochemical, and histochemical studies on 48 cases. Arch Pathol Lab Med 1986;110:212–8.
16. Kijner CH, Yousem SA. Systemic light chain deposition disease presenting as multiple pulmonary nodules. A case report and review of the literature. Am J Surg Pathol 1988;12:405–13.
17. Knapp MJ, Roggli VL, Kim J, Moore JO, Shelburne JD. Pleural amyloidosis. Arch Pathol Lab Med 1988;112:57–60.
18. Kobayashi H, Matsuoka R, Kitamura S, Tsunoda N, Saito K. Sjogren's syndrome with multiple bullae and pulmonary nodular amyloidosis. Chest 1988;94:438–40.
19. Koss MN, Hochholzer L, Langloss J, Wehunt WD, Lazarus AA. Lymphoid interstitial pneumonia: clinico-pathological and immunopathological findings in 18 cases. Pathology 1987;19:178–85.
20. _____, Hochholzer L, Nichols PW, Wehunt WD, Lazarus AA. Primary non-Hodgkin's lymphoma and pseudolymphoma of lung: a study of 161 patients. Hum Pathol 1983;14:1024–38.
21. Kradin R, Mark E. Benign lymphoid disorders of the lung, with a theory regarding their development. Hum Pathol 1983;14:857–67.
22. Laden SA, Cohen ML, Harley RA. Nodular pulmonary amyloidosis with extrapulmonary involvement. Hum Pathol 1984;15:594–7.
23. Mata JM, Caceres J, Senac JP, Giron J, Alegret X. General case of the day. Nodular amyloidosis of the lung. Radiographics 1991;11:716–8.
24. Morgan JE, McCaul DS, Rodriguez FH, Abernathy DA, deShazo RD, Banks DE. Pulmonary immunologic features of alveolar septal amyloidosis associated with multiple myeloma. Chest 1987;92:704–8.
25. Morinaga S, Watanabe H, Gemma A, et al. Plasmacytoma of the lung associated with nodular deposits of immunoglobulin. Am J Surg Pathol 1987;11:989–95.
26. Page DL, Isersky C, Harada M, Glenner GG. Immunoglobulin origin of localized nodular pulmonary amyloidosis. Res Exp Med 1972;159:75–86.
27. Pepys MB. Amyloidosis. Some recent developments. Q J Med 1988;67:283–98.
28. Polansky SM, Ravin CE. Nodular pulmonary infiltrate in a patient with Sjogren's syndrome. Chest 1980;77:411–2.
29. Richmond I, Hasleton PS, Samedian S. Systemic amyloid associated with carcinoma of the bronchus. Thorax 1990;45:156–7.
30. Saab SB, Burke J, Hopeman A, Almond C. Primary pulmonary amyloidosis. Report of two cases. J Thorac Cardiovasc Surg 1974;67:301–7.
31. Schuller H, Bolin H, Linder E, Stenram U. Tumor-forming amyloidosis of the lower respiratory system. Report of a case in the lung and a short review of the literature. Dis Chest 1962;42:58–67.
32. Stone MJ. Amyloidosis: A final common pathway for protein deposition in tissues. Blood 1990;75:531–45.
33. Strimlan CV, Rosenow EC III, Weiland LH, Brown LR. Lymphocytic interstitial pneumonitis. Review of 13 cases. Ann Int Med 1978;88:616–21.
34. Thompson PJ, Citron KM. Amyloid and the lower respiratory tract. Thorax 1983;38:84–7.
35. Wilson W, Sanders D, Delarue N. Intrathoracic manifestations of amyloid disease. Radiology 1976;120:283–9.
36. Yousem SA. Pulmonary adenosquamous carcinomas with amyloid-like stroma. Mod Pathol 1989;2:420–6.

Pulmonary Hyalinizing Granuloma

37. Case records of the Massachusetts General Hospital. Case 6-1989. N Engl J Med 1989;320:380–9.
38. Chalaoui J, Gregoire P, Sylvestre J, Lefebvre R, Amyot R. Pulmonary hyalinizing granuloma: a cause of pulmonary nodules. Radiology 1984;152:23–6.
39. Dent RG, Godden DJ, Stovin PG, Stark JE. Pulmonary hyalinizing granuloma in association with retroperitoneal fibrosis. Thorax 1983;38:955–6.
40. Engleman P, Liebow AA, Gmelich J, Friedman PJ. Pulmonary hyalinizing granuloma. Am Rev Resp Dis 1977;115:997–1008.

41. Gans SJ, van der Elst AM, Straks W. Pulmonary hyalinizing granuloma. Eur Respir J 1988;1:389–91.

42. Guccion JG, Rohatgi PK, Saini N. Pulmonary hyalinizing granuloma. Electron microscopic and immunologic studies. Chest 1984;85:571–3.

43. Ikard RW. Pulmonary hyalinizing granuloma. Chest 1988;93:871–2.

44. Patel Y, Ishikawa S, MacDonnell KF. Pulmonary hyalinizing granuloma presenting as multiple cavitary calcified nodules. Chest 1991;100:1720–1.

45. Schlosnagle DC, Check IJ, Sewell CW, Plummer A, York RM, Hunter RL. Immunologic abnormalities in two patients with pulmonary hyalinizing granuloma. Am J Clin Pathol 1982;78:231–5.

46. Ulbright T, Katzenstein A. Solitary necrotizing granulomas of the lung. Differentiating features and etiology. Am J Surg Pathol 1980;4:13-28.

47. Yousem SA, Hochholzer L. Pulmonary hyalinizing granuloma. Am J Clin Pathol 1987;87:1–6.

Pulmonary Malakoplakia

48. Byard R, Bourne A, Thorner P. Malacoplakia of the lung—a review. Surgical Pathology 1991;4:301–7.

49. Colby TV, Hunt S, Pelzmann K, Carrington CB. Malakoplakia of the lung: a report of two cases. Respiration 1980;39:295–9.

50. Crouch E, White V, Wright J, Churg A. Malakoplakia mimicking carcinoma metastatic to lung. Am J Surg Pathol 1984;8:151–6.

51. Damjanov I, Katz SM. Malakoplakia. Pathol Annu 1981;16:103–26.

52. Schwartz DA, Ogden PO, Blumberg HM, Honig E. Pulmonary malakoplakia in a patient with the acquired immunodeficiency syndrome. Differential diagnostic considerations. Arch Pathol Lab Med 1990;114:1267–72.

53. Shabtai M, Anaise D, Frei L, et al. Malakoplakia in renal transplantation: an expression of altered tissue reactivity under immunosuppression. Transplant Proc 1989;21:3725–7.

Rounded Atelectasis

54. Case records of the Massachusetts General Hospital. Case 24:1983. N Engl J Med 1983;308:1466–72.

55. Dernevik L, Gatzinsky P. Pathogenesis of shrinking pleuritis with atelectasis—rounded atelectasis. Eur J Respir Dis 1987;71:244–9.

56. Franzblau A. Asbestos-associated rounded atelectasis: a case report and review of the literature. Mt Sinai J Med 1989;56:321–5.

57. Hillerdal G. Rounded atelectasis. Clinical experience with 74 patients. Chest 1989;95:836–41.

58. Menzies R, Fraser R. Round atelectasis. Pathologic and pathogenetic features. Am J Surg Pathol 1987;11:674–81.

59. Mintzer RA, Cugell DW. The association of asbestos-induced pleural disease and rounded atelectasis. Chest 1982;81:457–60.

60. _____, Gore RM, Vogelzang RL, Holz S. Rounded atelectasis and its association with asbestos-induced pleural disease. Radiology 1981;139:567–70.

61. Szydlowski GW, Cohn HE, Steiner RM, Edie RN. Rounded atelectasis: a pulmonary pseudotumor. Ann Thorac Surg 1992;53:817–21.

Focal Organizing Pneumonia

62. Ackerman LV, Elliott GV, Alanis M. Localized organized pneumonia: its resemblance to carcinoma. AJR 1954;71:988–96.

63. Cordier JF, Loire R, Brune J. Idiopathic bronchiolitis obliterans organizing pneumonia. Definition of characteristic clinical profiles in a series of 16 patients. Chest 1989;96:999–1004.

✧✧✧

25

TUMORS METASTATIC TO THE LUNG

The lung is one of the most frequent sites of metastasis for extrathoracic tumors (Table 25-1). Between 20 to more than 50 percent of patients dying from extrapulmonary solid tumors develop metastases to lung (1,5,11,12,42). In 15 to 25 percent of these cases, lung involvement is the only manifestation of metastatic disease. Certain malignancies, namely malignant melanoma, some sarcomas, renal cell carcinoma, testicular tumors, uterine choriocarcinoma, breast carcinoma, and prostate and thyroid carcinoma show a particular tendency to metastasize to lung (Table 25-1). A variety of distinctive patterns of metastasis are recognized and discussed in the following section: multiple pulmonary nodules, and lymphangitic, endobronchial, embolic, solitary, and pleural metastases.

PATTERNS OF METASTASIS

Multiple Nodules

The most common presentation of pulmonary metastasis is in the form of multiple bilateral nodules or masses of varying sizes, ranging from miliary nodules to "cannonball" lesions (figs. 25-1–25-4). Grossly, the tumors are often well defined and variable in color. Thus, metastases with abundant associated fibrosis may be white or gray; metastatic malignant melanoma may be black or brown (fig. 25-3); vascular tumors may appear dark red or, when associated with considerable hemosiderin deposits, brown; and metastases containing abundant fat, such as renal cell carcinoma, adrenocortical carcinoma, or necrotic tumors, may appear yellow (fig. 25-2). Metastatic sarcomas and lymphomas typically have a pale, fish flesh appearance (fig. 25-4). Microscopically, the tumor nodules may be well demarcated from the surrounding parenchyma, with a pushing border, or they may invade the surrounding alveoli or interstitium (figs. 25-5, 25-6).

Metastatic nodules are most common in the lower lobes. Concomitant lymphangitic, endobronchial, or endovascular metastases may be present, producing a complicated gross appearance (fig. 25-1). The pattern of metastasis is only occasionally of aid in determining the primary site. In general, miliary nodules are particularly common in malignant melanoma, renal cell carcinoma, medullary carcinoma of the thyroid, and, on occasion, ovarian carcinoma. Cannonball metastases are most often seen in sarcomas, renal cell carcinoma, malignant melanoma, and colorectal carcinoma (11).

Lymphangitic Metastasis

When malignant cells extensively invade the pulmonary lymphatics, the term lymphangitic metastasis is used. Lymphangitic metastasis is fairly common, comprising 6 to 8 percent of all

Table 25-1

FREQUENCY OF METASTASES TO LUNG FOR SELECTED PRIMARY TUMORS*

Primary Tumor	Found at Autopsy (%)	Clinically Recognized Premortem (%)
Malignant melanoma	80	5 (2-5)**
Ewing sarcoma	77	18
Osteosarcoma	75	15
Germ cell tumors (testicular)	70-80	12
Choriocarcinoma (women)	70-100	60
Thyroid carcinoma	65	5-10
Breast carcinoma	60	5 (1-2)
Prostatic carcinoma	53	5
Rhabdomyosarcoma	55	21
Renal cell carcinoma	50-75	5-30
Colorectal carcinoma	40	5 (2)
Head and neck carcinoma[†]	40	5
Bladder carcinoma	30	5-10

*From references 8,10,14,15,24.
**Figures in parentheses refer to cases presenting clinically as a solitary pulmonary nodule.
[†]Tumors of the larynx, tonsil, and nasopharynx have a particularly high incidence of lung metastasis.

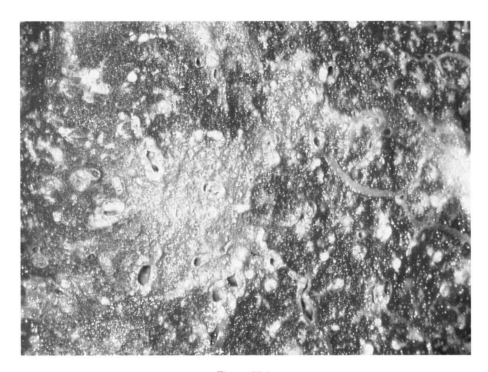

Figure 25-1
MILIARY AND LYMPHANGITIC METASTASIS

Numerous minute nodules, a larger area of ill-defined consolidation, and thickening of the walls of small blood vessels, interlobular septa, and airways are present.

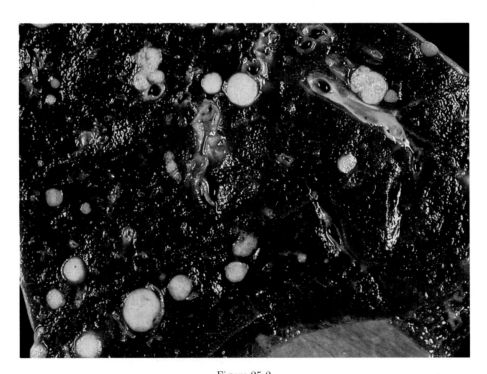

Figure 25-2
MULTINODULAR METASTASIS

The abundant fat content of the primary tumor, renal cell carcinoma, imparts a yellow appearance to the metastatic nodules.

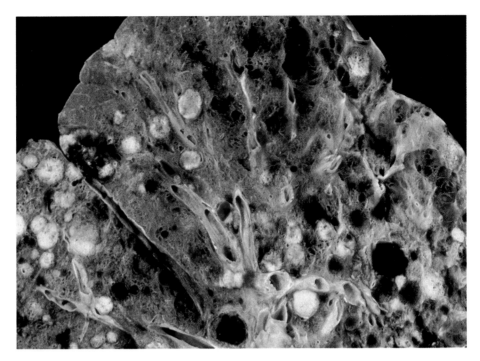

Figure 25-3
MULTINODULAR METASTASIS

The primary in this case was malignant melanoma. The abundant melanin pigment within the tumor produces a black appearance in some of the nodules.

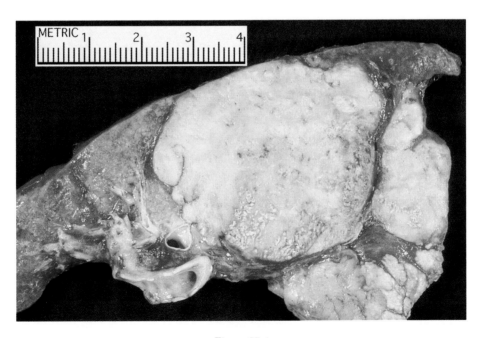

Figure 25-4
"CANNONBALL" METASTASIS

A variety of tumors, including sarcomas, renal cell carcinoma, malignant melanoma, and colorectal carcinoma produce this appearance. In this case, the primary tumor was osteogenic sarcoma.

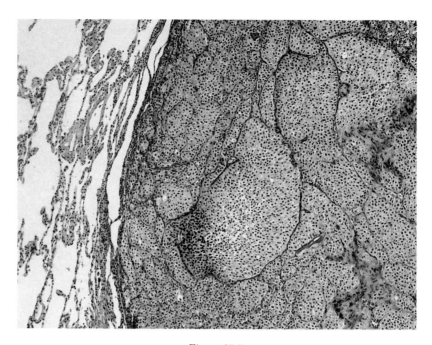

Figure 25-5
SHARPLY DEFINED NODULAR METASTASIS IN LUNG

The metastatic tumor, an alveolar soft part sarcoma, is well circumscribed with a pushing border. Metastases often have this appearance.

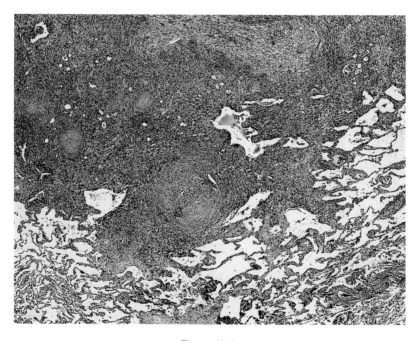

Figure 25-6
METASTASIS SHOWING IRREGULAR MARGIN

A nodule of metastatic leiomyosarcoma extends into the interstitium of the surrounding lung, producing this irregular border. A vessel has been overrun by the tumor in the center of the field.

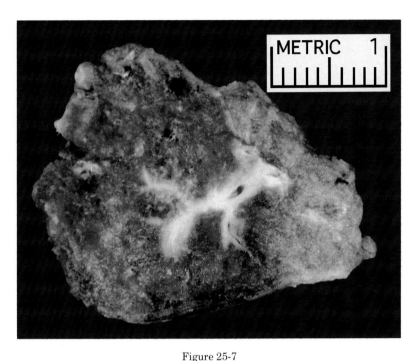

Figure 25-7
LYMPHANGITIC METASTASIS
The primary was a leiomyosarcoma. Note the arborizing pattern produced by tumor within perivascular lymphatics.

pulmonary metastases (42). Adenocarcinoma is the usual histologic subtype: 82 percent of cases in one study (42). The tumors are most often from lung, breast, gastrointestinal tract, or pancreas. The frequency of each primary site differs with the country and year of the study. For example, breast primaries are more common in North America whereas the stomach is a more common primary site in Japan. In addition, data from older studies may not reflect current demographic trends in the frequency of cancers or their metastases.

The presenting symptoms of lymphangitic metastasis are usually those of interstitial lung disease with dyspnea, nonproductive cough, and weight loss, sometimes without chest X-ray abnormalities (23,36). Computerized axial tomographic (CT) studies, particularly thin-section (1.5 mm) tomograms, are a more sensitive diagnostic tool than chest X ray (23). The prognosis is poor: 90 percent of patients die within 6 months (42).

Grossly, the lungs usually show diffuse linear and nodular thickening of the bronchovascular bundles, interlobular septa, and pleural and subpleural regions, i.e., the location of the pulmonary lymphatics (figs. 25-1, 25-7). The involve-

ment can be focal in early stages of disease or when the primary is bronchogenic carcinoma (23,36,42). There may or may not be associated parenchymal tumor nodules (fig. 25-1).

Microscopically, tumor cells are found in periarterial, peribronchial, or peribronchiolar lymphatics and in perivenous lymphatics both within and outside interlobular septa (figs. 25-8, 25-9). The fibrous connective tissue of the septa may be edematous early in the clinical course. Later, the tumor cells extend into the interstitium along the lymphatics or enter alveolar spaces to produce tumor nodules (fig. 25-9), sometimes with a striking desmoplastic response. Usually, this fibrous reaction comprises less than half of the resultant nodules (16). Sometimes, it is difficult to distinguish reactive alveolar hyperplasia in an area of pulmonary fibrosis from carcinoma. A striking variant of parenchymal involvement occurs when dyscohesive tumor cells fill alveoli to produce a tumoral "pneumonia" (fig. 25-10).

Localized areas of thickened pleura and sometimes underlying interlobular septa are typical of pleural disease (figs. 25-11, 25-21). Arterial tumor thrombi may also be found (16).

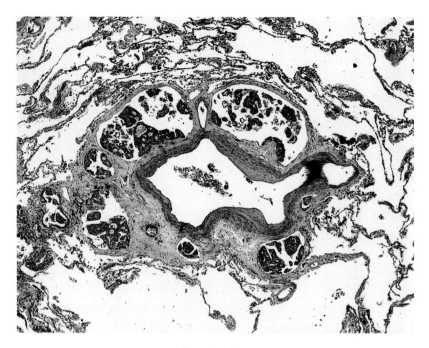

Figure 25-8
LYMPHANGITIC METASTASIS
The perivascular lymphatics are markedly dilated and filled with clumps of tumor cells, in this case metastatic breast carcinoma.

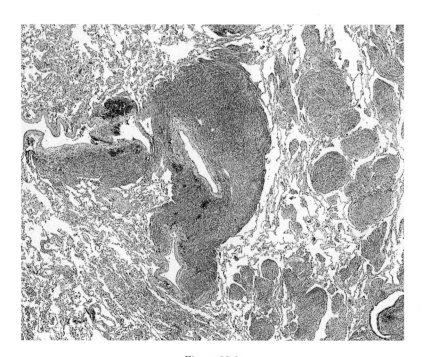

Figure 25-9
LYMPHANGITIC METASTASIS
Leiomyosarcoma encircles blood vessels and small airways in a lymphangitic pattern. The tumor has also extended into alveolar parenchyma in the form of multiple small nodules.

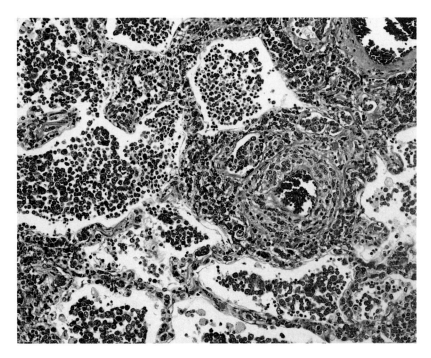

Figure 25-10
LYMPHANGITIC METASTASIS AND TUMORAL "PNEUMONIA"
The tumor involves not only the periarterial lymphatics but also extends into the vascular wall and the alveolar interstitium. Dyscohesive tumor cells have poured into the alveolar lumens, producing the low-power microscopic appearance of a pneumonia.

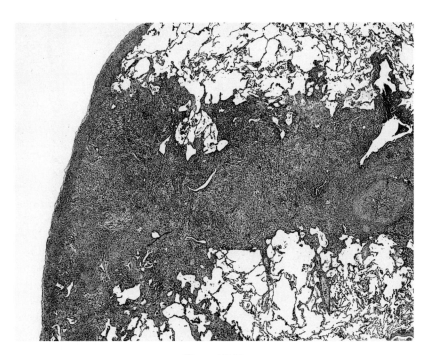

Figure 25-11
LYMPHANGITIC METASTASIS WITH PLEURAL INVOLVEMENT
The tumor, a metastatic leiomyosarcoma, thickens the visceral pleura and tracks along an underlying interlobular septum, an area rich in lymphatics, into lung. Note that the neoplasm has extended to involve a small artery and airway.

Because of the rich lymphatic supply of the bronchi, transbronchial biopsy is an effective means of diagnosing lymphangitic carcinoma (40). Still, the ease of diagnosis varies with the amount of tumor. There is usually no diagnostic problem in extensive disease when large groupings of cells distend the lymphatic channels in the bronchial walls, around bronchioles, and around arteries and veins (figs. 25-8, 25-9, 25-14). However, in some cases there may be only a few cells that are scarcely detectable by their atypical cytologic appearance and location within lymphatics. Malignant cells in the bronchial wall or in perivascular lymphatics can also be difficult to distinguish from pulmonary macrophages in tangentially cut alveolar spaces. Crush artefact or overstaining may also complicate interpretation of small numbers of cells within the bronchial wall. The intracytoplasmic particulate matter of macrophages usually aids in differential diagnosis. Step sections or mucin stains may also help.

Endobronchial Metastasis

Microscopic bronchial metastasis occurs in 18 to 51 percent of autopsied patients with extrapulmonary malignant tumors (5,11,26,27). Most cases result from invasion of the bronchus by tumor in nearby lung parenchyma or lymph nodes. Metastases involving only bronchus are unusual, seen in less than 5 percent of patients who die of solid tumors (11). The most common primary tumor sites are head and neck, breast, colon, rectum, and kidney (Table 25-2).

Rarely, endobronchial metastasis produces a clinical appearance that mimics primary lung cancer. Grossly visible metastases to a central or major bronchus from an extrathoracic solid tumor are found in 2 to 5 percent of autopsied cases and 1 to 2 percent of bronchoscopies of cancer patients (4,5,18,27). The most frequent primary tumors are breast, kidney, and colorectal carcinomas and sarcomas (8,27). In a series of thoracotomies for metastatic sarcoma, 4 percent of cases had clinically significant endobronchial involvement, most frequently due to metastatic leiomyosarcoma, but also caused by angiosarcoma, fibrosarcoma, osteogenic sarcoma, and malignant schwannoma (38).

Patients with a significant metastasis to bronchus develop symptoms and chest X-ray findings that closely mimic those of bronchogenic carci-

Table 25-2

FREQUENCY OF MICROSCOPIC ENDOBRONCHIAL METASTASIS AT AUTOPSY BY PRIMARY SITE*

Primary Site (Tumor Type)	%
Head and neck	31.0
Breast	14.0
Kidney	13.5
Large bowel	10.9
Uterus/cervix	7.8
Skin (malignant melanoma)	4.3
Soft tissues (sarcomas)	3.9
Thyroid	2.6
Urinary bladder	2.1
Ovary	1.7
Prostate	1.3
Esophagus	1.3
Testis	1.3
Pancreas	0.8
Adrenal	0.8
Stomach	0.4

*From reference 27.

noma. These include cough, hemoptysis, dyspnea, or chest pain, with a mass, infiltrate, or total or lobar collapse (4,8,12). Bronchoscopy may show a polypoid endobronchial mass.

Usually, endobronchial metastasis occurs late in the clinical course; only rarely does it produce symptoms. As expected, the prognosis is poor.

Grossly, the bronchus may appear concentrically narrowed or show a polypoid endobronchial nodule (figs. 25-12, 25-13). Histologically, metastatic tumor is most often seen in submucosal lymphatics; this may account for the low diagnostic yield of sputum cytologies (fig. 25-14) (27). In resection specimens, the most common pattern is infiltration of the bronchial wall from contiguous tumor in the lung, and occasionally there is invasion and replacement of the bronchial epithelial surface. As noted above, a polypoid mass may be the presenting finding, both in carcinomas and sarcomas (figs. 25-13).

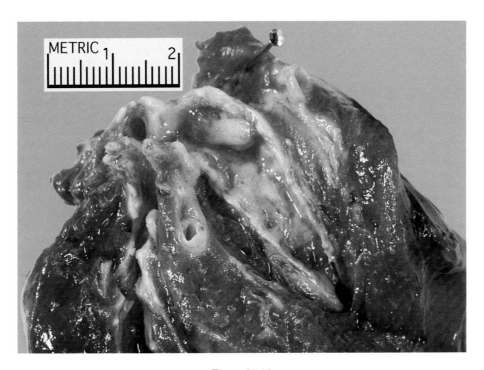

Figure 25-12
ENDOBRONCHIAL METASTASIS
A nodular lesion protrudes into the bronchial lesion. Microscopic examination revealed metastatic adrenocortical carcinoma.

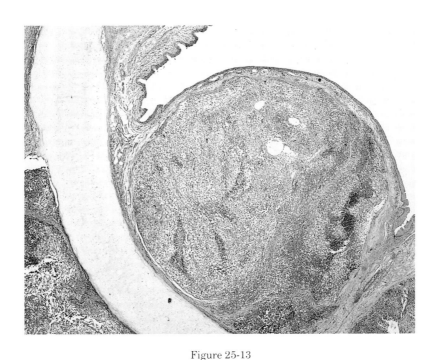

Figure 25-13
ENDOBRONCHIAL METASTASIS
A submucosal nodule of metastatic rhabdomyosarcoma produces nodular protrusion of the bronchial mucosa into the lumen.

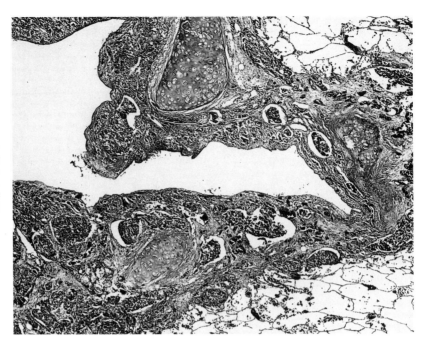

Figure 25-14
ENDOBRONCHIAL METASTASIS
Microscopic involvement of the airways is far more common than gross or clinically apparent involvement. A typical example is shown in this micrograph. Metastatic carcinoma dilates lymphatic channels within the submucosa of this cartilage-bearing bronchus.

Distinguishing endobronchial metastatic tumor from a lung primary is relatively easy if the patient has a known primary or multiple parenchymal nodules in lung (as is usually the case with metastatic disease); if slides of the extrapulmonary primary are available for comparison; or if the histologic appearance of the tumor is characteristic or incompatible with a lung primary (3,4). Problems arise when metastasis occurs a long time after excision of the primary tumor. For example, metastatic colorectal carcinoma to the airway has been described up to 16 years after the initial primary (8). Not only does a long interval raise the possibility of a new pulmonary primary, but slides of the primary tumor may not be available for review. Small sample size and poor differentiation or differentiation simulating a lung primary (e.g., mucinous adenocarcinoma or squamous cell carcinoma) cause difficulties (26). In problematic cases, the finding of in situ carcinoma in the bronchial epithelium points to lung cancer.

Metastatic Tumor Embolization

Tumor embolization of lung is common, occurring in 2 to 26 percent of autopsied patients with malignant neoplasms (11,19,31,41). The emboli can occur at any level of the arterial vasculature, and they range from a few scattered emboli to extensive embolization causing respiratory distress. Major tumor embolization may be defined as: 1) one or more emboli in segmental or larger arteries; 2) more than 5 emboli in elastic arteries of greater than 500 μm diameter; or 3) more than 15 tumor emboli in muscular vessels (up to 500 mm in diameter) (43). The affected vessels show emboli completely composed of tumor cells, tumor mixed with a fibrin thrombus, or organization of fibrin thrombi with eccentric subintimal fibrous cushions (31). While the diagnosis may be made by transbronchial biopsy, involvement of the microvasculature is more often diagnosed at autopsy. Cytologic examination of blood obtained by wedge pulmonary artery catheterization may be useful in making an antemortem diagnosis of microvascular metastasis (21).

Metastatic tumor emboli can occlude main or segmental pulmonary arteries; affect small muscular pulmonary arteries, arterioles, and capillaries; or affect distal vessels. Malignant emboli that occlude main or segmental arteries are rare (17,41). Renal cell carcinoma and hepatocellular carcinoma (neoplasms that invade veins) as well as chondrosarcoma, choriocarcinoma, and gastric adenocarcinoma are all known to produce this type of embolization (41,43). A rubbery red or pale tan clot is present within the affected artery, often producing a coiled snake-like appearance in larger

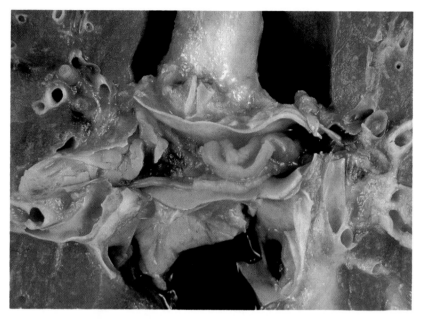

Figure 25-15
INTRA-ARTERIAL
METASTASIS TO
THE MAIN
PULMONARY ARTERY
The tumor embolus is coiled in worm-like fashion within the lumen of the artery.

arterial sites (fig. 25-15). The distal lung may show peripheral, localized zones of hemorrhage. Parenchymal tumor nodules are often absent. Microscopically, the tumor cells occur in solid clumps or masses, either alone or surrounded by fibrin or organizing fibrin, with resultant dilatation of the artery. Other complications include pulmonary infarction and acute cor pulmonale (43). There may not be parenchymal extension of the tumor in these cases (41).

The most common type of clinically significant embolization affects small muscular pulmonary arteries (less than 2 mm in diameter), arterioles, and, occasionally, capillaries. There may be simultaneous lymphangitic involvement and parenchymal tumor extension (35,41), or the tumor may be confined to the pulmonary arteries (31). The sources of clinically significant tumor emboli are shown in Table 25-3. Grossly, the pulmonary vasculature is often clear, but occasionally intraluminal webs reflecting organization of thrombi may be seen. The involvement can be focal in early stages of disease (23,36,42). Parenchymal tumor nodules may not be present. The tumor cells occur in clumps, usually surrounded by fibrin or organizing fibrin, within muscular pulmonary arteries and arterioles (figs. 25-16, 25-17). Pure tumor emboli are frequently seen in breast cancer, while admixed fibrin emboli are more common in gastric carcinoma (31).

Table 25-3

PRIMARY SITES IN 157 PATIENTS WITH NEOPLASTIC PULMONARY EMBOLI AND PULMONARY HYPERTENSION, SUBACUTE COR PULMONALE, OR DYSPNEA*

Primary Site	No. Patients	% Patients
Breast	40	25
Stomach	22	14
Placenta	20	13
Liver	17	11
Prostate	9	6
Cervix	7	4
Other	27	17

*From reference 31.

Extensive distal arterial tumor emboli can result in *thrombotic microangiopathy*, also termed *carcinomatous arteriopathy* or *carcinomatous pulmonary endarteritis* (19). Severe obliterative fibrointimal hyperplasia of arteries is characteristic, and clinical features of progressive dyspnea, pulmonary hypertension, and right ventricular failure are common. Tumor-induced

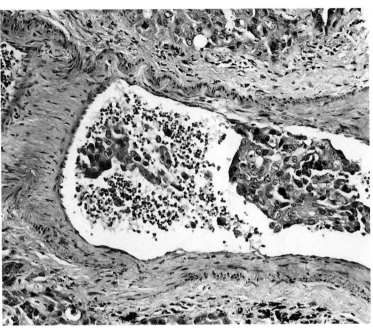

Figure 25-16
INTRA-ARTERIAL METASTASIS
A clump of neoplastic cells (carcinoma) is present within the lumen and may adhere to the wall of this muscular pulmonary artery in one area. Admixed fibrin is not appreciated. Tumor is also present in periarterial lymphatics.

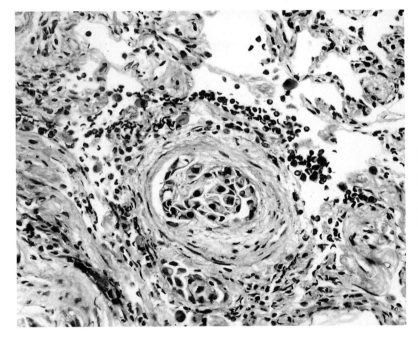

Figure 25-17
INTRA-ARTERIAL METASTASIS
A small pulmonary artery shows a carcinomatous embolus in its lumen. The tumor thrombus has undergone partial organization, resulting in eccentric fibrosis and narrowing of the vascular lumen. Neoplastic cells are entrapped within the organizing fibrous tissue and adhere to the vascular wall.

thrombotic microangiopathy is seen rarely in autopsies of patients with malignant neoplasms (29,35,39). It is produced most often by adenocarcinomas, usually gastric adenocarcinomas but also adenocarcinomas of breast and liver, and choriocarcinomas (19,39). Grossly, the lumens of small distal arteries may appear occluded or show webs, indicative of recanalization. Proximal arteries often have thickened walls. Pulmonary nodules may also be present. Small arteries have tumor cells in intraluminal clumps surrounded by fibrin or attached directly to the endothelium. Significant eccentric or concentric fibrocellular intimal proliferation occurs

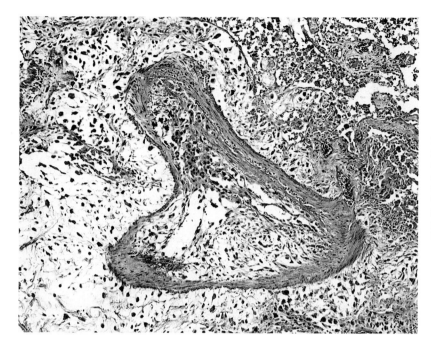

Figure 25-18
CARCINOMATOUS
ARTERIOPATHY
The patient had extensive organizing tumor emboli within vascular lumens. Here, there is focal fibrointimal narrowing of the vascular lumen. A cluster of neoplastic cells is also present within the vascular lumen, partially adherent to the vascular wall. An admixture of tumor cells and myxoid fibrous connective tissue is present in the surrounding parenchyma.

Figure 25-19
CARCINOMATOUS
ARTERIOPATHY
At times, occlusive arteriopathy may occur without tumor being readily apparent in the vascular lumen. The lumen of this artery is completely filled with fibromyxoid granulation tissue, but tumor is not noticeable within the vessel (although it is present in perivascular tissues). Same case as figure 25-18.

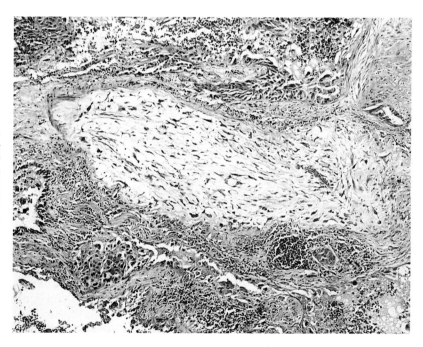

(fig. 25-18). In cases of profound vascular involvement, the resultant increase in vascular resistance may result in pulmonary hypertension; subacute or, rarely, acute cor pulmonale; and death. In some of these cases, there may be few malignant cells and the luminal fibrointimal proliferation is the dominant histologic finding

(fig. 25-19). A careful examination of multiple step sections may be necessary to demonstrate intraluminal malignant cells and exclude other causes of pulmonary hypertension.

As expected, the prognosis of patients with tumor emboli-induced hypertension is poor. The average survival ranges from 4 to 12 weeks (19,31).

The differential diagnosis of metastatic tumor emboli includes intravascular lymphoma and primary pulmonary artery sarcomas. Intravascular (angiotrophic) lymphoma is a rare form of systemic lymphoma consisting of cells with large, vesicular, deeply indented nuclei that aggregate within small vessels with resultant thrombosis. Pulmonary arteries can also show muscular hypertrophy, intraluminal thrombi, and eccentric or concentric intimal fibrous scars. The neoplastic cells are readily distinguished from usual embolic metastases because they express common leukocyte antigen (CD45) and other lymphocytic (and more specifically B-cell) markers.

Pulmonary artery sarcomas are discussed in chapter 20. Briefly, a variety of histologic types may be found, including leiomyosarcomas, fibrosarcomas, and undifferentiated sarcomas. On occasion, these tumors extend into the distal lung either directly or as emboli, producing an arteriopathy. The finding of a spindle cell sarcoma within pulmonary arterial lumens or walls should therefore raise this consideration. The pathological suspicion is supported by the presence of a mass involving the wall/lumen of the main pulmonary arterial trunk, the usual primary site, which may be visualized by chest X ray, computerized tomographic scan, or arteriogram.

The Solitary Pulmonary Metastasis

As noted above, when metastasis occurs to lung it is usually in the form of numerous nodules or masses. However, solitary metastasis does occur: 1 to 5 percent of all metastatic lesions are solitary (Table 25-1), and 3 to 9 percent of all solitary pulmonary nodules are caused by metastasis (11). The tumors that are most commonly associated with solitary metastasis include malignant melanoma; colon, breast, renal cell, and bladder carcinomas; sarcomas; and nonseminomatous testicular neoplasms (11,37). Although there is still debate about the therapeutic value of metastatectomy, resection of localized pulmonary metastasis can lead to improved survival in at least some patients with renal cell carcinoma, breast cancer, colon cancer, malignant melanoma, and sarcomas (2,15,20,24).

When a solitary mass is found in the lung in a patient with a history of malignancy elsewhere, a clinically and pathologically ambiguous situation arises in which the differential diagnosis is primary lung cancer versus solitary metastasis. In general, the overall incidence of a new lung primary in this setting is greater than that of a solitary metastasis (7). The location of the previous primary can sometimes aid in estimating the likelihood of metastasis clinically. In a patient older than 35 years who has a history of squamous cell carcinoma of the head and neck, a solitary lung mass is most likely a separate primary (6,11). By contrast, if the extrapulmonary primary is sarcoma from bone or soft tissue, or malignant melanoma, then the lung tumor will almost always be a metastasis (2,7). Finally, when the pulmonary nodule occurs in a patient with a history of extrapulmonary adenocarcinoma, clinical and radiographic features do not reliably separate a new primary from metastasis (2).

Microscopic findings can also help in diagnosing a solitary mass as primary versus secondary cancer. A few histologic subtypes, such as melanoma or some types of sarcoma, suggest an extrapulmonary primary (11). Multiplicity of lesions also favors metastasis, although bronchioloalveolar carcinoma can be multicentric. Histologic and sometimes histochemical and immunohistochemical comparison of the extrapulmonary primary and the pulmonary tumor provide the best way of establishing a tumor as a metastasis. Still, at times a shift in the histologic appearance of a tumor can be seen during treatment, causing confusion when the primary and metastasis are compared (9).

When the tumor is adenocarcinoma or squamous cell carcinoma, the histologic appearance is only occasionally useful for diagnosis. The presence of clear cells or colloid suggests metastatic renal cell or thyroid carcinoma, respectively, but these are exceptional instances. In general, metastatic adenocarcinoma tends to be more necrotic ("dirty necrosis") and pleomorphic than primary pulmonary adenocarcinomas (see Lepidic Growth Pattern) (13). A pulmonary primary is favored if there is carcinoma in situ in the vicinity of the tumor. Also, the presence of an infiltrating versus pushing border with normal lung may aid in the diagnosis (33).

Immunohistochemical staining is being systematically explored as a means of distinguishing adenocarcinomas of lung from metastases. Antibodies to pulmonary surfactant apoprotein or protein A stain about 50 percent of lung adenocarcinomas,

Table 25-4

PRIMARY TUMOR SITES ASSOCIATED WITH PLEURAL METASTASES*

Primary Site	No. Metastases/ Total Tumors	Pleural Metastasis (%)
Lung	32/459	7.0
Stomach	7/195	3.6
Breast	20/645	3.1
Ovary	9/303	2.9
Pancreas	3/NA**	–
Colon	3/NA	–
Prostate	2/NA	–
Uterus	2/NA	–

*From reference 11. Diagnosis by pleural biopsy or cytology of pleural effusion.
**NA=Data not available.

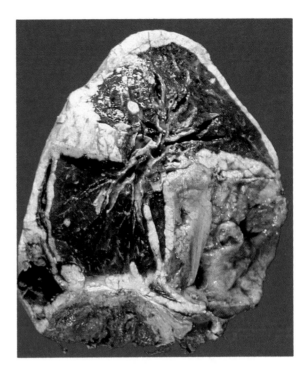

Figure 25-20
DIFFUSE PLEURAL METASTASIS
SIMULATING MESOTHELIOMA
A solid rind of neoplasm occupies the pleural surface and extends along the fissure between lobes. Several small parenchymal tumor nodules are also seen. The primary in this case was renal cell carcinoma.

but do not stain metastatic lung tumors (22,32). Monoclonal anti-carcinoembryonic antigen (CEA) helps identify pulmonary and enteric adenocarcinomas, if the pattern of reactivity is also taken into account (25). The presence of gross cystic disease fluid protein (GCDFP-15), estrogen receptor protein (ERP), or S-100 protein favors a breast primary over lung (2,25). In the future, molecular techniques, such as analysis for mutation in the p53 tumor suppressor gene, may help in distinguishing a primary from a metastasis (2).

Pleural Metastases

While pleural tumors are the subject of a separate Fascicle, it seems appropriate to briefly mention the histologic appearance of metastases in the pleura. Usually, pleural metastases occur in the setting of lymphangitic or vascular involvement. The primary sites that can lead to pleural involvement are shown in Table 25-4. Primary tumors from below the diaphragm that metastasize to pleura usually also involve the liver, a finding that has led to the hypothesis that the liver acts as a nidus for subsequent pleural seeding. Other mechanisms may also play a role: some cases of breast carcinoma may involve parietal pleura by direct extension through the chest wall. Cancers may also metastasize to pleura by retrograde lymphatic spread or, in some instances, direct invasion through the diaphragm.

The microscopic diagnosis of metastatic tumor in pleura can be made by effusion cytology or biopsy. The yield from cytologic examination is 66 percent while that of biopsy is 46 percent (28). The combination of the two techniques increases the yield to 73 percent; repeated cytology specimens and biopsies can also increase the yield. Grossly, the pleura may show scattered nodules, miliary nodules, a dominant mass, or, rarely, a solid rind of tumor of variable thickness that mimics mesothelioma (fig. 25-20). Microscopically, a number of patterns of pleural involvement can be seen (11). Frequently, there are small endolymphatic collections of tumor cells in the rich lymphatic network below the pleural surface. Fibrosis of the pleura, often extensive, results when the tumor cells invade the pleural connective tissues, producing the nodular appearance seen in some gross specimens (fig. 25-21). When fibrosis predominates, the neoplastic

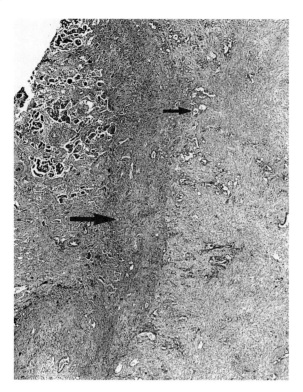

Figure 25-21
PLEURAL METASTASIS OF
ADENOCARCINOMA WITH
EXTENSIVE REACTIVE FIBROSIS

Small neoplastic glands (small arrow) are present within the abundant fibrous connective tissue on the visceral pleural surface. Tumor is also present in the subjacent lung. The original pleural demarcation with lung is denoted by the large arrow.

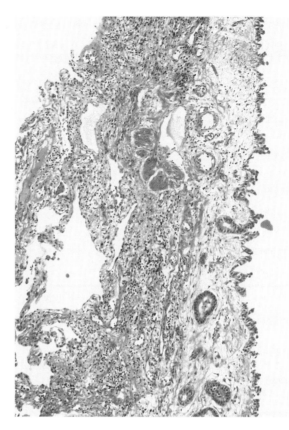

Figure 25-22
PLEURAL METASTASIS OF ADENOCARCINOMA
MIMICKING MESOTHELIOMA

The pleural surface (right) shows a diffuse growth of adenocarcinoma cells mimicking the growth pattern of a mesothelioma. The underlying lung tissue shows congestion and atelectasis.

cells may be reduced to small nests or files that may be easy to overlook.

The malignancy can invade the mesothelial surface, linearly replacing mesothelial cells, or producing sheets or papillary fronds that suggest mesothelioma (fig. 25-22). Prominent reactive mesothelial changes may also be seen in response to the accompanying fibrinous exudate, and the resultant cytologic atypia of these cells may cause additional confusion for the pathologist. Finally, the underlying lung may show either lymphangitic carcinomatosis or pulmonary arterial tumor emboli (or both). Any histologic pattern that can be seen in a primary tumor can be replicated in the pleural metastasis, from glands, solid nests, papillae, and tubules to squamous nests or spindle cells.

The main entity in the differential diagnosis of pleural metastatic tumors is malignant mesothelioma. When the metastatic tumor is adenocarcinoma, the distinction from mesothelioma can at times be difficult. In these cases, antibodies directed against carcinomatous epitopes such as pulmonary surfactant protein A (antibody PE-10), CEA, Ber-EP4, or Leu-M1 (CD15) can aid in diagnosis (22,30,32,34). If the tumor is mucin secreting, then the demonstration of neutral (periodic acid–Schiff-positive) mucin favors adenocarcinoma. Spindle cell sarcomas metastatic to pleura can simulate diffuse malignant fibrous mesothelioma. The presence of diffuse intense staining for keratin within the spindle cells supports a diagnosis of mesothelioma.

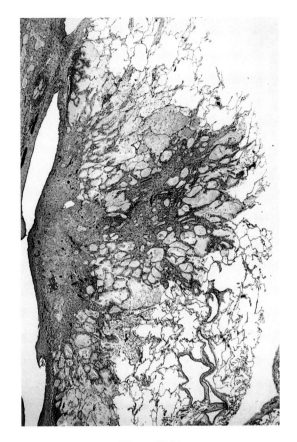

Figure 25-23
LEPIDIC GROWTH PATTERN IN
METASTATIC ADENOCARCINOMA

An area of pleural fibrosis (presumably tumor-induced) caps a well-differentiated, mucin-secreting adenocarcinoma that manifests lepidic growth along alveolar septa. In this case, the primary site was pancreas.

DISTINCTIVE HISTOLOGIC GROWTH PATTERNS

In some metastases, there are distinctive growth patterns or secondary changes. These include lepidic growth, interstitial spread, and cavitation.

Lepidic Growth Pattern

Metastatic adenocarcinoma in lung may grow along the alveolar septa in a lepidic or scale-like pattern, simulating bronchioloalveolar carcinoma. This usually occurs with metastatic colonic adenocarcinoma, and, rarely, with other adenocarcinomas (figs. 25-23, 25-24). In one study of pulmonary metastases in 41 patients with colonic cancer, 6 (15 percent) had metastases that resembled bronchioloalveolar carcinoma (50). The difficulty in distinguishing the two is increased by the fact that there

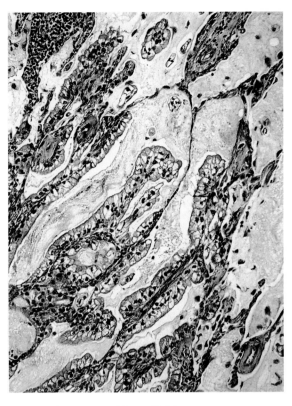

Figure 25-24
LEPIDIC GROWTH PATTERN IN
METASTATIC ADENOCARCINOMA

High magnification view of case shown in figure 25-23. This well-differentiated, mucin-secreting pancreatic adenocarcinoma shows the typical lepidic growth pattern of bronchioloalveolar carcinoma.

are mucinous bronchioloalveolar carcinomas with enteric differentiation, including Paneth cells (see chapter 13) (52).

Grossly, these tumors occur in lung as one or multiple soft to firm nodules or masses, similar to bronchioloalveolar carcinoma. Still, the tumors usually lack the pigmented central nidus present in many peripheral bronchioloalveolar carcinomas.

Microscopically, in addition to a lepidic growth pattern, metastatic adenocarcinoma may show papillary areas, variable mucin production and, on occasion, central foci of fibrosis. The last do not typically show anthracotic pigment. For colonic adenocarcinomas, the finding of multifocal areas of necrosis (dirty necrosis) in hematoxylin and eosin–stained sections, combined with diffuse strong staining with monoclonal antibody D-14, identifies most cases of metastasis, whereas negative staining for D-14 practically excludes a

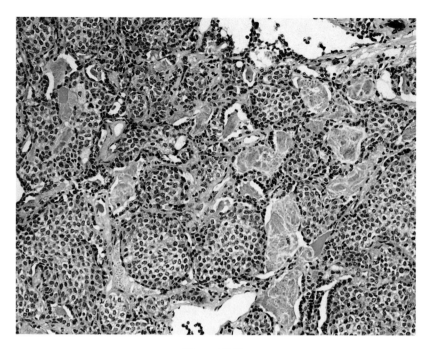

Figure 25-25
INTERSTITIAL GROWTH PATTERN IN METASTASIS
Interstitial metastasis of a thymic carcinoid tumor produces a nodular appearance, with alveolar lining cells overlying the nests of malignant cells.

colonic primary (47). Still, dirty tumor necrosis may also occur in some primary adenocarcinomas of lung (45). Other antibodies, such as PE-10 directed against surfactant apoprotein, may, if positive, point to a pulmonary primary (48).

Interstitial Spread

Solid metastases, particularly from sarcomas, often spread interstitially at their margins. Occasionally, the pulmonary interstitium is the principal site of involvement. This pattern can be caused by sarcomas, lymphomas, and malignant histiocytoses secondarily involving lung. Occasionally, we have seen malignant epithelial tumors such as carcinomas, carcinoids, and malignant melanoma display interstitial growth (fig. 25-25).

At low magnification, the tumor often has poorly circumscribed borders and a Medusa-head appearance as it infiltrates the surrounding lung (figs. 25-6, 25-26). The interstitium is expanded by the neoplastic cells, while the overlying alveolar lining cells show a variable degree of type 2 pneumocyte hyperplasia. The resultant appearance often incorrectly suggests a biphasic tumor, particularly when the interstitial cells are of

mesenchymal origin and have a spindled pattern of growth (fig. 25-27). Expansion into the alveolar lumens can create tumorous nodules.

Cavitation

About 4 percent of metastatic malignancies in lung cavitate or develop thin-walled cysts, compared to 2 to 16 percent of primary lung carcinomas (46,49). Rarely, rupture with spontaneous pneumothorax is the first clinical sign of cystic metastasis (51). Cavitation may occur spontaneously, as when a rapidly growing tumor outgrows its blood supply or impinges on its feeding arteries, or it may result from tumor necrosis induced by chemotherapy or radiation therapy. The histologic subtypes most likely to cavitate are of epithelial origin, and include squamous cell carcinoma, most often of head and neck and of cervix uteri, transitional cell carcinoma of bladder, and adenocarcinomas of colon and breast (Table 25-5) (46). Often, more than one nodule cavitates, usually in the upper lobes (49). The metastatic mesenchymal neoplasms that produce thin-walled cysts are leiomyosarcomas, malignant fibrous histiocytoma, fibrosarcomas, endometrial

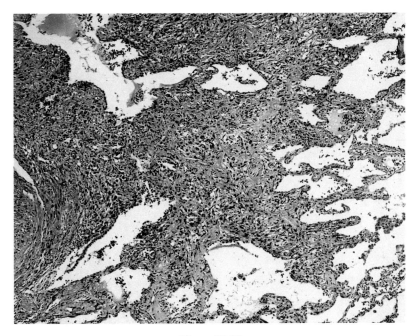

Figure 25-26
INTERSTITIAL GROWTH PATTERN IN METASTASIS
Metastatic sarcomas more commonly adopt an interstitial pattern than epithelial tumors. This view shows interstitial growth of metastatic leiomyosarcoma.

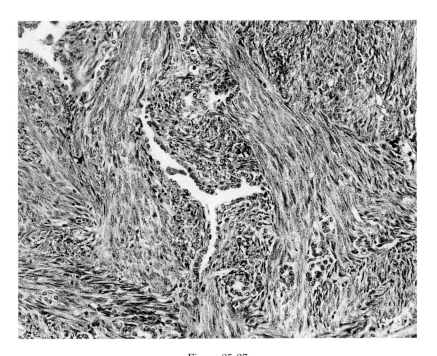

Figure 25-27
ENTRAPMENT OF ALVEOLAR EPITHELIUM WITHIN A METASTATIC SARCOMA
Slowly growing sarcomas not uncommonly entrap residual alveolar elements. Such a pattern may mistakenly suggest a biphasic tumor. Here, metastatic leiomyosarcoma is shown growing around a residual alveolar space.

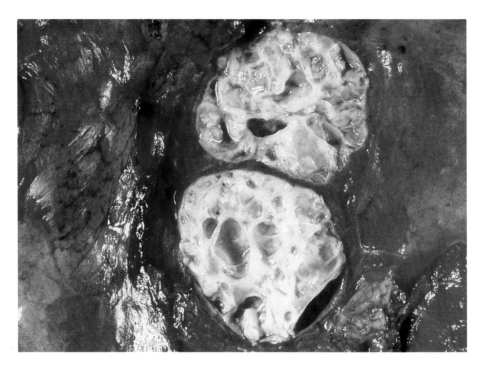

Figure 25-28
CAVITARY METASTASIS
In this case, the metastatic tumor was a teratoma from the testis, a neoplasm well documented to undergo cavitary changes when it metastasizes to lung.

Table 25-5

FREQUENCY OF CAVITARY PULMONARY METASTASES IN SELECTED CARCINOMAS BY PRIMARY SITE*

Primary Site	No. Metastases	% Cavitating
Oropharynx and larynx	24	17
Colon	16	19
Bladder	6	16
Cervix uteri	30	13
Breast	94	2

*From reference 46.

stromal sarcomas, dermatofibrosarcoma protuberans, synovial sarcoma, and angiosarcoma (44,51). Metastatic teratomas and lymphomas can cavitate or form thin-walled cysts, as can melanomas (fig. 25-28).

Grossly, these tumors have walls of varying thickness. While most of the cavitary walls are shaggy and thick, many thin-walled cysts are lined by capsules less than 1 mm in width and smooth in surface (figs. 25-28, 25-29) (46). They may be white, tan, gray, or red.

The cavity walls are usually composed of a mixture of tumor, granulation tissue, and fibrous connective tissue (fig. 25-30). In squamous cell carcinomas, the cavities are composed of multiple layers of cornified debris. Occasionally, only a thin rim of viable squamous cell carcinoma may be present, without central debris. Presumably, the absence of debris results from excavation of the semiliquid cavity contents via the airways. The cavities in other types of malignancies can be either thin walled (particularly in colonic adenocarcinoma) or thick walled. In adenocarcinoma of breast or colon, abundant mucin may be present.

The thin-walled cysts formed by metastatic mesenchymal tumors have central necrotic debris lined by variable amounts of tumor (fig. 25-30). In some, sections of the wall may also be lined by squamous metaplastic epithelium, by a narrow rim of inflammatory cells, or by compressed or atelectatic lung (46).

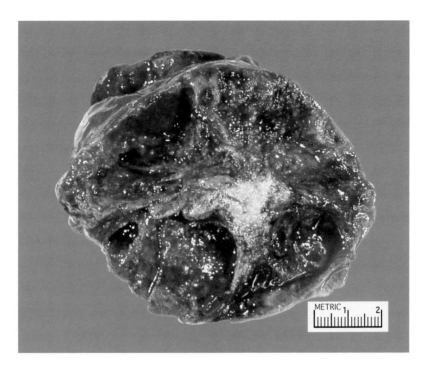

Figure 25-29
CAVITARY METASTASIS
The hemorrhagic tumor mass has undergone multifocal cavitation, with roughened walls of varying thickness.

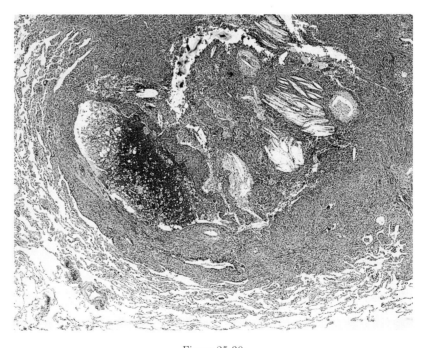

Figure 25-30
NECROSIS AND CYST FORMATION IN A METASTATIC SARCOMA
A relatively thin wall of granulation tissue, fibrous connective tissue, and tumor is present around the necrotic cyst contents (presumably necrotic tumor). Note the cholesterol clefts. The necrotic debris may be removed by expectoration if the cystic tumor makes contact with an airway, leaving behind an air-filled cyst.

Table 25-6

**IMMUNOHISTOCHEMICALLY DEMONSTRABLE ANTIGENS IN THE DIFFERENTIAL
DIAGNOSIS OF POORLY DIFFERENTIATED METASTATIC MALIGNANCIES***

Tumor Phenotype	Antigens
Carcinoma	Keratins, epithelial membrane antigen (EMA), carcinoembryonic antigen (CEA), Ber-EP4, Leu-M1(CD15), B72.3, +/- vimentin
Neuroendocrine	Neuron-specific enolase (NSE), chromogranin, synaptophysin, Leu-7, hormones
Malignant melanoma	S-100 protein, HMB-45, vimentin, NSE (+/- CEA, EMA)
Sarcomas	Vimentin
Leiomyosarcoma	Smooth muscle actin, desmin
Rhabdomyosarcoma	Desmin, myoglobin
Malignant schwannoma	S-100 protein, Leu-7
Clear cell sarcoma	S-100 protein, HMB-45**
Synovial sarcoma	Keratins, vimentin
Epithelioid sarcoma	Keratins, vimentin
Malignant vascular tumor	+/- Factor VIII–related antigen, *Ulex europaeus* agglutinin, CD34, CD31
Malignant fibrous histiocytoma	Alpha-1-antitrypsin, alpha-1-antichymotrypsin
Germ cell tumors	Keratins (+/- or negative in seminoma), placental alkaline phosphatase, alpha-1-antitrypsin, alpha-fetoprotein, human chorionic gonadotropin, and specific pregnancy beta-1-glycoprotein
Glial tumors	Glial fibrillary acidic protein, S-100 protein, +/- keratin, neurofilament protein
Meningiomas	EMA, vimentin, +/- keratin, S-100 protein
Peripheral neuroectodermal tumor	+/- NSE, +/- S-100 protein, + neurofilament protein, MIC-II (12E7, HBA 71)

*Modified from DeLellis (63,92).
**HMB-45 may also stain smooth muscle proliferations, such as those found in lymphangioleiomyomatosis.

SPECIAL TECHNIQUES AND THEIR APPLICATION IN THE DIAGNOSIS OF PULMONARY METASTASES

The diagnosis of metastases to lung is often challenging. For example, the yield of bronchoscopic biopsy, bronchial washings, and sputum cytology in diagnosing metastatic carcinoma in 1974 was only 12 percent as compared to 76 percent for diagnosing primary lung cancers (59). Today, there is an increasing emphasis on diagnosis of metastases in smaller fragments of tissue, particularly fine needle aspirates (69,74,95), and in cytology specimens varying from sputa and bronchial brushings to bronchoalveolar lavage and pleural effusions (87,96). While histologic and histochemical methods may suggest the correct diagnosis, immunohistochemical stains, electron microscopy, and, possibly in the future, molecular probes may help determine the phenotype of a tumor, occasionally pinpoint the site of origin and even aid in determining prognosis.

Immunohistochemistry

Immunohistochemistry is an important adjunct in determining the phenotype of poorly differentiated metastases in lung. It may also aid in specifying the site of origin when it is unclear that there is an extrapulmonary primary, when slides of a known extrapulmonary tumor are not available for study, or when the known extrathoracic primary appears histologically dissimilar to the lung neoplasm.

The differential diagnosis of poorly differentiated metastatic tumors in lung encompasses poorly differentiated carcinoma, malignant melanoma, sarcomas, germ cell tumors, and lymphomas (Table 25-6) (63). While the markers shown in Table 25-6 are useful in a general sense to sort out the phenotype of a tumor, experience has shown that antigen-tumor phenotype interrelations are more complicated than originally conceived and that many antigens are not necessarily restricted to a single tumor phenotype.

Some of the caveats that we and others have encountered are pointed out in the discussion below.

In general, the most important epithelial marker is cytokeratin. Many laboratories use cocktails or mixes of monoclonal antibodies to keratins of differing weight (AE1/AE3, MAK-6, CAM 5.2), ranging from 40-69 kD, to increase sensitivity. High molecular weight cytokeratins are present in squamous cell carcinomas, whereas low molecular weight keratins are found in adenocarcinomas. Most carcinomas, germ cell tumors (with the exception of seminomas), and certain sarcomas, such as epithelioid sarcoma, synovial sarcoma, and epithelioid angiosarcoma, diffusely express keratin (63,67,78). Still, some epithelial phenotypes, such as spindle cell carcinomas, demonstrate it weakly or not at all and certain undoubted mesenchymal tumors, such as smooth muscle tumors, localized fibrous tumors of pleura, and Schwann cell malignancies also focally express keratin.

Similarly, epithelial membrane antigen (EMA) stains most epithelial tumors (39) and some sarcomas with distinct epithelial differentiation such as epithelioid sarcomas or synovial sarcomas (67). However, as in the case of keratins, EMA may also stain spindle cell carcinoma weakly or not at all and it may focally stain some mesenchymal neoplasms, such as neural tumors and localized fibrous tumors, as well as some lymphomas and meningiomas.

More specific epithelial markers can help identify an epithelial phenotype in poorly differentiated metastases. Carcinoembryonic antigen (CEA) is expressed in gastrointestinal adenocarcinomas, pancreatic and gall bladder carcinomas, and teratomas, and as scattered cells of some embryonal carcinomas and yolk sac tumors. It is also a sensitive marker for lung adenocarcinomas. However, poorly differentiated carcinomas frequently fail to show immunoreactivity. Ber-EP4 appears to be a sensitive marker for adenocarcinomas from many sites (86). However, some carcinomas from certain organs, most notably kidney and breast, may fail to stain with the antibody (85). In general, if a metastatic epithelial neoplasm is suspected, it is best to use a battery of these epithelial markers.

The diagnosis of metastatic malignant melanoma can be facilitated by finding S-100 protein or HMB-45 in a keratin-negative, vimentin-positive malignancy. The sensitivity of S-100 protein is high, but its specificity is low: many other cell types such as Schwann cells, chondrocytes, lipocytes, myoepithelial cells, and Langerhans cells may stain with the antibody. Still, since these other cell types are usually easily distinguished by their histopathologic features, immunohistochemical study for S-100 protein remains useful. While antibody to HMB-45 has been considered to be more specific for melanocytic differentiation, it is also less sensitive than that to S-100 protein. It will also stain certain other cell types such as smooth muscle cells in renal angiomyolipoma, lymphangioleiomyomatosis, angiolipoma, cells of benign clear cell tumors of lung and breast, and breast and hepatocellular carcinomas (68). Some of this staining may be due to differences in antibody preparations (58).

Germ cell tumors may be pleomorphic or undifferentiated. Antibody to placental alkaline phosphatase (PLAP) is found diffusely on the cell surfaces of most seminomas, except for spermatocytic seminoma, and focally in other types of germ cell tumors. Some somatic tumors may also stain for PLAP (97). Other commonly sought antigens include alpha-1-antitrypsin (71) and alpha-fetoprotein (70), present within yolk sac tumors (and rarely, teratomas), and human chorionic gonadotropin (hCG) and pregnancy-specific beta-1-glycoprotein (71), found in syncytiotrophoblasts of choriocarcinoma and other malignant germ cell tumors. However, while hCG occurs in syncytiotrophoblasts of germ cell tumors metastatic to lung, it can also be present in some giant cell and undifferentiated large cell carcinomas of lung. In addition, alpha-fetoprotein is reported in primary pulmonary tumors showing a mixed yolk sac and blastomatous phenotype as well as pulmonary blastomas (88).

Metastatic sarcomas are often difficult to classify. Virtually all sarcomas are vimentin positive (but so are many carcinomas of lung). Smooth muscle actin and desmin can be helpful in the identification of muscle tumors; myoglobin and desmin may aid in diagnosis of rhabdomyosarcomas; and S-100 protein can be useful in the diagnosis of a malignant peripheral nerve sheath tumor as well as cartilaginous differentiation. Factor VIII–related antigen, CD34, CD31, and the lectin *Ulex europaeus* may be present in vascular tumors, such as Kaposi sarcoma and some angiosarcomas.

Table 25-7

IMMUNOHISTOCHEMICAL FINDINGS IN SELECTED CARCINOMAS BY PRIMARY SITE*

Primary Site/Phenotype	Antigen(s)
Prostate/adenocarcinoma	Prostate-specific antigen (PSA), prostatic acid phosphatase (PAP)
Breast	Gross cystic disease fluid protein-15, estrogen receptor protein, S-100 protein, MC5
Ovary/adenocarcinoma	Carcinoembryonic antigen, OC 125 (coelomic antigen), CA19-9, epithelial membrane antigen
Thyroid/follicular, papillary, and anaplastic carcinoma	Thyroglobulin, T3, T4, coexpression of keratin and vimentin
Thyroid/medullary carcinoma	Hormones (calcitonin, somatostatin), other neuroendocrine markers
Liver/hepatocellular carcinoma	Alpha-fetoprotein, alpha-1-antitrypsin, CEA (laminar pattern)
Pancreas/islet cell carcinoma	Hormones (insulin, glucagon, somatostatin, vasoactive intestinal peptide (VIP), other neuroendocrine markers, keratin, chromogranin, neuron-specific enolase (NSE)
Pancreas/acinar cell carcinoma	Amylase
Salivary gland/adenoid cystic carcinoma	S-100 protein, actin, low molecular weight keratins (such as CAM 5.2), vimentin
Salivary gland/acinic cell carcinoma	Amylase, alpha-1-antichymotrypsin
Skin/Merkel cell carcinoma (trabecular carcinoma)	Keratin, NSE, hormones (bombesin, calcitonin, VIP, ACTH, gastrin, leu-enkephalin, somatostatin), +/- chromogranin, +/- neurofilament antigen

*From reference 63.

However, it is important to realize that S-100 protein and the vascular differentiation antigens can also be absent in these tumors (92). Clear cell sarcomas of tendon sheath usually stain for S-100 protein and often for HMB-45 as well (60).

Epithelioid sarcomas typically demonstrate coexpression of both keratin and vimentin, as well as alpha-1-antitrypsin and alpha-1-antichymotrypsin (78). Finally, rhabdomyosarcomas most often stain for desmin, myoglobin, and actin (92).

Glial fibrillary acidic protein (GFAP) is a marker of astroglial differentiation that helps to distinguish metastatic central nervous system tumors. At the same time, GFAP has also been demonstrated in pleomorphic adenomas of salivary gland (where it marks myoepithelial cells), chordomas, peripheral nerve sheath tumors, pulmonary chondromas, renal cell carcinoma, and meningioma (98).

Antibody studies can also be useful for specific diagnostic problems. Their role in distinguishing adenocarcinoma of lung and bronchioloalveolar carcinoma from metastatic adenocarcinoma of colon or breast origin has already been pointed out (see Solitary Pulmonary Metastasis and Lepidic Growth Pattern, this chapter).

Immunohistochemistry can be of great use in separating benign clear cell tumor and metastatic renal cell carcinoma of lung. In particular, benign clear cell tumor (so-called sugar tumor) is often decorated by antibodies to HMB-45 but fails to stain for keratins, whereas renal cell carcinoma stains for keratins but not HMB-45 (68). While immunohistochemical studies are of less use in distinguishing benign clear cell tumor from metastatic clear cell sarcoma of tendon sheath because of similarity in antigenic profiles, this differential diagnosis is rarely encountered.

Finally, primary sites of adenocarcinoma can be suggested in a number of tumors by specific antibodies (Table 25-7). Prostate-specific antigen and prostatic acid phosphatase in combination are useful in identifying metastatic prostatic adenocarcinomas (79); alpha-fetoprotein in identifying hepatocellular carcinoma and yolk sac tumors; thyroglobulin for follicular, papillary, and anaplastic carcinomas of thyroid; gross cystic disease fluid protein-15, estrogen receptor

Table 25-8

ELECTRON MICROSCOPIC FEATURES IN THE DIFFERENTIAL DIAGNOSIS OF SELECTED METASTATIC MALIGNANCIES IN LUNG*

Tumor	EM Features
Anaplastic carcinoma	Desmosomes or junctional complexes infrequently present; microvilli or intracellular lumens may be present; tonofilaments may be present; neurosecretory, mucin, or zymogen granules may be present
Malignant melanoma	Desmosomes and junctional complexes absent; melanosomes present (but may be rare)
Malignant lymphoma	Simplified cytoplasm, no diagnostic cytoplasmic inclusions; desmosomes typically absent
Sarcomas	
Leiomyosarcoma	Subplasmalemmal aggregates of thin filaments; pinocytotic vesicles; basal lamina
Rhabdomyosarcoma	Abundant glycogen, Z-band material, thick and thin filaments; basal lamina
Malignant schwannoma	Often fibroblastic cells; may have complex cell processes with basal lamina
Synovial sarcoma	Glandular epithelial cells with desmosomes, microvilli, basal lamina around glands; spindle cells undifferentiated, or may show tonofilaments; basal lamina
Alveolar soft part sarcoma	Characteristic cytoplasmic crystalloid inclusions
Epithelioid sarcoma	Abundant whorled cytoplasmic filaments
Malignant vascular tumor	Vascular spaces lined by basal lamina; pericytes; Weibel-Palade bodies absent in malignant vascular tumors
Malignant fibrous histiocytoma	Myofibroblasts, macrophage-like cells, multinucleated cells, primitive mesenchymal cells

*From references 54,92.

protein, and MC5 (a monoclonal antibody produced against milk fat globule membrane) for metastatic breast carcinoma (62,83); and coelomic antigen (OC 125) for metastatic ovarian carcinoma (72). Still, alpha-fetoprotein is found in mixed blastomas-yolk sac tumors in lung, and OC 125 can occasionally be seen in primary lung cancers (72,73).

Electron Microscopy

As with immunohistochemistry, electron microscopic evaluation should be viewed as an adjunct to light microscopy, and performed with a knowledge of the clinical setting, history, and histopathology. Azar (54) has pointed out that electron microscopy of tumors offers few "truly specific or diagnostic features," so that correlation with light microscopic and immunohistochemical studies is essential. Electron microscopy can be of value in the determination of the underlying phenotype of poorly differentiated metastatic large cell malignancies or sarcomas in lung (Tables 25-8, 25-9).

Oncogenes

Malignant neoplasms appear to be composed of genetically heterogeneous populations of cells, some of which are better able to metastasize than others. A corollary is that tumor cell populations continually generate clones of cells with differing metastatic potential. Factors that may be responsible for metastasis include development of growth autonomy, loss of cell adherence, development of increased cell mobility, and production of proteolytic enzymes and angiogenic factors. These factors result in a multistep cascade of events leading to the development of viable tumor colonies in distant sites (75). Initiation of neoplasia is followed by tumor promotion and progression, uncontrolled proliferation, angiogenesis-induced local invasion, invasion of local blood and lymphatic vessels, and circulating tumor cell arrest and extravasation in the metastatic site. This is followed by formation of distant colonies and growth that evades host defenses or the effects of therapy.

Table 25-9

CORRELATION OF CERTAIN SPECIFIC ULTRASTRUCTURAL FEATURES WITH PHENOTYPE OF METASTATIC MALIGNANCIES

Phenotype	EM Features
Malignant melanoma	Melanosomes
Angiosarcoma	Weibel-Palade bodies (infrequently seen)
Histiocytosis X	Birbeck granules
Hairy cell leukemia	Numerous cytoplasmic projections; ribosomal lamellar complexes
Alveolar soft part sarcoma	Crystalloid cytoplasmic inclusions
Neuroendocrine tumors	Dense core granules; cell processes
Oncocytic cells of salivary gland tumors, renal cell carcinoma, Hurthle cells of thyroid tumors	Numerous mitochondria
Squamous cell carcinomas, other carcinomas, synovial carcinoma	Desmosomes (macula adherens)
"Rhabdoid" tumors	Whorled cytoplasmic aggregates of 10-nm intermediate filaments
Adenocarcinomas	Tight junctions (zonula occludens); intracellular lumens

The development of the metastatic cascade may involve abnormalities in many genes whose products are necessary for progression through each step of the cascade. Further, the specific genetic abnormalities may vary for different families of tumors. The concept that expression of oncogenes and their proteins may be predictors of metastasis or survival has opened up a whole new area of research for pathologists. This understanding has been coupled with important technical advances, such as polymerase chain reaction (PCR), DNA sequencing methods (direct sequencing, PCR single strand conformation polymorphism), and immunohistochemistry, to allow identification of genetic mutations and overexpressed gene products in frozen and formalin-fixed, paraffin-embedded sections of tumors (76). These methods are sensitive enough to be used even in small fragments of tissue, such as needle biopsies. In combination with other techniques, they are now being employed to link specific oncogene or tumor suppressor gene mutations with metastatic potential (65,66,75,76).

Some of the more important oncogenes and other genes now being studied include: epidermal growth factor receptor protein (EGRF), c-*erb*B-2; N-*myc*; p53; H-*ras*-1, K-*ras*-2, and N-*ras*; and *bcl*-2.

The c-*erb*B-2 (HER-2/*neu* or *neu*) oncogene produces a cytoplasmic protein product that is related to epidermal growth factor receptor (EGRF) (81). Both the *neu* oncogene protein and EGRF are tyrosine-specific kinases encoding growth factor receptors (56). Overamplification of the protein products of both the c-*erb*B-2 and EGRF genes have been linked to metastatic potential in breast cancer, specifically metastasis to lymph nodes, as well as high morphologic grade, low disease-free survival, and low overall survival (77,81,84,90). Monoclonal antibodies are now commercially available for both of these protein products. Other procedures, such as Southern, Northern, and Western blot analyses, can be used to detect the *neu* oncogene or its product, but the results may be confusing due to intermixing of nontumorous stroma (94).

Amplification of the N-*myc* oncogene is correlated with prognosis in neuroblastomas, but not other small cell sarcomas. Overexpression of the gene product is associated with translocation of the gene from chromosome 2 to 1 with resultant abnormalities of the short arm of chromosome 1 (1p deletions) and, in most cases, with multiple copies (more than 10) of the gene, as demonstrated by Southern blot analysis (94). Overexpression of the gene product can be shown by immunohistochemical methods on frozen sections, smears, or imprints of the tumor (89). Paraffin sections are less reliable.

The tumor suppressor gene p53, located on chromosome 17, is one whose product, a nuclear phosphoprotein, is ubiquitous in normal tissue. As the name indicates, p53 is not an oncogene; rather, point mutations, genomic rearrangement, or deletions, most frequently in codons 5 to 8 of the gene, result in loss of normal p53 tumor suppressor function and derepression of other oncogenes in the cell, and probably play a role in the development (and possibly prognosis) of a number of malignancies (61,93). These mutations, which have been described in a variety of tumors, result in abnormal proteins that lack biologic function and may accumulate within the cell. The protein can be detected within the nuclei of cells in paraffin sections by monoclonal antibodies, providing an initial screening technique for mutations of the gene, which can then be more specifically demonstrated by DNA analysis (57,94). In colon cancers, for example, it appears that these abnormalities are associated with the transition from benign to malignant states as well as the development of metastasis (55,64). In breast cancer, p53 protein accumulation in nuclei of cells, as demonstrated in paraffin tissue sections by immunohistochemical methods, appears to be an independent marker of poor prognosis (93). On the other hand, no correlation was found between p53 protein staining in squamous cell carcinomas of the head and neck and stage of disease or number of involved lymph nodes (80).

The oncogene K-*ras*-2 has also been associated with metastasis in colonic adenocarcinomas. Mutations of the gene occur early in the development of about 40 percent of sporadic colonic cancers (53). Significantly higher rates of single mutations in the gene, and more specifically in its codon 12, occur in colonic adenocarcinomas that metastasize (66). In addition, these mutations occur preferentially not only in the primary tumors but in their distant metastases, including those in lung. Solitary or limited metastases show normal K-*ras*-2 phenotypes, while disseminated and numerous metastases to lung, liver, and brain are associated with codon 12 point mutations: most frequently with a substitution in codon 12-aspartate (30). In summarizing their data, Finkelstein and associates (66) noted that specific mutation profiles seemed associated with different forms of clinical behavior: mutations in codon 13-aspartate and in codon 12-valine were found in indolent tumors, normal K-*ras*-2 was associated with locally aggressive tumors, while most cases of very aggressive behavior (distant hematogenous metastasis) were associated with codon 12-aspartate. It seems likely that identifying oncogene profiles in some tumors will be an important addition to currently used morphologic and clinical predictors of biologic behavior.

REFERENCES

Patterns of Metastasis

1. Abrams HL, Spiro R, Goldstein N. Metastases in carcinoma. Analysis of 1000 autopsied cases. Cancer 1950;3:74–85.
2. Askin FB. Something old? Something new? Second primary or pulmonary metastasis in the patient with known extrathoracic carcinoma. Am J Clin Pathol 1993;100:4–5.
3. Baumgartner WA, Mark JB. Metastatic malignancies from distant sites to the tracheobronchial tree. J Thorac Cardiovasc Surg 1980;79:499–503.
4. Bourke SJ, Henderson AF, Stevenson RD, Banham SW. Endobronchial metastases simulating primary carcinoma of the lung. Respir Med 1989;83:151–2.
5. Braman SS, Whitcomb ME. Endobronchial metastasis. Arch Intern Med 1975;135:543–7.
6. Cahan WG, Castro EB, Hajdu SI. Proceedings: the significance of a solitary lung shadow in patients with colon carcinoma. Cancer 1974;33:414–21.
7. _____, Shah JP, Castro EB. Benign solitary lung lesions in patients with cancer. Ann Surg 1978;187:241–4.
8. Carlin BW, Harrell JH II, Olson LK, Moser KM. Endobronchial metastases due to colorectal carcinoma. Chest 1989;96:1110–4.
9. Derstappen T, Roessner A, Muller KM, Grundmann E. Morphology of pulmonary metastases from osteosarcoma during chemotherapy. J Cancer Res Clin Oncol 1987;113:241–8.
10. Dinkel E, Mundinger A, Schopp D, Grosser G, Hauenstein KH. Diagnostic imaging in metastatic lung disease. Lung 1990;168(Suppl):1129–36.

11. Filderman AE, Coppage L, Shaw C, Matthay RA. Pulmonary and pleural manifestations of extrathoracic malignancies. Clin Chest Med 1989;10:747–887.
12. Fitzgerald RH Jr. Endobronchial metastases. South Med J 1977;70:440–1.
13. Flint A, Lloyd RV. Pulmonary metastases of colonic adenocarcinoma. Distinction from pulmonary adenocarcinoma. Arch Pathol Lab Med 1992;116:39–42.
14. Gilbert HA, Kagan AR. Metastases: incidence, detection and evaluation without histologic confirmation. In: Weiss L, ed. Fundamental aspects of metastases. Amsterdam: North-Holland Publishing Co., 1976.
15. Harpole DH Jr, Johnson CM, Wolfe WG, George SL, Seigler HF. Analysis of 945 cases of pulmonary metastatic melanoma. J Thorac Cardiovasc Surg 1992;103:743–50.
16. Janower ML, Blennerhassett JB. Lymphangitic spread of metastatic carcinoma to lung. A radiologic-pathologic classification. Radiology 1971;101:267–73.
17. Kane RD, Hawkins HK, Miller JA, Noce PS. Microscopic pulmonary tumor emboli associated with dyspnea. Cancer 1975;36:1473–82.
18. King DS, Castleman B. Bronchial involvement in metastatic pulmonary malignancy. J Thorac Surg 1943;12:305–15.
19. Kupari M, Laitinen L, Hekali P, Luomanmäki K. Cor pulmonale due to tumor cell embolization. Report of a case and a brief review of the literature. Acta Med Scand 1981;210:507–10.
20. Lanza L, Natarajan G, Roth JA, Putnam JB Jr. Long-term survival after resection of pulmonary metastases from carcinoma of the breast. Ann Thorac Surg 1992;54:244–7.
21. Masson RG, Ruggieri J. Pulmonary microvascular cytology. A new diagnostic application of the pulmonary artery catheter. Chest 1985;88:908–14.
22. Mizutani Y, Nakajima T, Morinaga S, et al. Immunohistochemical localization of pulmonary surfactant apoproteins in various lung tumors: special reference to nonmucus producing lung adenocarcinomas. Cancer 1988;61:532–7.
23. Munk PL, Muller NL, Miller RR, Ostrow DN. Pulmonary lymphangitic carcinomatosis: CT and pathologic findings. Radiology 1988;166:705–9.
24. Pogrebniak HW, Haas G, Lineham WM, Rosenberg SA, Pass HI. Renal cell carcinoma: resection of solitary and multiple metastases. Ann Thorac Surg 1992;54:33–8.
25. Raab SS, Berg LC, Swanson PE, Wick MR. Adenocarcinoma in the lung in patients with breast cancer. A prospective analysis of the discriminatory value of immunohistology. Am J Clin Pathol 1993;100:27–35.
26. Rosenblatt MB, Lisa JR, Trinidad S. Pitfalls in the clinical and histologic diagnosis of bronchogenic carcinoma. Dis Chest 1966;49:396–404.
27. Rovirosa Casino A, Bellmunt J, Salud A, et al. Endobronchial metastases in colorectal adenocarcinoma. Tumori 1992;78:270–3.
28. Sahn SA. Malignant pleural effusion. In: Fishman AP, ed. Pulmonary diseases and disorders. New York: McGraw-Hill, 1988.
29. Schriner RW, Ryu JH, Edwards WD. Microscopic pulmonary tumor embolism causing subacute cor pulmonale: a difficult antemortem diagnosis. Mayo Clin Proc 1991;66:143–8.
30. Sheibani K, Esteban JM, Bailey A, Battifora H, Weiss LM. Immunopathologic and molecular studies as an aid to the diagnosis of malignant mesothelioma. Hum Pathol 1992;23:107–16.
31. Shields DJ, Edwards WD. Pulmonary hypertension attributable to neoplastic emboli: an autopsy study of 20 cases and a review of literature. Cardiovasc Pathol 1992;1:279–87.
32. Shijubo N, Tsutahara S, Hirasawa M, Takahashi H, Honda Y, Suzuki A, et al. Pulmonary surfactant protein A in pleural effusions. Cancer 1992;69:2905–9.
33. Shirakusa T, Tsutsui M, Mononaga R, Ando K, Kusano T. Resection of metastatic lung tumor: the evaluation of histologic appearance in the lung. Am Surg 1988;54:655–8.
34. Singh G, Scheithauer BW, Katyal SL. The pathologic features of carcinomas of type II pneumocytes. An immunocytologic study. Cancer 1986;57:994–9.
35. Soares FA, Landell GA, de Oliveira JA. Pulmonary tumor embolism to alveolar septal capillaries. A prospective study of 12 cases. Arch Pathol Lab Med 1991;115:127–30.
36. Thurlbeck WM, Miller RR, Muller NL, Rosenow EC. Diffuse diseases of the lung: a team approach. Philadelphia: BC Decker, 1991:150.
37. Toomes H, Delphendahl A, Manke HG, Vogt-Moykopf I. The coin lesion of the lung. A review of 955 resected coin lesions. Cancer 1983;51:534–7.
38. Udelsman R, Roth JA, Lees D, Jelenich SE, Pass HI. Endobronchial metastases from soft tissue sarcoma. J Surg Oncol 1986;32:145–9.
39. von Herbay A, Illes A, Waldherr R, Otto HF. Pulmonary tumor thrombotic microangiopathy with pulmonary hypertension. Cancer 1990;66:587–92.
40. Wall CP, Gaensler EA, Carrington CB, Hayes JA. Comparison of transbronchial and open biopsies in chronic infiltrative lung diseases. Am Rev Respir Dis 1981;123:280–5.
41. Winterbauer RH, Elfenbein IB, Ball WC Jr. Incidence and clinical significance of tumor embolization to the lungs. Am J Med 1968;45:271–90.
42. Yang SP, Lin CC. Lymphangitic carcinomatosis of the lungs. The clinical significance of its roentgenologic classification. Chest 1972;62:170–87.
43. Yutani C, Imakita M, Ishibashi-Ueda H, Katsuragi M, Yoshioka T, Kunieda T. Pulmonary hypertension due to tumor emboli: a report of three autopsy cases with morphological correlations to radiological findings. Acta Pathol Jpn 1993;43:135–41.

Distinctive Histologic Growth Patterns

44. Abrams J, Talcott J, Corson JM. Pulmonary metastases in patients with low-grade endometrial stromal sarcoma. Clinicopathologic findings with immunohistochemical characterization. Am J Surg Pathol 1989;13:133–40.
45. Askin FB. Something old? Something new? Second primary or pulmonary metastasis in the patient with known extrathoracic carcinoma. Am J Clin Pathol 1993;100:4–5.
46. Dodd GD, Boyle JJ. Excavating pulmonary metastases. Amer J Roentgenol 1961;85:277–93.
47. Flint A, Lloyd RV. Pulmonary metastases of colonic adenocarcinoma. Distinction from pulmonary adenocarcinoma. Arch Pathol Lab Med 1992;116:39–42.

48. Mizutani Y, Nakajima T, Morinaga S, et al. Immunohisto-chemical localization of pulmonary surfactant apoproteins in various lung tumors. Special reference to nonmucus producing lung adenocarcinomas. Cancer 1988;61:532–7.

49. Pulmonary cavitary disease (clinical conference). NY State J Med 1992;92:193–8.

50. Rosenblatt MB, Lisa JR, Collier F. Primary and metastatic bronchiolo-alveolar carcinoma. Chest 1967;52:147–52.

51. Traweek T, Rotter AJ, Swartz W, Azumi N. Cystic pulmonary metastatic sarcoma. Cancer 1990;65:1805–11.

52. Tsao MS, Fraser RS. Primary pulmonary adenocarcinoma with enteric differentiation. Cancer 1991;68:1754–7.

Special Techniques and Their Application in the Diagnosis of Pulmonary Metastases

53. Aaltonen LA, Peltomaki P, Leach FS, et al. Clues to the pathogenesis of familial colorectal cancer. Science 1993;260:812–6.

54. Azar HA. Attributes of neoplasms: ultrastructural and functional considerations. In: Azar HA, ed. Pathology of human neoplasms. An atlas of diagnostic electron microscopy and immunohistochemistry. New York: Raven Press, 1988.

55. Baker SJ, Fearon ER, Nigro JM, et al. Chromosome 17 deletions and p53 gene mutations in colorectal carcinomas. Science 1989;244:217–21.

56. Bargmann CI, Hung MC, Weinberg RA. The neu oncogene encodes an epidermal growth factor receptor-related protein. Nature 1986;319:226–30.

57. Bartek J, Iggo R, Gannon J, Lane DP. Genetic and immunochemical analysis of mutant p53 in human breast cancer cell lines. Oncogene 1990;5:893–9.

58. Bonetti F, Pea M, Martignoni G, et al. False-positive immunostaining of normal epithelia and carcinomas with ascites fluid preparations of anti-melanoma monoclonal antibody HMB45. Am J Clin Pathol 1991;95:454–9.

59. Cahan WG, Castro EB, Hajdu SI. Proceedings: the significance of a solitary lung shadow in patients with colon carcinoma. Cancer 1974;33:414–21.

60. Chung EB, Enzinger FM. Malignant melanoma of soft parts. A reassessment of clear cell sarcoma. Am J Surg Pathol 1983;7:405–13.

61. Cossman J, Schlegel R. p53 in the diagnosis of human neoplasia. JNCI 1991;83:980–1.

62. de Almeida PC, Pestana CB. Immunohistochemical markers in the identification of metastatic breast cancer. Breast Cancer Res Treat 1992;21:201–10.

63. DeLellis RA, Dayal Y. Principles of immunohistochemistry as applied to the surgical pathology of neoplasms. In: Azar HA, ed. Pathology of human neoplasms. An atlas of diagnostic electron microscopy and immunohistochemistry. New York: Raven Press, 1988.

64. Fearon ER, Vogelstein B. A genetic model for colorectal tumorigenesis. Cell 1990;61:759–67.

65. Filderman AE, Coppage L, Shaw C, Matthay RA. Pulmonary and pleural manifestations of extrathoracic malignancies. Clin Chest Med 1989;10:747–807.

66. Finkelstein SD, Sayegh R, Christensen S, Swalsky PA. Genotypic classification of colorectal adenocarcinoma. Biologic behavior correlates with K-ras-2 mutation type. Cancer 1993;71:3827–38.

67. Fisher C. Synovial sarcoma: ultrastructural and immunohistochemical features of epithelial differentiation in monophasic and biphasic tumors. Hum Pathol 1986;17:996–1008.

68. Gal AA, Koss MN, Hochholzer L, Chejfec G. An immuno-histochemical study of benign clear cell (sugar) tumor of the lung. Arch Pathol Lab Med 1991; 115:1034–8.

69. Gattuso P, Reddy VB, Castelli MJ. Fine needle aspiration biopsy of paranasal chondrosarcoma metastatic to lung [Letter]. Acta Cytol 1990;34:102–4.

70. Jacobsen GK. Alpha-fetoprotein (AFP) and human chorionic gonadotropin (HCG) in testicular germ cell tumours. A comparison of histologic and serologic occurrence of tumour markers. Acta Pathol Microbiol Scand [A] 1983;91:183–90.

71. _____, Jacobsen M, Clausen PP. Distribution of tumor-associated antigens in the various histologic components of germ cell tumors of the testis. Am J Surg Pathol 1981;5:257–66.

72. Kabawat SE, Bast RC Jr, Bhan AK, Welch WR, Knapp RC, Colvin RB. Tissue distribution of a coelomic-epithelium-related antigen recognized by the monoclonal antibody OC125. Int J Gynec Pathol 1983;2:275–85.

73. _____, Bast RC, Welch WR, Knapp RC, Colvin RB. Immunopathologic characterization of a monoclonal antibody that recognizes common surface antigens of human ovarian tumors of serous, endometrioid, and clear cell types. Am J Clin Pathol 1983;79:98–104.

74. Landolt U, Zobeli L, Pedio G. Pleomorphic adenoma of the salivary glands metastatic to the lung: diagnosis by fine needle aspiration cytology [Letter]. Acta Cytol 1990;34:101–2.

75. Liotta L, Kohn E. Genetic regulation of invasion and metastasis. In: Fenoglio-Preisser CM, Willman CL, eds. Molecular diagnostics in pathology. Baltimore: Williams & Wilkins, 1991.

76. Marchetti A, Buttitta F, Merlo G, et al. p53 alterations in non-small cell lung cancers correlate with metastatic involvement of hilar and mediastinal lymph nodes. Cancer Res 1993;53:2846–51.

77. McCann AH, Dervan PA, O'Regan M, et al. Prognostic significance of c-erbB-2 and estrogen receptor status in human breast cancer. Cancer Res 1991;51:3296–303.

78. Mukai M, Torikata C, Iri H, et al. Cellular differentiation of epithelioid sarcoma. An electron-microscopic, enzyme-histochemical and immunohistochemical study. Am J Pathol 1985;119:44–56.

79. Nadji M, Tabei SZ, Castro A, et al. Prostatic specific antigen: an immunohistochemical marker for prostatic neoplasms. Cancer 1981;48:1229–32.

80. Pavelic ZP, Gluckman JL, Gapany M, et al. Improved immunohistochemical detection of p53 protein in paraffin-embedded tissues reveals elevated levels in most head and neck and lung carcinomas: correlation with clinicopathological parameters. Anticancer Res 1992;12:1389–94.

81. Poller DN, Ellis IO. Oncogenes and tumor morphology prediction. Mod Pathol 1993;6:376–7.

82. Przygodski R, Sayegh R, Bakker A, Swalsky P, Finkelstein S. Specific type of K-ras-2 mutation type predicts occurrence and extent of visceral metastasis in colorectal adenocarcinoma [Abstract]. Mod Pathol 1993;6:51A.

83. Raab SS, Berg LC, Swanson PE, Wick MR. Adenocarcinoma in the lung in patients with breast cancer. A prospective analysis of the discriminatory value of immunohistology. Am J Clin Pathol 1993;100:27–35.

84. Sainsbury JRC, Farndon JR, Needham GK, Malcolm AJ, Harris AL. Epidermal-growth-factor receptor status as predictor of early recurrence of and death from breast cancer. Lancet 1987;1:1398–402.

85. Sheibani K, Esteban JM, Bailey A, Battifora H, Weiss LM. Immunopathologic and molecular studies as an aid to the diagnosis of malignant mesothelioma. Hum Pathol 1992;23:107–16.

86. _____, Shin SS, Kezirian J, Weiss LM. Ber-EP4 antibody as a discriminant in the differential diagnosis of malignant mesothelioma versus adenocarcinoma. Am J Surg Pathol 1991;15:779–84.

87. Shijubo N, Tsutahara S, Hirasawa M, et al. Pulmonary surfactant protein A in pleural effusions. Cancer 1992;69:2905–9.

88. Siegel RJ, Bueso-Ramos C, Cohen C, Koss M. Pulmonary blastoma with germ cell (yolk sac) differentiation: report of two cases. Mod Pathol 1991;4:566–70.

89. Slamon DJ, Boone TC, Murdock DC, et al. Studies of the human c-myb gene and its product in human acute leukemias. Science 1986;233:347–51.

90. _____, Godolphin W, Jones LA, et al. Studies of the HER-2/neu proto-oncogene in human breast and ovarian cancer. Science 1989;244:707–12.

91. Sloane JP, Hughes F, Omerod MG. An assessment of the nature of epithelial membrane antigen and other epithelial markers in solving diagnostic problems in tumor pathology. Histochem J 1983;15:645–54.

92. Taxy JB. Soft tissue neoplasms. In: Azar HA, ed. Pathology of human neoplasms. An atlas of diagnostic electron microscopy and immunohistochemistry. New York: Raven Press, 1988.

93. Thor AD, Moore DH II, Edgerton SM, et al. Accumulation of p53 tumor suppressor gene protein: an independent marker of prognosis in breast cancers. JNCI 1992;84:845–55.

94. Triche TJ. Detection of genes, oncogenes and their products in tumour analysis. In: Bullock GR, Van Velzen V, Warhol MJ, eds. Techniques in diagnostic pathology. London: Academic Press Ltd., 1992.

95. Varma S, Amy RW. Adrenal cortical carcinoma metastatic to the lung: report of a case diagnosed by fine needle aspiration biopsy [Letter]. Acta Cytol 1990;34:104–5.

96. Verstraeten A, Sault MC, Wallaert B, Lemonnier P, Gosselin B, Tonnel AB. Metastatic prostatic adenocarcinoma—diagnosed by bronchoalveolar lavage and tumour marker determination. Eur Respir J 1991;4:1296–8.

97. Wick MR, Swanson PE, Manivel JC. Placental-like alkaline phosphatase reactivity in human tumors: an immunohistochemical study of 520 cases. Hum Pathol 1987;18:946–54

98. Wittchow R, Landas SK. Glial fibrillary acidic protein expression in pleomorphic adenoma, chordoma, and astrocytoma. A comparison of three antibodies. Arch Pathol Lab Med 1991;115:1030–3.

❖❖❖

Index*

*Numbers in boldface indicate table and figure pages.

✧✧✧